Paulo J. G. Bettencourt
Editor

Tuberculosis Vaccines

Springer

Editor
Paulo J. G. Bettencourt
Faculty of Medicine
Universidade Católica Portuguesa
Lisbon, Portugal

ISBN 978-3-031-94539-7 ISBN 978-3-031-94540-3 (eBook)
https://doi.org/10.1007/978-3-031-94540-3

This Springer imprint is published by the registered company Springer Nature Switzerland AG
The registered company address is: Gewerbestrasse 11, 6330 Cham, Switzerland

Contents

Part I

Introduction to Tuberculosis

1 Introduction to Tuberculosis and Mycobacteriology

Paulo J. G. Bettencourt

1.1 Brief History of Tuberculosis

It is estimated that, since the identification of the causative agent of tuberculosis (TB), *Mycobacterium tuberculosis* (*Mtb*), in 1882 by Robert Koch, the number of people that died from the disease is over one billion. In fact, TB has killed more people than plague, influenza, smallpox, cholera, HIV/AIDS, and malaria combined [1]. It is undoubtedly the biggest killer among all infectious diseases that afflicted mankind and still the greatest killer today, with more than one million deaths reported yearly by the World Health Organization (WHO), only surpassed by Sars-CoV-2, during the COVID-19 pandemic [2, 3].

TB has been in the collective memory of humanity since the beginning of time. This ancient disease decimated humans since the dawn of modern humans, as it is supported by 4000-year-old skeletons presenting characteristic visible lesions in the spine, known as Pott's disease, in different regions of the world, with particular relevance to Egyptian mummies [4]. Even though the integrity of this information may be occasionally challenged, bioarcheology has gained substantial support across the scientific community, with confirmed specimen findings across the world [5–7].

It has been postulated that there is co-evolution or co-adaptation between the human immune system and *Mtb* [8] far longer, perhaps since the beginning of agriculture, when humans started to organize larger communities and created the ideal conditions for *Mtb* transmission. Although this was 12,000 years ago, there are reports claiming that the disease originated 35,000 years ago infecting other

P. J. G. Bettencourt (✉)
Universidade Católica Portuguesa, Center for Interdisciplinary Research in Health, Lisbon, Portugal

Universidade Católica Portuguesa, Faculty of Medicine, Lisbon, Portugal
e-mail: pbettencourt@ucp.pt

P. J. G. Bettencourt (ed.), *Tuberculosis Vaccines*,
https://doi.org/10.1007/978-3-031-94540-3_1

mammalians, with phylogenetic and biogeographic models suggesting the origin to be 2.6 million years ago [9]. Even though it is difficult to establish the beginning of this host–pathogen interaction, *Mtb* has been extremely successful in infecting humans for a long time.

In ancient Greece, TB was described as "phthisis", meaning "consumption" [10], due to the severe wasting seen in affected individuals. In Europe, in the eighteenth and nineteenth centuries, the TB epidemic known as the "white plague" was the highest cause of death and thought to be driven by industrialization, poor housing, overcrowding, bad sanitation, and malnutrition [11].

The establishment of sanatoria in the nineteenth century, in the pre-chemotherapy era, to treat patients by providing fresh air, rest, and an improved diet, until self-cure or death, marked one of the first organized efforts to combat TB, in addition to surgery [12].

Early in the twentieth century, the development of the first and only vaccine against TB, by Calmette and Guérin, the BCG, still in use today, brought hope to control the epidemics. However, for some reasons that will be explored comprehensively throughout the book, the vaccine was partially successful, warranting the need for the development of more efficacious TB vaccines. In addition, the discovery of Streptomycin, in the mid-twentieth century, brought new hope to the fight against TB, but the development of resistance against antibiotics soon after was a disappointment, revealing the capacity of *Mtb* to adapt to new environments. The resistance to antibiotics is a major concern not only for TB but also against all infectious diseases treatable with antibiotics. This is not the theme of this book, and there is extensive literature on this subject [13–16]. Later in the end of the twentieth century, the HIV/AIDS epidemic aggravated the TB situation worldwide, offering a new and dramatic condition, the *Mtb*-HIV co-infection [11].

1.2 Tuberculosis Disease

TB affects primarily the lungs (pulmonary TB or PTB) with the majority of cases (about 90%) but can affect virtually every human tissue, being designated as extra-pulmonary TB (EPTB), such as pleural TB, cutaneous TB, urogenital TB, lymph node TB, bone TB (Pott's disease), and others. In fact, the same patient can have more than one form of TB simultaneously, for example, pulmonary and urogenital TB [17]. Strikingly, in late HIV/AIDS patients co-infected with *Mtb*, 50% of the cases are EPTB with the disseminated form of the disease, or miliary TB, more frequently reported [18].

The symptoms may vary depending on the site of infection. However, pulmonary TB is characterized by chronic cough, chest pain, fever, night sweats, and weight loss. These unspecific symptoms may be confounded with other pathologies. Hemoptysis can occur in the later stages of the disease. The diagnosis can take a long time to be conclusive and involves a combination of exams including radiologic imaging, sputum smear microscopy, tuberculin skin test (TST), molecular tests such as the Xpert MTB/RIF assay, and the gold standard IGRA assays. The treatment of drug-susceptible TB requires a combination of isoniazid, rifampicin, pyrazinamide, and ethambutol for 6 to 9 months. In the case of drug-resistant TB (DR-TB), multidrug-resistant TB (MDR-TB), or extensively drug-resistant TB (XDR-TB), there is the requirement for more complex and prolonged treatments with second-line antibiotics that can last up to 2 years, with HIV/AIDS co-infection presenting an additional layer of complexity and lower rates of treatment success. For further details on the diagnostics, treatment, and management of TB, refer to the literature [19, 20].

The transmission of *Mtb* occurs mostly through droplets containing bacteria. The susceptible recipient will inhale the bacterium, and two scenarios may occur:

1. The airway mucus layer of the respiratory system will capture the microorganism and expel it very efficiently. This is a mechanical clearance system that will eliminate most inhaled particulates and constitutes the first host defense system against *Mtb* [21].
2. The bacterium passes the mucus barrier and interacts with the lung epithelial cells, which are not merely bystander cells, as they are the first cells to have a direct sensing of the invading bacterium, respond to it by secreting cytokines, chemokines, and antimicrobials, initiating a cascade of events that eventually lead to the recruitment of the first innate immune cells, the alveolar macrophages [21, 22]. This initial host-pathogen interaction is a scientific field of its own right, with extensive literature available, even though the mechanisms involved have not been clearly described yet.
   (1) Once in the alveolar macrophages, the successful Mycobacteria are able to survive inside the cell, by accessing nutrients from the cell and surviving within it, enclosed in the early phagosome. This parasitic type of interaction is a key point for the success of *Mtb* in causing disease. *Mtb* has evolved strategies to survive within the host macrophages, including blocking the acidification of the early phagosome, the inhibition of phagosome-lysosome fusion, resistance to reactive oxygen and nitrogen species, and the ability to enter a dormant state where it can persist for years in a latent form. The model macrophage-mycobacteria is widely studied *in vivo* and *in vitro* as a surrogate of TB disease [23–26].
   (2) *Mtb*-infected alveolar macrophages initiate the immune response by secreting cytokines and chemokines to recruit other cell types to the site of infection. These include T-cells, B-cells, neutrophils, NK cells, and others that form an organized structure surrounding the infected macrophage. This is the granuloma, the hallmark of TB. The initial granuloma has a dual and contradictory function: on the one hand, it contains the infection and prevents the spread of bacteria; on the other hand, the bacteria remain in the lung indefinitely. Should the bacteria remain in the granuloma, not causing active disease, this is known as latent tuberculosis infection (LTBI). It has been postulated that the mycobacteria inside the LTBI granuloma are dormant and activate dormancy systems, such as the DosR regulon [27]. More recently, it has been recognized that these bacteria are metabolically active

and can change their metabolism by sensing the host health status. In fact, the TB granuloma has been shown to be highly heterogeneous temporally and spatially and in its cell distribution [28]. This supports the hypothesis that there is a state of continuum between both LTBI and active disease, rather than the two defined conditions. At the same time, T-cells that encounter antigens migrate to the local lymph nodes and start the adaptive immune response against *Mtb*. This response, however, is delayed by multiple mechanisms of immune evasion [29]. The immune response against *Mtb* infection, and particularly the response promoted by vaccines against TB, will be extensively discussed in the following chapters of the book.

Should *Mtb* start dividing and growing inside the granuloma, the structure will change and show a typical cheesy appearance, described as the caseating granuloma due to the accumulation of lipids, and, eventually, bursts leading to the spread of actively replicating bacteria, thus completing the transmission cycle of the disease.

Interestingly, a new hypothesis about *Mtb* transmission has been proposed. Digby Warner, Robin Wood, and colleagues studied the transmission of *Mtb* in a TB-endemic setting and detected the equivalent release of aerosols containing *Mtb* by confirmed TB patients and individuals without a TB diagnosis, indicating potential colonization by Mtb, differentiable from infection [30]. These are surprising observations that challenge the current paradigm of TB transmission, and could have implications when designing new vaccines against TB.

1.3 Biology of *Mtb*

Mtb is a facultative intracellular pathogen, considered to be an obligate aerobic and facultative anaerobic, meaning it requires oxygen to grow but can stand hypoxic environments [31]. In addition, it is nonmotile and can survive for weeks in harsh environments. Interestingly, growing *Mtb* culture requires a rich medium, and it is a slow-growing bacterium that divides every 18–24 h, in contrast, for example, with *Escherichia coli* that divides every 20 min [32]. *Mtb* does not follow the general Gram classification of bacteria. Instead, it is an acid-fast bacillus that can be stained with the Ziehl-Neelsen method, with some characteristics of Gram-positive bacteria, like the presence of ESX secretion systems [33–35] (Fig. 1.1). This is due to the thick and complex nature of the cell wall, rich in exquisite lipid structures that can change and adapt to new environments by synthesizing different lipids and obtaining its carbon from distinct carbon sources [36]. The *Mtb* cell wall lipids constitute about 40% of the dry mass, but this percentage can change in function of the growth conditions [37], and this remarkable metabolic flexibility allows to survive in nutrient-restricted conditions, such as within a macrophage's phagosome, in granulomas. In fact, *Mtb*'s flexibility to adapt to new environments makes it difficult to establish long-lasting successful therapies. For example, *Mtb* can form multibacterial structures known as cords due to the lipid composition of the outermost layer of the cell wall, including trehalose dimycolate (TDM), or cord-factor, which has the

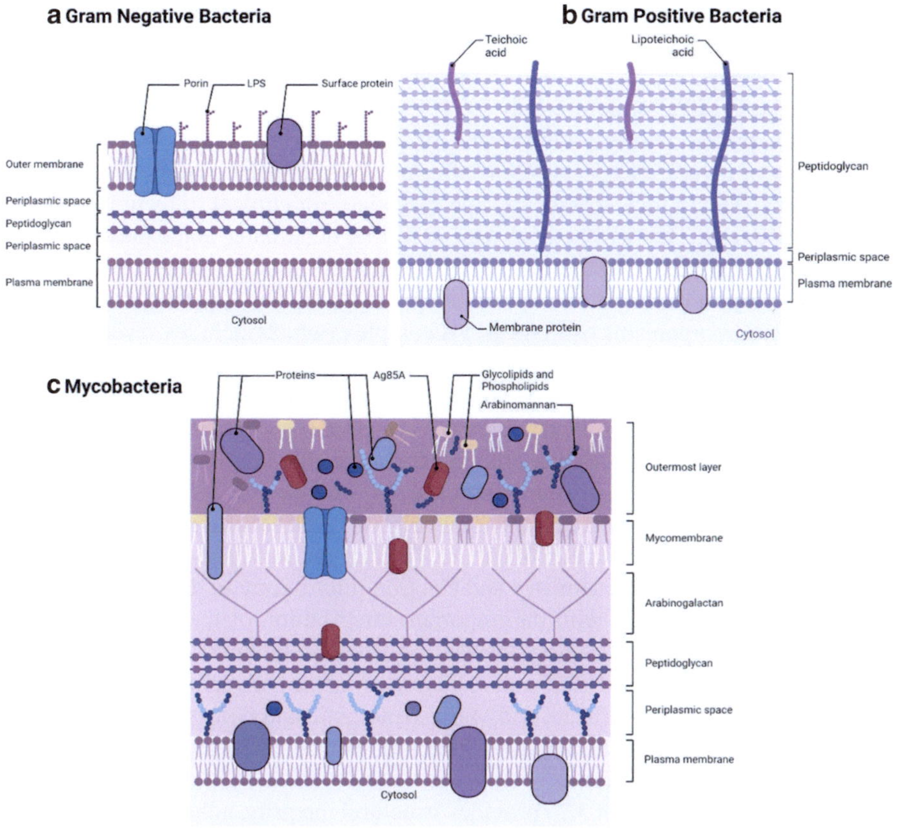

Fig. 1.1 Cell wall structure of bacteria. The cell wall of bacteria is located at the outer leaflet of the plasma membrane and is composed of rigid peptidoglycan, followed by the presence or absence of an outer membrane. (**a**) Cell wall of Gram-negative bacteria consists of a thin layer of peptidoglycan in the periplasmic space. The outer membrane contains lipopolysaccharides, and facilitate transport through channels such as porins. (**b**) Cell wall of Gram-positive bacteria is characterized by the presence of a thick peptidoglycan cell wall, teichoic, and lipoteichoic acid, and contrasts with the Gram-negative bacteria by lacking an outer membrane. (**c**) The plasma membrane of Mycobacteria has lipoarabinomannan (LAM) and arabinomannan (AM). The cell wall of mycobacteria consists of a thick layer of peptidoglycan and arabinogalactan, followed by a monolayer of mycolic acids, known as the mycomembrane. These are in contact with glycolipids, phospholipids, and include transmembrane proteins such as porins. Some authors refer to the presence of an outermost layer or capsule, outside of the mycomembrane, composed primarily of polysaccharide, including AM and LAM, protein, and lipid. Some proteins such as Ag85A are found in several locations on the cell wall. (Adapted from [34, 35]. Created in BioRender. Bettencourt, PJG. (2024) BioRender.com/h87n452)

capacity to suppress the innate immune system. Moreover, in the presence of antibiotics, bacteria in cords remain translationally active and can resume growth upon the removal of antibiotics [38]. In the absence of TDM, cords are not properly formed.

In 1998, the most common laboratory strain of *Mtb,* H37Rv, was sequenced, revealing that the genome consists of approximately 4.4 million base pairs, encodes about 4000 genes, and is rich in GC content. Strikingly, a new protein family was revealed, the PE/PPE protein family [39]. This absolute surprise created the hope that the new protein family could provide many answers for the unknown aspects of the biology of mycobacteria as well as offering new antigens to be included in vaccines against TB. In fact, several vaccine candidates in clinical trials today use PE and PPE antigens. This will be described in further detail later in the book.

Another important revelation is that *Mtb* differs from other bacteria by possessing a large proportion of genes involved in lipid metabolism [39]. This is also shared with other microorganisms from the MTB complex (which includes several closely related species that cause TB in humans and animals, namely *M. africanum, M. bovis, M. caprae, M. microti, M. mungi, M. orygis, M. pinnipedii,* and *M. canettii*). These lipids are part of the complex cell wall that is recognized as a major virulence factor of *Mtb.* Interestingly, the genetic variability in *Mtb* is relatively low compared to other bacteria, even though specific mutations can lead to drug resistance or influence virulence. Notably, the cell wall architecture is so complex that its clear definition is still a matter of debate. The current models took several decades of intense research in biochemistry and electron microscopy to define, particularly in the 1960's and 1970's, with the important contribution of the most prestigious laboratories in the world, namely the Patrick Brennan laboratory at the Colorado State University, US, David E. Minnikin laboratory at the University of Birmingham, UK, Cécile and Jean Asselineau, and Marie-Antoinette and Gilbert Lanéelle laboratories at the Université Paul Sabatier, Toulouse, France, and Hugo L. David at the Institut Pasteur in Paris, France.

The complex cell wall of *Mtb* provides structural integrity, adhesion to host cells, resistance to environmental stress including protection against host defense mechanisms, and the capacity of immune modulation of several defense mechanisms, including the inhibition of phagosome–lysosome fusion [40], leading to a delay in MHC-I and MHC-II presentation [41], autophagy [42], and induction of apoptosis, promoting the intracellular growth of bacteria [43]. In addition to the cord factor [44], some of the most studied cell wall lipids include LAM [45], tuberculostearic acid [46], mycolic acids [47], phosphatidyl inositol mannosides (PIM) [48], and the phenolic glycolipid, triglycosyl phenol phthiocerol di-mycocerosate (PGL-Tb1) [49]. The localization of the most representative lipids and antigens of mycobacteria is shown in Fig. 1.1.

The contribution of cell wall lipids and the secreted mycobacterial antigens consist of a fundamental weaponry utilized by *Mtb* to evade the host immune response. One of such examples includes mycobactins. These lipid-soluble siderophores are high-affinity iron-chelating compounds secreted by *Mtb* to sequester free iron from its surroundings and deliver to the phagosome-containing mycobacteria [50, 51]. These and others constitute a magnificent mechanism utilized by *Mtb* to survive and thrive in the harsh environment of the phagosome.

The lipid biochemistry of *Mtb* is very complex and can sometimes be confounded with the host lipid biochemistry [52]. *Mtb* utilizes several enzymes not found in other prokaryotes but in eukaryotes, such as the fatty acid synthase I involved in fatty acid elongation, and a pre-clinical vaccine candidate [53].

In addition to a plethora of complex lipids, *Mtb* has the ability to utilize host lipids as a nutrient source, which is crucial for persistence within the macrophage. Cholesterol, phospholipids, glycolipids, and fatty acids are abundant in the host environment and can be involved in both stimulatory and inhibitory signaling pathways, leading to opposing effects in the survival of *Mtb*. Different lipids, including the ω-6 arachidonic acid, were found to facilitate the killing of *Mtb* in phagosomes, by activating the actin assembly and phagosome maturation in infected macrophages. By contrast, other lipids such as the polyunsaturated ω-3 fatty acids, including the eicosapentaenoic acid (EPA), were shown to facilitate pathogen growth, thus revealing contradictory effects promoted by different dietary lipids in vitro [54] and in vivo [55]. Strikingly, the common dietary lipid oleic acid when conjugated in complex lipids can be utilized by *Mtb* as a carbon source [56]; however, in its free state, it directly kills *Mtb* [56, 57].

In addition to the inhibition of phagosome-lysosome fusion, with the consequent reduction of antigen presentation, *Mtb* actively employs other strategies to manipulate the host cell fate. These include the manipulation of the host innate immune response at the level of microRNA expression [58, 59], gene expression [60, 61], and consequently protein expression, and cytokine secretion, manipulating the host immune response to its own advantage [61]. In early infection, *Mtb* induces the expansion of regulatory T cells, leading to a delay in the adaptive immune response. T regs also play a role in reducing tissue inflammation-mediated damage, which can be beneficial to the host [62]. All these mechanisms combined and sequentially orchestrated offer *Mtb* an advantage to avoid immune clearance and establish long-term infections.

Another strategy employed by *Mtb* is the utilization of the Type VII secretion system ESX-1 that injects proteins into the cytoplasm of the infected macrophage. The 6 kDa early secreted antigenic target (ESAT-6) and the 10 kDa culture filtrate protein (CFP-10) are among these proteins, form a heterodimeric complex that contributes to virulence, and are known to modulate host cell functions promoting *Mtb* survival and replication. ESAT-6 was shown to induce rupture of the phagolysosome and translocation of *Mtb* to the cytoplasm [63], and necrosis of infected macrophages, to facilitate bacterial dissemination [64]. The heterodimer induces a strong T-cell-mediated immune response, which is the base of the most reliable diagnostic method, the IGRA assay [33]. Moreover, the BCG vaccine, which is an attenuated form of the pathogenic *Mycobacterium bovis*, lost a genetic region designated as the region of difference 1 (RD1) that includes part of the genes encoding the ESX-1 structural components, leading to an impairment of protein secretion into the infected macrophage. This suggests that the presence of the ESX-1 secretion system has a role in *Mtb* virulence, and its absence is partially responsible for the attenuation of BCG [65]. For all these reasons combined, some vaccine candidates in clinical trials use ESAT-6 and CFP-10 antigens, which will be discussed further in the book.

Remarkably, after more than a century of BCG's usage, one-third of its genes have undefined functions, and a large proportion are involved in intermediary metabolism and respiration, PE/PPE, lipid metabolism, and cell wall processes [61]. This is an urgent call on the necessity to better characterize the function of BCG and *Mtb* genes, to better inform vaccine design.

1.4 Complex Field of Mycobacteriology

Mycobacteriology is a multidisciplinary and highly specialized field of bacteriology that combines genetics, molecular biology, biochemistry (including lipid chemistry, enzymology, and metabolomics), physiology, immunology, and many others. In any of these disciplines, Mycobacteria are presented as the exception or the exotic element that brings curiosity and diversity to the subject matters. This is undoubtedly one of the most difficult scientific fields, demonstrated by the constant success of the pathogen. The profound understanding of *Mtb* requires the combination of all these disciplines, which can be a challenge to most scientists specialized in their own field of research. Multidisciplinary collaboration between scientists is fundamental for a better understanding of the pathogen, and this is paramount for the rational development of vaccines against TB.

Competing Interests The author(s) has no competing interests to declare that are relevant to the content of this manuscript.

Ethics Approval The author(s) declares that this manuscript does not include primary research with human participants.

References

1. Fauci AS. Addressing the tuberculosis epidemic: 21st century research for an ancient disease. JAMA. 2018;320(13):1315–6.
2. World Health Organization. Global tuberculosis report 2022. Geneva; 2022.
3. Schumacher AE, Kyu HH, Aali A, Abbafati C, Abbas J, Abbasgholizadeh R, et al. Global age-sex-specific mortality, life expectancy, and population estimates in 204 countries and territories and 811 subnational locations, 1950–2021, and the impact of the COVID-19 pandemic: a comprehensive demographic analysis for the Global Burden of Disease Study 2021. Lancet. 2024;403(10440):1989–2056.
4. Donoghue HD. 2016. Paleomicrobiology of Human Tuberculosis. Microbiol Spectr 4: https://doi.org/10.1128/microbiolspec.poh-0003-2014.
5. Donoghue HD, Hershkovitz I, Minnikin DE, Besra GS, Lee OYC, Galili E, et al. Biomolecular archaeology of ancient tuberculosis: response to "Deficiencies and challenges in the study of ancient tuberculosis DNA" by Wilbur et al. (2009). J Archaeol Sci. 2009;36(12):2797–804.
6. Roberts CA. Old World tuberculosis: evidence from human remains with a review of current research and future prospects. Tuberculosis. 2015;95:S117–21.
7. Daniel TM. The origins and precolonial epidemiology of tuberculosis in the Americas: can we figure them out? Int J Tuberc Lung Dis. 2000;4(5):395–400.

8. Phelan J, Gomez-Gonzalez PJ, Andreu N, Omae Y, Toyo-Oka L, Yanai H, et al. Genome-wide host-pathogen analyses reveal genetic interaction points in tuberculosis disease. Nat Commun. 2023;14(1):549.
9. Stone AC, Wilbur AK, Buikstra JE, Roberts CA. Tuberculosis and leprosy in perspective. Am J Phys Anthropol. 2009;140(Suppl 49):66–94.
10. Cilione M, Martini M, Zampieri F, Riccardi N, Brigo F, Gazzaniga V. Aristotle – Ἀριστοτέλης (ARISTOTÉLĒS, 384/3- 322/1 BCE) the revelation of tuberculosis in his zoological works. Pathog Glob Health. 2023;117(6):605–10.
11. Cole ST. Comparative and functional genomics of the *Mycobacterium tuberculosis* complex. Microbiology (Reading). 2002;148(Pt 10):2919–28.
12. Zwick ED, Pepperell CS. Tuberculosis sanatorium treatment at the advent of the chemotherapy era. BMC Infect Dis. 2020;20(1):831.
13. Tacconelli E, Carrara E, Savoldi A, Harbarth S, Mendelson M, Monnet DL, et al. Discovery, research, and development of new antibiotics: the WHO priority list of antibiotic-resistant bacteria and tuberculosis. Lancet Infect Dis. 2018;18(3):318–27.
14. Jassal M, Bishai WR. Extensively drug-resistant tuberculosis. Lancet Infect Dis. 2009;9(1):19–30.
15. Smith T, Wolff KA, Nguyen L. Molecular biology of drug resistance in *Mycobacterium tuberculosis*. Curr Top Microbiol Immunol. 2013;374:53–80.
16. Zhang Y, Vilchèze C, Jacobs WR. Mechanisms of drug resistance in *Mycobacterium tuberculosis*. In: Tuberculosis and the tubercle bacillus. Wiley; 2004. p. 115–40.
17. Zachoval R, Nencka P, Vasakova M, Kopecka E, Borovička V, Wallenfels J, et al. The incidence of subclinical forms of urogenital tuberculosis in patients with pulmonary tuberculosis. J Infect Public Health. 2018;11(2):243–5.
18. Sharma SK, Mohan A, Sharma A. Miliary tuberculosis: a new look at an old foe. J Clin Tuberc Other Mycobact Dis. 2016;3:13–27.
19. Lewinsohn DM, Leonard MK, LoBue PA, Cohn DL, Daley CL, Desmond E, et al. Official American Thoracic Society/Infectious Diseases Society of America/Centers for Disease Control and Prevention clinical practice guidelines: diagnosis of tuberculosis in adults and children. Clin Infect Dis. 2017;64(2):111–5.
20. Chegou NN, Hoek KGP, Kriel M, Warren RM, Victor TC, Walzl G. Tuberculosis assays: past, present and future. Expert Rev Anti-Infect Ther. 2011;9(4):457–69.
21. Torrelles JB, Schlesinger LS. Integrating lung physiology, immunology, and tuberculosis. Trends Microbiol. 2017;25(8):688–97.
22. de Waal AM, Hiemstra PS, Ottenhoff TH, Joosten SA, van der Does AM. Lung epithelial cells interact with immune cells and bacteria to shape the microenvironment in tuberculosis. Thorax. 2022;77(4):408–16.
23. Vergne I, Chua J, Singh SB, Deretic V. Cell biology of *Mycobacterium tuberculosis* phagosome. Annu Rev Cell Dev Biol. 2004;20:367–94.
24. Pires D, Marques J, Pombo JP, Carmo N, Bettencourt P, Neyrolles O, et al. Role of cathepsins in *Mycobacterium tuberculosis* survival in human macrophages. Sci Rep. 2016;6:32247.
25. Pires D, Bettencourt P, Carmo N, Bergant T, Jordao L, Anes E. Interference of *Mycobacterium tuberculosis* with the endocytic pathways on macrophages and dendritic cells from healthy donors: role of cathepsins. Drug Discov Today. 2010;15(23–24). A90. 1112.
26. Pires D, Bettencourt P, Carmo N, Niederweis M, Anes E. Role of *Mycobacterium tuberculosis* outer-membrane porins in bacterial survival within macrophages. Drug Discov Today. 2010;15(23–24). A91. 1112–1113.
27. Peddireddy V, Doddam SN, Ahmed N. Mycobacterial Dormancy Systems and Host Responses in Tuberculosis. Front Immunol. 2017;8:84.
28. Xu R, Xiao W, Ding G, Zeng J, Liu H, Cai Y, et al. The use of multiplex imaging techniques to characterize tuberculous granuloma heterogeneity. WIREs Mech Dis. 2023;15(3):e1601.
29. Ernst JD. Mechanisms of *M. tuberculosis* immune evasion as challenges to TB vaccine design. Cell Host Microbe. 2018;24(1):34–42.

30. Dinkele R, Gessner S, Patterson B, McKerry A, Hoosen Z, Vazi A, et al. Persistent *Mycobacterium tuberculosis* bioaerosol release in a tuberculosis-endemic setting. iScience. 2024;27(9):110731.
31. Sherman DR, Voskuil M, Schnappinger D, Liao R, Harrell MI, Schoolnik GK. Regulation of the *Mycobacterium tuberculosis* hypoxic response gene encoding α-crystallin. Proc Natl Acad Sci. 2001;98(13):7534–9.
32. Bettencourt P, Carmo N, Pires D, Timóteo P, Anes E. Mycobacterial infection of macrophages: the effect of the multiplicity of infection. In: Antimicrobial research: novel bioknowledge and educational programs; 2017. pp 651–664. Méndez-Vilas A (Ed.). Formatex Research Center, Badajoz, Spain.
33. Simeone R, Bottai D, Brosch R. ESX/type VII secretion systems and their role in host–pathogen interaction. Curr Opin Microbiol. 2009;12(1):4–10.
34. Brown L, Wolf JM, Prados-Rosales R, Casadevall A. Through the wall: extracellular vesicles in Gram-positive bacteria, mycobacteria and fungi. Nat Rev Microbiol. 2015;13(10):620–30.
35. Chiaradia L, Lefebvre C, Parra J, Marcoux J, Burlet-Schiltz O, Etienne G, et al. Dissecting the mycobacterial cell envelope and defining the composition of the native mycomembrane. Sci Rep. 2017;7(1):12807.
36. de Carvalho LPS, Fischer SM, Marrero J, Nathan C, Ehrt S, Rhee KY. Metabolomics of *Mycobacterium tuberculosis* reveals compartmentalized co-catabolism of carbon substrates. Chem Biol. 2010;17(10):1122–31.
37. Jackson M. The mycobacterial cell envelope – lipids. Cold Spring Harb Perspect Med. 2014;4(10):a021105.
38. Mishra R, Hannebelle M, Patil VP, Dubois A, Garcia-Mouton C, Kirsch GM, et al. Mechanopathology of biofilm-like *Mycobacterium tuberculosis* cords. Cell. 2023;186(23):5135–5150.e28.
39. Cole ST, Brosch R, Parkhill J, Garnier T, Churcher C, Harris D, et al. Deciphering the biology of *Mycobacterium tuberculosis* from the complete genome sequence. Nature. 1998;393(6685):537–44.
40. Goren MB, D'Arcy Hart P, Young MR, Armstrong JA. Prevention of phagosome-lysosome fusion in cultured macrophages by sulfatides of *Mycobacterium tuberculosis*. Proc Natl Acad Sci. 1976;73(7):2510–4.
41. Clemens DL, Horwitz MA. Characterization of the *Mycobacterium tuberculosis* phagosome and evidence that phagosomal maturation is inhibited. J Exp Med. 1995;181(1):257–70.
42. Gutierrez MG, Master SS, Singh SB, Taylor GA, Colombo MI, Deretic V. Autophagy is a defense mechanism inhibiting BCG and *Mycobacterium tuberculosis* survival in infected macrophages. Cell. 2004;119(6):753–66.
43. Keane J, Balcewicz-Sablinska MK, Remold HG, Chupp GL, Meek BB, Fenton MJ, et al. Infection by *Mycobacterium tuberculosis* promotes human alveolar macrophage apoptosis. Infect Immun. 1997;65(1):298–304.
44. Hunter RL, Venkataprasad N, Olsen MR. The role of trehalose dimycolate (cord factor) on morphology of virulent *M. tuberculosis* in vitro. Tuberculosis. 2006;86(5):349–56.
45. Schlesinger LS, Kaufman TM, Iyer S, Hull SR, Marchiando LK. Differences in mannose receptor-mediated uptake of lipoarabinomannan from virulent and attenuated strains of *Mycobacterium tuberculosis* by human macrophages. J Immunol. 1996;157(10):4568–75.
46. Traunmüller F, Alexander Zeitlinger M, Stoiser B, Lagler H, Abdulla Abdel Salam H, Presterl E, et al. Circulating tuberculostearic acid in tuberculosis patients. Scand J Infect Dis. 2003;35(11–12):790–3.
47. Verschoor JA, Baird MS, Grooten J. Towards understanding the functional diversity of cell wall mycolic acids of *Mycobacterium tuberculosis*. Prog Lipid Res. 2012;51(4):325–39.
48. Gilleron M, Quesniaux VFJ, Puzo G. Acylation state of the phosphatidylinositol hexamannosides from Mycobacterium bovis Bacillus Calmette Guérin and *Mycobacterium tuberculosis* H37Rv and its implication in toll-like receptor response. J Biol Chem. 2003;278(32):29880–9.
49. Papa F, Laszlo A, David HL. Specificity of *Mycobacterium tuberculosis* phenolic glycolipid (PGL-Tb1) antiserum. Ann Inst Pasteur Microbiol (1985). 1988;139(5):535–45.

50. Luo M, Fadeev EA, Groves JT. Mycobactin-mediated iron acquisition within macrophages. Nat Chem Biol. 2005;1(3):149–53.
51. Bosne S, Papa F, Clavel-Sérès S, Rastogi N. A simple and reliable EDDA method for mycobactin production in mycobacteria: optimal conditions and use in mycobacterial speciation. Curr Microbiol. 1993;26(6):353–8.
52. Teng O, Ang CKE, Guan XL. Macrophage–bacteria interactions—a lipid-centric relationship. Front Immunol. 2017;8:8.
53. Bettencourt P, Müller J, Nicastri A, Cantillon D, Madhavan M, Charles PD, et al. Identification of antigens presented by MHC for vaccines against tuberculosis. NPJ Vaccines. 2020;5(1):2.
54. Anes E, Kühnel MP, Bos E, Moniz-Pereira J, Habermann A, Griffiths G. Selected lipids activate phagosome actin assembly and maturation resulting in killing of pathogenic mycobacteria. Nat Cell Biol. 2003;5(9):793–802.
55. Jordao L, Lengeling A, Bordat Y, Boudou F, Gicquel B, Neyrolles O, et al. Effects of omega-3 and -6 fatty acids on *Mycobacterium tuberculosis* in macrophages and in mice. Microbes Infect. 2008;10(12–13):1379–86.
56. Minami K. Bactericidal action of oleic acid for tubercle bacilli. J Bacteriol. 1957;73(3):338–44.
57. Kondo E, Kanai K. The lethal effect of long-chain fatty acids on mycobacteria. Jpn J Med Sci Biol. 1972;25(1):1–13.
58. Bettencourt P, Marion S, Pires D, Santos LF, Lastrucci C, Carmo N, et al. Actin-binding protein regulation by micrornas as a novel microbial strategy to modulate phagocytosis by host cells: the case of N-Wasp and miR-142-3p. Front Cell Infect Microbiol. 2013;3:4(JUN).
59. Bettencourt P, Pires D, Anes E. Immunomodulating microRNAs of mycobacterial infections. Tuberculosis. 2016;97:1.
60. Tailleux L, Waddell SJ, Pelizzola M, Mortellaro A, Withers M, Tanne A, et al. Probing host pathogen cross-talk by transcriptional profiling of both *Mycobacterium tuberculosis* and infected human dendritic cells and macrophages. PLoS One. 2008;3(1):e1403.
61. Medley J, Goff A, Bettencourt PJG, Dare M, Cole L, Cantillon D, et al. Dissecting the Mycobacterium bovis BCG response to macrophage infection to help prioritize targets for anti-tuberculosis drug and vaccine discovery. Vaccines (Basel). 2022;10(1):113.
62. Larson RP, Shafiani S, Urdahl KB. Foxp3(+) regulatory T cells in tuberculosis. Adv Exp Med Biol. 2013;783:165–80.
63. Houben D, Demangel C, van Ingen J, Perez J, Baldeón L, Abdallah AM, et al. ESX-1-mediated translocation to the cytosol controls virulence of mycobacteria. Cell Microbiol. 2012;14(8):1287–98.
64. Welin A, Eklund D, Stendahl O, Lerm M. Human macrophages infected with a high burden of ESAT-6-expressing *M. tuberculosis* undergo Caspase-1- and Cathepsin B-independent necrosis. PLoS One. 2011;6(5):e20302.
65. Simeone R, Bottai D, Frigui W, Majlessi L, Brosch R. ESX/type VII secretion systems of mycobacteria: insights into evolution, pathogenicity and protection. Tuberculosis. 2015;95:S150–4.

Part II

Historical Perspectives on Bacillus Calmette-Guérin and Tuberculosis Vaccine Candidates

100 Years of BCG Against Tuberculosis and Other Diseases

2

Camille Locht

2.1 Introduction

In 1895, Albert Calmette, a trained marine physician and Director of the Pasteur Institute in Saigon, was appointed as the director of the newly founded Institut Pasteur de Lille, in Northern France [1]. His major mission was to produce anti-diphtheria antiserum according to the procedure developed by Emil Roux because diphtheria was a major public health issue in the North of France. However, Albert Calmette realized that, besides diphtheria, for which a treatment was now available, people in the North of France also suffered from another infectious disease, tuberculosis, for which no treatment was yet available. Therefore, Calmette created the Lille dispensary in 1901 (Fig. 2.1), where tuberculosis patients were diagnosed, triaged, trained in basic hygiene measures, and eventually sent to sanatoriums.

Camille Guérin, a veterinarian trained by Edmond Nocard at the veterinarian school d'Alfort, joined Albert Calmette in 1897 to work on tuberculosis, in particular on the mode of infection. A key question debated at that time was the route of infection, either the oral route or aerosol. The initial results using a goat model and milk contaminated with the bovine tubercle bacillus *Mycobacterium bovis* or the human bacillus *Mycobacterium tuberculosis* showed that goats could readily be infected orally by either organism and that the oral administration of the bovine bacillus induced tuberculous lesions in the lungs [2]. The conclusion Calmette and Guérin took from these initial studies was that in the vast majority of cases, pulmonary tuberculosis was acquired by ingestion and not by inhalation of the bacilli.

Importantly, a single oral infection of cattle with a low dose of *M. bovis* was found to induce lung lesions that healed spontaneously. This was accompanied by a

The original chapter was inadvertently published with spelling errors, missing "R" in "Revaccination" and "Mycobacterium" in Bibliography No. 44, which have now been corrected.

C. Locht (✉)
Univ. Lille, CNRS, Inserm, CHU Lille, Institut Pasteur de Lille,
U1019-UMR9017–CIIL – Centre for Infection and Immunity of Lille, Lille, France
e-mail: camille.locht@pasteur-lille.fr

P. J. G. Bettencourt (ed.), *Tuberculosis Vaccines*,
https://doi.org/10.1007/978-3-031-94540-3_2

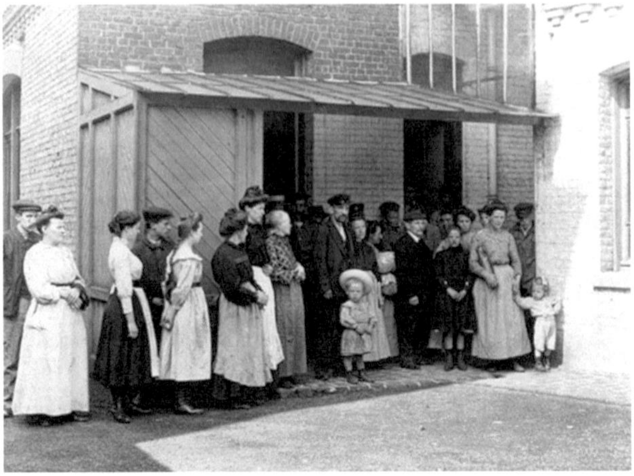

Fig. 2.1 Tuberculosis dispensary in Lille. The first French tuberculosis dispensary, opened in Lille in 1901, was available to general population in order to provide consultancies and hygiene recommendations. (With permission from General Director of Institut Pasteur de Lille)

positive result in the tuberculin skin test (TST), followed 2 months later by a negative TST result. Subsequently, these cattle became resistant to reinfection, even with a high challenging dose of *M. bovis* [3]. This observation opened the perspective of an antituberculosis vaccine.

2.2 Birth of BCG

Inspired by the success of Louis Pasteur in developing safe live vaccines by attenuation via various procedures, Calmette and Guérin started to use a variety of methods to attenuate the *M. bovis* strain, contained in contaminated milk supplied by Nocard, the "lait de Nocard". The first attempts to attenuate the *M. bovis* strain consisted in cultivating it over several passages at elevated temperatures [4], similar to Louis Pasteur's method used for the attenuation of the anthrax bacillus. However, eventually, repetitively cultivating the organism every 2 weeks on a glycerinated potato-based medium in the presence of ox bile resulted in gradual attenuation [5].

After 4 years of continued passaging, the strain had lost its virulence for cattle and guinea pigs but was still virulent for horses and rabbits. Finally, after 230 passages during 13 years, from 1908 to 1921, virulence was lost for all animal species tested, including sheep, dogs, rats, mice, as well as pigeons and chicken, even at very high doses [6]. This irreversibly attenuated *M. bovis* strain was consequently named Bacillus Calmette-Guérin (BCG) and was found to prevent bovine tuberculosis upon challenge with virulent *M. bovis* [7]. This was especially the case for neonatal calves, within the first 2 weeks of life.

On July 18, 1921, BCG was given for the first time to a human being. A newborn boy received three consecutive oral doses of BCG, mounting to a total of 2.4×10^8 bacilli, on days 3, 5, and 7 after birth at the hospital La Charité in Paris under the supervision of Dr. Benjamin Weill-Hallé [6]. The boy lived in close contact with his grandmother suffering from tuberculosis. and his mother had died from the disease a few hours after delivery. Under those conditions, the probability of dying from tuberculosis within the first year of life was about 25%. After vaccination, the boy suffered from no notable adverse events and remained free of tuberculosis.

In the following years, many additional studies were conducted by Weill-Hallé and his disciple Raymond Turpin, confirming a good safety profile in neonates, even with doses up to 1.2×10^9 bacilli, and remarkable efficacy against infant tuberculosis in high-risk families [8]. In July 1924, a BCG manufacturing laboratory was established at the Institut Pasteur in Paris, and BCG was distributed throughout France, free of charge, with the request that the receiving physicians provide feedback on adverse events and efficacy. From July 1924 to January 1926, 5183 neonates had been vaccinated without any reported vaccine-related adverse events. During that period, 1317 children were followed up for 6 to 18 months after vaccination, and 107 of them had died. Among them, only 11 might have died from suspected tuberculosis. The vaccine effectiveness calculated based on the epidemiological background situation was estimated to be 93% against tuberculosis-caused childhood mortality during the first year of life [6].

Soon after, BCG was provided to many countries, initially mostly in tropical areas under French Protectorat, including Senegal, Madagascar, Vietnam, and others, which all hosted a Pasteur Institute, as a member of the international Pasteur Institutes network. Rapidly, other countries, such as Belgium, Italy, Poland, Sweden, Argentina, Brazil, and many others, also had access to BCG, leading eventually to a world-wide use of BCG.

Although numerous studies have shown the efficacy and safety of BCG in children, doubts persisted about its safety and potential reversion to virulence [9]. Furthermore, the statistical rigor employed by Calmette was vehemently criticized by epidemiologists and statisticians [10]. These doubts were further fueled by the "Lübeck Disaster", an unfortunate event, in which 251 newborns in Lübeck were vaccinated during early 1930 with a preparation thought to be based on a BCG culture provided a few months earlier by the Institut Pasteur in Paris. Seventy-two children died with disseminated tuberculosis, 131 developed clinical tuberculosis, while the others showed no tuberculosis symptoms. This led to the Calmette trial in 1931, which eventually established that BCG was not responsible for these deaths but that the Lübeck preparation was inadvertently contaminated with the virulent tubercle bacillus.

Nevertheless, this incidence caused an important setback for BCG, and it took close to 20 years to regain the universal acceptance of BCG. Finally, at the first international Congress on BCG held in June 1948 (Fig. 2.2), the World Health Organization declared in 10 concise bullet points that BCG is safe in humans and effective in preventing tuberculosis, and therefore it is recommended for large-scale vaccination, especially in newborns. BCG vaccination was integrated into the UNICEF program on infant immunization in 1974, and today this vaccine is still globally the most widely used vaccine and the oldest vaccine still in use.

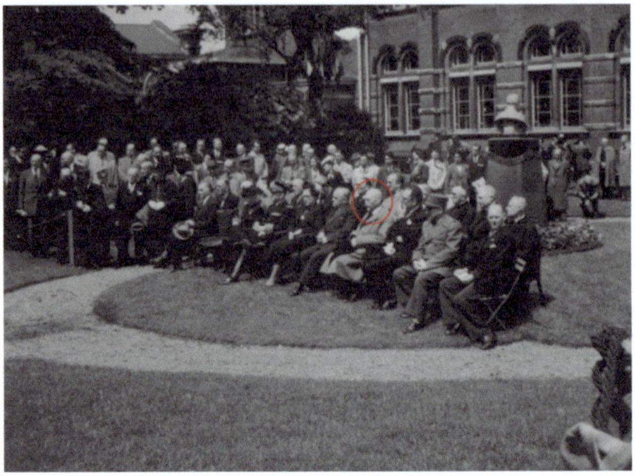

Fig. 2.2 First international BCG congress. In 1948 the first international BCG congress was held on the campus of the Institut Pasteur de Lille in the presence of Camille Guérin (circled in red). (With permission from General Director of Institut Pasteur de Lille)

2.3 BCG Substrains

As BCG was distributed throughout the world, associated with a precise protocol describing how to cultivate it, how to prepare it for vaccination, and how to deliver it [6], it has continued to evolve by continued culturing in different areas of the globe, at least until the 1960s, when finally archival seed lots were established. This has resulted in more than a dozen different daughter BCG strains displaying sometimes profound genetic heterogeneity [11].

The genome sequence of the BCG Pasteur 1173P2 strain became available in 2007 and could thus be compared to the genome sequences of *M. tuberculosis* and *M. bovis* [12]. These comparisons confirmed several important genomic differences between BCG and the other mycobacteria, including two large tandem duplications, which resulted in an increased genome size of BCG compared to *M. bovis*. More importantly, genome comparisons revealed 42 regions of difference (RD) between BCG and the other mycobacteria, most of which resulted in gene loss in BCG. Among them, one, named RD1, has been extensively studied and found to be a major contributor of attenuation which distinguishes BCG from the virulent mycobacteria [13]. RD1 contains part of the genes encoding the ESX-1 secretion system, responsible for the secretion of early secreted antigen target 6 (ESAT-6) and culture filtrate protein 10 (CFP-10), both involved in the virulence of *M. tuberculosis* by allowing the mycobacteria to egress from the phagosome into the cytosol [14]. However, ESAT-6 and CFP-10 are also considered protective antigens, and a BCG strain in which RD1 has been artificially introduced showed improved protection in rodent models as compared to the BCG mother strain [13]. Although the introduction of RD1 into the genome of BCG increased the BCG virulence, the virulence level remained still lower than that of *M. tuberculosis* [13], suggesting that additional changes in the genome of BCG might also contribute to attenuation.

Comparative genome analyses of the various daughter BCG strains revealed several single-nucleotide polymorphisms, as well as other genome rearrangements, such as genomic deletions, tandem duplications, and insertion sequences, which vary between the different daughter strains [15]. These polymorphisms have led to a subclassification of the various BCG strains into early strains, including BCG Russia, Moreau, Japan, Sweden, and Birkhaug, and late strains, including BCG Prague, Glaxo, Danish, Tice, Frappier, Connaught, Phipps, and Pasteur [16]. These genome polymorphisms also resulted in important variations in gene expression between early and late BCG strains, as well as within each group, which have also led to important differences in proteomic profiles between the different daughter strains [15].

Whether these genomic differences between the various BCG daughter strains have impact on the protective efficacy against tuberculosis is still a matter of debate. Although in use for more than 100 years now, the protective efficacy of BCG against tuberculosis varies tremendously between different clinical studies. A meta-analysis by Colditz et al. [17] concluded that BCG provides an overall protective efficacy of 50%, but it also showed large outcome variations between studies, some of which showed very low to no protective efficacy. While many reasons may be responsible for these variable outcomes between clinical studies, differences in strains used in the various settings have long been suspected to account for the differences in clinical outcomes [18]. A comprehensive study using murine models has compared the residual virulence and protective efficacy of 13 BCG strains and found that the late strains Phipps, Frappier, Pasteur, and Tice were more virulent in SCID mice than the early strains Sweden and Birkhaug, which was correlated with strain-specific DNA tandem duplications and deletions [19]. This study also found a general trend of greater effectiveness in a mouse protection assay with increased virulence, when reduction in the lung bacterial load was used as a measurement for protection.

However, considering the inherent limitations of the mouse models to predict the protective efficacy in humans, it is uncertain whether these conclusions can be extrapolated to protection in humans, and, as of today, there is no clear evidence that differences in BCG strains used in the vaccines may lead to differences in protective efficacy in humans. Only few studies have addressed this issue in humans, with inconclusive results. A randomized controlled study involving 209 infants immunized at birth with BCG Japan, BCG Russia, or BCG Denmark concluded that there were significant differences in immune responses induced by the three vaccines [20]. BCG Denmark, a late strain, and BCG Japan, an early strain, induced stronger immune responses, as evidenced by increased frequencies of mycobacteria-specific polyfunctional and cytotoxic T-cells and higher levels of Th1 cytokine production, than BCG Russia, another early strain. Transcriptomic studies have shown that genes involved in translation, including those coding for ribosomal proteins, were upregulated in BCG Denmark and BCG Japan compared to BCG Russia when grown in a liquid culture medium [15], suggesting increased protein synthesis, which may increase immunogenicity. However, as no immune correlate of protection against tuberculosis has yet been established, it is not clear whether and how these differences in immunogenicity may translate into differences in protection against tuberculosis in these infants. Furthermore, the three vaccines were produced and provided by three different manufacturers (Statens Serum Institute, Copenhagen;

BCG Laboratory, Tokyo and Bulbio; Sofia for BCG Danish, Japan, and Russia, respectively). Different manufacturing procedures may, therefore, also have had an impact on the immunogenicity of the vaccines.

2.4 Search for Immune Correlates of Protection

The variable efficacies seen in many of the BCG vaccine trials have prompted investigations to understand the reasons for these differences and to discover the immune correlates of protection in order to improve BCG vaccines. Several clinical studies have shown that BCG-mediated protection is higher in young children compared to other age groups and improves with the distance from the equator [21]. This has been suggested to be due to the likelihood of prior exposure to mycobacteria, including environmental, nontuberculous mycobacteria. These nontuberculous mycobacteria might have induced immunity against BCG and block BCG replication and, therefore, its immunogenicity [22]. However, a definitive proof of the involvement of environmental mycobacteria exposure in poor BCG-mediated protection is still lacking.

It is also possible that BCG protects better against some *M. tuberculosis* strains than against others. A case contact study conducted in Indonesia suggested that BCG protects better against infection by strains from a non-Beijing lineage than against strains from the Beijing lineage [23], a lineage that is most prevalent in Asia but is now spreading throughout the world.

BCG is today mostly given intradermally, and in most, albeit not all, cases, BCG vaccination induces a positive reaction in the TST. A negative TST result often motivates a second BCG vaccination. However, very early on, it was already recognized that there was no correlation between TST positivity and the protection induced by BCG [6], and the TST reaction can therefore not be used as a correlate of protection.

BCG is known to induce strong T- and B-cell responses. T-cell responses have long been recognized to be essential for the control of *M. tuberculosis* infection. Patients with reduced $CD4^+$ T-cell counts, such as AIDS patients, have a strongly increased risk of developing tuberculosis [24]. Neonatal BCG vaccination results in a strong Th1-type T-cell response and subjects with a genetic deficiency in the interferon-gamma signaling pathway have an increased risk to develop severe mycobacterial infections [25]. These observations establish the crucial importance of the Th1-type cytokines, such as interferon-gamma (IFN-γ), in protection against tuberculosis. These cytokines can activate macrophages to kill the intracellular *M. tuberculosis* bacteria.

However, we now know that the activation of the IFN-γ signaling pathway is not sufficient to provide protection against tuberculosis. An experimental tuberculosis vaccine designed to induce strong IFN-γ responses was found to provide no protection in a randomized placebo-controlled phase 2b trial in South Africa [26]. Furthermore, a study enrolling 5662 BCG-vaccinated infants did not find a significant difference in BCG-specific IFN-γ production between protected and unprotected children followed up for 2 years after vaccination [27]. There was also no difference in the frequencies of $CD4^+$, $CD8^+$, and $\gamma\delta$ T-cells in peripheral blood, nor in the expression of TNF-α, IL-2, and IL-17. The protective immune mechanism relies thus on more than the mere Th1 or Th17 immune responses, as can be measured in the blood.

Although disregarded initially because of the intracellular nature of *M. tuberculosis* infection, B-cell and antibody responses have more recently regained attention as the possible effectors of antituberculosis immunity. B-cells can function as antigen-presenting cells to T-cells, thereby enhancing the T-cell memory. Some of the BCG-induced anti-*M. tuberculosis* antibodies may also have protective potential [28].

A recent study comparing various routes of BCG vaccination in non-human primates has shown that the intravenous route of vaccination induced the strongest immunity against tuberculosis disease and provided near-sterile immunity against *M. tuberculosis* infection in most vaccinated animals [29]. Interestingly, this was associated with a strong induction of antigen-specific tissue-resident memory T-cells in the lungs, not seen when BCG was administered by other routes. Since tuberculosis is mostly, but not exclusively, a pulmonary disease, this observation might provide a mechanistic explanation for enhanced protection by intravenous BCG vaccination.

2.5 Nonspecific Effects of BCG

Shortly after the large-scale implementation of BCG vaccination in various countries, Calmette noted that among children vaccinated with BCG, the mortality rates during the first year of life due to causes other than tuberculosis was also significantly lower than what was observed among nonvaccinated children [30]. In a French study, vaccinated infants appeared to be generally more resistant to various infant infections, which suggested to Calmette that either *M. tuberculosis* infection plays a more important role in infant mortality than that previously assumed or that BCG confers "a special aptitude to resist those other infections which are so frequent in young children." [31] Similar observations were made by Carl Naeslund studying the overall mortality of 20,000 children between 0 and 4 years in Sweden. He concluded that "One could obviously seek to explain the lower mortality of vaccinated children by the idea that BCG causes a non-specific immunity." [32] This reduction in overall mortality and morbidity has subsequently been confirmed in many observational studies and randomized controlled trials [33].

These nonspecific protective effects are likely due to the ability of BCG to induce trained immunity of innate immune cells that are able to protect in an antigen-agnostic manner [34]. The concept of trained innate immunity induced by BCG has been extensively discussed during the last decade and was shown to rely on epigenetic changes and metabolic reprogramming of innate immune cells [35]. This leads to enhanced expression of activation markers, cytokine production, and enhanced effector functions of neutrophils, which may explain the nonspecific protective effects against heterologous infections.

However, BCG has also found many applications in conditions other than infectious diseases, as recently summarized at the Third International Symposium on BCG [36]. Since more than 50 years, BCG has been successfully used in the treatment of non-muscle-invasive bladder cancer [37]. Intravesical injection of BCG can eradicate and prevent the recurrence of superficial bladder tumors. Although the mechanism has not been fully elucidated yet, BCG can attach to urothelial cells and induce strong local inflammatory responses and apoptotic cell death of tumor cells.

In addition to the proinflammatory properties of BCG, potentially important for its effect against heterologous infectious diseases and bladder cancer, BCG also displays important anti-inflammatory properties and was shown to prevent or at least diminish the symptoms of a variety of inflammatory and auto-immune conditions [38], including atopy, multiple sclerosis, type 1 diabetes [39], and Alzheimer's disease [40].

2.6 A Glimpse at the Future

BCG was primarily designed as an antituberculosis vaccine, and as such, its protective effect against tuberculosis in newborns has largely been confirmed in numerous studies, with the rates of protection against laboratory-confirmed cases of an estimated average of 83% [41]. In contrast, protective rates against pulmonary tuberculosis in adolescents and adults are much more variable, and the average protective efficacy, as estimated by large meta-analyses, is approximately 50% [17]. Interestingly, Calmette already insisted that BCG be used very early in life, preferably immediately after birth [31]. There is thus room for improvement to enhance protection against pulmonary tuberculosis in adolescents and adults, who represent the most contagious patient groups.

BCG-induced immunity wanes over time, and Calmette recommended BCG revaccination at ages of 3, 7, and 15 years [31]. However, a large cluster-randomized trial carried out in Brazil in 761 schools involving more than 200,000 children aged 7–14 years randomized 1:1, all of which had received as single BCG vaccination as infants, showed no substantial additional protection against tuberculosis disease by revaccination [42]. This is somewhat in contrast to the results from a more recent study performed in South Africa with close to 1000 adolescents randomized 1:1:1 to receive placebo, BCG, or an experimental vaccine [43]. All had received neonatal BCG vaccination and were tested negative for *M. tuberculosis* infection at the time of enrolment. After a follow-up of 30 months, BCG was concluded to reduce sustained *M. tuberculosis* infection by 45.5% over placebo. A recent, larger placebo-controlled efficacy study, also conducted in South Africa could not confirm these initial results [44].

In addition to BCG revaccination studies, many efforts are deployed to improve the protective efficacy of BCG by genetic engineering. The first attempt to improve BCG consisted of over-producing one of the protective antigens, named Antigen

85B, in a recombinant BCG strain. In a guinea pig model of pulmonary tuberculosis, this strain reduced the bacterial load after infection with a highly virulent *M. tuberculosis* strain by 0.5–1 log more than the parental nonrecombinant BCG strain. This was paralleled by fewer and smaller lesions in the lung, spleen, and liver [44]. Despite these encouraging results, this vaccine has not reached clinical development.

The most advanced recombinant BCG vaccine strain is VPM1002. This vaccine was designed based on the assumption that a recombinant BCG strain inducing more $CD8^+$ T-cell responses than nonrecombinant BCG would also induce superior protection. Increased $CD8^+$ T-cell responses occur when antigens are targeted to the MHC I pathway in antigen-presenting cells, which is the preferred antigen-presenting mechanism for cytosolic antigens. By using a recombinant BCG strain that produces listeriolysin, meant to help BCG antigens to egress from the phagosome into the cytoplasm, and that lacks urease C in order to decrease the intraphagosomal pH to a range that is optimal for listeriolysin activity, mice were indeed better protected against *M. tuberculosis* challenge than after vaccination with nonrecombinant BCG [45]. Importantly, while nonrecombinant BCG showed poor protection against a Beijing strain in mice, vaccination with the recombinant strain resulted in significant protection against the same Beijing strain. Interestingly, the recombinant strain also proved to be safer in immune-compromised mice, as SCID mice survived significantly longer after the administration of the recombinant vaccine strain than after the administration of the nonrecombinant BCG.

This vaccine has now undergone several clinical trials in adults and in neonates. A phase 2, double-blind, randomized controlled trial in South African newborns showed less reactogenicity than BCG, in both HIV-exposed and unexposed babies [46]. However, immunogenicity, as measured by the percentages of multifunctional $CD4^+$ T-cells and $CD8^+$ T-cells, was lower for VPM1002 than for BCG. This vaccine is now in a head-to-head comparison study with BCG to evaluate the potential superiority in the prevention of tuberculosis disease.

A different vaccine, named MTBVAC, is based on the hypothesis that BCG, originated from *M. bovis*, may be less protective than an attenuated variant of *M. tuberculosis*. Although most antigens are conserved between the two species, *M. tuberculosis* produces additional protective antigens that are absent in *M. bovis*, such as ESAT-6, for example. MTBVAC is an attenuated mutant of the clinical isolate *M. tuberculosis* Mt103, engineered to lack the *fadD26* and *phoP* genes [47]. In preclinical studies, MTBVAC was at least as safe as BCG, including in immune-compromised mice, but outperformed BCG in its protective effect against *M. tuberculosis* challenge in various animal models, including nonhuman primates [48]. This vaccine has also entered clinical development, and several clinical trials have been completed in adults and in neonates, in Europe and South Africa, showing a safety profile comparable to that of BCG and a durable $CD4^+$ memory T-cell response that was superior to that induced by BCG [49]. A phase 3 trial is currently ongoing to compare the efficacy of MTBVAC to that of BCG in more than 7000 HIV-uninfected infants at various sites in Sub-Saharan Africa (NCT04975178). This study is planned to be completed in 2028.

Other live-attenuated or recombinant BCG vaccine candidates are being developed across the globe, such as recombinant BCG strains that produce human cytokines (e.g., Ref [50]) or that have the *M. tuberculosis* or *Mycobacterium marinum* RD1 region inserted into their chromosome [13, 51]. However, none of them have yet entered clinical evaluation. Some of these recombinant strains may also show enhanced performance in the nonspecific prophylactic or therapeutic effects, as has already been seen in preclinical models [52].

2.7 Conclusions

Although a centenary vaccine, BCG is today still the most widely used vaccine in the world, mainly to protect young infants from severe and deadly tuberculosis. Other applications have emerged over the last 50 years, the most important of which is the use of BCG for the treatment of non-muscle-invasive bladder cancer. However, other indications are also actively being pursued, such as for the treatment of type 1 diabetes. Many more may come in the future, as increasing numbers of studies are being conducted on a variety of inflammatory and autoimmune diseases, including neurodegenerative diseases, such as Alzheimer's disease. Despite these important developments, many basic questions on the mode of action as a vaccine against tuberculosis and of the nonspecific effects remain unanswered. These knowledge gaps are important hurdles for strategies to improve BCG. Tuberculosis is still one of the most important global causes of death due to infection, despite a wide BCG vaccination coverage. Whether a vaccine that is better than BCG against tuberculosis will ever become available is still an open question, and finding immune correlates of protection remains a major challenge. The reasons for the enormous variation in efficacy between the various clinical studies are still not elucidated, and it is still not clear whether different BCG substrains display different protective properties in humans. There are thus many questions for which we still seek answers, but the great potential of BCG in a wide range of applications will probably maintain a strong interest in this vaccine at least for the next 100 years to come.

Competing Interests The author(s) has no competing interests to declare that are relevant to the content of this manuscript.

Ethics Approval The author(s) declares that this manuscript does not include primary research with human participants.

References

1. Sakula A. BCG: who were Calmette and Guérin? Thorax. 1983;38:806–12.
2. Calmette A, Guérin C. Origine intestinale de la tuberculose pulmonaire. Ann Inst Pasteur. 1905;19:601–18.
3. Calmette A, Guérin C. Vaccination des bovidés contre la tuberculose par les voies digestives. Ann Inst Pasteur. 1907;21:525–32.

4. Calmette A, Guérin C. Sur la vaccination contre la tuberculose par les voies digestives. CR Acad Sci. 1906;142:1319–22.
5. Calmette A, Guérin C. Sur quelques propriétés du bacille tuberculeux d'origine bovine cultivé sur bile de bœuf glycérinée. CR Acad Sci. 1909;149:716–8.
6. Calmette A, Guérin C, Nègre L, et al. Prémunition des nouveau-nés contre la tuberculose par le vaccin BCG (1921 à 1926). Ann Inst Pasteur. 1926;40:89–133.
7. Calmette A, Guérin C. Vaccination des bovidés contre la tuberculose et méthode nouvelle de prophylaxie de la tuberculose bovine. Ann Inst Pasteur. 1924;38:371–98.
8. Camlette A, Guérin C, Weill-Hallé B, et al. Essais de prémunition par le BCG contre l'infection tuberculeuse de l'homme et des animaux. Bull Acad Med. 1924;91:787–96.
9. Petroff SA, Branch A, Steenken W. A study of Bacillus Calmette-Guérin (BCG). Biological characteristics, cultural "dissociation" and animal experimentation. Am Rev Tuberc. 1929;19:9–46.
10. Greenwood M. Professor Calmette's statistical study of B.C.G. vaccination. Br Med J. 1928;1:793–5.
11. Behr MA, et al. Comparative genomics of BCG vaccines by whole-genome DNA microarray. Science. 1999;284:1520–3.
12. Brosch R, Gordon SV, Garnier T, et al. Genome plasticity of BCG and impact on vaccine efficacy. Proc Natl Acad Sci USA. 2007;104:5596–601.
13. Pym AS, Brodin P, Majlessi L, et al. Recombinant BCG exporting ESAT-6 confers enhanced protection against tuberculosis. Nat Med. 2003;9:533–9.
14. Majlessi L, Brosch R. *Mycobacterium tuberculosis* meets the cytosol: the role of cGAS in antimycobacterial immunity. Cell Host Microb. 2015;17:733–5.
15. Abdallah MA, Hill-Cawthorne GA, Otto TD, et al. Genomic expression catalogue of a global collection of BCG vaccine strains show evidence for highly diverged metabolic and cell-wall adaptations. Sci Rep. 2015;5:15443.
16. Behr MA, Small PM. A historical and molecular phylogeny of BCG strains. Vaccine. 1999;17:915–22.
17. Colditz GA, Brewer TF, Berkey CS, et al. Efficacy of BCG vaccine in the prevention of tuberculosis. Meta-analysis of the published literature. JAMA. 1994;271:698–702.
18. Dubos RJ, Pierce CH. Differential characteristics in vitro and in vivo of several substrains of BCG. IV Immunizing effectiveness. Am Rev Tuberc. 1956;74:699–717.
19. Zhang L, Ru HW, Chen FZ, et al. Variable virulence and efficacy of BCG vaccine strains in mice and correlation with genome polymorphisms. Mol Ther. 2016;24:398–405.
20. Ritz N, Dutta B, Donath S, et al. The influence of Bacille Calmette-Guérin vaccine strain on the immune response against tuberculosis. Am J Respir Crit Care Med. 2012;185:213–22.
21. Mangtani P, Abubakar I, Ariti C, et al. Protection by BCG vaccine against tuberculosis: a systematic review of randomized controlled trials. Clin Infect Dis. 2014;58:470–80.
22. Palmer CE, Long MW. Effects of infection with atypical mycobacteria on BCG vaccination and tuberculosis. Am Rev Respir Dis. 1966;94:553–68.
23. Verrall AJ, Chaidir L, Ruesen C, et al. Lower bacillus Calmette-Guérin protection against *Mycobacterium tuberculosis* infection after exposure to Beijing strains. Am J Respir Crit Care Med. 2020;201:1152–5.
24. Getahun H, Gunneberg C, Granich R, et al. HIV infection-associated tuberculosis: the epidemiology and the response. Clin Infect Dis. 2009;50(Suppl 3):S201–7.
25. Altare F, Durandy A, Lammas D, et al. Impairment of mycobacterial immunity in human interleukin-12 receptor deficiency. Science. 1998;280:1432–5.
26. Tameris MD, Hatherill M, Landry BS, et al. Safety and efficacy of MVA85A, a new tuberculosis vaccine, in infants previously vaccinated with BCG: a randomized, placebo-controlled phase 2b trial. Lancet. 2013;381:1021–8.
27. Kagina BMN, Abel B, Scriba TJ, et al. Specific T cell frequency and cytokine expression profile do not correlate with protection against tuberculosis after bacillus Calmette-Guérin vaccination of newborns. Am J Respir Crit Care Med. 2010;182:1073–9.

28. Li H, Wang XX, Wang B, et al. Latently and uninfected healthcare workers exposed to TB make protective antibodies against *Mycobacterium tuberculosis*. Proc Natl Acad Sci USA. 2017;114:5023–8.
29. Darrah PA, Zeppa JJ, Maiello P, et al. Prevention of tuberculosis in macaques after intravenous BCG immunization. Nature. 2020;577:95–102.
30. Calmette A, Guérin C, Weill-Hallé B, Nègre L, Boquet A, Wilbert TR. Essais de prémunition par le BCG contre l'infection tuberculeuse de l'homme et des animaux. Bull. Acad Med. 1925;92:681–9.
31. Calmette A. Preventive vaccination against tuberculosis with BCG. Proc Royal Soc Med. 1931;24:1481–90.
32. Naeslund C. Résultats des expériences de vaccination par le BCG poursuivies dans le Norrbotten (Suède) [Septembre 1927-Décembre 1931]. Vaccine Prev Tuberc Rapp Doc Paris Inst Pasteur; 1932. p. 274–84.
33. Higgins JPT, Soares-Weiser K, López-López JA, et al. Association of BCG, DTP, and measles containing vaccines with childhood mortality: systematic review. BMJ. 2016;355:i5170.
34. Netea MG, van Crevel R. BCG-induced protection: effects on innate immune memory. Semin Immunol. 2014;26:512–7.
35. Kleinnijenhuis J, Quintin J, Preijers F, et al. Bacille Calmette-Guerin induces NOD2-dependent nonspecific protection from reinfection via epigenetic reprogramming of monocytes. Proc Natl Acad Sci USA. 2012;109:17537–42.
36. Locht C. Highlights of the 3rd international BCG symposium: 100th anniversary of the first administration of BCG. Microbes Infect. 2022;24:105043.
37. Lamm DL, Morales A. A BCG success story: from prevention of tuberculosis to optimal bladder cancer treatment. Vaccine. 2021;39:7308–18.
38. Kowalewicz-Kulbat M, Locht C. BCG and protection against inflammatory and auto-immune diseases. Exp Rev Vaccines. 2017;16:699–708.
39. Kühltreiber WM, Tran L, Kim T, et al. Long-term reduction in hyperglycemia in advanced type 1 diabetes: the value of induced aerobic glycolysis with BCG vaccinations. npj Vaccines. 2018;3:23.
40. Gofrit ON, Klein BY, Cohen IR, et al. Bacillus Calmette-Guérin (BCG) therapy lowers the incidence of Alzheimer's disease in bladder cancer patients. PLoS One. 2019;14:e0224433.
41. Colditz GA, Berkey CS, Mosteller F, et al. The efficacy of bacillus Calmette-Guérin vaccination of newborns and infants in the prevention of tuberculosis: meta-analysis of the published literature. Pediatrics. 1995;96:29–35.
42. Rodrigues LC, Pereira SM, Cunha SS, et al. Effect of BCG revaccination on incidence of tuberculosis in school-aged children in Brazil: the BCG-REVAC cluster-randomised trial. Lancet. 2005;366:1290–5.
43. Nemes E, Geldenhuys H, Rozot V, et al. Prevention of *M. tuberculosis* infection with H4:IC31 vaccine or BCG revaccination. N Engl J Med. 2018;379:138–49.
44. Schmidt AC, Fairlie L, Hellström E, et al. BCG Revaccination for the prevention of Mycobacterium tuberculosis infection. N Eng J Med 2025;392:1789–1800.
45. Horwitz MA, Harth G, Dillon BJ, et al. Recombinant bacillus Calmette-Guérin (BCG) vaccines expressing the *Mycobacterium tuberculosis* 30-kDa major secretory protein induce greater protective immunity against tuberculosis than conventional BCG vaccines in a highly susceptible animal model. Proc Natl Acad Sci USA. 2000;97:13853–8.
46. Grode L, Seiler P, Baumann S, et al. Increased vaccine efficacy against tuberculosis of recombinant *Mycobacterium bovis* bacilli Calmette-Guérin mutants that secrete listeriolysin. J Clin Invest. 2005;115:2472–9.
47. Cotton MF, Madhi SA, Luabeya AK, et al. Safety and immunogenicity of VPM1002 versus BCG in South African newborn babies: a randomized, phase 2 non-inferiority double-blind controlled trial. Lancet Infect Dis. 2022;22:1472–83.
48. Arbues A, Aguilo JI, Gonzalo-Asensio J, et al. Construction, characterization and preclinical evaluation of MTBVAC, the first live-attenuated *M. tuberculosis*-based vaccine to enter clinical trials. Vaccine. 2013;31:4867–73.

49. White AD, Sibley L, Sarfas C, et al. MTBVAC vaccination protects rhesus macaques against aerosol challenge with *M. tuberculosis* and induces immune signatures analogous to those observed in clinical studies. npj Vaccines. 2021;6:4.
50. Tameris M, Mearns H, Penn-Nicholson A, et al. Live-attenuated *Mycobacterium tuberculosis* vaccine MTBVAC versus BCG in adults and neonates: a randomized controlled, double-blind dose-escalation trial. Lancet Respir Med. 2019;7:757–70.
51. Szpakowski P, Biet F, Locht C, et al. Dendritic cell activity driven by recombinant *Mycobacterium bovis* BCG producing human IL-18, in healthy BCG vaccinated adults. J Immunol Res. 2015;2015:359153.
52. Gröschel MI, Sayes F, Shin SJ, et al. Recombinant BCG expressing ESX-1 of *Mycobacterium marinum* combines low virulence with cytosolic immune signaling and improved TB protection. Cell Rep. 2017;18:2752–65.
53. Kowalewicz-Kulbat M, Locht C. Recombinant BCG to enhance its immunomodulatory activities. Vaccine. 2022;10:827.

TB or Not TB: The Parallel Lives of BCG

3

Mayra Fernanda Martínez-López, Pedro Curto, Palmira Barreira-Silva, Rita Fior, and Pedro Moura-Alves

3.1 Parallel Lives of BCG

The Bacillus Calmette-Guérin (BCG) vaccine has been widely used for over a century. This enduring presence in vaccination programs is largely due to BCG's proven ability to protect newborns from severe forms of tuberculosis (TB), including TB meningitis and miliary TB, making it a staple in the immunization schedules of numerous countries for decades [1, 2]. BCG is one of the most widely administered vaccines globally, with over 100 million individuals receiving it each year [1]. This extensive use has generated substantial epidemiological evidence, indicating that infants vaccinated with BCG exhibit lower rates of all-cause mortality, benefit that extends beyond mere TB prevention [1, 2]. Studies, particularly with individuals

Mayra Fernanda Martínez-López, Pedro Curto and Palmira Barreira-Silva contributed equally with all other contributors.

M. F. Martínez-López · R. Fior (✉)
Champalimaud Research, Champalimaud Foundation, Av. Brasilia, Lisbon, Portugal
e-mail: rita.fior@neuro.fchampalimaud.org

P. Curto
i3S, Institute for Research and Innovation in Health, University of Porto, Porto, Portugal

IBMC, Institute for Molecular and Cell Biology, University of Porto, Porto, Portugal

CiBB, Centre for Innovative Biomedicine and Biotechnology, University of Coimbra, Coimbra, Portugal

P. Barreira-Silva · P. Moura-Alves (✉)
i3S, Institute for Research and Innovation in Health, University of Porto, Porto, Portugal

IBMC, Institute for Molecular and Cell Biology, University of Porto, Porto, Portugal
e-mail: pmouraalves@i3s.up.pt

P. J. G. Bettencourt (ed.), *Tuberculosis Vaccines*,
https://doi.org/10.1007/978-3-031-94540-3_3

from countries of the African continent, have demonstrated that BCG vaccination offers protection against respiratory viral diseases in children [3]. The vaccine's ability to boost immune system responses extends beyond childhood, protecting adolescents, adults, and the elderly against various infectious diseases, including respiratory tract infections (Fig. 3.1), puzzling, as it contrasts with its failure to protect against adult pulmonary TB [4–6]. Experimental models have also shown BCG's protective effects against yellow fever, malaria, and cancer (Fig. 3.1) [7–9]. In light of these findings, BCG has been tested in clinical trials involving elderly patients to assess its potential to prevent subsequent infections after hospital discharge [10]. Herein, we discuss multiple studies and applications of BCG to treat infections other than TB and other diseases, such as cancer, asthma, and neurological and metabolic diseases.

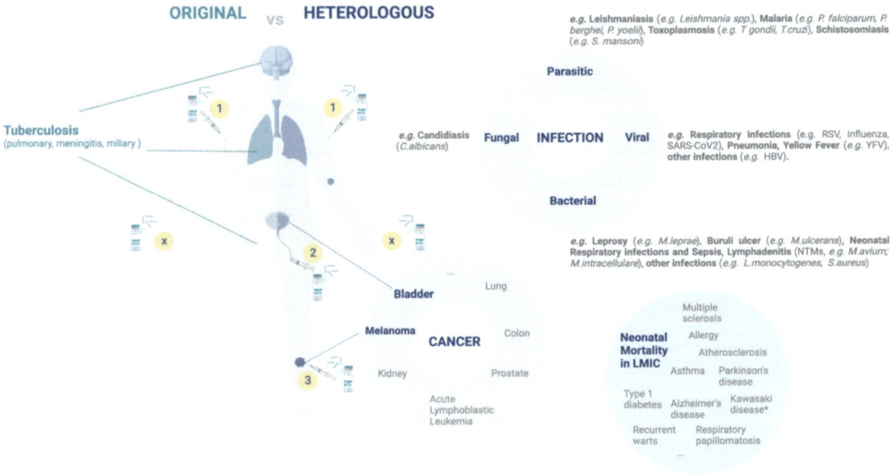

Fig. 3.1 The parallel lives of BCG. The efficacy and outcomes of BCG vaccination have been assessed in multiple diseases, other than its original purpose, preventing Tuberculosis. These span from infectious-related diseases (e.g., other bacterial infections, viral infections), cancer (e.g., bladder, melanoma), and others (e.g., asthma, multiple Sclerosis). Furthermore, BCG vaccination has also been proposed as a potential aid in diagnostic applications (e.g., Kawasaki disease). Furthermore, in addition to its major route of administration, intradermal (1), other routes of administration have also been evaluated and/or are in use (e.g., Intravesical instillation (2); Intratumoral injection (3); and others (X, e.g., oral or intranasal administration). * BCG as diagnostic tool Abbreviations: HBV Hepatitis B Virus, LMIC Lower-Middle Income Countries, RSV Respiratory Syncytial Virus, SARS-CoV2 Severe Acute Respiratory Syndrome Coronavirus 2, YFV Yellow Fever Virus. (Created in BioRender. Moura Alves, P. (2024) BioRender.com/t96i918)

3.1.1 BCG and Cancer Immunotherapy

History of Cancer Immunotherapy

Immunotherapy was termed by the scientific community as the "breakthrough of the year" more than a decade ago [11]. Nonetheless, as far back as 3000 years ago in ancient Egypt, there were already accounts of neoplastic-like diseases being cured following episodes of infection and fever. Throughout history, additional reports of neoplastic growths spontaneously regressing in patients after postoperative infections or the onset of diseases such as erysipelas and syphilis have surfaced [12].

In the nineteenth century, Dr. William Coley, a bone surgeon, became particularly intrigued by the observed effects of postoperative infections on cancer. At a time when surgical resection was the sole treatment option for cancer, and motivated by his own clinical experiences, Coley decided to inject *Streptococcus pyogenes* directly into the tumor of a patient with an inoperable sarcoma (Fig. 3.2). After 60 consecutive rounds of daily injections, which induced signs of infection, the patient was reportedly cured [13, 14]. Building on this success and aiming to

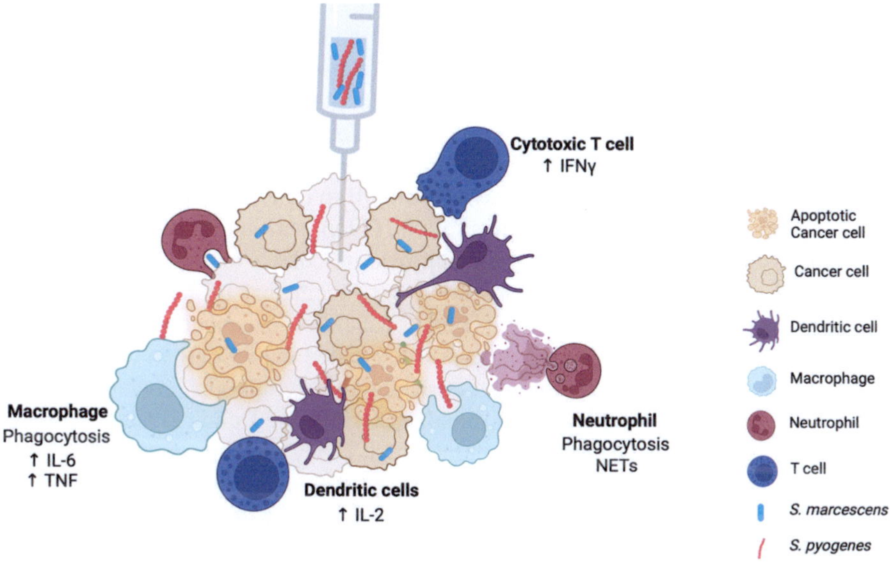

Fig. 3.2 Proposed anticancer effect of Coley's toxin. Following intratumoral administration, heat-inactivated *S. pyogenes* and *S. marcescens* are phagocytosed by tumor-associated macrophages and neutrophils. This initiates the production and release of proinflammatory cytokines, including TNF, which trigger apoptosis in cancer cells and recruit immune cells, such as cytotoxic T lymphocytes (CTLs). Concurrently, dendritic cells (DCs) recognize the bacterial components, present bacterial antigens to T-cells, and secrete IL-2. These combined actions lead to the induction of cancer cell apoptosis and contribute to tumor regression. Abbreviations: CTL cytotoxic T lymphocyte, DC dendritic cell, IFNγ interferon gamma, IL interleukin, NETs neutrophil extracellular traps, TNF tumor necrosis factor-alpha. (Figure adapted from [27]. Created in BioRender. Moura-Alves, P. (2024) BioRender.com/i88a580)

treat cancer patients more broadly, Dr. Coley developed a vaccine using heat-killed toxins from *Streptococcus pyogenes* and *Serratia marcescens* [14]. However, the vaccine eventually fell out of favor due to several factors: the unclear mechanism of action, the risk of systemic infections, inconsistent results, and the rise of chemotherapy and radiation therapy as new treatment options. It was not until nearly half a century later that those advancements in understanding the physiological processes of sepsis and infection began to reveal the underlying mechanisms behind the anticancer effects of Coley's toxins [13, 15, 16].

Anticancer Effects of Coley's Toxins

When Coley's toxins vaccine (Fig. 3.2) was developed, the complex cascade of inflammatory responses was not yet well understood [13, 14, 16]. Decades later, the critical role of cytokines in immune responses was finally elucidated [17]. It was discovered that the activation of the immune system, along with proinflammatory responses and fever, is regulated by the expression of interleukins (IL-1, IL-2, and IL-6), tumor necrosis factor (TNF), and interferon gamma (IFNγ) [17–19]. Furthermore, it was revealed that immune cells are not static; rather, they are dynamic, and their functions can be activated and modulated by both external and internal stimuli [20, 21]. This understanding led to the belief that Coley's toxins worked by triggering a proinflammatory activation of the immune system, which then polarized immune cells toward an antitumoral phenotype (Fig. 3.2). As a result, Coley's toxins are recognized as a form of nonspecific immunotherapy [15]. Unfortunately, there was no standardized method for producing this vaccine, resulting in multiple formulations and inconsistent clinical outcomes [22]. The lack of reproducible results and limited positive reports from other clinicians prompted the United States Food and Drug Administration (FDA), starting in 1963, to mandate rigorous testing in clinical trials for the approval of Coley's toxins in humans [22]. Since then, conducting human studies using this vaccine has been highly challenging, hindering further exploration of its biological effects in cancer patients. Despite these challenges, some researchers successfully tested the vaccine in clinical trials for various cancer types, including non-Hodgkin's lymphoma, melanoma, and hepatocellular carcinoma [23–25]. A notable 2012 Phase I clinical trial involving NY-ESO-1-expressing cancers demonstrated that Coley's vaccine significantly elevated serum cytokines, such as IL-6, in treated patients, accompanied by an increase in body temperature [26]—effects that closely mirrored Coley's original observations [14]. Remarkably, a patient with metastatic bladder cancer experienced a significant reduction in tumor size correlated with these immunological responses. This study underscored the potential of Coley's toxins as powerful immunomodulators in cancer treatment [22]. However, the financial and logistical challenges of developing this vaccine have made further research and exploration of Coley's toxins in cancer therapy difficult to achieve [22].

BCG Use in Cancer Immunotherapy

Heterologous immunotherapy functions by broadly activating the immune system through the induction of inflammatory responses. This approach does not directly target cancer cells; instead, they are eliminated as part of a wider, systemic reaction. To the best of the authors' knowledge, Coley's vaccine was the first nonspecific immunotherapy to be clinically utilized and documented. Although Coley's toxins vaccine is no longer in use, the BCG vaccine has emerged as a promising candidate in cancer immunotherapy.

In 1959, researchers demonstrated BCG's effectiveness in murine cancer models, revealing that mice inoculated with BCG exhibited increased resistance to tumor engraftment [28]. A decade later, *Zbar* et al. confirmed BCG's antitumoral effects in guinea pigs, where live BCG was directly injected into subcutaneous tumors [29]. The treated guinea pigs showed significant tumor rejection and were protected from metastasis. The researchers also identified several key factors for BCG's optimal efficacy: proximity to the tumor, an immunocompetent host, a sufficient number of viable mycobacteria, and a small tumor burden [29]. Building on the preclinical success of direct BCG injections in tumor regression, its potential for treating advanced prostate cancer was first explored in 1973. *Merrin* et al. reported that intraprostatic injections of BCG and PPD successfully induced tumor necrosis in an immunocompetent patient [30]. However, this effect was not observed in another patient with deficient lymphocyte function, underscoring the critical role of an intact immune system for the efficacy of this treatment [30]. This initial study was followed by further analysis involving a larger cohort of patients, with results presented in 1976 at the Workshop in Genitourinary Cancer Immunology held in Iowa City. The findings demonstrated that intratumoral injection of BCG, later termed intralesional administration, led to macrophage infiltration and granuloma formation, which in turn induced necrosis of prostate cancer cells [31]. Subsequent studies confirmed similar results, further validating the immunotherapeutic potential of BCG in prostate cancer [32]. However, the development of severe side effects, particularly granulomatous growths in other organs such as the intestine, has limited the widespread adoption of BCG treatment in prostate cancer [31].

The visible and accessible nature of cutaneous melanoma made it an ideal candidate for testing the efficacy of intralesional BCG therapy. In 1974, a 7-year study involving 151 melanoma patients treated with BCG, either as a standalone therapy or as an adjuvant to surgery, demonstrated that direct intralesional injection into metastatic melanoma lesions in the skin yielded the highest treatment efficacy, with 90% tumor regression [33]. Interestingly, abscopal responses were also observed in immunocompetent patients, with 17% of non-injected tumors showing regression. While these results were promising, BCG proved less effective when used as an adjuvant therapy or for treating subcutaneous or visceral tumors compared to direct injection [33]. Nevertheless, this study reinforced *Zbar* et al.'s assertion that BCG achieves maximum efficacy when in direct contact with the tumors [29]. The superior efficacy of intralesional administration was also underscored by studies using intradermal BCG, which aimed to induce a systemic immune response. These studies failed to produce significant tumor regression or disease-free survival in melanoma patients [34–36], demonstrating the importance of direct tumor engagement for therapeutic success. To date, although not a first-line treatment due to its side effects, intralesional BCG remains listed as an optional therapy for stage III in-transit cutaneous melanoma in the National Comprehensive Cancer Network (NCCN) guidelines [37]. These promising results established the efficacy of intratumoral BCG and set the stage for further research across various types of cancer.

In 1980, a pivotal trial involving 33 patients with lung cancer who received intratumoral BCG—26 of whom also underwent pulmonary resection—was published [38]. Consistent with the findings in other cancers, patients who responded positively to BCG treatment exhibited significant inflammation and immune cell infiltration within their tumors. Remarkably, at a median follow-up of 16 months, 85% of patients with bronchogenic carcinoma and 58% with metastatic cancer remained relapse-free, highlighting the potential of BCG as a valuable therapeutic strategy in lung cancer [38].

In the bladder, due to its unique anatomical characteristics, BCG treatment has shown greater success, as it allowed for intravesical administration, ensuring direct contact between the bacilli and the tumor cells (Fig. 3.3) [39]. In animal models, such as dogs treated with intravesical BCG, researchers observed an inflammatory

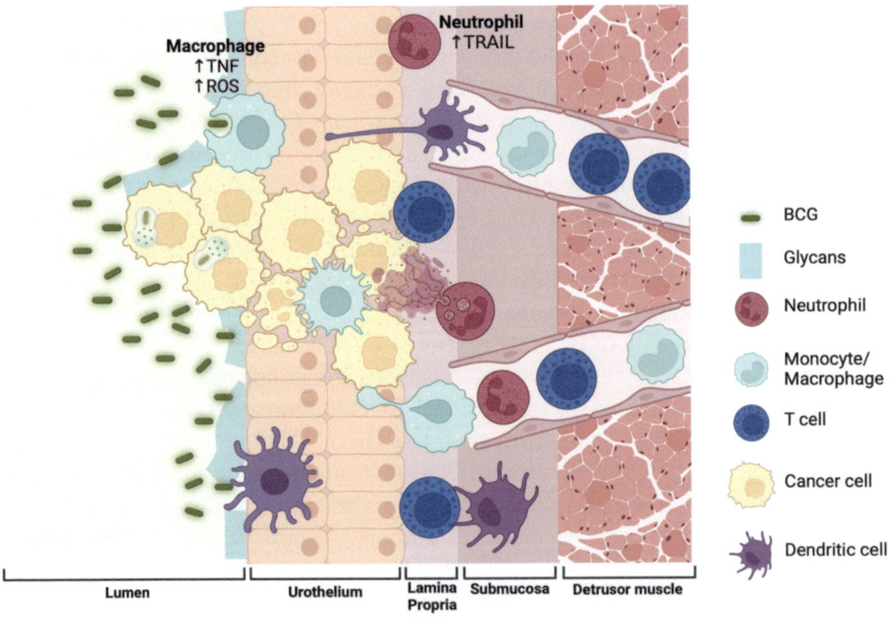

Fig. 3.3 BCG therapy in bladder cancer. Live BCG adheres to the urothelium via fibronectin and integrin α5b1 and is internalized by bladder cancer cells through macropinocytosis. Resident macrophages and dendritic cells phagocytose the bacteria. This process leads to increased expression of MHC II (on antigen-presenting cells and cancer cells) and presentation of tumor epitopes, facilitating the recruitment of T lymphocytes. Simultaneously, macrophages release cytokines and chemokines, attracting innate and adaptive immune cells from the circulation. These activated and recruited cells induce cancer cell apoptosis through direct cell-to-cell contact and by secreting cytotoxic agents such as nitric oxide (NO) and tumor necrosis factor (TNF). Abbreviations: BCG bacillus Calmette-Guérin, TNF tumor necrosis factor, ROS reactive oxygen species. (Figure adapted from [27]. Created in BioRender. Moura Alves, P. (2024) BioRender.com/q54h175)

Table 3.1 Treatment recommendations for bladder cancer according to risk classification

Classification	Treatment recommendation
NMIBC—Low risk	TURBT + One instillation of chemotherapy
NMIBC—Intermediate risk	TURBT + Several instillations of chemotherapy for 1 year max Or TURBT + 1 year of BCG instillations
NMIBC—High risk	TURBT + 1 to 3 years of BCG instillations
NMIBC BCG-resistant or MIBC	Radical cystectomy Trimodal therapy Immune checkpoint therapy Adjuvant therapy + partial cystectomy

Abbreviations: *NMIBC* non-muscle-invasive bladder cancer, *MIBC* muscle-invasive bladder cancer, *TURBT* transurethral resection of bladder tumor, *BCG* bacillus Calmette-Guérin. Based on the European Association of Urology Guidelines [55]

response in the bladder wall, which resolved within approximately 7 weeks [40]. These promising results led to a clinical study in 1976, introducing intravesical BCG therapy for non-muscle-invasive bladder cancer (NMIBC) [41]. This treatment has demonstrated significant success and continues to be widely used today (discussed in detail below; Table 3.1).

Alternative routes of administration for BCG immunotherapy have also been explored to enhance its efficacy (Fig. 3.1). For example, *Eriguchi* et al. investigated the use of oral BCG in patients with gastrointestinal cancer [42]. Oral administration of BCG successfully activated immune cells within the mesenteric lymph nodes, demonstrating a localized immune response. Notably, in patients with stage IV stomach cancer, those treated with oral BCG had a significantly higher 2-year survival rate (44.4%) compared to those who did not receive BCG (6.3%) [42]. However, this treatment approach was not further validated, and subsequent studies using BCG as an intradermal adjuvant for colorectal cancer yielded inconsistent results.

The effectiveness of BCG varied widely, depending on the cancer stage and the immunological status of the patients, leading to uncertainty about its overall efficacy in this context [43, 44]. A study evaluating the effects of intravenous BCG on acute myeloid leukemia (AML) found no significant difference in outcomes between patients who received BCG after remission and those who received no further treatment. However, patients who exhibited a stronger immunological response to BCG—marked by fever, purified protein derivative (PPD) test positivity, and inflammation—had higher survival rates compared to those who did not respond or did not receive BCG therapy [45]. Additionally, adjuvant intradermal BCG combined with chemotherapy was shown to induce a higher remission rate in AML patients compared to those who received chemotherapy alone [46, 47]. Furthermore, intradermal BCG proved effective in preventing central nervous system (CNS) leukemic infiltration in a study involving 32 AML patients [48]. In contrast, in a study involving 502 children, intradermal BCG used as an adjuvant therapy for preventing acute lymphocytic leukemia (ALL) remission demonstrated no additional efficacy, when compared to standard chemotherapy regimens or no treatment at all [49].

3.1.1.1 BCG in Bladder Cancer: A Success Story

In 2022, bladder cancer was diagnosed in approximately 614,298 people worldwide, making it the ninth most common malignant neoplasm. That same year, the disease resulted in 220,596 deaths. Currently, the high prevalence of bladder cancer means that over 1.9 million people are living with the disease globally [50]. The average age at diagnosis for bladder cancer is 70 years. Key risk factors include aging and environmental exposures such as cigarette smoking, aromatic amines found in dyes and petroleum products, and chronic bacterial or parasitic infections of the bladder [51]. Men are three to four times more likely than women to be diagnosed with bladder cancer, primarily due to lifestyle factors that increase their exposure to these risks. The early symptoms of bladder cancer often mimic those of urinary infections, which are more common in women. This similarity can lead to delayed diagnosis or misdiagnosis in women, resulting in the disease being detected at more advanced stages. As a result, women generally have a poorer prognosis and higher mortality rates compared to men. Additionally, recent studies indicate that differences in hormone receptors may also play a role in the variations in outcomes and mortality between sexes [51, 52].

Bladder Cancer Pathophysiology, Diagnosis, and Treatment

Bladder cancer primarily targets the umbrella cells that line the bladder lumen, representing approximately 95% of all urothelial carcinomas [52, 53]. Based on the extent of bladder wall invasion, tumors are categorized into two main groups with differing characteristics and clinical outcomes: NMIBC and muscle-invasive bladder cancer (MIBC) [51, 53, 54].

NMIBC is the most frequently diagnosed form of bladder cancer, accounting for about 70% of cases, and is characterized by significant biological heterogeneity [52–54]. Patients with NMIBC may present with low-risk tumors, which generally respond well to treatment and have a 5-year survival rate of over 90%. However, those with high-risk tumors face elevated risks of recurrence (50–70%), progression, and mortality. MIBC, which makes up approximately 20% of cases, has a poorer prognosis, with a 5-year survival rate of less than 50%, limited treatment options, and a high risk of metastasis. Unfortunately, survival rates for MIBC have remained stagnant over the past four decades [52–54].

When bladder cancer is suspected, patients typically undergo cystoscopy for confirmation. If a neoplastic malignancy is found, the recommended procedure is transurethral resection of the bladder tumor (TURBT) [55]. The different therapeutic approaches are listed in Table 3.1. In brief, TURBT is conducted to remove all visible tumors and to collect pathology specimens for accurate tumor staging [52]. When tumors are classified as low-risk NMIBC, a single dose of intravesical Mitomycin C (MMC) is administered within 24 h of TURBT to eliminate residual tumor cells. If MMC is unavailable or the patient cannot tolerate it due to side effects, alternative pharmacological treatments such as gemcitabine, valrubicin, or epirubicin are recommended [52, 55]. For tumors staged as intermediate or high-risk NMIBC, treatment typically involves intravesical BCG immunotherapy, initiated approximately 2 weeks after TURBT. BCG induction therapy consists of six weekly instillations, followed by maintenance therapy for 1 to 3 years, which is strongly recommended to prevent recurrence and progression [55]. In cases of high-risk NMIBC that does not respond to BCG therapy, or in patients with MIBC, radical cystectomy is considered the most effective treatment option [52, 54–56], involving the complete removal of the urinary bladder, along with the prostate and seminal vesicles in men, and the uterus, ovaries, and part of the vagina in women.

Mechanism(s) of Action of BCG in Bladder Cancer Immunotherapy
For bladder cancer treatment, BCG is administered directly into the patient's bladder via a sterile solution that remains in the bladder for approximately 2 h before being voided (Fig. 3.1, 2).

The Barrier The bladder's inner surface is lined with glycosaminoglycans (GAGs), which are polysaccharides that form a hydrophilic and sulfated barrier, protecting the bladder from harmful substances in the urine and preventing the attachment of microorganisms, including bacteria [57, 58]. The surface of BCG bacteria is also negatively charged, which typically prevents them from adhering to the bladder wall due to the repulsive force between the two negatively charged surfaces [58, 59]. This GAG barrier must be disrupted for BCG to successfully bind to the bladder lumen. Studies using electrocauterized mouse bladders have shown that BCG adheres more effectively to areas of the bladder that have been damaged and where a clot has formed [60]. This suggests that wounds caused by TURBT might similarly disrupt the GAG barrier, facilitating better BCG adherence. In addition, BCG expresses fibronectin attachment protein (FAP), which binds to fibrin in clots [60–62]. Research indicates that not only do changes in the bacterial membrane's charge assist BCG binding, but the interaction between FAP and fibronectin also allows BCG to closely interact with the urothelium in mice [60]. However, these results were not replicated in guinea pig models, where BCG did not adhere to the wounded bladder [63]. So far, it has not been possible to confirm whether this process occurs in humans, primarily because it is unsafe to perform bladder biopsies immediately after BCG immunotherapy due to the high risk of inducing a serious systemic infection [64]. Blocking clot formation, which in murine models was found to affect BCG binding to the bladder lumen [65], did not influence the recurrence-free survival of patients receiving BCG therapy [66].

While most BCG is expelled in the first urine pass in mice and patients within 2 h after instillation, live, culturable BCG has been detected in patient urine up to a week after treatment [67, 68]. Moreover, the immediate local effects of BCG on the urothelium [69] suggest that FAP binding might not be the only mechanism necessary for BCG adherence to the bladder.

BCG Uptake by Urothelial Cells It has been proposed that BCG interacts directly with urothelial cells through an integrin receptor ($\alpha 5\beta 1$) on the cell surface, which binds to the FAP on the bacteria [62]. Both in vitro and in vivo studies have demonstrated that normal and malignant urothelial cells can internalize BCG. In intact mouse bladders treated with BCG, mycobacteria were detected inside umbrella cells 24 h after instillation [70]. In vitro studies further revealed that this internalization process relies on the actin cytoskeleton and protein kinases within bladder cancer cells, as inhibiting these mechanisms significantly reduced BCG uptake [71].

BCG internalization also involves the activation of the Rac1/Cdc42/Pak1 genes, where silencing these genes inhibits BCG uptake, whereas their overexpression in BCG-resistant cell lines has the reverse impact on bacterial uptake [71]. Unlike phagocytosis, the internalization of BCG by malignant urothelial cells includes the uptake of the extracellular matrix and is independent of dectin-1. This suggests that BCG internalization in bladder cancer cells occurs through macropinocytosis [71], albeit not yet proven in vivo. Additionally, bladder cancer cells with PTEN mutations or Ras oncogenic activations are more likely to internalize BCG. Knockdown of PTEN or overactivation of Ras has been shown to enhance BCG uptake in bladder cancer cell lines [71]. Once internalized, the mycobacteria are stored and degraded in phagolysosomes [63]. Although it has been proposed that BCG treatment prompts bladder cancer cells to express antigens in the MHC-II context [72], this effect has not been consistent between studies. Furthermore, most animal models and human studies have primarily detected internalized BCG within immune cells, such as neutrophils and macrophages [63, 69, 73, 74].

BCG Immunomodulation Due to the bladder's anatomical structure, the initial cellular interactions following BCG treatment can only be observed through immunohistochemistry of postmortem samples in mammals and humans [73]. However, analyzing urinary samples from patients immediately after treatment can provide valuable insights into the presence of immune cells and the factors they secrete. Flow cytometry and Luminex analysis have shown that 4 h after instillation, the urine of treated patients contains elevated levels of CXCL-10 (C-X-C motif chemokine ligand 10, also known as IP-10), CCL4 (C-C motif chemokine ligand 4, also known as MIP-1β), IL-8, IL-6, IL-1β, IL-15, G-CSF (granulocyte colony-stimulating factor), GM-CSF (granulocyte-macrophage colony-stimulating factor), TNF (tumor necrosis factor), and TRAIL (TNF-related apoptosis-inducing ligand) [64, 75]. These cytokines and chemokines are mostly secreted by granulocytes and macrophages. In vitro stimulation of monocytes and granulocytes with BCG similarly leads to the upregulation of these cytokines, which plays a crucial role in inflammatory responses and immune cell recruitment [76].

The bladder contains resident macrophages and DCs [77], and upon interaction with BCG, these resident cells are thought to phagocytose the mycobacteria and secrete a variety of inflammatory mediators. These secreted factors then attract granulocytes and circulating monocytes, which subsequently differentiate into macrophages, amplifying the immune response [73].

An important feature of macrophages is their role in initiating granuloma formation, particularly in the bladder wall. Granulomas are immune aggregates characteristic of chronic inflammatory conditions such as mycobacterial infections. These structures are composed of macrophages, neutrophils, DCs, fibroblasts, and lymphocytes and encapsulate pathogens and debris [78, 79]. Interestingly, granulomas contain different types of macrophages, including epithelioid cells, giant cells, and foam cells [80]. Although granulomas are rare in cancers like lung cancer and do not become cancerous themselves [81], their presence is crucial for an effective response to BCG therapy in bladder cancer [82]. Retrospective observational studies have also correlated the granuloma presence with better survival outcomes in patients with breast cancer, melanoma, and lymphoma [83]. Within the granuloma and bladder wall, infiltrating immune cells encounter BCG, leading to an increased secretion of inflammatory molecules [84]. Granulocytes and macrophages not only release factors that stimulate inflammatory responses but also play a direct role in inducing cancer cell death [85, 86]. In vitro studies have shown that BCG-activated macrophages induce apoptosis in bladder cancer cell lines through direct cell contact and the release of cytotoxic factors such as nitric oxide (NO) and TNF [76, 86]. Recent findings have further elucidated the role of macrophages in vivo in BCG therapy. A study using zebrafish xenograft models showed that BCG induces the recruitment of macrophages to the tumor microenvironment (TME) and their polarization toward a proinflammatory phenotype, marked by TNF, IL-1β, and IL-6 production [87]. These macrophages directly induced apoptosis of cancer cells through TNF signaling, demonstrating that macrophages play an active role in tumor clearance beyond their traditional function in antigen presentation and cytokine secretion. The depletion of macrophages in this model completely abrogated the BCG-induced antitumor effects, highlighting their critical role in the therapeutic process [87].

Neutrophils stimulated with live or heat-killed BCG in vitro produce and release high levels of IL-8 and TRAIL [88, 89]. Notably, TRAIL and TRAIL-expressing neutrophils can be detected in the urine of patients immediately following BCG instillation. Urine from patients who respond to BCG treatment is capable of killing bladder cancer cells, whereas urine from nonresponders or healthy controls does not exhibit this effect—an action mediated by soluble TRAIL [75]. TRAIL interacts with its death receptors, TRAIL-R1 and TRAIL-R2, to induce apoptosis in malignant cells through a p53-independent pathway that activates caspase 8, subsequently triggering effector caspases 3 and 7 [90]. This mechanism appears to be specific to BCG, as TRAIL is not found in the urine of patients with urinary tract infections [75, 77]. BCG-activated neutrophils also recruit monocytes and macrophages, which further enhance the infiltration of CD4+ T-cells into the bladder [89].

The recruitment of T-cells is facilitated by the expression of MHC-II on DCs [89]. In vivo experiments in mice have demonstrated that approximately 1 week after BCG administration, CD4+ and CD8+ T cells are recruited to the TME [89]. Depletion of these T-cell subsets resulted in more than 80% of mice failing to reject tumors, even upon BCG treatment and IL-2 stimulation, demonstrating a major role for these cells in immune-mediated tumor rejection [91]. The influx of Th1-polarized T-cells has been strongly associated with improved outcomes in BCG immunotherapy. Analyses of cell populations in the bladders of BCG-treated patients reveal that those who respond to treatment exhibit higher infiltration of CD4+ T-cells and a higher CD4+/CD8+ ratio, correlating with better therapeutic outcomes [89].

Natural killer (NK) cells are known for their ability to recognize the loss of MHC-I expression in cancer cells and induce apoptosis through direct contact mechanisms and by activating cytotoxic T-cells [92]. In vitro studies have demonstrated that NK cell cytotoxicity can be activated by incubation with BCG, resulting in an increased expression of activation markers such as CD56 and enhanced proliferation [93]. However, the exact roles of NK cells in vivo during BCG immunotherapy remain not fully understood, as the depletion of NK cells in mice did not significantly impair BCG-mediated tumor rejection [94].

The adaptive immune system is crucial to BCG immunotherapy success. In an orthotopic mouse model of bladder cancer, it has been shown that prior parenteral vaccination with BCG significantly enhanced the inflammatory antitumor response when tumors were subsequently introduced [67]. Along the same line, high-risk NMIBC patients receiving BCG immunotherapy were stratified based on their PPD status before treatment. A positive PPD test indicates prior infection with one of several mycobacterium strains, including *Mycobacterium tuberculosis*, *Mycobacterium bovis*, or *M. bovis* BCG, and the development of adaptive immunological memory [95]. Patients with a positive PPD test had higher recurrence-free survival compared to those with a negative PPD test [67]. Similarly, patients who converted to a positive PPD test after intravesical BCG immunotherapy had better outcomes and prognosis than those who did not [96]. These findings suggest that previous exposure to BCG, such as through intradermal vaccination, may enhance the response to BCG immunotherapy in bladder cancer patients. While the initial effects of BCG are localized, they can eventually manifest systemically in patients [73].

Trained Immunity

BCG treatment for NMIBC involves weekly instillations during the induction phase, followed by a maintenance phase that can extend up to 3 years. The innate immune system's response to BCG treatment is known to intensify as the therapy progresses [9, 73, 74, 97]. This escalation, along with the broad nonspecific effects of BCG, is partly attributed to a phenomenon known as trained immunity. BCG vaccination has been shown to induce epigenetic and transcriptional changes in the hematopoietic stem and progenitor cells of healthy individuals, leading to trained immunity in monocytes and granulocytes, which exhibit heightened responsiveness to bacterial and fungal pathogens up to 90 days after vaccination [9, 98–101]. Although data on trained immunity specifically related to BCG treatment in bladder cancer is limited, the observed systemic increase in inflammatory cytokine and chemokine production during therapy suggests that trained immunity may play a significant role in the effectiveness of BCG immunotherapy for bladder cancer. Additionally, BCG treatment of bladder cancer zebrafish xenografts showed a skewing of the hematopoietic progenitor cells toward the myeloid lineage [87]. In just 3 days after the initial injection, it was already possible to observe an increase in myeloid markers in the hematopoietic tail region (equivalent to the bone marrow) of the xenografts, accompanied by the systemic induction of *tnfa*, *il1b*, *il6,* and *il10* expression [87].

BCG Intravesical Immunotherapy: Challenges and Side Effects

While BCG intravesical immunotherapy is an effective treatment, it is also highly invasive and presents several common side effects stemming from the method of administration [102–104]. The procedure involves inserting a catheter through the urethra, which can potentially injure the delicate tissues of the urethra and bladder, causing significant pain and discomfort for patients [55]. This process, particularly the filling and voiding of the bladder, can also lead to bladder hyperactivity, a condition that is especially prevalent in elderly patients [105, 106]. These effects lead to a percentage of discontinuation of treatment of about 35% [107]. Additionally, because BCG is a live bacterium, it often induces symptoms similar to those of a urinary tract infection due to the inflammatory response it triggers. There is a risk that these side effects may worsen over time, making it difficult for patients to continue treatment. Furthermore, BCG is contraindicated in immunosuppressed patients and individuals with bladder lesions. In these cases, the risk of systemic infection and sepsis is heightened, which can severely compromise the prognosis of patients who are ineligible for this treatment [108, 109].

Several alternatives to BCG are available for treating NMIBC, particularly for patients who cannot tolerate BCG or when it proves ineffective, nonetheless, they have all proven to be less effective than BCG [110, 111]. Intravesical chemotherapy options, such as Mitomycin C, Gemcitabine, and Doxorubicin, are frequently used in BCG-refractory cases due to their ability to inhibit DNA synthesis [112–114]. Immunotherapy alternatives like Pembrolizumab, an immune checkpoint inhibitor, and interferon-α offer viable options, especially for those patients ineligible for cystectomy [115, 116]. Device-assisted therapies, including hyperthermic intravesical chemotherapy and electromotive drug administration, enhance chemotherapy efficacy by applying heat or electrical currents [117–119]. Additionally, photodynamic therapy, which involves a photosensitizing agent activated by light to selectively induce tumor cell death, presents another, albeit less common, alternative [120]. For high-risk NMIBC patients who are unresponsive to BCG, radical cystectomy may be considered, though a more invasive approach [55].

VPM1002 is a promising alternative to BCG for treating NMIBC. This recombinant mycobacterial vaccine, derived from the *M. bovis* BCG strain, has been genetically engineered to enhance both safety and immunogenicity, making it particularly suitable for immunocompromised patients [121, 122]. By deleting the urease C gene to reduce virulence and incorporating the listeriolysin O gene to boost the immune response, VPM1002 aims to improve the therapeutic outcomes of bladder cancer treatment [121, 122]. Early clinical trials suggest that VPM1002 could match or even surpass the efficacy of traditional BCG, with a significantly better safety profile, making it a viable option for patients who are unresponsive to BCG or unable to tolerate its side effects [123, 124].

3.1.2 Heterologous Use of BCG in Infectious Diseases

Besides protecting against *M. tuberculosis* infection, increasing evidence has also pointed toward the protective role of BCG against different infectious diseases, including other tuberculosis and nontuberculosis mycobacterial (NTM) infections, as well as other bacterial, fungi, parasitic, and viral infections [125–128]. Indeed, several studies have reported the beneficial impact of BCG for all-cause infections [129–131]. In a double-blind, randomized clinical trial to evaluate BCG-mediated protection against infection in elderly patients, BCG has been found to increase the time to first infection and decrease the incidence of new infections with a major impact on the incidence of respiratory tract infections [10].

Mycobacteria Other Than Mycobacterium tuberculosis

In the late 1930s, it was observed that BCG immunization resulted in a positive skin reaction following intradermal injection of heat-killed *Mycobacterium leprae* [126]. Since then, several cohort and case–control trials have shown that BCG immunization is associated with a reduction in the incidence of leprosy [132–135]. More recently, a meta-analysis study that included seven experimental and 19 observational studies reported an overall 26% protective effect of BCG against *M. leprae* [136]. Similarly, BCG vaccination has also been found to protect against *Mycobacterium ulcerans* (causative agent of Buruli ulcer), *Mycobacterium avium*, and *Mycobacterium intracellulare* [137–142]. In France, an increase in culture-confirmed cases of nontuberculous mycobacterial cervical lymphadenitis has been observed after the discontinuation of the mandatory BCG vaccination [143]. These results are aligned with other surveillance studies from Finland [144], Sweden [145], and Czech Republic [146] and a meta-analysis-based study that reported higher risk of nontuberculous mycobacterial lymphadenitis in unvaccinated children compared with BCG-immunized counterparts [147]. Together, these data support the hypothesis that BCG confers cross-protection against infection with other mycobacteria (e.g., *M. leprae*) and NTM disease in humans., Therefore, the protective effect of the BCG vaccine against other infectious agents should be taken into consideration when considering universal BCG vaccination programs.

Other Bacteria and Fungi

In addition to mycobacterial infections, which share many common antigens with BCG, heterologous immunity of BCG has also been demonstrated for other bacterial agents (e.g., *Listeria monocytogenes*, *Staphylococcus aureus,* and *Rickettsia tsutsugamushi*) and fungi (e.g., *Candida albicans*). In the 1960s, two seminal studies performed by *Mackaness* showed that BCG-immunized mice become highly resistant to *L. monocytogenes* infection [148, 149]. Later, in the 1970s, other studies further explored the BCG-induced cross-protection against *L. monocytogenes* [150, 151]. In the 1980s, it was demonstrated that macrophages isolated from BCG-immunized mice are more resistant to *R. tsutsugamushi* infection [152]. Another study also showed that macrophages from BCG-immunized mice have an increased ability to kill *C. albicans* intracellularly [153]. More recently, the protective effects of BCG against other bacterial and fungal infections have also been demonstrated in humans[154]. It was shown that BCG immunization of healthy individuals results in an enhanced function of circulating monocytes, characterized by increased production of proinflammatory cytokines in response to *S. aureus* and *C. albicans* stimuli [154]. These enhanced functions were induced through the NOD2 receptor and epigenetic reprogramming of innate immune cells, which were accompanied by an increase in the expression of activation markers such as CD11b and Toll-like receptor 4 [154]. Besides macrophages, NK cells have also been shown to play a role in BCG heterologous immunity. Vaccination of healthy volunteers with BCG resulted in an increased production of proinflammatory cytokines by NK cells in response to *S. aureus* and *C. albicans* stimuli [155]. These results were further confirmed in a murine model of disseminated candidiasis, where BCG vaccination led to increased survival of SCID mice, which was partially dependent on NK cells [155].

Parasites

Several reports have shown that BCG immunization can protect against parasites. In the 1970s, a study demonstrated that BCG-immunized mice presented fewer trypomastigotes in circulation when compared to non-immunized mice, which suggested BCG-mediated protection against *Trypanosoma cruzi* infection [156]. More recently, other studies showed that BCG confers partial protection against *Plasmodium yoelii 17XNL* infection in mice [157, 158]. BCG administration has also demonstrated beneficial effects against leishmaniasis [159]. Intravenous administration of BCG exhibited both prophylactic and therapeutic effects, with BCG-immunized mice showing reduced parasite burdens in the spleen and liver [160]. The beneficial effects of BCG in controlling leishmaniasis have also been explored in several human studies, which described improved clinical outcomes of patients with severe forms of tegumentary leishmaniasis after BCG administration [161–166]. Conversely, in malaria, a randomized controlled phase 1 clinical trial revealed that BCG-vaccinated volunteers presented earlier and more severe clinical adverse events to *Plasmodium falciparum* infection [8]. Hence, these opposing results indicate that more studies are needed to better understand the heterologous impact of BCG in parasitic infections.

Viruses

The effect of BCG vaccination on viral infections has also been studied and comprehensively reviewed [125–127]. In mice models, BCG-induced protection was shown for Herpes simplex virus (HSV) [167, 168], Influenza A virus [168–171], Hepatitis B virus [172], Japanese encephalitis virus [173], Encephalomyocarditis virus [174, 175], Ectromelia virus [176, 177], Vaccina [178, 179], severe acute respiratory syndrome coronavirus-2 (SARS-CoV2) [171, 180–184], and Ebola virus [185], among others. The beneficial impact of BCG immunization in viral infections has also been demonstrated in humans. In a randomized controlled trial, it was reported that BCG immunization leads to protection against experimental infection with an attenuated yellow fever virus (YFV) vaccine strain by inducing genome-wide epigenetic reprogramming of monocytes [7]. Another example is a case-control study performed in young children in Guinea-Bissau, showing that BCG vaccination may reduce the incidence of acute lower respiratory tract infections caused by respiratory syncytial virus (RSV) [3]. During the COVID-19 pandemic, several studies reported that countries with ongoing BCG vaccination programs have lower SARS-CoV-2 incidence and death rates [186–188]. However, these comparisons are limited to the wide-ranging differences between countries [189], and, not all these studies indicate a beneficial impact of BCG in COVID-19 prevention [190, 191]. Moreover, several clinical trials have also found that BCG vaccination did not affect the incidence of COVID-19 or other clinically relevant respiratory tract infections [192–194].

In addition to providing prophylactic protection against infections, BCG has also demonstrated effectiveness as a nonspecific therapy in several virus-associated clinical conditions, such as cutaneous and genital warts caused by human papillomavirus (HPV) [195–198] and recurrent episodes of HSV infection [199, 200]. Furthermore, BCG administration has been shown to enhance the immune response to vaccines against viral infections, as evidenced by increased antibody titters against the 2009 pandemic influenza A virus (H1N1) strain [201] and HBV [202, 203].

3.1.3 Heterologous Use of BCG in Noncommunicable Diseases

In addition to its proinflammatory effects that enhance immunity against various infections and cancers, BCG vaccination also induces immunotolerance, contributing to neuroprotection and the attenuation of autoimmune and inflammatory diseases [125, 204].

Alzheimer's Disease

Different cohort studies associated the use of intravesical BCG to treat bladder cancer with a decreased risk for Alzheimer's disease [205–209], which have been compiled in recent systematic reviews and meta-analyses [210, 211]. Moreover, BCG administration to APP/PS1 mice reversed the cognitive decline and reduced the neuroinflammation characteristic of this Alzheimer's disease model [212]. However, no alterations were observed in the Aβ burden in APP/PS1 mice treated with BCG compared with those untreated [212], suggesting that BCG had no impact on the accumulation of Aβ deposits.

Parkinson's Disease

In a multicenter retrospective cohort study, the use of intravesical BCG during bladder cancer treatment was associated with a decreased risk for Parkinson's disease (PD) [207]. In experimental mice models, intraperitoneal administration of live or freeze-dried BCG before the induction of the PD phenotype (by treatment with the toxin 1-methyl-4-phenyl-1,2,3,6-tetrahydropyridine, MPTD) resulted in increased neuroprotection, consisting of higher levels of dopamine and dopamine transporter ligand binding in the striatum and decreased numbers of activated microglia in the substantia nigra, compared to unvaccinated mice [213, 214]. Similar results were observed in the rat model of PD (induced by treatment with rotenone), where BCG-vaccinated rats presented higher neuroprotection with decreased inflammatory markers, increased neurotransmitters, and restoration of motor deficits [215].

Multiple Sclerosis

A Norwegian population-based cohort study showed that a strong tuberculin skin test (TST). In the BCG for cancer we refer to the PPD the PPD which is the substance injected in the TST, should we keep them as different or use only one. As they basically mean the same after BCG vaccination was associated with a lower risk of developing multiple sclerosis (MS) over a 30-year period [216]. The authors linked this phenomenon to a possible deviation of the T-cell-mediated immunity preceding MS onset. The use of BCG as an MS disease modifier was first reported in 1999, when individuals with relapsing-remitting MS exhibited a reduction in magnetic resonance imaging (MRI)-active lesions, including fewer new enhancing lesions and fewer evolving black holes, following intracutaneous administration of BCG [217, 218]. Another study showed that early BCG vaccination following disease onset may prove beneficial. Individuals who received BCG vaccination after the first demyelinating episode showed fewer cumulative lesions and a lower likelihood of progressing to clinically definite MS or requiring disease-modifying therapies, compared to those who were not vaccinated [219]. Using the experimental autoimmune encephalomyelitis (EAE) model of MS, it was shown that BCG inactivated by extended freeze-drying may be used as a potential immunomodulating therapy during MS [220]. This study showed that mice subcutaneously injected with extended freeze-drying BCG developed attenuated EAE, and presented decreased inflammation in the periphery and central nervous system, associated with increased regulatory T-cells (Treg) induced by plasmacytoid dendritic cells (pDC) [220]. Additionally, intracerebral injection of BCG has been shown to suppress the development of EAE [221].

Atherosclerosis

The impact of BCG immunization on atherosclerosis has been the subject of different studies. Using the New Zealand white rabbit as a model, BCG immunization was shown to enhance peripheral leukocyte activation and aortic monocyte recruitment, leading to pro-atherogenic effects in cholesterol-fed animals [222]. Conversely, in two strains of atherosclerosis-prone mice (*Ldlr*$^{-/-}$ and *Apoe* $^{-/-}$), BCG immunization reduced atherosclerosis by increasing IL-10 levels and inducing Treg expansion, both known to control inflammation during atherogenesis [223, 224]. Furthermore, in hyperlipidemic mice (*APOE*3-Leiden.CETP*) BCG markedly reduced plasma cholesterol levels and foam cell formation, delaying atherosclerosis progression and reducing lesion severity [225]. In a different study using the hyperlipidemic *Ldlr*$^{-/-}$ mice, BCG led to the expansion of CD4^{+} T-cells and Ly6C^{low} monocytes and aggravated atherosclerosis formation in the aortas [226]. These contradictory results highlight the need for further research to better understand the impact of BCG on atherosclerosis. Notably, the mouse studies referenced employed different BCG administration routes, underscoring the importance of investigating how the route of delivery influences outcomes in future studies.

Asthma and Allergies

Numerous studies have elucidated the role of BCG vaccination in asthma and other allergic and atopic disorders (reviewed in [227]). However, the conclusions lack consensus. Systematic reviews and meta-analyses were performed to compile human data from different studies showing a potential protective effect of BCG vaccination early in life against asthma [228, 229]. However, many studies demonstrated methodological limitations, and the outcome measures varied widely accross reports, which rendered them challenging to combine. A later systematic review and meta-analysis, which included additional studies, found no association between BCG vaccination and asthma, indicating that if a benefic role for BCG exists, it must be transient [230]. Looking into the therapeutic effect of BCG in adults, a study involving asthmatic patients showed that treatment with percutaneous BCG led to increased lung function and decreased medication use. Nonetheless, although BCG suppressed the Th2-type immune response and eosinophil influx, no changes were observed in the asthma symptoms score [231]. Additional doses of BCG seemed to improve the beneficial effects against asthma, as evidenced by enhanced lung function and increased IFNγ/IL-4 ratio after vaccination [232]. In agreement, another study reported that asthmatic patients treated with three BCG administrations presented lower eosinophilia and IL-4 levels, along with reduced asthma symptoms and use of medication, compared with those receiving only one dose of BCG [233]. Although significant progress has been made, a the full extent of the clinical benefit of BCG vaccination against asthma is yet to be fully understood.

Even though the anti-asthma effect of BCG in humans has been ambiguous between studies, the use of mouse models clearly showed a prophylactic and therapeutic effect of BCG against asthma. In mouse models of allergic asthma, BCG vaccination administered before allergen sensitization unveiled that the short-term protective role of BCG against this disease is mainly due to the induction of a Th1-type immune response, a reduced IL-5 and IL-4 production, and impaired Th2 and eosinophils homing to the lungs (reviewed in [227]). On the other hand, the long-term effect of BCG-mediated protection against asthma seems to be independent of this Th1/Th2 balance [234, 235] and more related to IL-10 and IL-17 production [235–237]. It is important to note that the protective effect of BCG against allergic asthma was found to vary accross experimental models, BCG strains, and route of administration (reviewed in [227]). For instance, the use of BCG as a therapeutic against allergic asthma, by administration after sensitization, reverted the allergic response. This included reduced eosinophil infiltration, lung pathology, and mucus production, correlated with decreased specific IgE, IgG1, and Th2-type response and increased IL-10 production and M1 alveolar macrophages [238–240].

Diabetes

BCG vaccination has demonstrated potential as a therapeutic strategy against diabetes. Several studies have already evaluated the impact of BCG on disease progression, early disease treatment, and disease reversal of advanced cases. Using the nonobese diabetic mouse model, it was shown that BCG suppresses insulitis and prevents the development of diabetes [241–244]. In humans, it was also observed that a single low dose of BCG in patients with late-stage pre-diabetes successfully induced clinical remission in 65% of the cases [245]. Moreover, neonatal BCG vaccination has been associated with reduced autoantibodies associated with type 1 diabetes (T1D) [246]. Conversely, other studies in humans have failed to confirm that neonatal BCG vaccination or administration in newly diagnosed T1D patients reduces the progression of diabetes and insulin requirements [247–249]. However, in patients with long-standing T1D, BCG vaccination showed beneficial antidiabetic effects by selectively eliminating autoreactive T-cells, inducing beneficial Tregs, transiently increasing fasting C-peptide levels, and reducing the hemoglobin A1c to near-normal levels [250–252]. Mechanistically, the BCG-induced long-term reduction of hyperglycemia has been attributed to the reprogramming in the glucose metabolism away from oxidative phosphorylation to aerobic glycolysis, which is the mechanism of action of metformin, one of the most effective and commonly used drugs for type 2 diabetes (T2D) [253–256]. Although several studies have already reported that BCG protects T2D mice against tuberculosis [257, 258], studies evaluating the impact of BCG on T2D are still needed. Interestingly, in a study performed by *Radhakrishnan* et al., it was noted that BCG vaccination enhanced the survival of T2D mice [258].

Kawasaki Disease

BCG has also been described as a valuable tool in Kawasaki disease (KD) diagnosis. During the acute phase of KD, patients who received BCG vaccination developed erythema, induration, or crusting at the BCG inoculation site [259–262]. The BCG hyper-responsiveness observed in KD patients was attributed to the cross-reactivity between mycobacterial and human proteins [263, 264]. This reaction is characterized by small vessel dilation in the dermis, with $CD4^{+}$T lymphocytes and $CD13^{+}$ macrophage infiltration and increased levels of IL-1α, TNF, IFNγ, and IL-2 [265]. Several studies have been conducted to investigate the epidemiologic features of KD patients with changes at the BCG inoculation site and to evaluate the specificity of this sign for KD diagnosis. A study performed in Japan identified redness and crust formation at the BCG inoculation site in 49.9% of KD patients, with a particularly high prevalence (70%) in children aged 3 to 20 months [266]. However, a different study performed in Mexico reported that only 24.3% of KD patients presented the BCG reaction at the inoculation site [267]. Differences in ethnicity and the strain of BCG vaccine used have been postulated as the cause of such variability in sensitivity, which limits its applicability as a widespread diagnostic tool. The BCG reaction at the inoculation site has also been reported for other medical conditions (e.g., HSV type 6 infection and measles), hampering the use of this reaction as a diagnostic marker [268, 269]. Despite its limitations, the BCG inoculation site reaction shows promise as an important diagnostic marker for KD, particularly in countries with universal BCG vaccination programs. Hence, it serves as a visible and early sign in the acute phase of KD, especially in cases where classic KD symptoms are not yet fully present.

3.2 Conclusions

The heterologous effects of BCG vaccination extend far beyond its original purpose, TB prevention. This chapter explored the diverse and often surprising roles of BCG in modulating immune responses across a spectrum of diseases, including cancer (focusing on bladder cancer), other infectious diseases, autoimmune disorders, and neurodegenerative conditions. The ability of BCG to reprogram innate and adaptive immune responses through mechanisms such as trained immunity has opened new avenues for therapeutic interventions, with the potential to reshape our approach to a variety of diseases. However, further research is urgently needed to fully elucidate the BCG potential in preventing and treating different diseases. It is critical to unravel the precise mechanisms by which BCG exerts its broad-spectrum effects and to translate these findings into effective clinical applications, such as those in bladder cancer immunotherapy. The legacy of BCG, one of the oldest vaccines in use, may yet be redefined in the twenty-first century as a versatile tool for enhancing human health beyond its original role in fighting TB.

Acknowledgments Mayra Martínez-López acknowledges the support of the Portuguese Foundation for Science and Technology (FCT) PhD fellowship (PD/BD/138203/2018). Rita Fior and Mayra Martínez-López acknowledge funding from the Champalimaud Foundation and CRI-Cancer Research Institute- Technology Impact Award. Pedro Curto is partly financed by national funds through Portuguese "FCT – Foundation for Science and Technology, I.P.," within the scope of the project—https://doi.org/10.54499/2022.02702.PTDC. Pedro Moura-Alves, Palmira Barreira-Silva, and Pedro Curto acknowledge funding from the European Union's Horizon 2020 research and innovation program under grant agreement No 951921.

Competing Interests The author(s) has no competing interests to declare that are relevant to the content of this manuscript.

Ethics Approval The author(s) declares that this manuscript does not include primary research with human participants.

References

1. Lalvani A, Sridhar S. BCG vaccination: 90 years on and still so much to learn. Thorax. 2010;65(12):1036–8.
2. Dockrell HM, Smith SG. What have we learnt about BCG vaccination in the last 20 years? Front Immunol. 2017;8:1134.
3. Stensballe LG, Nante E, Jensen IP, Kofoed PE, Poulsen A, Jensen H, et al. Acute lower respiratory tract infections and respiratory syncytial virus in infants in Guinea-Bissau: a ben-

eficial effect of BCG vaccination for girls community based case-control study. Vaccine. 2005;23(10):1251–7.
4. Ohrui T, Nakayama K, Fukushima T, Chiba H, Sasaki H. Prevention of elderly pneumonia by pneumococcal, influenza and BCG vaccinations. Nihon Ronen Igakkai Zasshi. 2005;42(1):34–6.
5. Nemes E, Geldenhuys H, Rozot V, Rutkowski KT, Ratangee F, Bilek N, et al. Prevention of M. tuberculosis infection with H4:IC31 vaccine or BCG revaccination. N Engl J Med. 2018;379(2):138–49.
6. Wardhana DEA, Sultana A, Mandang VV, Jim E. The efficacy of Bacillus Calmette-Guerin vaccinations for the prevention of acute upper respiratory tract infection in the elderly. Acta Med Indones. 2011;43(3):185–90.
7. Arts RJW, Moorlag S, Novakovic B, Li Y, Wang SY, Oosting M, et al. BCG vaccination protects against experimental viral infection in humans through the induction of cytokines associated with trained immunity. Cell Host Microbe. 2018;23(1):89–100 e5.
8. Walk J, de Bree LCJ, Graumans W, Stoter R, van Gemert GJ, van de Vegte-Bolmer M, et al. Outcomes of controlled human malaria infection after BCG vaccination. Nat Commun. 2019;10(1):874.
9. van Puffelen JH, Keating ST, Oosterwijk E, van der Heijden AG, Netea MG, Joosten LAB, et al. Trained immunity as a molecular mechanism for BCG immunotherapy in bladder cancer. Nat Rev Urol. 2020;17(9):513–25.
10. Giamarellos-Bourboulis EJ, Tsilika M, Moorlag S, Antonakos N, Kotsaki A, Dominguez-Andres J, et al. Activate: randomized clinical trial of BCG vaccination against infection in the elderly. Cell. 2020;183(2):315–23 e9.
11. Couzin-Frankel J. Breakthrough of the year 2013. Cancer immunotherapy. Science. 2013;342(6165):1432–3.
12. Dobosz P, Dzieciatkowski T. The intriguing history of cancer immunotherapy. Front Immunol. 2019;10:2965.
13. McCarthy EF. The toxins of William B. Coley and the treatment of bone and soft-tissue sarcomas. Iowa Orthop J. 2006;26:154–8.
14. Coley WB. The treatment of inoperable sarcoma by bacterial toxins (the mixed toxins of the streptococcus erysipelas and the Bacillus prodigiosus). Proc R Soc Med. 1910;3(Surg Sect):1–48.
15. Nauts HC, Swift WE, Coley BL. The treatment of malignant tumors by bacterial toxins as developed by the late William B. Coley, M.D., reviewed in the light of modern research. Cancer Res. 1946;6:205–16.
16. Nauts HC, Fowler GA, Bogatko FH. A review of the influence of bacterial infection and of bacterial products (Coley's toxins) on malignant tumors in man; a critical analysis of 30 inoperable cases treated by Coley's mixed toxins, in which diagnosis was confirmed by microscopic examination selected for special study. Acta Med Scand Suppl. 1953;276:1–103.
17. Dinarello CA. Historical insights into cytokines. Eur J Immunol. 2007;37 Suppl 1(Suppl 1):S34–45.
18. Conti B, Tabarean I, Andrei C, Bartfai T. Cytokines and fever. Front Biosci. 2004;9:1433–49.
19. Evans SS, Repasky EA, Fisher DT. Fever and the thermal regulation of immunity: the immune system feels the heat. Nat Rev Immunol. 2015;15(6):335–49.
20. Rossi JF, Lu ZY, Massart C, Levon K. Dynamic immune/inflammation precision medicine: the good and the bad inflammation in infection and cancer. Front Immunol. 2021;12:595722.
21. Garg AD. The dynamic interface of genetics and immunity: toward future horizons in health & disease. Genes Immun. 2023;24(4):155–8.
22. Carlson RD, Flickinger JC Jr, Snook AE. Talkin' toxins: from Coley's to modern cancer immunotherapy. Toxins (Basel). 2020;12(4):241.
23. Tang ZY, Zhou HY, Zhao G, Chai LM, Zhou M, Lu JZ, et al. Preliminary result of mixed bacterial vaccine as adjuvant treatment of hepatocellular carcinoma. Med Oncol Tumor Pharmacother. 1991;8(1):23–8.

24. Kempin S, Cirrincione C, Straus D, Gee T, Arlin Z, Koziner B, et al., editors. Improved remission rate and duration in nodular non-Hodgkin lymphoma (NNHL) with the use of mixed bacterial vaccine (MBV). Proceedings of the American Association for Cancer Research; 1981: Amer Assoc Cancer Research 615 Chestnut St, 17th Floor, Philadelphia, PA.
25. Kölmel K, Vehmeyer K, Göhring E, Kuhn B, Wieding J. Treatment of advanced malignant melanoma by a pyrogenic bacterial lysate. A pilot study. Oncol Res Treat. 1991;14(5):411–7.
26. Karbach J, Neumann A, Brand K, Wahle C, Siegel E, Maeurer M, et al. Phase I clinical trial of mixed bacterial vaccine (Coley's toxins) in patients with NY-ESO-1 expressing cancers: immunological effects and clinical activity. Clin Cancer Res. 2012;18(19):5449–59.
27. López MFM. Zebrafish avatars as a model for immunotherapy response in bladder cancer [PhD]. Lisbon, Portugal: Universidade Nova de Lisboa; 2022.
28. Old LJ, Clarke DA, Benacerraf B. Effect of Bacillus Calmette-Guerin infection on transplanted tumours in the mouse. Nature. 1959;184(Suppl 5):291–2.
29. Zbar B, Tanaka T. Immunotherapy of cancer: regression of tumors after intralesional injection of living Mycobacterium bovis. Science. 1971;172(3980):271–3.
30. Merrin C, Han T, Klein E, Murphy GP. Immunotherapy of prostatic cancer with Bacillus Calmette-Guerin and purified protein derivative. Preliminary results. Urology. 1973;2(6):651–4.
31. Robinson MR, Rigby CC, Pugh RC, Dumonde DC. Prostate carcinoma: intratumor BCG immunotherapy. Natl Cancer Inst Monogr. 1978;49:351–3.
32. Guinan P, Crispen R, Baumgartner G, Rao R, Totonchi E, Ablin R, et al. Adjuvant immunotherapy with Bacillus Calmette-Guerin in prostatic cancer. Urology. 1979;14(6):561–5.
33. Morton DL, Eilber FR, Holmes EC, Hunt JS, Ketcham AS, Silverstein MJ, et al. BCG immunotherapy of malignant melanoma: summary of a seven-year experience. Ann Surg. 1974;180(4):635–43.
34. Sterchi JM, Wells HB, Case LD, Spurr CL, White DR, Richards F, et al. A randomized trial of adjuvant chemotherapy and immunotherapy in Stage I and Stage II cutaneous melanoma. An interim report. Cancer. 1985;55(4):707–12.
35. Paterson AH, Willans DJ, Jerry LM, Hanson J, McPherson TA. Adjuvant BCG immunotherapy for malignant melanoma. Can Med Assoc J. 1984;131(7):744–8.
36. Paterson AH, Willans D, Jerry LM, McPherson TA. Malignant melanoma (stage 1): a clinical trial of adjuvant BCG immunotherapy. Recent Results Cancer Res. 1978;68:387–92.
37. National Comprehensive Cancer Network [Internet]. 2024 [Available from: https://www.nccn.org/guidelines/guidelines-detail?category=1&id=1492.
38. Holmes EC. BCG immunotherapy of lung cancer. Jpn J Surg. 1980;10(1):1–6.
39. deKernion JB, Golub SH, Gupta RK, Silverstein M, Morton DL. Successful transurethral intralesional BCG therapy of a bladder melanoma. Cancer. 1975;36(5):1662–7.
40. Bloomberg SD, Brosman SA, Hausman MS, Cohen A, Battenberg JD. The effects of BCG on the dog bladder. Investig Urol. 1975;12(6):423–7.
41. Morales A, Eidinger D, Bruce AW. Intracavitary Bacillus Calmette-Guerin in the treatment of superficial bladder tumors. J Urol. 1976;116(2):180–3.
42. Eriguchi M, Fujii G. Oral administration of BCG as a local immunotherapy of gastrointestinal cancer. J Surg Oncol. 1984;26(2):100–6.
43. Harris JE, Ryan L, Hoover HC Jr, Stuart RK, Oken MM, Benson AB 3rd, et al. Adjuvant active specific immunotherapy for stage II and III colon cancer with an autologous tumor cell vaccine: Eastern Cooperative Oncology Group Study E5283. J Clin Oncol. 2000;18(1):148–57.
44. Uyl-de Groot CA, Vermorken JB, Hanna MG Jr, Verboom P, Groot MT, Bonsel GJ, et al. Immunotherapy with autologous tumor cell-BCG vaccine in patients with colon cancer: a prospective study of medical and economic benefits. Vaccine. 2005;23(17–18):2379–87.
45. Whittaker JA, Slater AJ. The immunotherapy of acute myelogenous leukaemia using intravenous BCG. Br J Haematol. 1977;35(2):263–73.
46. Powles RL, Crowther D, Bateman CJ, Beard ME, McElwain TJ, Russell J, et al. Immunotherapy for acute myelogenous leukaemia. Br J Cancer. 1973;28(5):365–76.

47. Crowther D, Powles RL, Bateman CJ, Beard ME, Gauci CL, Wrigley PF, et al. Management of adult acute myelogenous leukaemia. Br Med J. 1973;1(5846):131–7.
48. Summerfield GP, Gibbs TJ, Bellingham AJ. Immunotherapy using BCG during remission induction and as the sole form of maintenance in acute myeloid leukaemia. Br J Cancer. 1979;40(5):736–42.
49. Heyn RM, Joo P, Karon M, Nesbit M, Shore N, Breslow N, et al. BCG in the treatment of acute lymphocytic leukemia. 1975. p. 431. American Society of Hematology - Blood, 2021 L St. NW, Suite 900, Washington DC 20036-4929, USA.
50. World Cancer Research Fund International [Internet]. 2022 [Available from: https://www.wcrf.org/cancer-trends/bladder-cancer-statistics/.
51. Berdik C. Unlocking bladder cancer. Nature. 2017;551(7679):S34–S5.
52. Lenis AT, Lec PM, Chamie K, Mshs MD. Bladder cancer: a review. JAMA. 2020;324(19):1980–91.
53. Knowles MA, Hurst CD. Molecular biology of bladder cancer: new insights into pathogenesis and clinical diversity. Nat Rev Cancer. 2015;15(1):25–41.
54. Jordan B, Meeks JJ. T1 bladder cancer: current considerations for diagnosis and management. Nat Rev Urol. 2019;16(1):23–34.
55. Babjuk M, Burger M, Capoun O, Cohen D, Comperat EM, Dominguez Escrig JL, et al. European Association of Urology guidelines on non-muscle-invasive bladder cancer (Ta, T1, and Carcinoma in Situ). Eur Urol. 2022;81(1):75–94.
56. Witjes JA, Bruins HM, Cathomas R, Comperat EM, Cowan NC, Gakis G, et al. European Association of Urology guidelines on muscle-invasive and metastatic bladder cancer: summary of the 2020 guidelines. Eur Urol. 2021;79(1):82–104.
57. Casale J, Crane JS. Biochemistry, Glycosaminoglycans. Treasure Island: StatPearls; 2024.
58. Schamhart DH, De Boer EC, Vleeming R, Kurth KH. Theoretical and experimental evidence on the use of glycosaminoglycans in BCG-mediated immunotherapy of superficial bladder cancer. Semin Thromb Hemost. 1994;20(3):301–9.
59. Ayala-Torres C, Hernández N, Galeano A, Novoa-Aponte L, Soto C-Y. Zeta potential as a measure of the surface charge of mycobacterial cells. Ann Microbiol. 2014;64(3):1189–95.
60. Ratliff TL, Palmer JO, McGarr JA, Brown EJ. Intravesical Bacillus Calmette-Guerin therapy for murine bladder tumors: initiation of the response by fibronectin-mediated attachment of Bacillus Calmette-Guerin. Cancer Res. 1987;47(7):1762–6.
61. Abou-Zeid C, Ratliff TL, Wiker HG, Harboe M, Bennedsen J, Rook GA. Characterization of fibronectin-binding antigens released by Mycobacterium tuberculosis and Mycobacterium bovis BCG. Infect Immun. 1988;56(12):3046–51.
62. Zhao W, Schorey JS, Bong-Mastek M, Ritchey J, Brown EJ, Ratliff TL. Role of a Bacillus Calmette-Guérin fibronectin attachment protein in BCG-induced antitumor activity. Int J Cancer. 2000;86(1):83–8.
63. Teppema JS, de Boer EC, Steerenberg PA, van der Meijden AP. Morphological aspects of the interaction of Bacillus Calmette-Guerin with urothelial bladder cells in vivo and in vitro: relevance for antitumor activity? Urol Res. 1992;20(3):219–28.
64. Bisiaux A, Thiounn N, Timsit MO, Eladaoui A, Chang HH, Mapes J, et al. Molecular analyte profiling of the early events and tissue conditioning following intravesical bacillus calmette-guerin therapy in patients with superficial bladder cancer. J Urol. 2009;181(4):1571–80.
65. Kavoussi LR, Brown EJ, Ritchey JK, Ratliff TL. Fibronectin-mediated Calmette-Guerin bacillus attachment to murine bladder mucosa. Requirement for the expression of an antitumor response. J Clin Invest. 1990;85(1):62–7.
66. Lipsky MJ, Badalato GM, Motamedinia P, Hruby GW, McKiernan JM. The effect of fibrin clot inhibitors on the immunomodulatory efficacy of Bacillus Calmette-Guerin therapy for non-muscle-invasive bladder cancer. Urology. 2013;81(6):1273–8.
67. Biot C, Rentsch CA, Gsponer JR, Birkhauser FD, Jusforgues-Saklani H, Lemaitre F, et al. Preexisting BCG-specific T cells improve intravesical immunotherapy for bladder cancer. Sci Transl Med. 2012;4(137):137ra72.

68. Durek C, Richter E, Basteck A, Rusch-Gerdes S, Gerdes J, Jocham D, et al. The fate of Bacillus Calmette-Guerin after intravesical instillation. J Urol. 2001;165(5):1765–8.
69. Prescott S, Jackson AM, Hawkyard SJ, Alexandroff AB, James K. Mechanisms of action of intravesical bacille Calmette-Guerin: local immune mechanisms. Clin Infect Dis. 2000;31(Suppl 3):S91–3.
70. Saban MR, Simpson C, Davis C, Wallis G, Knowlton N, Frank MB, et al. Discriminators of mouse bladder response to intravesical Bacillus Calmette-Guerin (BCG). BMC Immunol. 2007;8:6.
71. Redelman-Sidi G, Iyer G, Solit DB, Glickman MS. Oncogenic activation of Pak1-dependent pathway of macropinocytosis determines BCG entry into bladder cancer cells. Cancer Res. 2013;73(3):1156–67.
72. Prescott S, James K, Busuttil A, Hargreave TB, Chisholm GD, Smyth JF. HLA-DR expression by high grade superficial bladder cancer treated with BCG. Br J Urol. 1989;63(3):264–9.
73. Pettenati C, Ingersoll MA. Mechanisms of BCG immunotherapy and its outlook for bladder cancer. Nat Rev Urol. 2018;15(10):615–25.
74. Simons MP, O'Donnell MA, Griffith TS. Role of neutrophils in BCG immunotherapy for bladder cancer. Urol Oncol. 2008;26(4):341–5.
75. Ludwig AT, Moore JM, Luo Y, Chen X, Saltsgaver NA, O'Donnell MA, et al. Tumor necrosis factor-related apoptosis-inducing ligand: a novel mechanism for Bacillus Calmette-Guerin-induced antitumor activity. Cancer Res. 2004;64(10):3386–90.
76. Luo Y, Chen X, O'Donnell MA. Role of Th1 and Th2 cytokines in BCG-induced IFN-gamma production: cytokine promotion and simulation of BCG effect. Cytokine. 2003;21(1):17–26.
77. Ingersoll MA, Albert ML. From infection to immunotherapy: host immune responses to bacteria at the bladder mucosa. Mucosal Immunol. 2013;6(6):1041–53.
78. Williams O, Fatima S. Granuloma. Treasure Island: StatPearls; 2024.
79. Flynn JL, Chan J, Lin PL. Macrophages and control of granulomatous inflammation in tuberculosis. Mucosal Immunol. 2011;4(3):271–8.
80. Herrtwich L, Nanda I, Evangelou K, Nikolova T, Horn V, Sagar, et al. DNA damage signaling instructs polyploid macrophage fate in granulomas. Cell. 2016;167(5):1264–80 e18.
81. Dagaonkar RS, Choong CV, Asmat AB, Ahmed DB, Chopra A, Lim AY, et al. Significance of coexistent granulomatous inflammation and lung cancer. J Clin Pathol. 2017;70(4):337–41.
82. Jallad S, Goubet S, Symes A, Larner T, Thomas P. Prognostic value of inflammation or granuloma after intravesival BCG in non-muscle-invasive bladder cancer. BJU Int. 2014;113(5b):E22–7.
83. Murthi M, Yoshioka K, Cho JH, Arias S, Danna E, Zaw M, et al. Presence of concurrent sarcoid-like granulomas indicates better survival in cancer patients: a retrospective cohort study. ERJ Open Res. 2020;6(4):00061.
84. Pagan AJ, Ramakrishnan L. The formation and function of granulomas. Annu Rev Immunol. 2018;36:639–65.
85. Luo Y, Knudson MJ. Mycobacterium bovis Bacillus Calmette-Guerin-induced macrophage cytotoxicity against bladder cancer cells. Clin Dev Immunol. 2010;2010:357591.
86. Pryor K, Goddard J, Goldstein D, Stricker P, Russell P, Golovsky D, et al. Bacillus Calmette-Guerin (BCG) enhances monocyte- and lymphocyte-mediated bladder tumour cell killing. Br J Cancer. 1995;71(4):801–7.
87. Martinez-Lopez MF, de Almeida CR, Fontes M, Mendes RV, Kaufmann SHE, Fior R. Macrophages directly kill bladder cancer cells through TNF signaling as an early response to BCG therapy. Dis Model Mech. 2024;17(8):dmm050693.
88. Kemp TJ, Ludwig AT, Earel JK, Moore JM, Vanoosten RL, Moses B, et al. Neutrophil stimulation with Mycobacterium bovis Bacillus Calmette-Guerin (BCG) results in the release of functional soluble TRAIL/Apo-2L. Blood. 2005;106(10):3474–82.
89. Suttmann H, Riemensberger J, Bentien G, Schmaltz D, Stockle M, Jocham D, et al. Neutrophil granulocytes are required for effective Bacillus Calmette-Guerin immunotherapy of bladder cancer and orchestrate local immune responses. Cancer Res. 2006;66(16):8250–7.

90. Wang S, El-Deiry WS. TRAIL and apoptosis induction by TNF-family death receptors. Oncogene. 2003;22(53):8628–33.
91. Ratliff TL, Ritchey JK, Yuan JJ, Andriole GL, Catalona WJ. T-cell subsets required for intravesical BCG immunotherapy for bladder cancer. J Urol. 1993;150(3):1018–23.
92. Mocikat R, Braumuller H, Gumy A, Egeter O, Ziegler H, Reusch U, et al. Natural killer cells activated by MHC class I(low) targets prime dendritic cells to induce protective CD8 T cell responses. Immunity. 2003;19(4):561–9.
93. Esteso G, Aguilo N, Julian E, Ashiru O, Ho MM, Martin C, et al. Natural killer anti-tumor activity can be achieved by in vitro incubation with heat-killed BCG. Front Immunol. 2021;12:622995.
94. Ratliff TL, Shapiro A, Catalona WJ. Inhibition of murine bladder tumor growth by bacille Calmette-Guerin: lack of a role of natural killer cells. Clin Immunol Immunopathol. 1986;41(1):108–15.
95. Center for Disease Control and Prevention [Internet]. 2020 [Available from: https://www.cdc.gov/tb/publications/factsheets/testing/Tuberculin_Skin_Testing_Information_for_Health_Care_Providers.pdf.
96. Kelley DR, Haaff EO, Becich M, Lage J, Bauer WC, Dresner SM, et al. Prognostic value of purified protein derivative skin test and granuloma formation in patients treated with intravesical Bacillus Calmette-Guerin. J Urol. 1986;135(2):268–71.
97. Redelman-Sidi G, Glickman MS, Bochner BH. The mechanism of action of BCG therapy for bladder cancer – a current perspective. Nat Rev Urol. 2014;11(3):153–62.
98. Cirovic B, de Bree LCJ, Groh L, Blok BA, Chan J, van der Velden W, et al. BCG vaccination in humans elicits trained immunity via the hematopoietic progenitor compartment. Cell Host Microbe. 2020;28(2):322–34 e5.
99. Lobo N, Brooks NA, Zlotta AR, Cirillo JD, Boorjian S, Black PC, et al. 100 years of Bacillus Calmette-Guerin immunotherapy: from cattle to COVID-19. Nat Rev Urol. 2021;18(10):611–22.
100. Moorlag S, Rodriguez-Rosales YA, Gillard J, Fanucchi S, Theunissen K, Novakovic B, et al. BCG vaccination induces long-term functional reprogramming of human neutrophils. Cell Rep. 2020;33(7):108387.
101. Liu K, Sun E, Lei M, Li L, Gao J, Nian X, et al. BCG-induced formation of neutrophil extracellular traps play an important role in bladder cancer treatment. Clin Immunol. 2019;201:4–14.
102. Lamm DL, van der Meijden PM, Morales A, Brosman SA, Catalona WJ, Herr HW, et al. Incidence and treatment of complications of Bacillus Calmette-Guerin intravesical therapy in superficial bladder cancer. J Urol. 1992;147(3):596–600.
103. Li R, Sundi D, Zhang J, Kim Y, Sylvester RJ, Spiess PE, et al. Systematic review of the therapeutic efficacy of bladder-preserving treatments for non-muscle-invasive bladder cancer following intravesical Bacillus Calmette-Guerin. Eur Urol. 2020;78(3):387–99.
104. Brausi M, Oddens J, Sylvester R, Bono A, van de Beek C, van Andel G, et al. Side effects of Bacillus Calmette-Guerin (BCG) in the treatment of intermediate- and high-risk Ta, T1 papillary carcinoma of the bladder: results of the EORTC genito-urinary cancers group randomised phase 3 study comparing one-third dose with full dose and 1 year with 3 years of maintenance BCG. Eur Urol. 2014;65(1):69–76.
105. Bourlotos G, Baigent W, Hong M, Plagakis S, Grundy L. BCG induced lower urinary tract symptoms during treatment for NMIBC-mechanisms and management strategies. Front Neurosci. 2023;17:1327053.
106. Liu Y, Lu J, Huang Y, Ma L. Clinical spectrum of complications induced by intravesical immunotherapy of Bacillus Calmette-Guerin for bladder cancer. J Oncol. 2019;2019:6230409.
107. Sun K, Wang D, Wu G, Ma J, Wang T, Wu J, et al. Mirabegron improves the irritative symptoms caused by BCG immunotherapy after transurethral resection of bladder tumors. Cancer Med. 2021;10(21):7534–41.
108. Lamm DL, Stogdill VD, Stogdill BJ, Crispen RG. Complications of Bacillus Calmette-Guerin immunotherapy in 1,278 patients with bladder cancer. J Urol. 1986;135(2):272–4.

109. Guven AT, Demiroglu YZ, Kocer NE. Systemic Bacillus Calmette-Guerin (BCG) infection and accompanying warm autoimmune haemolytic anaemia following intravesical BCG immunotherapy. Eur J Case Rep Intern Med. 2023;10(9):004009.
110. Passarelli R, Packiam VT. Contemporary treatment of NMIBC-is it time to move on from BCG? J Clin Med. 2024;13(14):4112.
111. Matulewicz RS, Steinberg GD. Non-muscle-invasive bladder cancer: overview and contemporary treatment landscape of neoadjuvant chemoablative therapies. Rev Urol. 2020;22(2):43–51.
112. Oosterlinck W, Kurth KH, Schroder F, Bultinck J, Hammond B, Sylvester R. A prospective European Organization for Research and Treatment of Cancer Genitourinary Group randomized trial comparing transurethral resection followed by a single intravesical instillation of epirubicin or water in single stage Ta, T1 papillary carcinoma of the bladder. J Urol. 1993;149(4):749–52.
113. Han MA, Maisch P, Jung JH, Hwang JE, Narayan V, Cleves A, et al. Intravesical gemcitabine for non-muscle invasive bladder cancer. Cochrane Database Syst Rev. 2021;6(6):CD009294.
114. Shelley MD, Mason MD, Kynaston H. Intravesical therapy for superficial bladder cancer: a systematic review of randomised trials and meta-analyses. Cancer Treat Rev. 2010;36(3):195–205.
115. O'Donnell MA, Krohn J, DeWolf WC. Salvage intravesical therapy with interferon-alpha 2b plus low dose Bacillus Calmette-Guerin is effective in patients with superficial bladder cancer in whom Bacillus Calmette-Guerin alone previously failed. J Urol. 2001;166(4):1300–4. discussion 4-5.
116. Bellmunt J, de Wit R, Vaughn DJ, Fradet Y, Lee JL, Fong L, et al. Pembrolizumab as second-line therapy for advanced urothelial carcinoma. N Engl J Med. 2017;376(11):1015–26.
117. Di Stasi SM, Giannantoni A, Stephen RL, Capelli G, Navarra P, Massoud R, et al. Intravesical electromotive mitomycin C versus passive transport mitomycin C for high risk superficial bladder cancer: a prospective randomized study. J Urol. 2003;170(3):777–82.
118. Tan WS, Panchal A, Buckley L, Devall AJ, Loubiere LS, Pope AM, et al. Radiofrequency-induced thermo-chemotherapy effect versus a second course of Bacillus Calmette-Guerin or institutional standard in patients with recurrence of non-muscle-invasive bladder cancer following induction or maintenance Bacillus Calmette-Guerin therapy (HYMN): a phase III, open-label, randomised controlled trial. Eur Urol. 2019;75(1):63–71.
119. Arends TJ, Nativ O, Maffezzini M, de Cobelli O, Canepa G, Verweij F, et al. Results of a randomised controlled trial comparing intravesical chemohyperthermia with mitomycin C versus Bacillus Calmette-Guerin for adjuvant treatment of patients with intermediate- and high-risk non-muscle-invasive bladder cancer. Eur Urol. 2016;69(6):1046–52.
120. Alvarez N, Sevilla A. Current advances in photodynamic therapy (PDT) and the future potential of PDT-combinatorial cancer therapies. Int J Mol Sci. 2024;25(2):1023.
121. Grode L, Seiler P, Baumann S, Hess J, Brinkmann V, Nasser Eddine A, et al. Increased vaccine efficacy against tuberculosis of recombinant Mycobacterium bovis bacille Calmette-Guerin mutants that secrete listeriolysin. J Clin Invest. 2005;115(9):2472–9.
122. Loxton AG, Knaul JK, Grode L, Gutschmidt A, Meller C, Eisele B, et al. Safety and immunogenicity of the recombinant Mycobacterium bovis BCG vaccine VPM1002 in HIV-unexposed newborn infants in South Africa. Clin Vaccine Immunol. 2017;24(2):e00439-16.
123. Grode L, Ganoza CA, Brohm C, Weiner J 3rd, Eisele B, Kaufmann SH. Safety and immunogenicity of the recombinant BCG vaccine VPM1002 in a phase 1 open-label randomized clinical trial. Vaccine. 2013;31(9):1340–8.
124. Rentsch CA, Thalmann GN, Lucca I, Kwiatkowski M, Wirth GJ, Strebel RT, et al. A phase 1/2 single-arm clinical trial of recombinant Bacillus Calmette-Guerin (BCG) VPM1002BC immunotherapy in non-muscle-invasive bladder cancer recurrence after conventional BCG therapy: SAKK 06/14. Eur Urol Oncol. 2022;5(2):195–202.
125. Singh AK, Netea MG, Bishai WR. BCG turns 100: its nontraditional uses against viruses, cancer, and immunologic diseases. J Clin Invest. 2021;131(11):e148291.

126. Fritschi N, Curtis N, Ritz N. Bacille Calmette Guerin (BCG) and new TB vaccines: specific, cross-mycobacterial and off-target effects. Paediatr Respir Rev. 2020;36:57–64.
127. Moorlag S, Arts RJW, van Crevel R, Netea MG. Non-specific effects of BCG vaccine on viral infections. Clin Microbiol Infect. 2019;25(12):1473–8.
128. Lange C, Aaby P, Behr MA, Donald PR, Kaufmann SHE, Netea MG, et al. 100 years of Mycobacterium bovis bacille Calmette-Guerin. Lancet Infect Dis. 2022;22(1):e2–e12.
129. Aaby P, Roth A, Ravn H, Napirna BM, Rodrigues A, Lisse IM, et al. Randomized trial of BCG vaccination at birth to low-birth-weight children: beneficial nonspecific effects in the neonatal period? J Infect Dis. 2011;204(2):245–52.
130. Biering-Sorensen S, Aaby P, Napirna BM, Roth A, Ravn H, Rodrigues A, et al. Small randomized trial among low-birth-weight children receiving Bacillus Calmette-Guerin vaccination at first health center contact. Pediatr Infect Dis J. 2012;31(3):306–8.
131. Biering-Sorensen S, Aaby P, Lund N, Monteiro I, Jensen KJ, Eriksen HB, et al. Early BCG-Denmark and neonatal mortality among infants weighing <2500 g: a randomized controlled trial. Clin Infect Dis. 2017;65(7):1183–90.
132. Lombardi C, Pedrazzani ES, Pedrazzani JC, Filho PF, Zicker F. Protective efficacy of BCG against leprosy in Sao Paulo. Bull Pan Am Health Organ. 1996;30(1):24–30.
133. Ponnighaus JM, Fine PE, Sterne JA, Wilson RJ, Msosa E, Gruer PJ, et al. Efficacy of BCG vaccine against leprosy and tuberculosis in northern Malawi. Lancet. 1992;339(8794):636–9.
134. Fine PE, Ponnighaus JM, Maine N, Clarkson JA, Bliss L. Protective efficacy of BCG against leprosy in Northern Malawi. Lancet. 1986;2(8505):499–502.
135. Stanley SJ, Howland C, Stone MM, Sutherland I. BCG vaccination of children against leprosy in Uganda: final results. J Hyg (Lond). 1981;87(2):233–48.
136. Setia MS, Steinmaus C, Ho CS, Rutherford GW. The role of BCG in prevention of leprosy: a meta-analysis. Lancet Infect Dis. 2006;6(3):162–70.
137. BCG vaccination against mycobacterium ulcerans infection (Buruli ulcer). First results of a trial in Uganda. Lancet. 1969;1(7586):111–5.
138. Smith PG, Revill WD, Lukwago E, Rykushin YP. The protective effect of BCG against Mycobacterium ulcerans disease: a controlled trial in an endemic area of Uganda. Trans R Soc Trop Med Hyg. 1976;70(5–6):449–57.
139. Nackers F, Dramaix M, Johnson RC, Zinsou C, Robert A, DE Biurrun Bakedano E, et al. BCG vaccine effectiveness against Buruli ulcer: a case-control study in Benin. Am J Trop Med Hyg. 2006;75(4):768–74.
140. Phillips RO, Phanzu DM, Beissner M, Badziklou K, Luzolo EK, Sarfo FS, et al. Effectiveness of routine BCG vaccination on buruli ulcer disease: a case-control study in the Democratic Republic of Congo, Ghana and Togo. PLoS Negl Trop Dis. 2015;9(1):e3457.
141. Pittet LF, Tebruegge M, Dutta B, Donath S, Messina N, Casalaz D, et al. Mycobacterium ulcerans-specific immune response after immunisation with Bacillus Calmette-Guerin (BCG) vaccine. Vaccine. 2021;39(4):652–7.
142. Dow CT. Proposing BCG vaccination for Mycobacterium avium ss. paratuberculosis (MAP) associated autoimmune diseases. Microorganisms. 2020;8(2):212.
143. Lacroix A, Piau C, Lanotte P, Carricajo A, Guillouzouic A, Peuchant O, et al. Emergence of nontuberculous mycobacterial lymphadenitis in children after the discontinuation of mandatory Bacillus Calmette and GuErin immunization in France. Pediatr Infect Dis J. 2018;37(10):e257–e60.
144. Kontturi A, Soini H, Ollgren J, Salo E. Increase in childhood nontuberculous mycobacterial infections after Bacille Calmette-Guerin coverage drop: a nationwide, population-based retrospective study, Finland, 1995-2016. Clin Infect Dis. 2018;67(8):1256–61.
145. Romanus V, Hallander HO, Wahlen P, Olinder-Nielsen AM, Magnusson PH, Juhlin I. Atypical mycobacteria in extrapulmonary disease among children. Incidence in Sweden from 1969 to 1990, related to changing BCG-vaccination coverage. Tuber Lung Dis. 1995;76(4):300–10.
146. Trnka L, Dankova D, Svandova E. Six years' experience with the discontinuation of BCG vaccination. 4. Protective effect of BCG vaccination against the Mycobacterium avium intracellulare complex. Tuber Lung Dis. 1994;75(5):348–52.

147. Zimmermann P, Finn A, Curtis N. Does BCG vaccination protect against nontuberculous mycobacterial infection? A systematic review and meta-analysis. J Infect Dis. 2018;218(5):679–87.
148. Mackaness GB. The influence of immunologically committed lymphoid cells on macrophage activity in vivo. J Exp Med. 1969;129(5):973–92.
149. Mackaness GB. The immunological basis of acquired cellular resistance. J Exp Med. 1964;120(1):105–20.
150. Ruitenberg EJ, Steerenberg PA. Stimulation of the non-specific resistance by Corynebacterium parvum and Bacillus Calmette Guerin. Tijdschr Diergeneeskd. 1976;101(14):775–8.
151. Jespersen A. Acquired resistance of BCG-vaccinated red mice to infection with Listeria monocytogenes. Acta Pathol Microbiol Scand B. 1976;84B(5):265–72.
152. Nacy CA, Meltzer MS. Macrophages in resistance to rickettsial infections: protection against lethal Rickettsia tsutsugamushi infections by treatment of mice with macrophage-activating agents. J Leukoc Biol. 1984;35(4):385–96.
153. van't Wout JW, Poell R, van Furth R. The role of BCG/PPD-activated macrophages in resistance against systemic candidiasis in mice. Scand J Immunol. 1992;36(5):713–9.
154. Kleinnijenhuis J, Quintin J, Preijers F, Joosten LA, Ifrim DC, Saeed S, et al. Bacille Calmette-Guerin induces NOD2-dependent nonspecific protection from reinfection via epigenetic reprogramming of monocytes. Proc Natl Acad Sci USA. 2012;109(43):17537–42.
155. Kleinnijenhuis J, Quintin J, Preijers F, Joosten LA, Jacobs C, Xavier RJ, et al. BCG-induced trained immunity in NK cells: role for non-specific protection to infection. Clin Immunol. 2014;155(2):213–9.
156. Ortiz-Ortiz L, Gonzalez-Mendoza A, Lamoyi E. A vaccination procedure against Trypanosoma cruzi infection in mice by nonspecific immunization. J Immunol. 1975;114(4):1424–5.
157. Parra M, Liu X, Derrick SC, Yang A, Tian J, Kolibab K, et al. Molecular analysis of non-specific protection against murine malaria induced by BCG vaccination. PLoS One. 2013;8(7):e66115.
158. Matsumoto S, Yukitake H, Kanbara H, Yamada H, Kitamura A, Yamada T. Mycobacterium bovis Bacillus Calmette-Guerin induces protective immunity against infection by Plasmodium yoelii at blood-stage depending on shifting immunity toward Th1 type and inducing protective IgG2a after the parasite infection. Vaccine. 2000;19(7–8):779–87.
159. Dos Santos JC, Vilela Teodoro Silva M, Ribeiro-Dias F, Joosten LAB. Non-specific effects of BCG in protozoal infections: tegumentary leishmaniasis and malaria. Clin Microbiol Infect. 2019;25(12):1479–83.
160. Smrkovski LL, Larson CL. Effect of treatment with BCG on the course of visceral leishmaniasis in BALB/c mice. Infect Immun. 1977;16(1):249–57.
161. Pereira LI, Dorta ML, Pereira AJ, Bastos RP, Oliveira MA, Pinto SA, et al. Increase of NK cells and proinflammatory monocytes are associated with the clinical improvement of diffuse cutaneous leishmaniasis after immunochemotherapy with BCG/Leishmania antigens. Am J Trop Med Hyg. 2009;81(3):378–83.
162. Convit J, Castellanos PL, Ulrich M, Castes M, Rondon A, Pinardi ME, et al. Immunotherapy of localized, intermediate, and diffuse forms of American cutaneous leishmaniasis. J Infect Dis. 1989;160(1):104–15.
163. Convit J, Ulrich M, Polegre MA, Avila A, Rodriguez N, Mazzedo MI, et al. Therapy of Venezuelan patients with severe mucocutaneous or early lesions of diffuse cutaneous leishmaniasis with a vaccine containing pasteurized Leishmania promastigotes and Bacillus Calmette-Guerin: preliminary report. Mem Inst Oswaldo Cruz. 2004;99(1):57–62.
164. Mayrink W, Botelho AC, Magalhaes PA, Batista SM, Lima Ade O, Genaro O, et al. Immunotherapy, immunochemotherapy and chemotherapy for American cutaneous leishmaniasis treatment. Rev Soc Bras Med Trop. 2006;39(1):14–21.
165. Alimohammadian MH, Khamesipour A, Darabi H, Firooz A, Malekzadeh S, Bahonar A, et al. The role of BCG in human immune responses induced by multiple injections of autoclaved Leishmania major as a candidate vaccine against leishmaniasis. Vaccine. 2002;21(3–4):174–80.

166. Mahmoodi M, Khamesipour A, Dowlati Y, Rafati S, Momeni AZ, Emamjomeh M, et al. Immune response measured in human volunteers vaccinated with autoclaved Leishmania major vaccine mixed with low dose of BCG. Clin Exp Immunol. 2003;134(2):303–8.
167. Starr SE, Visintine AM, Tomeh MO, Nahmias AJ. Effects of immunostimulants on resistance of newborn mice to herpes simplex type 2 infection. Proc Soc Exp Biol Med. 1976;152(1):57–60.
168. Floc'h F, Werner GH. Increased resistance to virus infections of mice inoculated with BCG (Bacillus Calmette-Guerin). Ann Immunol (Paris). 1976;127(2):173–86.
169. Spencer JC, Ganguly R, Waldman RH. Nonspecific protection of mice against influenza virus infection by local or systemic immunization with Bacille Calmette-Guerin. J Infect Dis. 1977;136(2):171–5.
170. Mukherjee S, Subramaniam R, Chen H, Smith A, Keshava S, Shams H. Boosting efferocytosis in alveolar space using BCG vaccine to protect host against influenza pneumonia. PLoS One. 2017;12(7):e0180143.
171. Tran KA, Pernet E, Sadeghi M, Downey J, Chronopoulos J, Lapshina E, et al. BCG immunization induces CX3CR1(hi) effector memory T cells to provide cross-protection via IFN-gamma-mediated trained immunity. Nat Immunol. 2024;25(3):418–31.
172. Scheid A, Borriello F, Pietrasanta C, Christou H, Diray-Arce J, Pettengill MA, et al. Adjuvant effect of Bacille Calmette-Guerin on Hepatitis B vaccine immunogenicity in the preterm and term newborn. Front Immunol. 2018;9:29.
173. Kulkarni S, Mukherjee S, Pandey A, Dahake R, Padmanabhan U, Chowdhary AS. Bacillus Calmette-Guerin confers neuroprotection in a murine model of Japanese encephalitis. Neuroimmunomodulation. 2016;23(5–6):278–86.
174. Lodmell DL, Ewalt LC. Enhanced resistance against encephalomyocarditis virus infection in mice, induced by a nonviable Mycobacterium tuberculosis oil-droplet vaccine. Infect Immun. 1978;19(1):225–30.
175. Lodmell DL, Ewalt LC. Induction of enhanced resistance against encephalomyocarditis virus infection of mice by nonviable Mycobacterium tuberculosis: mechanisms of protection. Infect Immun. 1978;22(3):740–5.
176. Suenaga T, Okuyama T, Yoshida I, Azuma M. Effect of Mycobacterium tuberculosis BCG infection on the resistance of mice to ectromelia virus infection: participation of interferon in enhanced resistance. Infect Immun. 1978;20(1):312–4.
177. Sakuma T, Suenaga T, Yoshida I, Azuma M. Mechanisms of enhanced resistance of Mycobacterium bovis BCG-treated mice to ectromelia virus infection. Infect Immun. 1983;42(2):567–73.
178. Ikeda S, Negishi T, Nishimura C. Enhancement of non-specific resistance to viral infection by muramyldipeptide and its analogs. Antivir Res. 1985;5(4):207–15.
179. Mathurin KS, Martens GW, Kornfeld H, Welsh RM. CD4 T-cell-mediated heterologous immunity between mycobacteria and poxviruses. J Virol. 2009;83(8):3528–39.
180. Ramirez MA, Loaiza RA, Martinez-Balboa Y, Bruneau N, Ramirez E, Gonzalez PA, et al. Co-administration of recombinant BCG and SARS-CoV-2 proteins leads to robust antiviral immunity. Vaccine. 2024;42(23):126203.
181. Hilligan KL, Namasivayam S, Clancy CS, Baker PJ, Old SI, Peluf V, et al. Bacterial-induced or passively administered interferon gamma conditions the lung for early control of SARS-CoV-2. Nat Commun. 2023;14(1):8229.
182. Hilligan KL, Namasivayam S, Sher A. BCG mediated protection of the lung against experimental SARS-CoV-2 infection. Front Immunol. 2023;14:1232764.
183. Zhang BZ, Shuai H, Gong HR, Hu JC, Yan B, Yuen TT, et al. Bacillus Calmette-Guerin-induced trained immunity protects against SARS-CoV-2 challenge in K18-hACE2 mice. JCI Insight. 2022;7(11):e157393.
184. Hilligan KL, Namasivayam S, Clancy CS, O'Mard D, Oland SD, Robertson SJ, et al. Intravenous administration of BCG protects mice against lethal SARS-CoV-2 challenge. J Exp Med. 2022;219(2):e20211862.

185. Ng TW, Furuyama W, Wirchnianski AS, Saavedra-Avila NA, Johndrow CT, Chandran K, et al. A viral vaccine design harnessing prior BCG immunization confers protection against Ebola virus. Front Immunol. 2024;15:1429909.
186. Berg MK, Yu Q, Salvador CE, Melani I, Kitayama S. Mandated Bacillus Calmette-Guerin (BCG) vaccination predicts flattened curves for the spread of COVID-19. Sci Adv. 2020;6(32):eabc1463.
187. Gursel M, Gursel I. Is global BCG vaccination-induced trained immunity relevant to the progression of SARS-CoV-2 pandemic? Allergy. 2020;75(7):1815–9.
188. Covian C, Retamal-Diaz A, Bueno SM, Kalergis AM. Could BCG vaccination induce protective trained immunity for SARS-CoV-2? Front Immunol. 2020;11:970.
189. Escobar LE, Molina-Cruz A, Barillas-Mury C. BCG vaccine protection from severe coronavirus disease 2019 (COVID-19). Proc Natl Acad Sci USA. 2020;117(30):17720–6.
190. Lindestam Arlehamn CS, Sette A, Peters B. Lack of evidence for BCG vaccine protection from severe COVID-19. Proc Natl Acad Sci USA. 2020;117(41):25203–4.
191. Hamiel U, Kozer E, Youngster I. SARS-CoV-2 rates in BCG-vaccinated and unvaccinated young adults. JAMA. 2020;323(22):2340–1.
192. Koekenbier EL, Fohse K, van de Maat JS, Oosterheert JJ, van Nieuwkoop C, Hoogerwerf JJ, et al. Bacillus Calmette-Guerin vaccine for prevention of COVID-19 and other respiratory tract infections in older adults with comorbidities: a randomized controlled trial. Clin Microbiol Infect. 2023;29(6):781–8.
193. Moorlag S, Taks E, Ten Doesschate T, van der Vaart TW, Janssen AB, Muller L, et al. Efficacy of BCG vaccination against respiratory tract infections in older adults during the coronavirus disease 2019 pandemic. Clin Infect Dis. 2022;75(1):e938–e46.
194. Pittet LF, Noble CCA, Messina NL, Curtis N. Using BCG vaccination to protect against COVID-19: when reality fails to meet expectation. Nat Rev Immunol. 2024;24(2):83–4.
195. Salem A, Nofal A, Hosny D. Treatment of common and plane warts in children with topical viable Bacillus Calmette-Guerin. Pediatr Dermatol. 2013;30(1):60–3.
196. Podder I, Bhattacharya S, Mishra V, Sarkar TK, Chandra S, Sil A, et al. Immunotherapy in viral warts with intradermal Bacillus Calmette-Guerin vaccine versus intradermal tuberculin purified protein derivative: a double-blind, randomized controlled trial comparing effectiveness and safety in a tertiary care center in Eastern India. Indian J Dermatol Venereol Leprol. 2017;83(3):411.
197. Jaisinghani AK, Dey VK, Suresh MS, Saxena A. Bacillus Calmette-Guerin immunotherapy for recurrent multiple warts: an open-label uncontrolled study. Indian J Dermatol. 2019;64(2):164.
198. Daulatabad D, Pandhi D, Singal A. BCG vaccine for immunotherapy in warts: is it really safe in a tuberculosis endemic area? Dermatol Ther. 2016;29(3):168–72.
199. Pittet LF, Moore CL, McDonald E, Barry S, Bonten M, Campbell J, et al. Bacillus Calmette-Guerin vaccination for protection against recurrent herpes labialis: a nested randomised controlled trial. EClinicalMedicine. 2023;64:102203.
200. Pittet LF, Curtis N. Does Bacillus Calmette-Guerin vaccine prevent herpes simplex virus recurrences? A systematic review. Rev Med Virol. 2021;31(1):1–9.
201. Leentjens J, Kox M, Stokman R, Gerretsen J, Diavatopoulos DA, van Crevel R, et al. BCG vaccination enhances the immunogenicity of subsequent influenza vaccination in healthy volunteers: a randomized, placebo-controlled pilot study. J Infect Dis. 2015;212(12):1930–8.
202. Ritz N, Mui M, Balloch A, Curtis N. Non-specific effect of Bacille Calmette-Guerin vaccine on the immune response to routine immunisations. Vaccine. 2013;31(30):3098–103.
203. Ota MO, Vekemans J, Schlegel-Haueter SE, Fielding K, Sanneh M, Kidd M, et al. Influence of Mycobacterium bovis Bacillus Calmette-Guerin on antibody and cytokine responses to human neonatal vaccination. J Immunol. 2002;168(2):919–25.
204. Yamazaki-Nakashimada MA, Unzueta A, Berenise Gamez-Gonzalez L, Gonzalez-Saldana N, Sorensen RU. BCG: a vaccine with multiple faces. Hum Vaccin Immunother. 2020;16(8):1841–50.

205. Gofrit ON, Klein BY, Cohen IR, Ben-Hur T, Greenblatt CL, Bercovier H. Bacillus Calmette-Guerin (BCG) therapy lowers the incidence of Alzheimer's disease in bladder cancer patients. PLoS One. 2019;14(11):e0224433.
206. Kim JI, Zhu D, Barry E, Kovac E, Aboumohamed A, Agalliu I, et al. Intravesical Bacillus Calmette-Guerin treatment is inversely associated with the risk of developing Alzheimer disease or other dementia among patients with non-muscle-invasive bladder cancer. Clin Genitourin Cancer. 2021;19(6):e409–e16.
207. Klinger D, Hill BL, Barda N, Halperin E, Gofrit ON, Greenblatt CL, et al. Bladder cancer immunotherapy by BCG is associated with a significantly reduced risk of Alzheimer's disease and Parkinson's disease. Vaccines (Basel). 2021;9(5):491.
208. Makrakis D, Holt SK, Bernick C, Grivas P, Gore JL, Wright JL. Intravesical BCG and incidence of Alzheimer disease in patients with bladder cancer: results from an administrative dataset. Alzheimer Dis Assoc Disord. 2022;36(4):307–11.
209. Weinberg MS, Zafar A, Magdamo C, Chung SY, Chou WH, Nayan M, et al. Association of BCG vaccine treatment with death and dementia in patients with non-muscle-invasive bladder cancer. JAMA Netw Open. 2023;6(5):e2314336.
210. Han C, Wang J, Chen YL, Guan CP, Zhang YA, Wang MS. The role of Bacillus Calmette-Guerin administration on the risk of dementia in bladder cancer patients: a systematic review and meta-analysis. Front Aging Neurosci. 2023;15:1243588.
211. Umar TP, Jain N, Stevanny B, Javed B, Priandhana A, Siburian R, et al. Protective role of Bacillus Calmette-Guerin vaccine in Alzheimer's disease progression: a systematic review and meta-analysis. Heliyon. 2024;10(5):e27425.
212. Zuo Z, Qi F, Yang J, Wang X, Wu Y, Wen Y, et al. Immunization with Bacillus Calmette-Guerin (BCG) alleviates neuroinflammation and cognitive deficits in APP/PS1 mice via the recruitment of inflammation-resolving monocytes to the brain. Neurobiol Dis. 2017;101:27–39.
213. Yong J, Lacan G, Dang H, Hsieh T, Middleton B, Wasserfall C, et al. BCG vaccine-induced neuroprotection in a mouse model of Parkinson's disease. PLoS One. 2011;6(1):e16610.
214. Lacan G, Dang H, Middleton B, Horwitz MA, Tian J, Melega WP, et al. Bacillus Calmette-Guerin vaccine-mediated neuroprotection is associated with regulatory T-cell induction in the 1-methyl-4-phenyl-1,2,3,6-tetrahydropyridine mouse model of Parkinson's disease. J Neurosci Res. 2013;91(10):1292–302.
215. Yedke NG, Soni D, Kumar P. Effect of Bacille-Calmette-Guerin vaccine against rotenone-induced Parkinson's disease: role of neuroinflammation and neurotransmitters. Fundam Clin Pharmacol. 2024;38(3):538–49.
216. Nakken O, Holmoy T, Stigum H, Myhr KM, Dahl J, Heldal E, et al. Strong tuberculin response after BCG vaccination is associated with low multiple sclerosis risk: a population-based cohort study. Int J Epidemiol. 2022;51(5):1637–44.
217. Ristori G, Buzzi MG, Sabatini U, Giugni E, Bastianello S, Viselli F, et al. Use of Bacille Calmette-Guerin (BCG) in multiple sclerosis. Neurology. 1999;53(7):1588–9.
218. Paolillo A, Buzzi MG, Giugni E, Sabatini U, Bastianello S, Pozzilli C, et al. The effect of Bacille Calmette-Guerin on the evolution of new enhancing lesions to hypointense T1 lesions in relapsing remitting MS. J Neurol. 2003;250(2):247–8.
219. Ristori G, Romano S, Cannoni S, Visconti A, Tinelli E, Mendozzi L, et al. Effects of Bacille Calmette-Guerin after the first demyelinating event in the CNS. Neurology. 2014;82(1):41–8.
220. Lippens C, Garnier L, Guyonvarc'h PM, Santiago-Raber ML, Hugues S. Extended freeze-dried BCG instructed pDCs induce suppressive tregs and dampen EAE. Front Immunol. 2018;9:2777.
221. Lee J, Reinke EK, Zozulya AL, Sandor M, Fabry Z. Mycobacterium bovis bacille Calmette-Guerin infection in the CNS suppresses experimental autoimmune encephalomyelitis and Th17 responses in an IFN-gamma-independent manner. J Immunol. 2008;181(9):6201–12.
222. Lamb DJ, Eales LJ, Ferns GA. Immunization with Bacillus Calmette-Guerin vaccine increases aortic atherosclerosis in the cholesterol-fed rabbit. Atherosclerosis. 1999;143(1):105–13.

223. Ovchinnikova OA, Berge N, Kang C, Urien C, Ketelhuth DF, Pottier J, et al. Mycobacterium bovis BCG killed by extended freeze-drying induces an immunoregulatory profile and protects against atherosclerosis. J Intern Med. 2014;275(1):49–58.
224. Bekkering S, Singh K, Lu H, Limawan AP, Nold-Petry CA, Wallace MJ, et al. Neonatal subcutaneous BCG vaccination decreases atherosclerotic plaque number and plaque macrophage content in ApoE(−/−) mice. Biology (Basel). 2022;11(10):1511.
225. van Dam AD, Bekkering S, Crasborn M, van Beek L, van den Berg SM, Vrieling F, et al. BCG lowers plasma cholesterol levels and delays atherosclerotic lesion progression in mice. Atherosclerosis. 2016;251:6–14.
226. Huaman MA, Qualls JE, Jose S, Schmidt SM, Moussa A, Kuhel DG, et al. Mycobacterium bovis Bacille-Calmette-Guerin infection aggravates atherosclerosis. Front Immunol. 2020;11:607957.
227. Kowalewicz-Kulbat M, Locht C. BCG for the prevention and treatment of allergic asthma. Vaccine. 2021;39(50):7341–52.
228. Arnoldussen DL, Linehan M, Sheikh A. BCG vaccination and allergy: a systematic review and meta-analysis. J Allergy Clin Immunol. 2011;127(1):246–53, 53 e1–21.
229. El-Zein M, Parent ME, Benedetti A, Rousseau MC. Does BCG vaccination protect against the development of childhood asthma? A systematic review and meta-analysis of epidemiological studies. Int J Epidemiol. 2010;39(2):469–86.
230. Linehan MF, Nurmatov U, Frank TL, Niven RM, Baxter DN, Sheikh A. Does BCG vaccination protect against childhood asthma? Final results from the Manchester Community Asthma Study retrospective cohort study and updated systematic review and meta-analysis. J Allergy Clin Immunol. 2014;133(3):688–95 e14.
231. Choi IS, Koh YI. Therapeutic effects of BCG vaccination in adult asthmatic patients: a randomized, controlled trial. Ann Allergy Asthma Immunol. 2002;88(6):584–91.
232. Choi IS, Koh YI. Effects of BCG revaccination on asthma. Allergy. 2003;58(11):1114–6.
233. Datau EA, Mewengkang H, Matheos JC, Purnawan I, Wibisono M, Wongdjaja K, et al. Clinical efficacy and laboratory improvement of Bacillus Calmette-Guerin vaccination on adult atopic asthma: a cohort study. World Allergy Organ J. 2008;1(4):63–9.
234. Shen H, Huang H, Wang J, Ye S, Li W, Wang K, et al. Neonatal vaccination with Bacillus Calmette-Guerin elicits long-term protection in mouse-allergic responses. Allergy. 2008;63(5):555–63.
235. Li R, Yang X, Wang L, Liu E. Respiratory syncytial virus infection reversed anti-asthma effect of neonatal Bacillus Calmette-Guerin vaccination in BALB/c mice. Pediatr Res. 2006;59(2):210–5.
236. Deng Y, Chen W, Zang N, Li S, Luo Y, Ni K, et al. The antiasthma effect of neonatal BCG vaccination does not depend on the Th17/Th1 but IL-17/IFN-gamma balance in a BALB/c mouse asthma model. J Clin Immunol. 2011;31(3):419–29.
237. Deng Y, Li W, Luo Y, Wang LJ, Xie XH, Luo J, et al. Inhibition of IFN-gamma promotes anti-asthma effect of Mycobacterium bovis Bacillus Calmette-Guerin neonatal vaccination: a murine asthma model. Vaccine. 2014;32(18):2070–8.
238. Yang X, Fan Y, Wang S, Han X, Yang J, Bilenki L, et al. Mycobacterial infection inhibits established allergic inflammatory responses via alteration of cytokine production and vascular cell adhesion molecule-1 expression. Immunology. 2002;105(3):336–43.
239. Gouveia AC, Brugiolo AS, Alves CC, Silva FM, Mesquita FP, Gameiro J, et al. Th2 responses in OVA-sensitized BALB/c mice are down-modulated by Mycobacterium bovis BCG treatment. J Clin Immunol. 2013;33(1):235–45.
240. Tarancon R, Mata E, Uranga S, Gomez AB, Marinova D, Otal I, et al. Therapeutic efficacy of pulmonary live tuberculosis vaccines against established asthma by subverting local immune environment. EBioMedicine. 2021;64:103186.
241. Yagi H, Matsumoto M, Kishimoto Y, Makino S, Harada M. Possible mechanism of the preventive effect of BCG against diabetes mellitus in NOD mouse. II. Suppression of pathogenesis by macrophage transfer from BCG-vaccinated mice. Cell Immunol. 1991;138(1):142–9.

242. Harada M, Kishimoto Y, Makino S. Prevention of overt diabetes and insulitis in NOD mice by a single BCG vaccination. Diabetes Res Clin Pract. 1990;8(2):85–9.
243. Sadelain MW, Qin HY, Lauzon J, Singh B. Prevention of type I diabetes in NOD mice by adjuvant immunotherapy. Diabetes. 1990;39(5):583–9.
244. Lakey JR, Singh B, Warnock GL, Rajotte RV. BCG immunotherapy prevents recurrence of diabetes in islet grafts transplanted into spontaneously diabetic NOD mice. Transplantation. 1994;57(8):1213–7.
245. Shehadeh N, Calcinaro F, Bradley BJ, Bruchim I, Vardi P, Lafferty KJ. Effect of adjuvant therapy on development of diabetes in mouse and man. Lancet. 1994;343(8899):706–7.
246. Sanjeevi CB, Das AK, Shtauvere-Brameus A. BCG vaccination and GAD65 and IA-2 autoantibodies in autoimmune diabetes in southern India. Ann N Y Acad Sci. 2002;958:293–6.
247. Huppmann M, Baumgarten A, Ziegler AG, Bonifacio E. Neonatal Bacille Calmette-Guerin vaccination and type 1 diabetes. Diabetes Care. 2005;28(5):1204–6.
248. Allen HF, Klingensmith GJ, Jensen P, Simoes E, Hayward A, Chase HP. Effect of Bacillus Calmette-Guerin vaccination on new-onset type 1 diabetes. A randomized clinical study. Diabetes Care. 1999;22(10):1703–7.
249. Pozzilli P. BCG vaccine in insulin-dependent diabetes mellitus. IMDIAB Group. Lancet. 1997;349(9064):1520–1.
250. Faustman DL. Benefits of BCG-induced metabolic switch from oxidative phosphorylation to aerobic glycolysis in autoimmune and nervous system diseases. J Intern Med. 2020;288(6):641–50.
251. Faustman DL. TNF, TNF inducers, and TNFR2 agonists: a new path to type 1 diabetes treatment. Diabetes Metab Res Rev. 2018;34(1).
252. Faustman DL, Wang L, Okubo Y, Burger D, Ban L, Man G, et al. Proof-of-concept, randomized, controlled clinical trial of Bacillus-Calmette-Guerin for treatment of long-term type 1 diabetes. PLoS One. 2012;7(8):e41756.
253. Kuhtreiber WM, Faustman DL. BCG therapy for type 1 diabetes: restoration of balanced immunity and metabolism. Trends Endocrinol Metab. 2019;30(2):80–92.
254. Kuhtreiber WM, Tran L, Kim T, Dybala M, Nguyen B, Plager S, et al. Long-term reduction in hyperglycemia in advanced type 1 diabetes: the value of induced aerobic glycolysis with BCG vaccinations. NPJ Vaccines. 2018;3:23.
255. Stienstra R, Netea MG. Firing up glycolysis: BCG vaccination effects on type 1 diabetes mellitus. Trends Endocrinol Metab. 2018;29(12):813–4.
256. Andrzejewski S, Gravel SP, Pollak M, St-Pierre J. Metformin directly acts on mitochondria to alter cellular bioenergetics. Cancer Metab. 2014;2:12.
257. Segura-Cerda CA, Marquina-Castillo B, Lozano-Ordaz V, Mata-Espinosa D, Barrios-Payan JA, Lopez-Torres MO, et al. BCG and BCGDeltaBCG1419c protect type 2 diabetic mice against tuberculosis via different participation of T and B lymphocytes, dendritic cells and pro-inflammatory cytokines. NPJ Vaccines. 2020;5(1):21.
258. Radhakrishnan RK, Thandi RS, Tripathi D, Paidipally P, McAllister MK, Mulik S, et al. BCG vaccination reduces the mortality of Mycobacterium tuberculosis-infected type 2 diabetes mellitus mice. JCI Insight. 2020;5(5):e133788.
259. Kawasaki T. Two cases with acute febrile mucocutaneous lymph node syndrome possibly induced by vaccinia or measles vaccination. Jpn J Pediatr. 1970;23:657–62.
260. Kuniyuki S, Asada M. An ulcerated lesion at the BCG vaccination site during the course of Kawasaki disease. J Am Acad Dermatol. 1997;37(2):303–4.
261. Diniz LMO, Castanheira RG, Giampietro YG, Silva MS, Nogueira FD, Pessoa PD, et al. Diagnostic value of the reaction at the Bacillus Calmette-Guerin vaccination site in Kawasaki disease. Rev Paul Pediatr. 2021;39:e2019338.
262. Novais C, Fortunato F, Bicho A, Preto L. Bacillus Calmette-Guerin reactivation as a sign of incomplete Kawasaki disease. BMJ Case Rep. 2016;2016:bcr2015213875.
263. Fujieda M, Karasawa R, Takasugi H, Yamamoto M, Kataoka K, Yudoh K, et al. A novel anti-peroxiredoxin autoantibody in patients with Kawasaki disease. Microbiol Immunol. 2012;56(1):56–61.

264. Sireci G, Dieli F, Salerno A. T cells recognize an immunodominant epitope of heat shock protein 65 in Kawasaki disease. Mol Med. 2000;6(7):581–90.
265. Sato N, Sagawa K, Sasaguri Y, Inoue O, Kato H. Immunopathology and cytokine detection in the skin lesions of patients with Kawasaki disease. J Pediatr. 1993;122(2):198–203.
266. Uehara R, Igarashi H, Yashiro M, Nakamura Y, Yanagawa H. Kawasaki disease patients with redness or crust formation at the Bacille Calmette-Guerin inoculation site. Pediatr Infect Dis J. 2010;29(5):430–3.
267. Garrido-Garcia LM, Castillo-Moguel A, Vazquez-Rivera M, Cravioto P, Fernando G. Reaction of the BCG scar in the acute phase of Kawasaki disease in Mexican children. Pediatr Infect Dis J. 2017;36(10):e237–e41.
268. Muthuvelu S, Lim KS, Huang LY, Chin ST, Mohan A. Measles infection causing Bacillus Calmette-Guerin reactivation: a case report. BMC Pediatr. 2019;19(1):251.
269. Kakisaka Y, Ohara T, Katayama S, Suzuki T, Sasai S, Hino-Fukuyo N, et al. Human herpes virus type 6 can cause skin lesions at the BCG inoculation site similar to Kawasaki disease. Tohoku J Exp Med. 2012;228(4):351–3.

Induction of Trained Immunity and Nonspecific Protective Effects Against Heterologous Diseases by BCG Vaccination

4

Somnath Shee and William Bishai

4.1 Introduction

Bacillus Calmette-Guérin (BCG) is a live-attenuated strain of *Mycobacterium bovis*. BCG was derived from a virulent *M. bovis* strain that underwent significant genomic alterations, accumulating ≈16 deletions in various regions of the chromosome [1]. BCG administration is effective in preventing disseminated forms of pediatric tuberculosis (TB) including meningitis and miliary TB with an estimated efficacy of ≈70% [2–5]. However, its effectiveness in preventing pulmonary TB in adults varies widely, ranging from 0% to 80% [2]. Due to its efficacy in children, the World Health Organization (WHO) recommends a single dose of BCG vaccination at birth for all infants in countries with a high burden of TB [6]. Administered to over 120 million infants worldwide annually, the BCG vaccine stands as one of the most extensively utilized vaccines in human history [7] (reviewed in [8]). However, despite the availability of BCG for more than a century, TB still caused approximately 1.3 million deaths annually in 2022, with approximately one-fourth of humans believed to be latently infected with *Mycobacterium tuberculosis* (*Mtb*) [9, 10].

While originally developed as a vaccine against TB, a growing body of evidence from epidemiological studies, clinical trials, and preclinical animal models has revealed the beneficial effects of BCG for diseases that are unrelated to TB. In other words, BCG shows protective or therapeutic properties against heterologous or nonmycobacterial diseases, beyond its TB prevention capabilities alone (Fig. 4.1). The presence of these BCG-dependent protective heterologous effects (PHEs) was first reported in Sweden, just 3 years after the vaccine's introduction into the general population in 1931 [11], and since then, BCG vaccination has been associated with

S. Shee (✉) · W. Bishai (✉)
Johns Hopkins School of Medicine, Baltimore, MD, USA
e-mail: sshee1@jhmi.edu; wbishai1@jhmi.edu

P. J. G. Bettencourt (ed.), *Tuberculosis Vaccines*,
https://doi.org/10.1007/978-3-031-94540-3_4

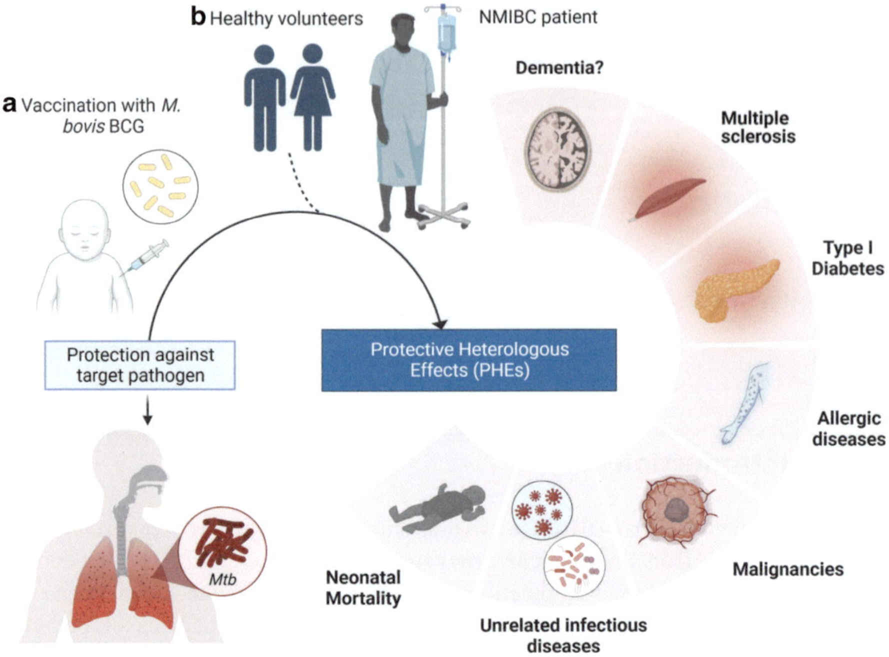

Fig. 4.1 BCG-induced protective heterologous effects (PHEs). Epidemiological studies, RCTs, and retrospective data analysis on (**a**) neonates and (**b**) volunteers/NMIBC patients provide evidence that BCG vaccination can induce PHEs against several unrelated pathogens and immune disorders, other than its intended target of prevention of TB

protecting both children and adults against a diverse range of diseases, including nonmycobacterial infections, immunologic disorders, and certain malignancies. In this chapter, we shall discuss these studies, our current understanding of BCG's mechanisms of action for these PHEs, and unanswered questions in the field.

4.2 Evidence of BCG-Induced Heterologous Immunity

4.2.1 All-Cause Mortality and Morbidity

4.2.1.1 All-Cause Mortality

The first study documenting the heterologous benefits of BCG vaccination in humans dates back to 1931 when a notable decrease in childhood mortality was observed among BCG-vaccinated children in Sweden [11]. Between 1927 and 1929, BCG vaccine provided strong protection against deaths from all diseases (infectious and non-infectious) with a relative risk (RR) of 0.09 (95% confidence interval (CI) = 0.02–0.36). This dramatic protection (>90%) may have stemmed from certain selection biases for study inclusion. However, in the period from 1930 to 1931, BCG was linked to a decrease in non-TB infectious deaths, with an RR of

0.75 (95% CI = 0.58–0.97). Two-thirds of these deaths were attributed to respiratory infections, where the BCG-vaccinated/unvaccinated RR was 0.61 (95% CI = 0.43–0.84) [11]. In addition to this, a similar study by researchers at the Institute Pasteur (Paris) in 1932 concluded that the mortality rate was 7.9% among BCG-vaccinated and 15.3% among nonvaccinated children [12]. Since the 1930s, similar beneficial effects of BCG against all-cause neonatal mortality were also noted in large observational studies and randomized, controlled trials in Asia, Africa, and America (reviewed in [12]). Interestingly, the mounting evidence prompted the WHO to commission a review of studies assessing BCG's impact on childhood mortality in 2014 [13]. The resulting meta-analysis, encompassing five clinical trials and nine observational studies, identified a BCG-associated 30% reduction in all-cause mortality in children under 5 years in clinical trials and a 53% reduction in observational studies [13].

Importantly, some studies report that BCG vaccination does not affect neonatal mortality. For example, early clinical trials among native American populations in Canada [14] and the United States [15] showed minimal BCG vaccination effects on all-cause mortality (6–9% reduction). Similarly, an observational study in Greenland, where the BCG vaccination program started in 1955, found no impact on hospitalization rates between BCG-vaccinated and BCG-unvaccinated children during a transient halt in vaccination from 1991 to 1996 [16]. In sum, these data emphasize the need for further research on BCG-induced PHEs, preferably through randomized controlled trials (RCTs) in settings beyond the high-mortality, low-income regions where most of the evidence for a beneficial BCG effect was generated.

4.2.1.2 General Infectious Morbidity Studies

In addition to neonatal mortality, BCG vaccination has been shown to decrease the frequency and severity of diseases in children. A large retrospective study in Spain, covering 464,611 pediatric hospitalizations, indicated a 41% lower risk of serious respiratory infection and a 53% lower risk of sepsis unrelated to TB in BCG-vaccinated children [17]. On the contrary, a study in Greenland with 19,363 children reported that BCG vaccination did not offer protection against infections requiring hospitalization in children aged 3 months to 3 years, although there was benefit during the first 3 months of life [16, 18]. Two large RCTs in high-income countries like Denmark (The Danish Calmette Study) [19] and Australia (The Melbourne Infant Study: BCG for Allergy and Infection Reduction or MISBAIR) [20] aimed to explore potential BCG benefits in settings with lower infectious disease burdens. While the MISBAIR study (following 1272 neonates) is ongoing, the Danish Calmette study (which monitored 4192 children, half of whom received BCG within 7 days of birth, for parent-reported infectious illnesses at 3 and 13 months of age) indeed found that BCG-vaccinated infants demonstrated a reduced number of infectious disease episodes and hospitalizations compared to their unvaccinated counterparts with an incidence rate ratio of 0.62 (95% CI = 0.39–0.98) [19]. However, this effect was only seen if the mother was BCG-vaccinated. This is intriguing and important because most previous studies demonstrating a BCG benefit were conducted in regions with high maternal BCG vaccination rates. Whether some degree of BCG-mediated protection may be transferred from mother to child remains an open question in this field.

BCG vaccination has also been explored for its potential to protect elderly individuals against all-cause infections. A double-blind, Phase 3 RCT known as the ACTIVATE trial in 198 Greek patients aged 65 or older found that BCG vaccination significantly delayed the time to the first infection by 5 weeks, decreased the incidence of new infection (25% relative to 42.3% in the unvaccinated group), and offered significant protection against viral respiratory tract infections (hazard ratio = 0.21, $p = 0.013$) [21]. A subsequent RCT of over 2000 Dutch patients over the age of 60 who were followed for 12 months failed to observe a lower incidence of respiratory tract infections in the BCG-vaccinated arm [22]. One difference is that the Netherlands does not routinely vaccinate infants, while Greek children receive it at 5–13 years of age, so it is possible that re-vaccination with BCG provides a benefit not seen with only a single dose.

4.2.1.3 Organ-Specific Infectious Morbidity

The protective effects of BCG vaccination have been documented in numerous animal studies demonstrating efficacy against a wide range of pathogens, including bacteria (e.g., *Shigella flexneri* [23], *Listeria monocytogenes* [24, 25], fungi (e.g., *Candida albicans*) [26], and protozoa (e.g., *Plasmodium* spp.) [27] (reviewed in [28])). The data from animal models is consistent with several human studies involving either high or low infant mortality settings. For example, Stensballe et al. reported a >twofold increased risk of acute lower respiratory tract infections (ALRTI) in unvaccinated infants relative to BCG recipients in a study involving 386 infants in Guinea-Bissau [29]. Interestingly, the protective effect was more prominent in females [29]. Similar findings were reported in a population-based retrospective analysis involving over 40,000 children, where BCG vaccination was associated with a 37% decrease in the development of ALRTI compared to non-BCG-vaccinated children [30].

4.2.2 Infectious Diseases

4.2.2.1 Viral Infections

In addition to bacterial and fungal infections, several preclinical and clinical datasets have demonstrated the PHEs of BCG vaccination against viral infections and disease severity. In 2020, a meta-analysis on BCG for herpes simplex virus (HSV) involving eight human (301 patients) and eight animal studies revealed that BCG exposure reduced the frequency and severity of HSV recurrences in humans, and in animal studies, it increased the survival rates by 1.9- to 5.5-fold in mice [31]. Further evidence demonstrating PHEs of BCG is provided by human studies against yellow fever virus (YFV) in an RCT (reduced viremia [32]), human papillomavirus (topical BCG treatment [33–35]), influenza A (increased and rapid antibody production against H1N1 virus [36]), and respiratory syncytial virus [29]. Moreover, BCG vaccination at birth also enhanced the antibody responses to routine childhood vaccines (pneumococcal, *Haemophilus influenzae* type B, and tetanus toxoid vaccines) given subsequently [37]. Detailed reviews on BCG-mediated effects against viral infections have been previously published [8, 38–40]. It is important to note that BCG-mediated benefits are not universally observed against viral infections. For example, animal studies have shown conflicting results in protection against influenza A virus, with one study showing no protection [41] in mice and another showing significant protection [42].

With the advent of COVID-19, there was early enthusiasm that BCG might be valuable to prevent or reduce the severity of SARS-CoV-2 infection. Initial studies reported that countries with existing BCG vaccination programs showed lower rates of COVID-19 incidence and death [43, 44]. Similarly, a retrospective study of 6679 healthcare workers in Los Angeles revealed that a history of BCG vaccination was linked to reduced COVID-19 symptoms and lower seroprevalence of anti-SARS-CoV-2 IgG with an odds ratio of 0.76 (95% CI = 0.57–0.99; p = 0.048) [45]. In contrast, some human observational studies in 2020 refuted the idea that BCG is beneficial for COVID-19 [46, 47]. Animal studies also showed that BCG given subcutaneously failed to protect against COVID-19 [42, 48], although intravenous BCG vaccination (not approved for human use) was shown to successfully reduce viral titers and disease severity in mice and hamsters [48–50]. However, at this point, numerous prospective human studies evaluating the efficacy of BCG for COVID-19 prevention in humans have been published, and there is a general consensus that BCG does not reduce the incidence of SARS-CoV-2 infections. For example, an RCT involving 2014 Dutch patients aged 60 or above showed no protection against SARS-CoV-2 or other respiratory tract infections, although BCG vaccination led to higher antibody titers after COVID-19 infection [22]. More recently, the BRACE Phase 3 multinational RCT of 3988 healthcare workers monitored for 12 months observed a 14.7% risk of symptomatic COVID-19 among BCG recipients and a 12.3% risk in unvaccinated controls (p = 0.13), with no significant differences in disease severity or rate of hospitalizations between the two groups [51, 52]. While the majority of human studies have not found that BCG reduces the incidence of COVID-19, it is worth noting that several studies have shown modest benefits in disease severity reduction or boosted antibody titers with BCG (reviewed in [53, 54]).

4.2.2.2 Nontuberculous Mycobacteria (NTM) Infections

Members of the genus *Mycobacteria* share numerous closely related antigenic proteins, lipids, glycoproteins, and glycolipids, so some degree of cross-immunity conferred by BCG against NTM infections is to be expected. While only a handful of mycobacterial species are innate human pathogens and cause bona fide tuberculosis (*M. tuberculosis*, *M. bovis*, *M. africanum*, and *M. microti*), some of the remaining members of the *Mycobacteria* genus, which comprise ~195 separate species [55], are opportunistic human pathogens and termed NTM, with *M. avium, M. intracellulare,* and *M. abscessus* being the most clinically important. In this context, it is interesting to note that in developed countries (United States, Canada, and Western Europe) where BCG vaccination is not commonly employed, there has been a consistent rise in pulmonary NTM infections caused by *M. avium, M. intracellulare,* and *M. abscessus* and related species over the past decades [56]. For instance, in France, the discontinuation of mandatory neonatal BCG vaccination in 2007 led to a ≈sixfold increase in the incidence of culture-confirmed NTM cervical lymphadenitis in children through 2013 [57]. Similarly, in Finland, childhood NTM infections (incidence rate ratio = 19.03 (95% CI = 8.8–41.07; $p < 0.001$) increased significantly since 2006 when the universal BCG vaccination policy was changed to be used in selective groups only [58]. A meta-analysis of 10 studies encompassing nearly 12 million subjects found that BCG-vaccinated children had a significantly lower risk ratio for NTM lymphadenitis of 0.04 (95% CI = 0.01–0.21), or in other words a 96% reduction in the relative risk, compared to unvaccinated controls [59].

Beyond its impact on the NTM disease caused by *M. avium, M. intracellulare,* and *M. abscessus*, BCG administration also appears to protect against leprosy (*M. leprae*) (for reviews, see [60]), and it may have some degree of efficacy against Buruli ulcer (*M. ulcerans*). A meta-analysis evaluating 28 clinical studies (observational trials, cohort studies, and case-control studies, but no RCTs) estimated that BCG confers 60% protection against human leprosy (95% CI = 0.51–0.7) [61]. Similar protective effects are observed for Buruli ulcer, where a cohort of 8856 Ugandan subjects were followed (half receiving BCG vaccination) during the 1970s, and BCG was found to be ≈47% protective against *M. ulcerans* infections [62, 63]. However, a significant challenge associated with this cross-protection is the limited duration of the immune response which is estimated to last only about 1 year [62, 63]. Despite early studies showing benefit, in a more recent case-control study comprising 401 positive cases with laboratory-confirmed Buruli ulcer and 826 controls (based on the presence or absence of a BCG scar) in Ghana, Togo, and Congo, no protective effect of BCG was found against the risk for developing Buruli ulcer [64]. Factors such as the rapidly waning protection and variable efficacy of different BCG strains may have contributed to the lack of observed efficacy in this study [64], and this requires further investigation.

4.2.3 Malignancies

The earliest connection between exposure to mycobacteria and cancer comes from a 1928 study at Johns Hopkins University where a two- to threefold lower incidence of malignant tumors was reported among inactive TB patients [65]. The concept gained significant credibility when Benacerraf and colleagues published a Nature paper in 1959 demonstrating that mice infected with BCG were more resistant to transplanted tumors than control animals [66]. Subsequently, human retrospective studies and RCTs evaluating the impact of BCG vaccination against several types of cancer began to appear and are discussed below.

4.2.3.1 Non-Muscle-Invasive Bladder Cancer

A total of 70,000 to 80,000 new cases of bladder cancer (BC) are reported annually in the United States [67], and among these cases, approximately 30% are categorized as muscle-invasive bladder cancer (MIBC), while the remaining 70% are non-muscle-invasive bladder cancer (NMIBC) [67]. NMIBC is commonly associated with a high rate of recurrences [67]. In a seminal work by Morales et al. in 1976 [68], it was discovered that the instillation of liquid suspensions of $\approx 1 \times 10^8$ CFU of BCG directly into the human bladder (intravesically) by catheterization had potent immunotherapeutic effects against pre-existing NMIBC. Indeed, for bladder cancer, the use of BCG as a first-line immunotherapy has now been clearly established [69–75]. Standard management involves an initial transurethral resection of bladder tumor (TURBT) [76], followed by repeated intravesical BCG treatments (typically 15 times over the course of 1 year), and under these conditions, BCG immunotherapy for high-risk NMIBC yields a 10-year progression-free survival rate of ~78% [77]. The mechanism of BCG action in NMIBC involves its entry into phagocytic cells in the bladder lumen, including tumor cells. This process triggers a proinflammatory response, turning a "cold" tumor (fibrotic lesions, high levels of immunosuppressive Treg cells, and myeloid-derived suppressor cells) into a "hot" one with increased infiltration of effector T-cells (reviewed in [75]). On the flip side, malignant cells develop mechanisms to evade immune recognition by upregulating cell surface molecules like programmed death ligand-1 (PD-L1). PD-L1, a ligand of the coinhibitory receptor PD1 on T-cells, has also been linked to resistance to BCG therapy [78]. Therefore, current research is evaluating a combinatorial therapy consisting of anti-PD-L1 and BCG immunotherapy for better treatment outcomes.

4.2.3.2 Melanoma

BCG has been studied for melanoma both as an intralesional therapy [79–81] and as a systemic therapy [82, 83]. For intralesional therapy, Tan et al. reported a pooled analysis from 15 prior studies and concluded that this form of BCG immunotherapy produced complete responses in 19% of patients with stage III disease and that it extended survival in 13% [84]. As a result of this and other studies, the use of intralesional BCG is recommended as a treatment option against inoperable stage III in-transit melanoma by the National Comprehensive Cancer Network (NCCN) guidelines [85]. When BCG is given systemically (typically intradermal vaccination) as an immune adjuvant alongside other therapies, it has been more difficult to discern an impact in melanoma outcomes [82, 83]. However, a correlative study on a cohort of 542 melanoma patients across seven countries in Europe and the Middle East evaluated melanoma survival in the context of vaccination histories with BCG and vaccinia (smallpox vaccine). The authors reported that BCG treatment resulted in a reduced melanoma hazard ratio (HR) of 0.69 (CI = 0.49–0.98) and that the recipients of both BCG and vaccinia had a melanoma HR of 0.41 (CI = 0.25–0.69) [86]. Similarly, a case control study of 1230 subjects found that vaccination with BCG plus vaccinia resulted in a lower risk of developing melanoma with an odds ratio (OR) of 0.44 (95% CI 0.26–0.72) [87].

4.2.3.3 Other Malignancies

A retrospective study published in 1970 indicated a 50% reduction in the incidence of acute leukemia with neonatal BCG vaccination in Quebec, Canada [88].

Additionally, a recent meta-analysis involving 12 studies examining the effect of BCG on childhood leukemia established significant protection with a 27% reduced risk [89]. One noteworthy study of BCG and cancer followed 2963 subjects for 60 years of follow-up after childhood BCG vaccination and found a significant reduction in the incidence of lung cancer with 18.2 cases per 100,000 person-years in BCG recipients as opposed to 45.4 in controls [90]. Similar beneficial effects of BCG have also been reported in prostate cancer [91, 92]. However, long-term studies using TB prevention cohorts which have assessed BCG against all-cause malignancies have yielded mixed results, with some studies showing no protective effects [93, 94]. Nevertheless, BCG continues to be studied as a cancer immunotherapy, and currently there are several active efforts to test it in combination immune checkpoint inhibitor monoclonal antibodies [95, 96] or to develop recombinant BCG strains with enhanced immunogenicity (reviewed in [97]).

4.2.4 Autoimmune Disorders

Human clinical trials as well as animal studies have suggested that BCG vaccination may prevent autoimmune disorders including Type I diabetes mellitus (T1D) [98] and multiple sclerosis (MS) [99–101]. T1D is a chronic autoimmune condition characterized by the destruction of pancreatic β cells by autoreactive CD8+ T-cells that primarily target islet cell autoantigens. Early research using the non-obese diabetic (NOD) murine model revealed that the BCG vaccination or injection of complete Freund's adjuvant (CFA; which includes killed BCG) can impede T1D disease progression and, remarkably, even cause disease reversal of advanced murine diabetes in certain models [102–106]. In agreement with these findings, CFA or BCG therapy prevented the destruction of pancreatic β cells in a small human trial [107]. Interestingly, neonatal BCG vaccination decreased the abundance of autoantibodies associated with T1D by ≈twofold ($p < 0.001$) [108] and was associated with a lower risk of T1D after age 30 [109]. Recent investigations have highlighted the potential antidiabetic effects of BCG administration in adults with long-standing T1D. These effects include a transient increase in C-peptide secretion (biomarker for insulin production), and the death of autoreactive T-cells, along with the expansion of Tregs (thought to be immune tolerizing) to restore the immune balance against autoreactive T-cells [110, 111]. A recent randomized 8-year-long human study at Massachusetts General Hospital involving 282 T1D patients found that BCG administration normalized the hemoglobin A1c levels [98]. At the same time, CD4+ T-cells from BCG-treated adults with T1D exhibited alterations in chromatin topology and gene expression, consistent with enhanced Treg activity [98]. In contrast to much of the existing BCG literature where BCG has proinflammatory effects, these findings suggest that BCG may also have an immunotolerizing effect, enhancing the Treg function.

4.2.5 Allergic Diseases

BCG has also been evaluated in the context of allergic and atopic conditions including allergic asthma, eczema/atopic dermatitis, and allergic rhinoconjunctivitis. Since this class of diseases is associated with increased Th2 immune responses [112], and mycobacteria including BCG are known to be Th1-polarizing [112, 113], BCG immunization early in life may shift host immunity away from a Th2-allergic pathway. Indeed, protective effects of BCG have been reported against atopic skin reactions [114–116] and allergic reactive airway disease/asthma [117, 118]. A meta-analysis involving 23 human studies estimated a 14% reduction in asthma occurrences among BCG recipients [119]. However, it must be noted that a number of these analyses were retrospective and reliant upon the presence of a BCG scar (which can be misleading). In addition, other studies have failed to detect the protective benefits of BCG against allergic disorders (discussed in [120]).

4.2.6 Dementia

Five clinical studies have evaluated BCG exposure and the risk of Alzheimer's or Parkinson's dementia and found a 20–75% reduction in the incidence of dementia in BCG recipients [121–125]. All of these studies were performed in bladder cancer patients who were typically beyond their fifth decade of life and received multiple intravesical instillations of BCG. A meta-analysis of these five studies calculated the protective effect to be a risk reduction of 45% [126]. At least three murine studies using APP/PS1 mice which are genetically predisposed to develop β-amyloid brain lesions have shown that BCG reduces disease progression in this model [127–129]. However, a clear mechanism of action for such BCG-mediated protection against dementia has not been established.

4.3 Immunological Responses by the Host to BCG Vaccination

Vaccination with live BCG, injected intradermally, is widely given to newborns for TB prevention, either as a national policy for all or special groups [7]. Studies show that the immunological effects post-vaccination are evident within days to weeks and can be sustained for years; this implies that the downstream signaling mechanisms post-BCG administration are both fast-acting and long-lasting [20, 130]. The immune response triggered by BCG is initiated at the site of inoculation, where the myeloid cells, including tissue-resident macrophages, neutrophils, and dendritic cells (DCs), first encounter the bacillus (reviewed in [131]). Later on, lymphoid cells receive antigen-specific activation signals from the myeloid cells.

4.3.1 Myeloid Cells

Immunologic recognition of BCG is mediated by the interaction of pattern recognition receptors (PRRs) on immune cells with pathogen-associated molecular patterns (PAMPs) such as peptidoglycan, arabinogalactan, and mycolic acids which comprise the mycobacterial outer envelope of the bacteria. For example, Toll-like receptor-2 (TLR2) recognizes mycobacterial cell wall lipoglycans known as lipomannan (LM) and lipoarabinomannan (LAM), and TLR4-signaling is triggered by mycobacterial heat shock proteins and glycoproteins [132–136]. Other PRRs that are implicated in BCG recognition and phagocytosis are complement receptors CR3 and CR4, C-type lectin family receptors such as the mannose receptor (MR), and the DC-specific ICAM-3 grabbing nonintegrin (DC-SIGN, CD209) which recognizes manLAM (mannose-capped LAM) [137–139]. Once BCG has been phagocytosed and degraded by the macrophages and DCs, a specific component of the cell wall (N-glycolyl muramyl dipeptide; MDP) activates the cytosolic PRR known as nucleotide-binding oligomerization domain-like receptor-2 (NOD-2), and the released DNA (CpG DNA) triggers the activation of cytosolic TLR9 [26, 140]. Such PRR-mediated interactions stimulate the maturation of macrophages and DCs, elevate the expression of cell surface markers of activation (CD11b, CD14, TLR4, MR), and promote the secretion of proinflammatory cytokines. In addition to this, increased expression and abundance of costimulatory molecules (MHC II, CD40, CD44, CD80, CD83, and CD86) on dendritic cells, and the enhanced production of proinflammatory cytokines (IL-1β, TNF-α, IL-6, IL-12), and chemokines (MCP-1, IL-8, MIP-1α, EGF, PDGF) by myeloid cells are also documented. This inflammatory milieu leads to the recruitment of additional macrophages, DCs, and neutrophils and provides maturation signals to them [131, 141–144].

4.3.2 Lymphoid Cells

The activation of the adaptive T- and B-cell responses follows traditional, established pathways with multiple recent studies adding to our understanding of BCG-mediated engagement of lymphoid cells (reviewed in [131]). Antigen-presenting macrophages and DCs migrate to nearby secondary lymphoid tissue or the spleen where they present BCG-specific peptides on MHC molecules to prime the resident T-cells. This is accompanied by the release of TNF-α, IL-6, and IL-12 by antigen presenting cells (APCs), and it results in the activation of both CD4+ helper (Th) and CD8+ cytotoxic T-cells [145–149]. The Th cells then differentiate mainly into Th1 cells (IFN-γ, TNF-α, and IL-2-secreting) [150] and Th17 cells (IL-17A-secreting) [145]. To a lesser extent, other subsets such as Th2 (IL-4+, IL-5+, IL-10 + -secreting) [151, 152], Treg [153, 154], CD1-restricted T-cells [155], innate-like MR1 (nonclassical MHC-1b)-restricted CD8+ T-cells (MAIT cells) [156], and polyfunctional T-cells (TNFα, IFNγ, IL-17A, and IL-2-secreting) [157–159] are also detected post-BCG vaccination. Mycobacteria-specific CD8+ T-cells proliferate in the peripheral blood where they secrete IFN-γ and express granzymes and perforins [160, 161]. In the later phases of the immune response (months after vaccination), BCG-specific CD4+, CD8+ T-cells [162, 163], and γδ T-cells [164] transition to a memory phenotype, secreting IFN-γ and contributing to a robust lymphoproliferative response to TB antigens. Between 4 and 8 weeks post-BCG vaccination, a B-cell response induces IgG production [165] and the development of long-lived memory B-cells [166]. These IgG molecules enhance phagocytosis and inhibit intracellular bacterial growth by opsonizing BCG [165]. Additionally, secreted antibodies complexed with the bacteria lead to enhanced antigen processing and presentation by APCs to CD4+ T-cells [167, 168]. Consequently, there is an increase in CD8+ T-cell activation and cytotoxic responses against live mycobacteria.

It is noteworthy that the antibody response varies depending on the route of administration of the BCG vaccine in both humans and preclinical animal models [169, 170]. Mucosal BCG vaccination via the intranasal or intrabronchial route (an experimental route studied in clinical research but not approved for general use) generates airway-resident memory T-cells [171], and giving BCG intranasally has been shown to result in CD4+ IL-17A+ T-cells as well as IgA in bronchoalveolar lavage (BAL) fluid [172]. While subcutaneous BCG enhances blood IgG, there is evidence that stimulating an IgA response via mucosal administration of BCG may provide better protection against respiratory infection with *Mtb* [172, 173]. B-cells also have a regulatory role during BCG vaccination, influencing IL-17 responses and impacting Th1 immune responses. Recent research has uncovered a non-antibody-mediated role of B-cells, specifically through their stimulation of T follicular helper cells (TFH). These CD4+ T-cells, located near B-cell follicles, play an important role in selecting and supporting B-cells, guiding their transformation into plasma cells and memory B-cells [174, 175]. Notably, TFH cells have been identified as significant contributors to BCG-mediated immunity as demonstrated by the studies of the recombinant BCG vaccine known as VPM1002 (BCG *ΔureC::hly* vaccine), which is currently in Phase 3 clinical trials. In animal models, VPM1002 and the closely related derivatives offer enhanced TB protection which correlates with the increased levels of central memory T-cells and TFH cells [176, 177].

4.4 Molecular Mechanisms Underlying BCG-Induced Heterologous Immunity

Traditionally, vaccines are developed to create specific immunity against target pathogens through the activation of adaptive immune responses involving T-cells and B-cells, with adjuvants playing a role in enhancing these responses (Fig. 4.2a). However, BCG vaccination, as discussed in earlier sections, not only confers protection against its target pathogen *Mtb* but also may protect against unrelated pathogens and noninfectious diseases. Mechanistically, this phenomenon seems to be driven by newly defined processes of setpoint elevation among cells traditionally considered part of the innate immune system or "trained innate immunity". These setpoint elevations among innate immune cells such as myeloid cells may also lead to enhanced functional levels among adaptive immune cells such as lymphoid cells.

4.5 Trained Immunity or the Innate Immune Memory

The immune system comprises innate and adaptive components that work together to combat microbial infections and establish long-lasting immunity. While adaptive immunity responds to specific immunogens (Fig. 4.2a), taking days to weeks for an efficient humoral and cellular response that also establishes immunologic memory, innate immunity provides rapid, preprogrammed responses to various microbial PAMPs without forming immunologic memory. However, recent evidence challenges this paradigm and suggests the innate arm also exhibits "memory" characteristics (Fig. 4.2b). Innate immune memory, also known as "trained immunity (TI)" [178, 179], involves long-term changes in innate immune cells resulting in an enhanced functional of antimicrobial responses which include cytokine/chemokine production, respiratory burst, phagocytosis, and antigen presentation. Beyond immune cells, nonimmune cells like endothelial or epithelial cells have also been identified to display trained immune phenotypes [180–182]. While adaptive memory relies on gene recombination and clonal expansion within T- and B-cells, TI uses different mechanisms to establish memory as described below [178, 179].

TI has been described following exposure to numerous antigenic stimuli or live pathogens themselves; these include fungal-derived β-glucan, peptidoglycan-derived muramyl dipeptide, or live *C. albicans*; however, live BCG is one of the best-studied stimulators of trained immunity [183]. For example, BCG-vaccinated mice can be shown to resist a lethal injection with *C. albicans,* and the effect is seen not only in wild-type mice but also in SCID (lacking both functional T- and B-cells) or NSG mice (lacking T, B, NK cells) [184]. These observations underscore the existence of a "memory"-equipped immune response that is independent of lymphocytes. Beyond lethal challenge studies in animal models, TI can be demonstrated readily in BCG-vaccinated versus nonvaccinated human subjects by subjecting peripheral blood mononuclear cells (PBMCs) to a heterologous antigen and then measuring cytokine responses. For example, a study in Guinea Bissau revealed that infants who received the BCG vaccine at birth exhibited heightened production of cytokines, including IL-1β, IL-6, TNF-α, and IFN-γ, in response to stimulation with the unrelated immunogen PMA (phorbol 12-myristate 13-acetate) or Pam3CSK4 (a synthetic triacylated lipopeptide and a TLR2/TLR1 agonist) [185]. Similarly, increased secretion of IL-1β, TNF-α, and IFN-γ was detected in monocytes from BCG-vaccinated healthy adults after stimulation with *S. aureus* or *C. albicans* [26, 130].

The mechanisms underlying TI may be classified based on the location: (1) "central TI" where bone marrow precursor cells exhibit memory or (2) "peripheral TI" where effector cells in tissues or circulation including macrophages, monocytes, DCs, Natural Killer (NK) cells, neutrophils, and innate lymphoid cells (ILCs) show immune memory (reviewed in [183]). Innate immune memory, lasting several months to a year, has a shorter duration to adaptive immune memory (the entire human lifespan in some cases), and it is influenced by factors such as the route of vaccine administration [186], genetics [187], host microbiome [188], age [189], sex [190], and other environmental factors.

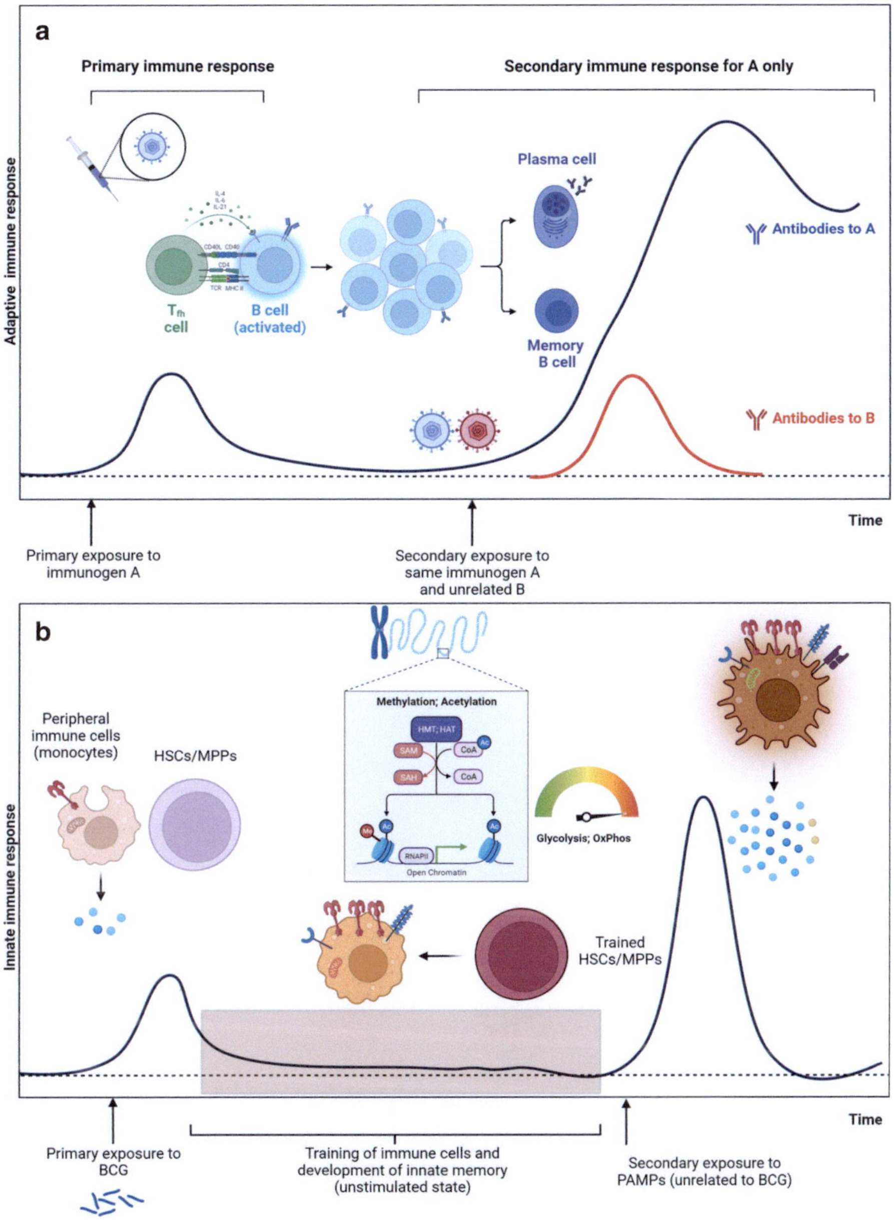

Fig. 4.2 BCG-induced trained innate immunity is different from adaptive immune memory. (**a**) Adaptive immune memory leads to specific protection against a target immunogen by producing antibodies and long-lived memory lymphocytes. (**b**) Innate immune memory contributes to unspecific protection provided by BCG against unrelated pathogens by an immunological process termed "trained immunity". Trained immunity results in functional reprogramming of innate immune cells that lead to enhanced innate immune responses (cytokines secretion, microbial killing, increased surface activation markers, and PRRs) upon secondary exposure to infections caused by pathogens after cells return to a nonactivated state. (HAT histone acetyltransferase, HMT histone methyltransferase, HSCs hematopoietic stem cells, MPPs multipotent progenitor cells, SAM S-adenosylmethionine, OxPhos oxidative phosphorylation)

4.5.1 Mechanisms of Trained Innate Immunity: Epigenetic Reprogramming

The molecular mechanisms underlying the induction of TI by BCG vaccination are not understood comprehensively. However, epigenetic reprogramming via alterations in chromatin topology that include covalent modifications of DNA itself (methylation) and/or nucleic acid-binding histones (methylation and acetylation) appears to play a causal role (Fig. 4.3). The differentiation of monocytes into macrophages requires large-scale epigenetic and transcriptional changes that define their heightened immune activity. For example, macrophage activity against a pathogen was thought to be determined by their primed epigenetic mark H3K4me1 (histone H3, lysine-4, monomethylation) or activation mark H3K27ac (histone H3, Lysine-27, acetylation) which correspond to chromatin states at the gene-enhancer regions in the chromosome marked by the PU.1 transcription factor [191]. However,

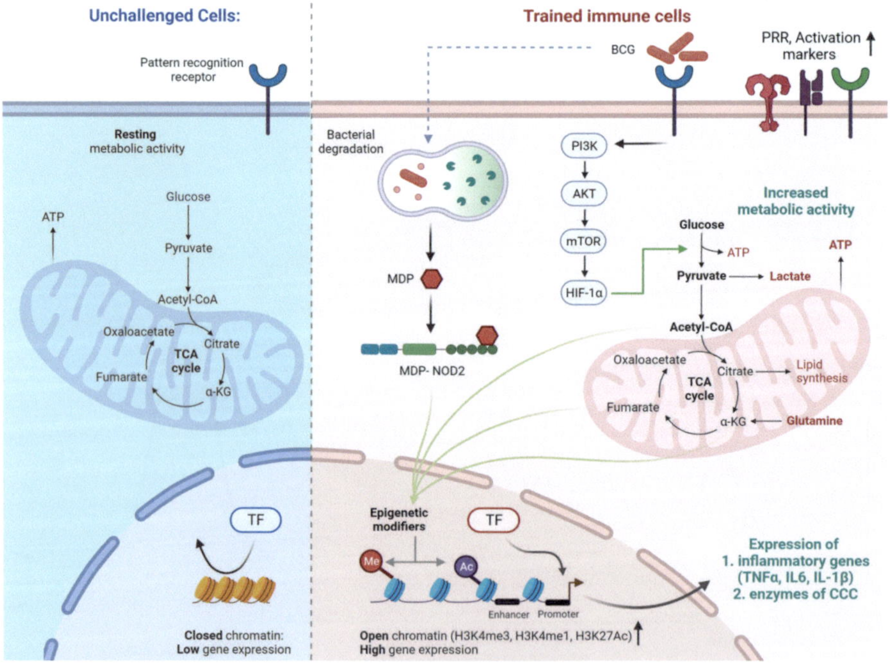

Fig. 4.3 Metabolic changes, epigenetic modification, and their crosstalk underlie the BCG-induced trained immunity or innate memory. Untrained immune cells exhibit basal metabolic fluxes and chromatin topology. On the other hand, BCG-trained immune cells undergo significant alterations in their chromatin architecture and metabolic rate. Glycolysis, oxidative phosphorylation, and glutaminolysis are enhanced in a PI3K/AKT-dependent manner. The TCA cycle intermediates can enhance the activity of several methyltransferases and acetyltransferases, leading to more open chromatin topology by methylation or acetylation of histones (H3K4me3, H3K4me1, and H3K27Ac) and increased expression of several inflammatory genes. Epigenetic reprogramming is also induced by MDP-NOD2 signaling in innate immune cells. (CCC central carbon metabolism)

a study by Ostuni et al. discovered "latent" enhancers in mouse macrophages exposed to LPS (lipopolysaccharide). These enhancers accumulate H3K27ac at distal gene regions not initially marked by H3K4me1 [192], and they lose the H3K27ac mark after stimulus removal. At the same time, these genetic elements retain the longer half-life H3K4me1 mark, and upon re-exposure to LPS, faster H3K27ac accumulation occurs. This novel finding suggests that innate immune cells may gain new distal gene regulatory chromatin elements upon exposure to environmental signals shaping their phenotype and response to future exposure [192]. In agreement with this, treatment of human monocytes with an inhibitor of histone methyltransferases (5′-methyl-thioadenosine or MTA) results in a reduced training effect manifested by decreased secretion of IL-6 and TNF-α from MTA-treated and primed human monocytes after induction by *S. cerevisiae* and its chitin [193]. This observation implies that the elicited TI response was dependent on histone methylation.

4.5.1.1 Activating Histone Modifications

BCG-mediated TI is associated with increases in activating epigenetic changes, as outlined in Fig. 4.3 [194–196]. Following BCG vaccination, peripheral blood monocytes display increased H3K4me3 and H3K27ac histone modifications, both of which are activating histone marks associated with increased transcriptional accessibility. These epigenetic changes are specifically localized in the promoters of genes encoding proinflammatory cytokines (IL-6, TNF-α), PRRs (TLRs, C-type lectin receptors, NOD-like receptors, and RIG-I-helicases), chemokine receptors (CCR2 and CXCR4), and costimulatory and/or signaling molecules (CD43, CD14, and CD40) [32, 197]. Elevated expression levels of TLRs, C-type lectin receptors, NOD-like receptors, and chemokine receptors lead to stimulation of T-cells, angiogenesis, and wound healing. Importantly, this response appears to be highly dependent on the NOD2 receptor, Rip2 (receptor-interacting protein kinase 2) [26], and autophagy-related proteins (*ATG2B and ATG5*) [187]. In contrast to monocytes from healthy individuals, BCG-trained monocytes derived from an individual lacking NOD2 were unable to secrete proinflammatory cytokines (IL-6 and TNF-α) upon stimulation with LPS [26]. Similarly, genetic polymorphisms in the autophagy protein ATG2B are associated with nonresponsiveness to BCG intravesical instillation for NMIBC patients [187].

4.5.1.2 Repressive Histone Modifications

BCG training also suppresses repressive histone marks associated with decreased transcriptional accessibility such as H3K9me3. And, like the aforementioned activating marks, the reduced repressive marks appear in the promoter regions of proinflammatory genes such as *il1β, il6, and tnfα* [32, 198]. The mechanism by which these activating (e.g., H3K4me3) and repressive (e.g., H3K9me3) marks are directed to specific gene promoters remains incompletely understood. However, initial data suggest that BCG and/or β-glucan training leads to the enhanced expression of a class of immune-priming long noncoding RNA (lncRNAs) or IPLs such as UMLILO (upstream master LncRNA of the inflammatory chemokine locus) and IPL-IL1 (IPL targeting interleukin-1) [199]. These IPLs are believed to engage with

SAM-dependent methyltransferases to direct H3K4me3 epigenetic priming to key target genes.

Apart from monocytes and macrophages, neutrophils [200] also exhibit trained immunological memory associated with H3K4me3 modification after BCG vaccination and subsequent heterologous restimulation. Specifically, neutrophils display increased activation, ROS production, and cytokine secretion [200]. Notably, when neutrophils derived from BCG-vaccinated human study participants were categorized into high and low responders based on their killing capacity (of *C. albicans*), IPL expression correlated strongly with the responder status [199, 200]. Additionally, innate lymphoid cells (ILCs), especially natural killer (NK) cells, from BCG-vaccinated individuals also show an elevated cytokine response upon heterologous stimulation [184].

4.5.1.3 Methylation of DNA

Recent studies suggest that DNA methylation patterns may differentiate individuals into BCG "responders" and "nonresponders". Responders—those showing enhanced containment of *Mtb* replication post-BCG vaccination—exhibited widespread loss of DNA methylation in gene promoters associated with immune pathways that were absent in nonresponders [195]. Subsequent studies identified 43 genes with distinct methylation patterns in BCG-naive responders [201]. As these studies focused on BCG-mediated *Mtb* killing and not the effects of secondary stimulation, it remains unclear whether similar DNA methylation patterns govern trained immunity responses and therefore needs to be investigated.

4.5.2 Mechanisms of Trained Innate Immunity: Metabolic Reprogramming

Myeloid cells that have undergone BCG-mediated TI demonstrate a unique metabolic profile with heightened glycolysis and oxidative phosphorylation (OxPhos) [198, 202] (Fig. 4.3). The mechanism is believed to require BCG engagement with the dectin-1 receptor which then initiates a signaling cascade with the PI3K (phosphoinositide 3 kinase)-AKT-mTOR (mammalian target of rapamycin)-HIF-1α (hypoxia-inducible factor-1α) pathway [198]. Activation of this pathway is associated with several metabolic changes: (1) a shift toward aerobic glycolysis and (2) increased glutaminolysis to replenish tricarboxylic acid cycle substrates. Increased glycolysis in BCG-trained monocytes has been shown to correlate with a significant increase in H3K4me3 modifications in the promoter regions of mTOR, hexokinase (HK2), and phosphofructokinase (PFKP). Similarly, increased glutaminolysis is associated with a decrease in the H3K9me3 repressive mark at the promoters of glutaminase (GLS) and glutamate dehydrogenase (GLUD) [198]. Significantly, this metabolic reprogramming increases the production of metabolites that can potentially act as cofactors for chromatin modifier enzymes (acetyltransferases and methyltransferases) [203] (Fig. 4.3). Indeed, pharmacological inhibition of BCG training with metabolic inhibitors targeting glutamine metabolism (e.g., BPTES) or mTOR/

glycolysis (e.g., rapamycin/metformin) reversed the H3K4me3 modification at the *il6* and/or *tnfα* promoters to the baseline status [198, 202], while myeloid-specific deletion of the phosphatase SHIP-1 (which is a PI3K/AKT inhibitor) enhanced the TI phenotype [204]. Therefore, shifts in key metabolite levels in BCG-trained monocytes likely represent a mechanism which links the metabolic and epigenetic programs during TI.

While the glycolytic shift in BCG-primed monocytes has been shown to induce proinflammatory cytokines, a recent study with T1D patients revealed the immunotolerizing effects of BCG [98]. CD4+ T-cells from BCG-vaccinated adults with T1D displayed epigenetic changes in genes associated with Treg function such as *foxp3, tnfrsf18, il2ra, ikzf2, ikzf4,* and *ctla4*. This suggests that under certain conditions BCG may also mediate an enhancement in Treg generation and function to balance this autoimmune disorder [98, 205].

In addition to the above alterations of central carbon metabolism, growing evidence suggests a critical role in the metabolism of lipid molecules in BCG-mediated TI [206–208]. Mass spectrometry-based metabolomic analysis of blood samples from BCG-vaccinated infants in Guinea-Bissau and Gambia revealed elevated plasma levels of free fatty acids with significant changes—both increased and decreased levels—of glycerophospholipids (GPLs), phospholipids, and sphingolipids. Importantly, changes in lipid concentrations strongly correlated with the levels of the proinflammatory cytokines IL-6, TNFα, and IFNγ. These data suggest that alteration in GPLs may contribute to BCG immunogenicity [207].

Additionally, monocytes with BCG-mediated TI phenotype exhibited increased biosynthesis of prostaglandins, eicosanoids, and leukotrienes. These lipid mediators which are the oxidation products of polyunsaturated fatty acids (PUFA) and further modified by cyclooxygenases (COX), lipoxygenases (LOX), and epoxygenases (CP450 enzymes) may play important roles in immune cell acquisition of TI [206]. Indeed, pharmacological inhibition of polyunsaturated fatty acid desaturase 2 (FADS2; short-chain PUFA desaturase required for the synthesis of PUFA) led to decreased production of TNF-α and IL-6 in BCG-primed macrophages after LPS stimulation. Additionally, SNPs in the LOX pathway gene *lox12* as well as in *fads2* influenced the induction of trained immunity (TNF-α and IL-6 production) in healthy human volunteers after BCG vaccination [206]. In sum, these studies indicate that bioactive lipids contribute to the mechanistic basis of TI.

4.5.3 Heightened Immune Responsiveness Among T-Cells

Antigen cross-reactivity due to molecular mimicry may explain certain aspects of BCG-mediated PHEs. In this context, BCG has demonstrated the ability to trigger heterologous lymphocyte responses with heightened immune responses against unrelated infectious agents [209]. For instance, BCG-vaccinated mice subsequently challenged with vaccinia virus showed increased CD4+ T-cell-mediated IFN-γ production [210]. Similarly, cytokines associated with Th1 lymphocytes were found to be elevated in human BCG recipients [185, 211]. In addition, it has been shown that neonatal BCG vaccination in humans induces IFN-γ production primarily by γδ T-cells [212]. The activated γδ T-cell receptors (TCR) appear to recognize diverse, unrelated immunogens through spatially distinct complementarity-determining regions (CDR1–CDR3), allowing discrimination between nonclonal agonist selection elements and clone-specific ligands [213]. This γδ T-cell response involves the activation and expansion of both CD4+ and CD8+ memory cells [164, 214] which may be specific to nontargeted antigens or antigen-independent bystander cells [215, 216], and it is thought that these γδ T-cells may influence Th1 and Th17 responses to nonmycobacterial secondary infections. Indeed, in human volunteers, BCG vaccination resulted in nonspecific Th1 and Th17 responses for at least a year after vaccination [130]. In addition to this, neonatal BCG vaccination exhibited a heightened antibody response to the hepatitis B vaccine [211], and the pneumococcal conjugate vaccine [37] compared to the nonvaccinated controls, indicating heightened humoral response due to potential T-cell cross-reactivity.

4.5.4 Central and Peripheral Trained Immunity

TI was initially believed to operate exclusively through mature myeloid cells such as monocytes and DCs. However, since these mature myeloid cells have a short lifespan of approximately 5–7 days [217–219], the month-long durability of trained innate immune changes remained unexplained. Recent research has shed light on this issue by demonstrating that TI can be induced not only in blood monocytes and tissue-resident macrophages (peripheral TI) but also in the bone marrow progenitor cells (central TI). Intravenous BCG vaccination in mice induces IFN-γ-dependent reprogramming of hematopoietic stem cells (HSCs) and multipotent progenitor cells (MPP) (Fig. 4.2), resulting in enhanced myelopoiesis [220]. This reprogramming of HSCs is regulated by lineage-specific transcription factors and includes significant transcriptomic and epigenetic changes such as increased H3K27ac and H3K4me3 histone modifications near the genes for antimicrobial responses [220]. Interestingly, a study of adult BCG recipients revealed that intradermal BCG administration did not alter the rate of myelopoiesis at 90 days post-infection [221]. However, the same study detected clear imprints of persistent transcriptomic myeloid bias in human HSC-granulocyte activation and neutrophil-mediated immunity were the top deregulated pathways; the study also detected increased TI-associated secretion of cytokines and epigenetic modifications. Thus, TI signals from the bone marrow appear to be successfully transmitted to peripheral CD14+ monocytes [221]. Another study with subcutaneous neonatal BCG vaccination observed the rapid generation of peripheral neutrophils within 3 days—so-called emergency granulopoiesis (EG)—in a G-CSF (granulocyte colony-stimulating factor)-dependent manner [222]. The same study found that EG was instrumental in conferring protection against neonatal sepsis [222]. Interestingly, emergency granulopoiesis (early response within 3 days) and myelopoiesis (delayed; > 3 months) have been hypothesized to be a continuum of the same effect cascade that may mediate central TI [223]. In sum, several studies now indicate that the route of BCG administration determines the extent of the development of TI in HSCs and that intravenous BCG may more profoundly alter immune set-points in the myeloid precursors in the marrow (reviewed in [223]).

4.6 Conclusions and Future Directions

Over the past century, BCG vaccination studies in humans and animals have produced substantial evidence for protective heterologous effects (PHE) mediated by BCG and have contributed to the emergence of the "trained innate immunity" concept. This chapter presents evidence supporting the idea that BCG vaccination induces protective heterologous effects against immune disorders and unrelated infections, particularly those of viral origin. Recent findings suggest that BCG vaccination may serve as both a heterologous protective vaccine and also an adjuvant that boosts the activity of disease-specific vaccines. Despite recent large clinical trials generating excitement, crucial questions persist regarding the precise identity of immune cells involved, the duration of BCG-induced TI specific to certain diseases, and the underlying molecular mechanisms. The unexpected lack of infection prevention in the Danish Calmette Study evaluating BCG unless there was maternal BCG vaccination has raised several questions and prompted considerations of geographical differences, exposure variations, environmental conditions, and genetic diversity in BCG-mediated PHEs. The fact that specific protection was observed only in children of BCG-vaccinated mothers raises the fascinating question of whether trained innate immunity is epigenetically transmitted via the germline. Future work will undoubtedly focus on refining the vaccine design to enhance TI, understanding the duration and modulating factors of BCG-induced cross-immune protection, and exploring variations in inducing TI among populations. Additionally, a key knowledge gap to establish biomarkers for BCG efficacy needs to be addressed. Ongoing clinical trials and research on next-generation BCG candidates as well as the potential applications of TI as a therapy against chronic diseases such as inflammatory bowel disease, gout, allergy, atherosclerosis, and dementia underscore the dynamic landscape of BCG and innate trained immunity research.

Acknowledgments The authors gratefully acknowledge the support of NIAID, NIH grants AI 167750, 155602, 155346, and 152688. Images were made with BioRender software. The authors acknowledge the use of the BioRender commercial software package in the preparation of the figures.

Competing Interests The author(s) has no competing interests to declare that are relevant to the content of this manuscript.

Ethics Approval The author(s) declares that this manuscript does not include primary research with human participants.

References

1. Brosch R, Gordon SV, Pym A, Eiglmeier K, Garnier T, Cole ST. Comparative genomics of the mycobacteria. Int J Med Microbiol. 2000;290:143–52.
2. Mangtani P, Abubakar I, Ariti C, et al. Protection by BCG vaccine against tuberculosis: a systematic review of randomized controlled trials. Clin Infect Dis. 2014;58:470–80.
3. Trunz BB, Fine P, Dye C. Effect of BCG vaccination on childhood tuberculous meningitis and miliary tuberculosis worldwide: a meta-analysis and assessment of cost-effectiveness. Lancet. 2006;367:1173–80.
4. Colditz GA, Brewer TF, Berkey CS, Wilson ME, Burdick E, Fineberg HV, Mosteller F. Efficacy of BCG vaccine in the prevention of tuberculosis. Meta-analysis of the published literature. JAMA. 1994;271:698–702.
5. Roy A, Eisenhut M, Harris RJ, et al. Effect of BCG vaccination against Mycobacterium tuberculosis infection in children: systematic review and meta-analysis. BMJ. 2014;349:g4643.
6. World Health Organization (WHO) (2015/2016). Implementing the end TB strategy: the essentials. WHO reference number: WHO/HTM/TB/2015.31.
7. Zwerling A, Behr MA, Verma A, Brewer TF, Menzies D, Pai M. The BCG World Atlas: a database of global BCG vaccination policies and practices. PLoS Med. 2011;8:e1001012.
8. Singh AK, Netea MG, Bishai WR. BCG turns 100: its nontraditional uses against viruses, cancer, and immunologic diseases. J Clin Invest. 2021;131(11):e148291.
9. World Health Organization (WHO) (2023). Global tuberculosis report 2023. Geneva: World Health Organization; 2023. Licence: CC BY-NC-SA 3.0 IGO.
10. Houben RMGJ, Dodd PJ. The global burden of latent tuberculosis infection: a re-estimation using mathematical modelling. PLoS Med. 2016;13:e1002152.
11. Schaltz-Buchholzer F, Kjær Sørensen M, Benn CS, Aaby P. The introduction of BCG vaccination to neonates in Northern Sweden, 1927-31: re-analysis of historical data to understand the lower mortality among BCG-vaccinated children. Vaccine. 2022;40:1516–24.
12. Netea MG, van Crevel R. BCG-induced protection: effects on innate immune memory. Semin Immunol. 2014;26:512–7.
13. Higgins JPT, Soares-Weiser K, López-López JA, Kakourou A, Chaplin K, Christensen H, Martin NK, Sterne JAC, Reingold AL. Association of BCG, DTP, and measles containing vaccines with childhood mortality: systematic review. BMJ. 2016;355:i5170.
14. Ferguson R, Simes A. BCG vaccination of Indian infants in Saskatchewan: a study carried out with financial assistance from the National Research Council of Canada. Tubercle. 1949;30:5–11.
15. Aronson JD. Protective vaccination against tuberculosis with special reference to BCG vaccination. Am Rev Tuberc. 1948;58:255–81.
16. Haahr S, Michelsen SW, Andersson M, Bjorn-Mortensen K, Soborg B, Wohlfahrt J, Melbye M, Koch A. Non-specific effects of BCG vaccination on morbidity among children in Greenland: a population-based cohort study. Int J Epidemiol. 2016;45:2122–30.
17. De Castro MJ, Pardo-Seco J, Martinón-Torres F. Nonspecific (heterologous) protection of neonatal BCG vaccination against hospitalization due to respiratory infection and sepsis. Clin Infect Dis. 2015;60:1611–9.
18. Benn CS, Sørup S. Commentary: BCG has no beneficial non-specific effects on Greenland. An answer to the wrong question? Int J Epidemiol. 2016;45:2131–3.
19. Kjærgaard J, Birk NM, Nissen TN, et al. Nonspecific effect of BCG vaccination at birth on early childhood infections: a randomized, clinical multicenter trial. Pediatr Res. 2016;80:681–5.
20. Freyne B, Donath S, Germano S, et al. Neonatal BCG vaccination influences cytokine responses to toll-like receptor ligands and heterologous antigens. J Infect Dis. 2018;217:1798–808.
21. Giamarellos-Bourboulis EJ, Tsilika M, Moorlag S, et al. Activate: randomized clinical trial of BCG vaccination against infection in the elderly. Cell. 2020;183:315–323.e9.

22. Moorlag SJCFM, Taks E, Ten Doesschate T, et al. Efficacy of BCG vaccination against respiratory tract infections in older adults during the coronavirus disease 2019 pandemic. Clin Infect Dis. 2022;75:e938–46.
23. Nakamura M, Cross WR. Susceptibility of rabbits immunized with Mycobacterium bovis (BCG) or Mycobacterium phlei to Shigella Keratoconjunctivitis. Infect Immun. 1972;6:1025–30.
24. Mackaness GB. The immunological basis of acquired cellular resistance. J Exp Med. 1964;120:105–20.
25. Mackaness GB. The influence of immunologically committed lymphoid cells on macrophage activity in vivo. J Exp Med. 1969;129:973–92.
26. Kleinnijenhuis J, Quintin J, Preijers F, et al. Bacille Calmette-Guerin induces NOD2-dependent nonspecific protection from reinfection via epigenetic reprogramming of monocytes. Proc Natl Acad Sci USA. 2012;109:17537–42.
27. Parra M, Liu X, Derrick SC, Yang A, Tian J, Kolibab K, Kumar S, Morris SL. Molecular analysis of non-specific protection against murine malaria induced by BCG vaccination. PLoS One. 2013;8:e66115.
28. Freyne B, Marchant A, Curtis N. BCG-associated heterologous immunity, a historical perspective: intervention studies in animal models of infectious diseases. Trans R Soc Trop Med Hyg. 2015;109:52–61.
29. Stensballe LG, Nante E, Jensen IP, Kofoed P-E, Poulsen A, Jensen H, Newport M, Marchant A, Aaby P. Acute lower respiratory tract infections and respiratory syncytial virus in infants in Guinea-Bissau: a beneficial effect of BCG vaccination for girls community based case-control study. Vaccine. 2005;23:1251–7.
30. Hollm-Delgado MG, Stuart EA, Black RE. Acute lower respiratory infection among Bacille Calmette-Guérin (BCG)–vaccinated children. Pediatrics. 2014;133:e73–81.
31. Pittet LF, Curtis N. Does bacillus Calmette-Guérin vaccine prevent herpes simplex virus recurrences? A systematic review. Rev Med Virol. 2021;31:1–9.
32. Arts RJW, Moorlag SJCFM, Novakovic B, et al. BCG vaccination protects against experimental viral infection in humans through the induction of cytokines associated with trained immunity. Cell Host Microbe. 2018;23:89–100.e5.
33. Salem A, Nofal A, Hosny D. Treatment of common and plane warts in children with topical viable Bacillus Calmette-Guerin. Pediatr Dermatol. 2013;30:60–3.
34. Podder I, Bhattacharya S, Mishra V, et al. Immunotherapy in viral warts with intradermal Bacillus Calmette-Guerin vaccine versus intradermal tuberculin purified protein derivative: a double-blind, randomized controlled trial comparing effectiveness and safety in a tertiary care center in Eastern India. Indian J Dermatol Venereol Leprol. 2017;83:411.
35. Daulatabad D, Pandhi D, Singal A. BCG vaccine for immunotherapy in warts: is it really safe in a tuberculosis endemic area? Dermatol Ther. 2016;29:168–72.
36. Leentjens J, Kox M, Stokman R, Gerretsen J, Diavatopoulos DA, van Crevel R, Rimmelzwaan GF, Pickkers P, Netea MG. BCG vaccination enhances the immunogenicity of subsequent influenza vaccination in healthy volunteers: a randomized, placebo-controlled pilot study. J Infect Dis. 2015;212:1930–8.
37. Ritz N, Mui M, Balloch A, Curtis N. Non-specific effect of Bacille Calmette-Guérin vaccine on the immune response to routine immunisations. Vaccine. 2013;31:3098–103.
38. O'Neill LAJ, Netea MG. BCG-induced trained immunity: can it offer protection against COVID-19? Nat Rev Immunol. 2020;20:335–7.
39. Moorlag SJCFM, Arts RJW, van Crevel R, Netea MG. Non-specific effects of BCG vaccine on viral infections. Clin Microbiol Infect. 2019;25:1473–8.
40. Taks EJM, Moorlag SJCFM, Netea MG, van der Meer JWM. Shifting the immune memory paradigm: trained immunity in viral infections. Annu Rev Virol. 2022;9:469–89.
41. de Bree LCJ, Marijnissen RJ, Kel JM, et al. Bacillus Calmette–Guérin-induced trained immunity is not protective for experimental influenza A/Anhui/1/2013 (H7N9) infection in mice. Front Immunol. 2018;9:869.

42. Kaufmann E, Khan N, Tran KA, et al. BCG vaccination provides protection against IAV but not SARS-CoV-2. Cell Rep. 2022;38:110502.
43. Berg MK, Yu Q, Salvador CE, Melani I, Kitayama S. Mandated Bacillus Calmette-Guérin (BCG) vaccination predicts flattened curves for the spread of COVID-19. Sci Adv. 2020;6:eabc1463.
44. Covián C, Retamal-Díaz A, Bueno SM, Kalergis AM. Could BCG vaccination induce protective trained immunity for SARS-CoV-2? Front Immunol. 2020;11:970.
45. Rivas MN, Ebinger JE, Wu M, Sun N, Braun J, Sobhani K, Van Eyk JE, Cheng S, Arditi M. BCG vaccination history associates with decreased SARS-CoV-2 seroprevalence across a diverse cohort of health care workers. J Clin Invest. 2021;131(2):e145157.
46. Lindestam Arlehamn CS, Sette A, Peters B. Lack of evidence for BCG vaccine protection from severe COVID-19. Proc Natl Acad Sci. 2020;117:25203–4.
47. Hamiel U, Kozer E, Youngster I. SARS-CoV-2 rates in BCG-vaccinated and unvaccinated young adults. JAMA. 2020;323:2340.
48. Hilligan KL, Namasivayam S, Clancy CS, et al. Intravenous administration of BCG protects mice against lethal SARS-CoV-2 challenge. J Exp Med. 2022;219(2):e20211862.
49. Singh AK, Wang R, Lombardo KA, et al. Intravenous BCG vaccination reduces SARS-CoV-2 severity and promotes extensive reprogramming of lung immune cells. iScience. 2023;26:107733.
50. Zhang B-Z, Shuai H, Gong H-R, et al. Bacillus Calmette-Guérin-induced trained immunity protects against SARS-CoV-2 challenge in K18-hACE2 mice. JCI Insight. 2022;7:e213800.
51. Pittet LF, Messina NL, Orsini F, et al. Randomized trial of BCG vaccine to protect against Covid-19 in health care workers. N Engl J Med. 2023;388:1582–96.
52. No authors listed. Hopes fizzle that a TB vaccine also fends off COVID. Nature. 2023;617:10.
53. Li J, Zhan L, Qin C. The double-sided effects of Mycobacterium Bovis bacillus Calmette-Guérin vaccine. NPJ Vaccines. 2021;6:14.
54. Netea MG, Ziogas A, Benn CS, et al. The role of trained immunity in COVID-19: lessons for the next pandemic. Cell Host Microbe. 2023;31:890–901.
55. Armstrong DT, Eisemann E, Parrish N. A brief update on mycobacterial taxonomy, 2020 to 2022. J Clin Microbiol. 2023;61(4):e0033122.
56. Ratnatunga CN, Lutzky VP, Kupz A, Doolan DL, Reid DW, Field M, Bell SC, Thomson RM, Miles JJ. The rise of non-tuberculosis mycobacterial lung disease. Front Immunol. 2020;11:507325.
57. Lacroix A, Piau C, Lanotte P, et al. Emergence of nontuberculous mycobacterial lymphadenitis in children after the discontinuation of mandatory Bacillus Calmette and GuÉrin immunization in France. Pediatr Infect Dis J. 2018;37:e257–60.
58. Kontturi A, Soini H, Ollgren J, Salo E. Increase in childhood nontuberculous mycobacterial infections after Bacille Calmette-Guérin coverage drop: a Nationwide, population-based retrospective study, Finland, 1995–2016. Clin Infect Dis. 2018;67:1256–61.
59. Zimmermann P, Finn A, Curtis N. Does BCG vaccination protect against nontuberculous mycobacterial infection? A systematic review and meta-analysis. J Infect Dis. 2018;218:679–87.
60. Ali L. Leprosy vaccines—a voyage unfinished. J Skin Sex Transmit Dis. 2021;3:40.
61. Merle CSC, Cunha SS, Rodrigues LC. BCG vaccination and leprosy protection: review of current evidence and status of BCG in leprosy control. Expert Rev Vaccines. 2010;9:209–22.
62. Smith PG, Revill WDL, Lukwago E, Rykushin YP. The protective effect of BCG against Mycobacterium ulcerans disease: a controlled trial in an endemic area of Uganda. Trans R Soc Trop Med Hyg. 1976;70:449–57.
63. The Uganda Buruli Group. BCG vaccination against Mycobacterium ulcerans infection (Buruli ulcer). First results of a trial in Uganda. Lancet. 1969;1:111–5.
64. Phillips RO, Phanzu DM, Beissner M, et al. Effectiveness of routine BCG vaccination on Buruli ulcer disease: a case-control study in the Democratic Republic of Congo, Ghana and Togo. PLoS Negl Trop Dis. 2015;9:e3457.

65. Pearl R. On the pathological relations between cancer and tuberculosis. Exp Biol Med. 1928;26:73–5.
66. Old LJ, Clarke DA, Benacerraf B. Effect of Bacillus Calmette-Guérin infection on transplanted Tumours in the mouse. Nature. 1959;184:291–2.
67. Matulewicz RS, Steinberg GD. Non-muscle-invasive bladder cancer: overview and contemporary treatment landscape of neoadjuvant chemoablative therapies. Rev Urol. 2020;22:43–51.
68. Morales A, Eidinger D, Bruce AW. Intracavitary Bacillus Calmette-Guerin in the treatment of superficial bladder tumors. J Urol. 1976;116:180–3.
69. Larsen ES, Joensen UN, Poulsen AM, Goletti D, Johansen IS. Bacillus Calmette-Guérin immunotherapy for bladder cancer: a review of immunological aspects, clinical effects and BCG infections. APMIS. 2020;128:92–103.
70. Redelman-Sidi G, Glickman MS, Bochner BH. The mechanism of action of BCG therapy for bladder cancer – a current perspective. Nat Rev Urol. 2014;11:153–62.
71. Sylvester RJ, van der Meijden APM, Lamm DL. Intravesical Bacillus Calmette-Guerin reduces the risk of progression in patients with superficial bladder cancer: a meta-analysis of the published results of randomized clinical trials. J Urol. 2002;168:1964–70.
72. Lobo N, Brooks NA, Zlotta AR, et al. 100 years of Bacillus Calmette–Guérin immunotherapy: from cattle to COVID-19. Nat Rev Urol. 2021;18:611–22.
73. van Puffelen JH, Keating ST, Oosterwijk E, van der Heijden AG, Netea MG, Joosten LAB, Vermeulen SH. Trained immunity as a molecular mechanism for BCG immunotherapy in bladder cancer. Nat Rev Urol. 2020;17:513–25.
74. Lamm DL, Morales A. A BCG success story: from prevention of tuberculosis to optimal bladder cancer treatment. Vaccine. 2021;39:7308–18.
75. Pettenati C, Ingersoll MA. Mechanisms of BCG immunotherapy and its outlook for bladder cancer. Nat Rev Urol. 2018;15:615–25.
76. Jiang S, Redelman-Sidi G. BCG in bladder cancer immunotherapy. Cancers (Basel). 2022;14:3073.
77. Williams SB, Howard LE, Foster ML, Klaassen Z, Sieluk J, De Hoedt AM, Freedland SJ. Estimated costs and long-term outcomes of patients with high-risk non–muscle-invasive bladder cancer treated with Bacillus Calmette-Guérin in the veterans affairs health system. JAMA Netw Open. 2021;4:e213800.
78. Inman BA, Sebo TJ, Frigola X, Dong H, Bergstralh EJ, Frank I, Fradet Y, Lacombe L, Kwon ED. PD-L1 (B7-H1) expression by urothelial carcinoma of the bladder and BCG-induced granulomata: associations with localized stage progression. Cancer. 2007;109:1499–505.
79. Seigler HF, Shingleton WW, Metzgar RS, Buckley CE, Bergoc PM, Miller DS, Fetter BF, Phaup MB. Non-specific and specific immunotherapy in patients with melanoma. Surgery. 1972;72:162–74.
80. Nathanson L. Regression of intradermal malignant melanoma after intralesional injection of Mycobacterium bovis strain BCG. Cancer Chemother Rep. 1972;56:659–65.
81. Morton DL, Eilber FR, Joseph WL, Wood WC, Trahan E, Ketcham AS. Immunological factors in human sarcomas and melanomas: a rational basis for immunotherapy. Ann Surg. 1970;172:740–9.
82. Benitez MLR, Bender CB, Oliveira TL, Schachtschneider KM, Collares T, Seixas FK. Mycobacterium bovis BCG in metastatic melanoma therapy. Appl Microbiol Biotechnol. 2019;103:7903–16.
83. Kremenovic M, Schenk M, Lee DJ. Clinical and molecular insights into BCG immunotherapy for melanoma. J Intern Med. 2020;288:625–40.
84. Tan JK, Ho VC. Pooled analysis of the efficacy of Bacille Calmette-Guerin (BCG) immunotherapy in malignant melanoma. J Dermatol Surg Oncol. 1993;19:985–90.
85. Coit DG, Thompson JA, Albertini MR, et al. Cutaneous melanoma, version 2.2019, NCCN clinical practice guidelines in oncology. J Natl Compr Cancer Netw. 2019;17:367–402.
86. Kölmel KF, Grange JM, Krone B, et al. Prior immunisation of patients with malignant melanoma with vaccinia or BCG is associated with better survival. An European Organization

for Research and Treatment of Cancer cohort study on 542 patients. Eur J Cancer. 2005;41:118–25.
87. Pfahlberg A, Kölmel KF, Grange JM, et al. Inverse association between melanoma and previous vaccinations against tuberculosis and smallpox: results of the FEBIM study. J Invest Dermatol. 2002;119:570–5.
88. Davignon L, Robillard P, Lemonde P, Frappier A. B.C.G. vaccination and leukemia mortality. Lancet. 1970;2:638.
89. Morra ME, Kien ND, Elmaraezy A, et al. Early vaccination protects against childhood leukemia: a systematic review and meta-analysis. Sci Rep. 2017;7:15986.
90. Usher NT, Chang S, Howard RS, Martinez A, Harrison LH, Santosham M, Aronson NE. Association of BCG vaccination in childhood with subsequent cancer diagnoses: a 60-year follow-up of a clinical trial. JAMA Netw Open. 2019;2:–e1912014.
91. Guinan P, Toronchi E, Shaw M, Crispin R, Sharifi R. Bacillus Calmette-Guerin (BCG) adjuvant therapy in stage D prostate cancer. Urology. 1982;20:401–3.
92. Guinan P, Crispen R, Baumgartner G, Rao R, Totonchi E, Ablin R, John T. Adjuvant immunotherapy with bacillus Calmette-Guérin in prostatic cancer. Urology. 1979;14:561–5.
93. Snider DE, Comstock GW, Martinez I, Caras GJ. Efficacy of BCG vaccination in prevention of cancer: an update: brief communication. J Natl Cancer Inst. 1978;60:785–8.
94. Kendrick MA, Comstock GW. BCG vaccination and the subsequent development of cancer in humans. J Natl Cancer Inst. 1981;66:431–7.
95. Da Gama Duarte J, Parakh S, Andrews MC, Woods K, Pasam A, Tutuka C, Ostrouska S, Blackburn JM, Behren A, Cebon J. Autoantibodies may predict immune-related toxicity: results from a phase I study of Intralesional Bacillus Calmette-Guérin followed by Ipilimumab in patients with advanced metastatic melanoma. Front Immunol. 2018;9:411.
96. Steinberg GD, Shore ND, Redorta JP, et al. CREST: phase III study of sasanlimab and Bacillus Calmette-Guérin for patients with Bacillus Calmette-Guérin-naïve high-risk non-muscle-invasive bladder cancer. Future Oncol. 2024;20:891. https://doi.org/10.2217/fon-2023-0271.
97. Singh AK, Srikrishna G, Bivalacqua TJ, Bishai WR. Recombinant BCGs for tuberculosis and bladder cancer. Vaccine. 2021;39:7321–31.
98. Kühtreiber WM, Tran L, Kim T, et al. Long-term reduction in hyperglycemia in advanced type 1 diabetes: the value of induced aerobic glycolysis with BCG vaccinations. NPJ Vaccines. 2018;3:23.
99. Ristori G, Buzzi MG, Sabatini U, et al. Use of Bacille Calmette-Guèrin (BCG) in multiple sclerosis. Neurology. 1999;53:1588–9.
100. Brenner SR. Effects of Bacille Calmette-Guérin after the first demyelinating event in the CNS. Neurology. 2014;83:380–1.
101. Lee J, Reinke EK, Zozulya AL, Sandor M, Fabry Z. Mycobacterium bovis Bacille Calmette-Guérin infection in the CNS suppresses experimental autoimmune encephalomyelitis and Th17 responses in an IFN-gamma-independent manner. J Immunol. 2008;181:6201–12.
102. Sadelain MW, Qin HY, Lauzon J, Singh B. Prevention of type I diabetes in NOD mice by adjuvant immunotherapy. Diabetes. 1990;39:583–9.
103. McInerney MF, Pek SB, Thomas DW. Prevention of insulitis and diabetes onset by treatment with complete Freund's adjuvant in NOD mice. Diabetes. 1991;40:715–25.
104. Kodama S, Kühtreiber W, Fujimura S, Dale EA, Faustman DL. Islet regeneration during the reversal of autoimmune diabetes in NOD mice. Science. 2003;302:1223–7.
105. Ryu S, Kodama S, Ryu K, Schoenfeld DA, Faustman DL. Reversal of established autoimmune diabetes by restoration of endogenous beta cell function. J Clin Invest. 2001;108:63–72.
106. Harada M, Kishimoto Y, Makino S. Prevention of overt diabetes and insulitis in NOD mice by a single BCG vaccination. Diabetes Res Clin Pract. 1990;8:85–9.
107. Shehadeh N, Calcinaro F, Bradley BJ, Bruchim I, Vardi P, Lafferty KJ. Effect of adjuvant therapy on development of diabetes in mouse and man. Lancet. 1994;343:706–7.
108. Sanjeevi CB, Das AK, Shtauvere-Brameus A. BCG vaccination and GAD65 and IA-2 autoantibodies in autoimmune diabetes in southern India. Ann N Y Acad Sci. 2002;958:293–6.

109. Corsenac P, Parent M-É, Mansaray H, Benedetti A, Richard H, Stäger S, Rousseau M-C. Early life Bacillus Calmette-Guerin vaccination and incidence of type 1, type 2, and latent autoimmune diabetes in adulthood. Diabetes Metab. 2022;48:101337.
110. Faustman DL, Wang L, Okubo Y, et al. Proof-of-concept, randomized, controlled clinical trial of Bacillus-Calmette-Guerin for treatment of long-term type 1 diabetes. PLoS One. 2012;7:e41756.
111. Faustman DL. TNF, TNF inducers, and TNFR2 agonists: a new path to type 1 diabetes treatment. Diabetes Metab Res Rev. 2018;34:e2941.
112. Erb KJ, Holloway JW, Sobeck A, Moll H, Le Gros G. Infection of mice with Mycobacterium bovis-Bacillus Calmette-Guérin (BCG) suppresses allergen-induced airway eosinophilia. J Exp Med. 1998;187:561–9.
113. Marchant A, Goetghebuer T, Ota MO, et al. Newborns develop a Th1-type immune response to Mycobacterium bovis bacillus Calmette-Guérin vaccination. J Immunol. 1999;163:2249–55.
114. Pittet LF, Messina NL, Gardiner K, et al. Prevention of infant eczema by neonatal Bacillus Calmette-Guérin vaccination: the MIS BAIR randomized controlled trial. Allergy. 2022;77:956–65.
115. Thøstesen LM, Kjaergaard J, Pihl GT, et al. Neonatal BCG vaccination and atopic dermatitis before 13 months of age: a randomized clinical trial. Allergy. 2018;73:498–504.
116. Aaby P, Shaheen SO, Heyes CB, Goudiaby A, Hall AJ, Shiell AW, Jensen H, Marchant A. Early BCG vaccination and reduction in atopy in Guinea-Bissau. Clin Exp Allergy. 2000;30:644–50.
117. Arnoldussen DL, Linehan M, Sheikh A. BCG vaccination and allergy: a systematic review and meta-analysis. J Allergy Clin Immunol. 2011;127:246–253.e21.
118. Marks GB, Ng K, Zhou J, Toelle BG, Xuan W, Belousova EG, Britton WJ. The effect of neonatal BCG vaccination on atopy and asthma at age 7 to 14 years: an historical cohort study in a community with a very low prevalence of tuberculosis infection and a high prevalence of atopic disease. J Allergy Clin Immunol. 2003;111:541–9.
119. El-Zein M, Parent M-E, Benedetti A, Rousseau M-C. Does BCG vaccination protect against the development of childhood asthma? A systematic review and meta-analysis of epidemiological studies. Int J Epidemiol. 2010;39:469–86.
120. Rousseau M-C, Parent M-E, St-Pierre Y. Potential health effects from non-specific stimulation of the immune function in early age: the example of BCG vaccination. Pediatr Allergy Immunol. 2008;19:438–48.
121. Makrakis D, Holt SK, Bernick C, Grivas P, Gore JL, Wright JL. Intravesical BCG and incidence of Alzheimer disease in patients with bladder cancer. Alzheimer Dis Assoc Disord. 2022;36:307–11.
122. Kim JI, Zhu D, Barry E, Kovac E, Aboumohamed A, Agalliu I, Sankin A. Intravesical Bacillus Calmette-Guérin treatment is inversely associated with the risk of developing Alzheimer disease or other dementia among patients with non–muscle-invasive bladder cancer. Clin Genitourin Cancer. 2021;19:e409–16.
123. Klinger D, Hill BL, Barda N, Halperin E, Gofrit ON, Greenblatt CL, Rappoport N, Linial M, Bercovier H. Bladder cancer immunotherapy by BCG is associated with a significantly reduced risk of Alzheimer's disease and Parkinson's disease. Vaccines (Basel). 2021;9:491.
124. Gofrit ON, Klein BY, Cohen IR, Ben-Hur T, Greenblatt CL, Bercovier H. Bacillus Calmette-Guérin (BCG) therapy lowers the incidence of Alzheimer's disease in bladder cancer patients. PLoS One. 2019;14:e0224433.
125. Weinberg MS, Zafar A, Magdamo C, et al. Association of BCG vaccine treatment with death and dementia in patients with non-muscle-invasive bladder cancer. JAMA Netw Open. 2023;6:e2314336.
126. Han C, Wang J, Chen Y-L, Guan C-P, Zhang Y-A, Wang M-S. The role of Bacillus Calmette-Guérin administration on the risk of dementia in bladder cancer patients: a systematic review and meta-analysis. Front Aging Neurosci. 2023;15:1243588.

127. Zuo Z, Qi F, Yang J, Wang X, Wu Y, Wen Y, Yuan Q, Zou J, Guo K, Bin YZ. Immunization with Bacillus Calmette-Guérin (BCG) alleviates neuroinflammation and cognitive deficits in APP/PS1 mice via the recruitment of inflammation-resolving monocytes to the brain. Neurobiol Dis. 2017;101:27–39.
128. Zuo Z, Qi F, Xing Z, Yuan L, Yang Y, He Z, Zhou L, Yao Z. Bacille Calmette-Guérin attenuates vascular amyloid pathology and maximizes synaptic preservation in APP/PS1 mice following active amyloid-β immunotherapy. Neurobiol Aging. 2021;101:94–108.
129. Li Q, Wang X, Wang ZH, et al. Changes in dendritic complexity and spine morphology following BCG immunization in APP/PS1 mice. Hum Vaccin Immunother. 2022;18:2121568.
130. Kleinnijenhuis J, Quintin J, Preijers F, et al. Long-lasting effects of BCG vaccination on both heterologous Th1/Th17 responses and innate trained immunity. J Innate Immun. 2014;6:152–8.
131. Moliva JI, Turner J, Torrelles JB. Immune responses to Bacillus Calmette-Guérin vaccination: why do they fail to protect against Mycobacterium tuberculosis? Front Immunol. 2017;8:407.
132. Bulut Y, Michelsen KS, Hayrapetian L, Naiki Y, Spallek R, Singh M, Arditi M. Mycobacterium tuberculosis heat shock proteins use diverse Toll-like receptor pathways to activate pro-inflammatory signals. J Biol Chem. 2005;280:20961–7.
133. Kim K, Sohn H, Kim J-S, Choi H-G, Byun E-H, Lee K-I, Shin SJ, Song C-H, Park J-K, Kim H-J. Mycobacterium tuberculosis Rv0652 stimulates production of tumour necrosis factor and monocytes chemoattractant protein-1 in macrophages through the Toll-like receptor 4 pathway. Immunology. 2012;136:231–40.
134. Godaly G, Young DB. Mycobacterium bovis Bacille Calmette Guerin infection of human neutrophils induces CXCL8 secretion by MyD88-dependent TLR2 and TLR4 activation. Cell Microbiol. 2005;7:591–601.
135. Jung S-B, Yang C-S, Lee J-S, et al. The mycobacterial 38-kilodalton glycolipoprotein antigen activates the mitogen-activated protein kinase pathway and release of proinflammatory cytokines through Toll-like receptors 2 and 4 in human monocytes. Infect Immun. 2006;74:2686–96.
136. Quesniaux VJ, Nicolle DM, Torres D, Kremer L, Guérardel Y, Nigou J, Puzo G, Erard F, Ryffel B. Toll-like receptor 2 (TLR2)-dependent-positive and TLR2-independent-negative regulation of proinflammatory cytokines by mycobacterial lipomannans. J Immunol. 2004;172:4425–34.
137. Sendide K, Reiner NE, Lee JSI, Bourgoin S, Talal A, Hmama Z. Cross-talk between CD14 and complement receptor 3 promotes phagocytosis of mycobacteria: regulation by phosphatidylinositol 3-kinase and cytohesin-1. J Immunol. 2005;174:4210–9.
138. Nigou J, Zelle-Rieser C, Gilleron M, Thurnher M, Puzo G. Mannosylated lipoarabinomannans inhibit IL-12 production by human dendritic cells: evidence for a negative signal delivered through the mannose receptor. J Immunol. 2001;166:7477–85.
139. Gagliardi MC, Teloni R, Giannoni F, Pardini M, Sargentini V, Brunori L, Fattorini L, Nisini R. Mycobacterium bovis Bacillus Calmette-Guerin infects DC-SIGN- dendritic cell and causes the inhibition of IL-12 and the enhancement of IL-10 production. J Leukoc Biol. 2005;78:106–13.
140. Li J, Fu L, Wang G, Subbian S, Qin C, Zhao A. Unmethylated CpG motif-containing genomic DNA fragment of Bacillus Calmette-Guerin promotes macrophage functions through TLR9-mediated activation of NF-κB and MAPKs signaling pathways. Innate Immun. 2020;26:183–203.
141. Tsuji S, Matsumoto M, Takeuchi O, Akira S, Azuma I, Hayashi A, Toyoshima K, Seya T. Maturation of human dendritic cells by cell wall skeleton of Mycobacterium bovis bacillus Calmette-Guérin: involvement of toll-like receptors. Infect Immun. 2000;68:6883–90.
142. Sendide K, Deghmane A-E, Pechkovsky D, Av-Gay Y, Talal A, Hmama Z. Mycobacterium bovis BCG attenuates surface expression of mature class II molecules through IL-10-dependent inhibition of cathepsin S. J Immunol. 2005;175:5324–32.
143. Covián C, Fernández-Fierro A, Retamal-Díaz A, Díaz FE, Vasquez AE, Lay MK, Riedel CA, González PA, Bueno SM, Kalergis AM. BCG-induced cross-protection and development of trained immunity: implication for vaccine design. Front Immunol. 2019;10:2806.

144. Suttmann H, Lehan N, Böhle A, Brandau S. Stimulation of neutrophil granulocytes with Mycobacterium bovis bacillus Calmette-Guérin induces changes in phenotype and gene expression and inhibits spontaneous apoptosis. Infect Immun. 2003;71:4647–56.
145. Prezzemolo T, Guggino G, La Manna MP, Di Liberto D, Dieli F, Caccamo N. Functional signatures of human CD4 and CD8 T cell responses to Mycobacterium tuberculosis. Front Immunol. 2014;5:83298.
146. Humphreys IR, Stewart GR, Turner DJ, Patel J, Karamanou D, Snelgrove RJ, Young DB. A role for dendritic cells in the dissemination of mycobacterial infection. Microbes Infect. 2006;8:1339–46.
147. Su H, Peng B, Zhang Z, Liu Z, Zhang Z. The Mycobacterium tuberculosis glycoprotein Rv1016c protein inhibits dendritic cell maturation, and impairs Th1 /Th17 responses during mycobacteria infection. Mol Immunol. 2019;109:58–70.
148. Bizzell E, Sia JK, Quezada M, Enriquez A, Georgieva M, Rengarajan J. Deletion of BCG Hip1 protease enhances dendritic cell and CD4 T cell responses. J Leukoc Biol. 2018;103:739–48.
149. Bollampalli VP, Harumi Yamashiro L, Feng X, Bierschenk D, Gao Y, Blom H, Henriques-Normark B, Nylén S, Rothfuchs AG. BCG skin infection triggers IL-1R-MyD88-dependent migration of EpCAMlow CD11bhigh skin dendritic cells to draining lymph node during CD4+ T-cell priming. PLoS Pathog. 2015;11:e1005206.
150. Soares AP, Scriba TJ, Joseph S, et al. Bacillus Calmette-Guérin vaccination of human newborns induces T cells with complex cytokine and phenotypic profiles. J Immunol. 2008;180:3569–77.
151. Power CA, Wei G, Bretscher PA. Mycobacterial dose defines the Th1/Th2 nature of the immune response independently of whether immunization is administered by the intravenous, subcutaneous, or intradermal route. Infect Immun. 1998;66:5743–50.
152. Hussey GD, Watkins MLV, Goddard EA, Gottschalk S, Hughes EJ, Iloni K, Kibel MA, Ress SR. Neonatal mycobacterial specific cytotoxic T-lymphocyte and cytokine profiles in response to distinct BCG vaccination strategies. Immunology. 2002;105:314–24.
153. Luo Y, Jiang W, Da Z, et al. Subunit vaccine candidate AMM down-regulated the regulatory T cells and enhanced the protective immunity of BCG on a suitable schedule. Scand J Immunol. 2012;75:293–300.
154. Jaron B, Maranghi E, Leclerc C, Majlessi L. Effect of attenuation of Treg during BCG immunization on anti-mycobacterial Th1 responses and protection against Mycobacterium tuberculosis. PLoS One. 2008;3:e2833.
155. Kawashima T, Norose Y, Watanabe Y, et al. Cutting edge: major CD8 T cell response to live Bacillus Calmette-Guérin is mediated by CD1 molecules. J Immunol. 2003;170:5345–8.
156. Jiang J, Wang X, An H, et al. Mucosal-associated invariant T-cell function is modulated by programmed death-1 signaling in patients with active tuberculosis. Am J Respir Crit Care Med. 2014;190:329–39.
157. Hawkridge T, Scriba TJ, Gelderbloem S, et al. Safety and immunogenicity of a new tuberculosis vaccine, MVA85A, in healthy adults in South Africa. J Infect Dis. 2008;198:544–52.
158. Bhatt K, Verma S, Ellner JJ, Salgame P. Quest for correlates of protection against tuberculosis. Clin Vaccine Immunol. 2015;22:258–66.
159. Boer MC, Prins C, van Meijgaarden KE, van Dissel JT, Ottenhoff THM, Joosten SA. Mycobacterium bovis BCG vaccination induces divergent proinflammatory or regulatory T cell responses in adults. Clin Vaccine Immunol. 2015;22:778–88.
160. Murray RA, Mansoor N, Harbacheuski R, et al. Bacillus Calmette Guerin vaccination of human newborns induces a specific, functional CD8+ T cell response. J Immunol. 2006;177:5647–51.
161. Hanekom WA. The immune response to BCG vaccination of newborns. Ann N Y Acad Sci. 2005;1062:69–78.
162. Silva CL, Bonato VL, Lima VM, Faccioli LH, Leão SC. Characterization of the memory/activated T cells that mediate the long-lived host response against tuberculosis after bacillus Calmette-Guérin or DNA vaccination. Immunology. 1999;97:573–81.

163. Soares AP, Kwong Chung CKC, Choice T, et al. Longitudinal changes in CD4+ T-cell memory responses induced by BCG vaccination of newborns. J Infect Dis. 2013;207:1084–94.
164. Hoft DF, Brown RM, Roodman ST. Bacille Calmette-Guérin vaccination enhances human γδ T cell responsiveness to mycobacteria suggestive of a memory-like phenotype. J Immunol. 1998;161:1045–54.
165. Chen T, Blanc C, Eder AZ, et al. Association of human antibodies to arabinomannan with enhanced mycobacterial opsonophagocytosis and intracellular growth reduction. J Infect Dis. 2016;214:300–10.
166. Sebina I, Cliff JM, Smith SG, Nogaro S, Webb EL, Riley EM, Dockrell HM, Elliott AM, Hafalla JCR, Cose S. Long-lived memory B-cell responses following BCG vaccination. PLoS One. 2012;7:e51381.
167. Kumar SK, Singh P, Sinha S. Naturally produced opsonizing antibodies restrict the survival of Mycobacterium tuberculosis in human macrophages by augmenting phagosome maturation. Open Biol. 2015;5:150171.
168. Lu LL, Chung AW, Rosebrock TR, et al. A functional role for antibodies in tuberculosis. Cell. 2016;167:433–443.e14.
169. Ritz N, Dutta B, Donath S, Casalaz D, Connell TG, Tebruegge M, Robins-Browne R, Hanekom WA, Britton WJ, Curtis N. The influence of Bacille Calmette-Guerin vaccine strain on the immune response against tuberculosis: a randomized trial. Am J Respir Crit Care Med. 2012;185:213–22.
170. Davids V, Hanekom WA, Mansoor N, et al. The effect of Bacille Calmette-Guérin vaccine strain and route of administration on induced immune responses in vaccinated infants. J Infect Dis. 2006;193:531–6.
171. Perdomo C, Zedler U, Kühl AA, Lozza L, Saikali P, Sander LE, Vogelzang A, Kaufmann SHE, Kupz A. Mucosal BCG vaccination induces protective lung-resident memory T cell populations against tuberculosis. MBio. 2016;7(6):e01686–16.
172. Uranga S, Marinova D, Martin C, Aguilo N. Protective efficacy and pulmonary immune response following subcutaneous and intranasal BCG administration in mice. J Vis Exp. 2016;115:54440.
173. Hansen IS, Baeten DLP, den Dunnen J. The inflammatory function of human IgA. Cell Mol Life Sci. 2019;76:1041–55.
174. Crotty S. T follicular helper cell differentiation, function, and roles in disease. Immunity. 2014;41:529–42.
175. Ma CS, Deenick EK, Batten M, Tangye SG. The origins, function, and regulation of T follicular helper cells. J Exp Med. 2012;209:1241–53.
176. Vogelzang A, Perdomo C, Zedler U, Kuhlmann S, Hurwitz R, Gengenbacher M, Kaufmann SHE. Central memory CD4+ T cells are responsible for the recombinant Bacillus Calmette-Guérin ΔureC::hly vaccine's superior protection against tuberculosis. J Infect Dis. 2014;210:1928–37.
177. Gengenbacher M, Nieuwenhuizen N, Vogelzang A, Liu H, Kaiser P, Schuerer S, Lazar D, Wagner I, Mollenkopf H-J, Kaufmann SHE. Deletion of nuoG from the vaccine candidate Mycobacterium bovis BCG ΔureC::hly improves protection against tuberculosis. MBio. 2016;7(3):e00679–16.
178. Netea MG, Joosten LAB, Latz E, Mills KHG, Natoli G, Stunnenberg HG, O'Neill LAJ, Xavier RJ. Trained immunity: a program of innate immune memory in health and disease. Science. 2016;352:aaf1098.
179. Netea MG, Quintin J, van der Meer JWM. Trained immunity: a memory for innate host defense. Cell Host Microbe. 2011;9:355–61.
180. Bigot J, Guillot L, Guitard J, Ruffin M, Corvol H, Chignard M, Hennequin C, Balloy V. Respiratory epithelial cells can remember infection: a proof of concept study. J Infect Dis. 2019;221:1000–5.
181. Naik S, Larsen SB, Gomez NC, Alaverdyan K, Sendoel A, Yuan S, Polak L, Kulukian A, Chai S, Fuchs E. Inflammatory memory sensitizes skin epithelial stem cells to tissue damage. Nature. 2017;550:475–80.

182. Sohrabi Y, Lagache SMM, Voges VC, Semo D, Sonntag G, Hanemann I, Kahles F, Waltenberger J, Findeisen HM. OxLDL-mediated immunologic memory in endothelial cells. J Mol Cell Cardiol. 2020;146:121–32.
183. Netea MG, Domínguez-Andrés J, Barreiro LB, et al. Defining trained immunity and its role in health and disease. Nat Rev Immunol. 2020;20:375–88.
184. Kleinnijenhuis J, Quintin J, Preijers F, Joosten LAB, Jacobs C, Xavier RJ, van der Meer JWM, van Crevel R, Netea MG. BCG-induced trained immunity in NK cells: role for non-specific protection to infection. Clin Immunol. 2014;155:213–9.
185. Jensen KJ, Larsen N, Biering-Sørensen S, et al. Heterologous immunological effects of early BCG vaccination in low-birth-weight infants in Guinea-Bissau: a randomized-controlled trial. J Infect Dis. 2015;211:956–67.
186. Vierboom MPM, Dijkman K, Sombroek CC, et al. Stronger induction of trained immunity by mucosal BCG or MTBVAC vaccination compared to standard intradermal vaccination. Cell Rep Med. 2021;2:100185.
187. Buffen K, Oosting M, Quintin J, et al. Autophagy controls BCG-induced trained immunity and the response to intravesical BCG therapy for bladder cancer. PLoS Pathog. 2014;10:e1004485.
188. Stražar M, Mourits VP, Koeken VACM, de Bree LCJ, Moorlag SJCFM, Joosten LAB, van Crevel R, Vlamakis H, Netea MG, Xavier RJ. The influence of the gut microbiome on BCG-induced trained immunity. Genome Biol. 2021;22:275.
189. Angelidou A, Diray-Arce J, Conti M-G, Netea MG, Blok BA, Liu M, Sanchez-Schmitz G, Ozonoff A, van Haren SD, Levy O. Human newborn monocytes demonstrate distinct BCG-induced primary and trained innate cytokine production and metabolic activation in vitro. Front Immunol. 2021;12:674334.
190. Koeken VA, de Bree LCJ, Mourits VP, et al. BCG vaccination in humans inhibits systemic inflammation in a sex-dependent manner. J Clin Invest. 2020;130:5591–602.
191. Ghisletti S, Barozzi I, Mietton F, et al. Identification and characterization of enhancers controlling the inflammatory gene expression program in macrophages. Immunity. 2010;32:317–28.
192. Ostuni R, Piccolo V, Barozzi I, Polletti S, Termanini A, Bonifacio S, Curina A, Prosperini E, Ghisletti S, Natoli G. Latent enhancers activated by stimulation in differentiated cells. Cell. 2013;152:157–71.
193. Rizzetto L, Ifrim DC, Moretti S, et al. Fungal chitin induces trained immunity in human monocytes during cross-talk of the host with Saccharomyces cerevisiae. J Biol Chem. 2016;291:7961–72.
194. Hole CR, Wager CML, Castro-Lopez N, Campuzano A, Cai H, Wozniak KL, Wang Y, Wormley FL. Induction of memory-like dendritic cell responses in vivo. Nat Commun. 2019;10:2955.
195. Verma D, Parasa VR, Raffetseder J, Martis M, Mehta RB, Netea M, Lerm M. Anti-mycobacterial activity correlates with altered DNA methylation pattern in immune cells from BCG-vaccinated subjects. Sci Rep. 2017;7:1–10.
196. Butkeviciute E, Jones CE, Smith SG. Heterologous effects of infant BCG vaccination: potential mechanisms of immunity. Future Microbiol. 2018;13:1193–208.
197. Arts RJW, Blok BA, Aaby P, Joosten LAB, de Jong D, van der Meer JWM, Benn CS, van Crevel R, Netea MG. Long-term in vitro and in vivo effects of γ-irradiated BCG on innate and adaptive immunity. J Leukoc Biol. 2015;98:995–1001.
198. Arts RJW, Carvalho A, La Rocca C, et al. Immunometabolic pathways in BCG-induced trained immunity. Cell Rep. 2016;17:2562–71.
199. Fanucchi S, Fok ET, Dalla E, et al. Immune genes are primed for robust transcription by proximal long noncoding RNAs located in nuclear compartments. Nat Genet. 2019;51:138–50.
200. Moorlag SJCFM, Rodriguez-Rosales YA, Gillard J, et al. BCG vaccination induces long-term functional reprogramming of human neutrophils. Cell Rep. 2020;33:108387.
201. Das J, Verma D, Gustafsson M, Lerm M. Identification of DNA methylation patterns predisposing for an efficient response to BCG vaccination in healthy BCG-naïve subjects. Epigenetics. 2019;14:589–601.

202. Cheng S-C, Quintin J, Cramer RA, et al. mTOR- and HIF-1α-mediated aerobic glycolysis as metabolic basis for trained immunity. Science. 2014;345:1250684.
203. Arts RJW, Netea MG. Epigenetic rewiring of monocytes in BCG vaccination. In: The value of BCG and TNF in autoimmunity, Second Edition. Elsevier; 2018. p. 109–20.
204. Saz-Leal P, del Fresno C, Brandi P, Martínez-Cano S, Dungan OM, Chisholm JD, Kerr WG, Sancho D. Targeting SHIP-1 in myeloid cells enhances trained immunity and boosts response to infection. Cell Rep. 2018;25:1118–26.
205. De Rosa V, Galgani M, Porcellini A, et al. Glycolysis controls the induction of human regulatory T cells by modulating the expression of FOXP3 exon 2 splicing variants. Nat Immunol. 2015;16:1174–84.
206. Ferreira AV, Alarcon-Barrera JC, Domínguez-Andrés J, et al. Fatty acid desaturation and lipoxygenase pathways support trained immunity. Nat Commun. 2023;14:7385.
207. Diray-Arce J, Angelidou A, Jensen KJ, et al. Bacille Calmette-Guérin vaccine reprograms human neonatal lipid metabolism in vivo and in vitro. Cell Rep. 2022;39:110772.
208. Sohrabi Y, Lagache SMM, Schnack L, Godfrey R, Kahles F, Bruemmer D, Waltenberger J, Findeisen HM. mTOR-dependent oxidative stress regulates oxLDL-induced trained innate immunity in human monocytes. Front Immunol. 2019;9:420330.
209. Goodridge HS, Ahmed SS, Curtis N, Kollmann TR, Levy O, Netea MG, Pollard AJ, van Crevel R, Wilson CB. Harnessing the beneficial heterologous effects of vaccination. Nat Rev Immunol. 2016;16:392–400.
210. Mathurin KS, Martens GW, Kornfeld H, Welsh RM. CD4 T-cell-mediated heterologous immunity between mycobacteria and poxviruses. J Virol. 2009;83:3528–39.
211. Ota MOC, Vekemans J, Schlegel-Haueter SE, et al. Influence of Mycobacterium bovis bacillus Calmette-Guérin on antibody and cytokine responses to human neonatal vaccination. J Immunol. 2002;168:919–25.
212. Gela A, Murphy M, Rodo M, et al. Effects of BCG vaccination on donor unrestricted T cells in two prospective cohort studies. EBioMedicine. 2022;76:103839.
213. Melandri D, Zlatareva I, Chaleil RAG, et al. The γδTCR combines innate immunity with adaptive immunity by utilizing spatially distinct regions for agonist selection and antigen responsiveness. Nat Immunol. 2018;19:1352–65.
214. Libraty DH, Zhang L, Woda M, Acosta LP, Obcena A, Brion JD, Capeding RZ. Neonatal BCG vaccination is associated with enhanced T-helper 1 immune responses to heterologous infant vaccines. Trials Vaccinol. 2014;3:1–5.
215. Berg RE, Crossley E, Murray S, Forman J. Memory CD8+ T cells provide innate immune protection against Listeria monocytogenes in the absence of cognate antigen. J Exp Med. 2003;198:1583–93.
216. Lertmemongkolchai G, Cai G, Hunter CA, Bancroft GJ. Bystander activation of CD8+ T cells contributes to the rapid production of IFN-γ in response to bacterial pathogens. J Immunol. 2001;166:1097–105.
217. Yona S, Kim K-W, Wolf Y, et al. Fate mapping reveals origins and dynamics of monocytes and tissue macrophages under homeostasis. Immunity. 2013;38:79–91.
218. Patel AA, Zhang Y, Fullerton JN, et al. The fate and lifespan of human monocyte subsets in steady state and systemic inflammation. J Exp Med. 2017;214:1913–23.
219. Merad M, Sathe P, Helft J, Miller J, Mortha A. The dendritic cell lineage: ontogeny and function of dendritic cells and their subsets in the steady state and the inflamed setting. Annu Rev Immunol. 2013;31:563–604.
220. Kaufmann E, Sanz J, Dunn JL, et al. BCG educates hematopoietic stem cells to generate protective innate immunity against tuberculosis. Cell. 2018;172:176–190.e19.
221. Cirovic B, de Bree LCJ, Groh L, et al. BCG vaccination in humans elicits trained immunity via the hematopoietic progenitor compartment. Cell Host Microbe. 2020;28:322–334.e5.
222. Brook B, Harbeson DJ, Shannon CP, et al. BCG vaccination-induced emergency granulopoiesis provides rapid protection from neonatal sepsis. Sci Transl Med. 2020;12:4517.
223. Andualem H, Hollams E, Kollmann TR, Amenyogbe N. BCG-induced immune training: interplay between trained immunity and emergency granulopoiesis. J Mol Biol. 2023;435:168169.

Part III

Pre-clinical Vaccines Against Tuberculosis

New Vaccine Strategies to Improve, Boost, or Replace BCG

5

Louis Torracinta, Beatrice Nassanga, and Rachel Tanner

5.1 Introduction

Bacille Calmette-Guérin (BCG) is a live attenuated vaccine that was developed at the Institut Pasteur in France by Albert Calmette and Camille Guérin through 200–240 re-seedings of initially virulent *Mycobacterium bovis* (*M. bovis*) in a glycerinated potato medium saturated with ox bile: a painstaking process that took over a decade [1]. Calmette and Guérin were ultimately successful in creating an attenuated vaccine, demonstrating safety and protective efficacy in animal models, followed by the first human immunization in 1921 [2].

Loss in virulence of the early "bacille bilié" strain is thought to be attributable to the removal of a 9.5 kb region of DNA—the "region of difference 1" (RD1), which codes for two key immunogenic antigens, ESAT-6 and CFP-10, plus several parts of the secretion system ESX-1 [3]. Loss of RD1 is understood to cause disruption of

L. Torracinta
Medical Sciences Division, University of Oxford, Oxford, UK
e-mail: louis.torracinta@gtc.ox.ac.uk

B. Nassanga
Jenner Institute, Nuffield Department of Medicine, University of Oxford, Oxford, UK

Department of Biology, University of Oxford, Oxford, UK

Department of Immunology and Molecular Biology, School of Biomedical Sciences, College of Health Sciences, Makerere University, Kampala, Uganda
e-mail: beatrice.francis@ndm.ox.ac.uk

R. Tanner (✉)
Department of Biology, University of Oxford, Oxford, UK
e-mail: rachel.tanner@biology.ox.ac.uk

P. J. G. Bettencourt (ed.), *Tuberculosis Vaccines*,
https://doi.org/10.1007/978-3-031-94540-3_5

the phagolysosome within host-infected macrophages [4]. Other studies indicate that unintentional variations, tandem duplications, and deletions exist between various early (pre-1927) and later (post-1927) BCG strains, potentially caused by arbitrary early decisions made by Calmette and colleagues regarding the composition of the culture medium, such as the inclusion of glycerol. Some have suggested that these differences may cause slight variations in the efficacy and reactogenicity of the present-day BCG vaccine strains descended from these early examples [5], although purported efficacy differences between BCG strains remain a matter of active debate [6, 7].

To date, BCG has been administered to over four billion people, making it one of the most widely used vaccines in history. The favorable safety profile is well-established, with correct intradermal (ID) administration generally resulting in a minor local reaction and any systemic adverse events associated almost exclusively with immunosuppression [8]. Other advantages include its consistently high efficacy against TB meningitis and disseminated disease in infants [9–11], cross-reactive protection against leprosy and Buruli ulcer disease (BUD) [12–17], and nonspecific effects reducing all-cause infant mortality [18, 19].

However, the protection BCG confers against pulmonary TB, the most common form of the disease, is highly variable, ranging from >70% in the UK, Denmark, and Norway to <20% in Southern India, Malawi, and Colombia [12, 20–26]. Efficacy is lowest in many TB-endemic regions most in need of a protective vaccine, and duration of protection may be limited [27]. Furthermore, BCG can interfere with the tuberculin skin test (TST) that is still widely used in the diagnosis of *Mycobacterium tuberculosis* (*M.tb*) in resource-limited settings [28, 29]. As it is a live replicating bacterium, the use of BCG is contraindicated for individuals with immunosuppression, including those who are HIV-positive and infants in high-prevalence areas until HIV status has been confirmed.

Due to these limitations, a more effective TB vaccine is urgently needed if the World Health Organization (WHO) End TB Strategy targets of a 95% reduction in TB mortality and 90% reduction of TB incidence worldwide by 2035 are to be realized. New regimens should be non-inferior to BCG in both the specific and nonspecific protection conferred, and thus many focus on improving or boosting BCG, while others aim to replace BCG with other live attenuated or inactivated mycobacterial strains or with more advanced DNA or RNA vaccines (Table 5.1) (Fig. 5.1).

Table 5.1 Vaccine candidates discussed in this chapter

Strategy		Vaccine	Description	Phase	Ref.
Improving BCG	Recombinant BCG strains	VPM1002	BCG expressing listeriolysin and lacking urease C	Phase III	[34–39]
		rBCG30	BCG TICE overexpressing Ag85B encoded by *fbpB* genes	Phase I, currently paused	[40–42]
		BCGΔzmp1	BCG Pasteur with deletion of the *Rv0198c* gene leading to deficiency of zinc metalloprotease 1 (Zmp1)	Preclinical	[43, 44]
		BCGΔBCG1419c	BCG Pasteur with removal of the *BCG1419c* gene resulting in attenuated intracellular replication	Preclinical	[45–49]
		ESX-1 inclusion rBCG candidates	BCG with reinserted genes of the ESAT-6 protein family secretion system-1 (ESX-1) from the RD1 region	Preclinical	[50–53]
		BCGΔsapM	BCG with the deletion of *SapM* with additional capping of cell wall LAM with a-1,2-oligomannosides (ManLAM)	Preclinical	[54–56]
	Different routes of administration	Aerosol BCG	Administered by the inhaled aerosol route	Phase I	[61, 62]
		Intravenous BCG	Administered by the IV route	Preclinical	[60, 63]
Boosting BCG	BCG revaccination	BCG	Homologous prime-boost with BCG	Phase IIb	[65–74]
	Protein/ adjuvant candidates	M72/AS01$_E$	Mtb32A and Mtb39A immunogenic fusion proteins with AS01$_E$ as an adjuvant	Phase IIb	[78]
		ID93 + GLA-SE	Rv2608, Rv2619, Rv3620 and Rv1813 antigens with GLA-SE adjuvant	Phase IIa	[79]
		H56:IC31	Ag85B, ESAT-6 and Rv2660c protein fusion antigens with IC31 adjuvant	Phase IIb, currently paused	[71]
		GamTBvac	Combines ESAT-6, CFP10 and Ag85A antigens with the novel adjuvant dextran/CpG	Phase III	[80]
		AEC/BC02	Ag85B and ESAT-6-CFP-10 proteins and the complex adjuvant system BC02	Phase IIa	[81]
		H107/CAF01	PPE68, ESAT-6, EspI, EspC, EspA, MPT64, MPT70, and MPT83, formulated in a liposome-based Cationic Adjuvant Formulation 1	Phase I	[82]
		LT70	ESAT-6, Ag85B, MPT64, M.tb8.4, HSPX and Rv2626c, in DDA and Poly I:C adjuvant	Preclinical	[84–86]
		CysVac2/ Advax	Fusion protein comprising Ag85B and CysD antigens with Advax adjuvant	Preclinical	[87–89, 92]
		CFMO-DMT	Rv0577, Rv2875, Rv3044 and Rv2073c expressed as a single protein and formulated in DMT adjuvant	Preclinical	[93]
	Recombinant vectors	ChAdOx1.85A MVA85A Aerosol / IM	ChAdOx1 and/or MVA vectors expressing Ag85A	Phase IIa	[97]
		Ad5Ag85A	Recombinant replication-deficient human Ad5 vector expressing Ag85A	Phase I	[100]
		ChAdOx1.5Ag/ MVA.5Ag	Recombinant ChAdOx1 prime and MVA boost vectors both expressing a fusion of Ag85A, PE8, PPE-15, EsxI and EsxJ	Preclinical	[101]
		Tri:ChAd:TB	Chimpanzee adenovirus serotype 68 vector expressing Ag85A, TB10.4 and RpfB	Preclinical	[106]
		RhCMV/TB	Rhesus CMV vector expressing ESAT-6, Ag85A, Ag85B, Rv3407, Rv1733, Rv2626, Rpf A, Rpf C and Rpf D	Preclinical	[107]
		Various novel vectors	Lentivirus, Sendai virus, VSV, Parainfluenza virus, Lactobacillus and Listeria-based vectors engineered to express *M.tb* antigens	Preclinical	[108–115]

(continued)

Table 5.1 (continued)

Strategy		Vaccine	Description	Phase	Ref.
Replacing BCG	Live attenuated *M.tb* strains	MTBVAC	Derivative of the clinical *M.tb* isolate Mt103, rationally attenuated by deletions in the *phoP* and *fadD26* genes	Phase III	[118–124]
		Various novel mutants	*M.tbΔsigH, M.tbΔlpqS, M.tbΔmosR, M.tbΔechR, M.tb Δmms, M. tb ΔsigE ΔfadD26,* GC1237 Rv1503c::Tn*ΔphoPR*	Preclinical	[125–128, 130–134]
	Naturally attenuated strains of other mycobacteria	Various	*M. smegmatis, M. vaccae, M. terrae, M. phlei, M. trivial, M. tb* H37Ra, *M. paragordonae*	Preclinical	[135, 136]
	Recombinant strains of other mycobacteria	mc^2-CMX	Recombinant *M. smegmatis* engineered to express Ag85C, MPT-51, and HspX	Preclinical	[137]
	Inactivated mycobacteria	MIP	Heat-inactivated *M. indicus pranii*	Phase III	[139]
		M.vaccae	Heat-killed *M. vaccae*	Phase III	[140]
		DAR-901	BCG booster vaccine manufactured from the same seed strain as SRL-172	Phase IIb	[141, 142]
		RUTI	Cell wall fragments of *M.tb* in a liposome suspension	Phase IIb	[143, 144] [129]
	Virus-like particles (VLPs)	Various	Influenza A VLPs displaying a 20aa sequence from *M.tb* ESAT-6, entire ESAT-6 protein inserted into HBV core particles, HPV VLPs as a carrier for *M.tb* Ag85B	Preclinical	[147–150]
	DNA vaccines	FnBPA+pValac:Ag85A	*Lactococcus lactis* modified to FnBPA genes from *Staphylococcus aureus* and a pValac plasmid vector [154] carrying Ag85A	Preclinical	[155, 156]
		Various	DNA constructs encoding Ag85B and MPT64, Hsp65 and Hsp70, ESAT-6 and CFP-10 among others	Preclinical	[157–159]
	RNA vaccines	BNT164a1 and BNT164b1	Unknown	Phase I	n/a
		M.tb MPT83	RNA encoding *M.tb* MPT83	Preclinical	[163]
		M.leprae Hsp65	mRNA encoding the Hsp65 protein from *M.leprae*	Preclinical	[164]
		ID91 repRNA	ID91 (encoding a fusion protein of Rv3619, Rv2389, Rv3478, and Rv1886) produced as a repRNA formulated in a nanostructured lipid	Preclinical	[162, 166]

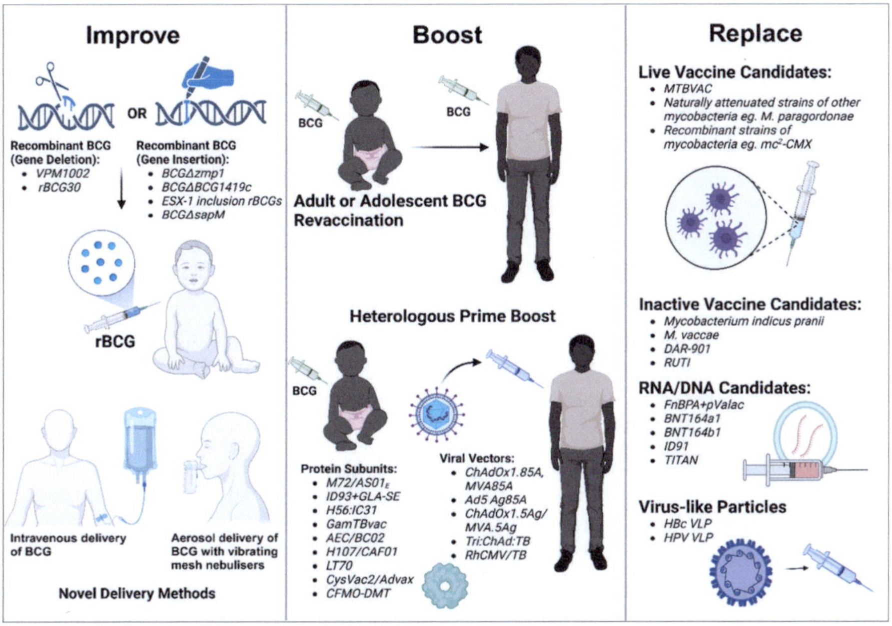

Fig. 5.1 Summary of vaccine strategies to improve, boost, or replace BCG. (Created in BioRender. Tanner, R. (2025) https://BioRender.com/j8ccbqr)

5.2 Improving BCG

5.2.1 Recombinant BCG Vaccine Candidates

Given the spartan approach to the invention of BCG over a century ago, and the vast developments in genetics, vaccinology, and technology since that time, it seems reasonable to suggest that thoughtful, targeted genetic modifications to BCG (resulting in "recombinant BCG" or "rBCG" strains) could improve upon Calmette and Guérin's pioneering work, perhaps extending its protection to new populations, to disseminated pulmonary TB, or to other diseases altogether. On the other hand, the polygenic drivers behind TB susceptibility may indicate that there are as yet unknown natural genetic barriers that make it difficult to improve upon the protection BCG confers in certain populations [30]. In any case, rBCG vaccines pose distinct advantages over subunit or other non-live candidate vaccines because they maintain broad antigen composition, including a complete repertoire of proteins, lipids, and carbohydrates that are likely to induce a correspondingly broader host immune response across both lymphoid and myeloid cell lineages, and might also be more likely to retain the nonspecific effects and relatively long-lasting immune memory associated with BCG [31]. In simple terms, a strong argument in favor of rBCG strategies for improvement is that live attenuated vaccines against TB (i.e., BCG itself) have worked well in the past, which cannot yet be said of any other TB vaccine platform.

Currently, a handful of rBCG vaccine candidates are in various stages of development, including VPM1002, *rBCG30, BCGΔzmp1, BCGΔESAT6-PE25SS,* and *BCGΔsapM*, although none have cleared phase II/III trials. To reach licensure, the WHO contends that future TB vaccine candidates must be (either in heterologous combination or on their own) at least as safe as BCG and/or more effective prophylactically [32]. It has been suggested that rBCG vaccines could ultimately be targeted to specific populations, for example, used to revaccinate adolescents with latent *M.tb* infection (but with a similar side effect profile) or to provide an equally effective but safer alternative to BCG for use in HIV-positive or exposed individuals [31]. Importantly, modeling studies indicate that there is likely to be significantly greater impact from a novel adolescent/adult vaccine versus an improved infant vaccine candidate as this population remains underserved currently and traditionally has the highest transmission burden of TB [33].

5.2.1.1 VPM1002

VPM1002 is the most progressed of the rBCG vaccines and the first to reach a phase III multicenter trial for prevention of infection (POI) in infants (NCT04351685). The primary alteration in VPM1002 is the replacement of the urease C gene with listeriolysin O (LLO)-encoding gene (*hly*) from *Listeria monocytogenes* [34]. Listeriolysin is a nonenzymatic cytolysin that has been known since the late 1980s to perforate the phagosomal membrane under specific acidic conditions (pH of 5.5) [35]. Simultaneously, deletion of the urease C subunit–encoding gene (*ureC*) in VPM1002 reduces acidification of the phagosomal compartment, creating the ideal conditions within which listeriolysin can operate. In combination, alterations in VPM1002 therefore allow enhanced release of BCG-derived antigens to break out of the phagosome and into the cytosol, facilitating antigen processing through MHC class I pathways and inducing proinflammatory conditions that result in elevated IL-1β and IL-18 cytokine secretion, apoptosis, and autophagy [36]. Ultimately, this process better mimics the immune response induced by *M.tb* infection itself. Listeriolysin degrades rapidly in the cytosol through ubiquitination of its proline-glutamate-serine-threonine (PEST) amino acid sequence, and its activity is thus restricted to the phagosome, providing an important in-built safety mechanism that avoids detrimental effects on surrounding cell membranes [37].

VPM1002 has been demonstrably safe and immunogenic when tested across a range of preclinical models as well as clinical trials in healthy adults and infants over the past decade [38]. Most recently, a phase II non-inferiority double-blind controlled trial was published that compared outcomes between HIV exposed–uninfected (HEU) and unexposed infants in South Africa (NCT02391415), finding that VPM1002 was less reactogenic than BCG but also conferred slightly reduced immunogenicity after 6 weeks [36]. Further research in HIV-positive and -exposed populations will be important in determining the safety profile of rBCG candidates given that up to 30% of the children in TB-endemic areas such as South Africa may be HIV-exposed, and HIV exposure is known to cause impaired T-cell proliferation and lower levels of IFN-γ production in response to BCG over time, thus representing a key driver of TB-related morbidity [39]. Results are also anticipated for a recently completed phase II/III trial on the efficacy and safety of VPM1002 in preventing pulmonary TB recurrence in exposed South Indian adults, the age demographic for which VPM1002 would likely have the greatest impact compared to BCG (NCT03152903).

5.2.1.2 *rBCG30*

rBCG30 was the first rBCG to be designed specifically to improve upon BCG and demonstrated improved immunogenicity in mice and guinea pig models. rBCG30 was modified to overexpress the immunodominant antigen 85B (Ag85B) encoded by *fbpB* genes and thought to stimulate IFN-γ secretion from CD4+ T-cells [40]. However, work on rBCG30 is currently paused as other more attenuated rBCG candidates proved more immunogenic [41]. Development of a separate vaccine candidate, AERAS-422, that combined the approaches of rBCG30 and VPM1002, was also terminated due to two adverse events, whereby varicella-zoster virus was activated in otherwise healthy patients [42].

5.2.1.3 *BCGΔzmp1*

BCGΔzmp1 is an rBCG in which deletion of the *Rv0198c* gene leads to deficiency of zinc metalloprotease 1 (Zmp1), resulting in enhanced phagosome maturation. When activated and overexpressed, Zmp1 prevents inflammasome activation in infected cells by inhibiting both caspase 1 and IL-1β activities. Deletion of the *Rv0198c* gene is thought to restrict the activation of Zmp1, thus enhancing bacterial processing and antigen presentation [43]. *BCGΔzmp1* has been tested in both healthy and immunocompromised mice as well as guinea pig and bovine models, in which it was well-tolerated even in immunocompromised conditions and demonstrated improved immunogenicity compared with BCG [44].

5.2.1.4 *BCGΔBCG1419c*

BCGΔBCG1419c is a separate deletion-based rBCG with the removal of the *BCG1419c* gene that has resulted in intentionally attenuated intracellular replication in murine macrophages and changes to the expression of its antigenic proteins [45]. This is likely mediated by the possible role of *BCG1419c* in the pellicle mode of growth of *M.tb* that has been equated to an "*in vitro* biofilm" that allows *M.tb* to persist within the host [46]. In C57BL/6 mice, *BCGΔBCG1419c* vaccination is associated with reduced lung pathology and IL-6 levels compared with its BCG Pasteur parent strain. A reduction in TNF-α and IL-10 production has also been observed in *BCGΔBCG1419c*-vaccinated mice compared with nonvaccinated controls at 6 months following *M.tb* challenge [47]. In another study, *BCGΔBCG1419c* showed improved induction of memory T-cells following intratracheal vaccination in mice compared to BCG, and subsequent challenge studies resulted in lower bacterial loads in the spleen and lungs of those vaccinated mice, particularly at 120 days post-infection [48]. Early assessments of *BCGΔBCG1419c* in alternative guinea pig models indicate transient reductions of the hematogenous spread of *M.tb* to the spleen while conferring equivalent protection in the lungs as measured by histopathology. Taken in combination, these studies suggest further investigations into the potential benefits of *BCGΔBCG1419c* are likely warranted [49].

5.2.1.5 ESX-1 Inclusion rBCG

Contrary to the above-described rBCGs that are based on gene deletions, several rBCG candidates have been constructed by re-inserting and enhancing the synthesis of specific proteins, such as the ESAT-6 protein family secretion system-1 (ESX-1) that comprises much of the RD1 region that was originally lost. However, a difficulty with such recombinants is that although the family of *BCG::RD1* strains are clearly more immunogenic than BCG in animal models, they may be less safe and are often associated with prolonged persistence and increased virulence in immunocompromised hosts [50]. A recent study that systematically compared 24 different vaccination approaches using three BCG strains and a variety of delivery combinations determined that two doses of parenteral *BCG::RD1* expressing ESX-1 *M.tb* antigens demonstrated the greatest efficacy against *M.tb* challenge in murine models and appears a promising approach provided it can maintain a safety profile similar to BCG [51]. Fully functional ESAT-6 protein seems to be required not only for the noncognate production of IFN-γ *in vivo* but also for the generation of a robust T-cell (including TRM) response against ESX-1-secreted effectors.

To avoid the safety difficulties associated with ESX-1 while retaining its immunogenic effects, the candidate vaccine *BCG::ESAT6-PE25SS* was designed such that it secretes full-length ESAT-6 via the ESX-5 secretion system. This recombination strategy has several advantages including the induction of ESAT-6-specific T-cells and conferred protection against TB but retains lower virulence and a more robust safety profile in both immunocompetent and immunocompromised animal hosts, as ESX-5 was retained in traditional BCG [52]. Additionally, compared with both *BCG::ESX1Mtb* and parental BCG, the mucosal administration of *BCG::ESAT6-PE25SS* seems to be associated with more rapid clearance of *M.tb* in the lungs of infected mice [45]. Other ESX-related rBCGs such as *BCG::ESAT-L28A/L29S* have also shown promise in guinea pig models of subcutaneous vaccination [53]. In combination, the ESX family of insertion rBCGs warrant further development (possibly via mucosal or novel routes of delivery) but have yet to be tested in human clinical trials.

5.2.1.6 *BCGΔsapM*

The rBCG candidate *BCGΔsapM* was created by the removal of secreted acid phosphatase *SapM* with additional capping of the cell wall lipoarabinomannan with a-1,2-oligomannosides (ManLAM). *SapM* was initially selected for deletion within an rBCG as it is implicated in the continuous removal of phosphatidylinositol-3-phosphate (PI3P) from the membranes of phagosomes surrounding mycobacteria, ultimately reducing the fusion with late endosomes and contributing to the blocking of phagosome maturation [54]. In initial guinea pig models, deletion of *sapM*, as expected, produced increased maturation of *M.tb*-containing phagosomes in THP-1 cells and decreased virulence [55]. However, in separate mouse trials, *BCGΔsapM* inoculation had no effect on stopping phagosome maturation in murine macrophages but still showed improved long-term protection against TB and improved survival rates, likely mediated by the enhancement of dendritic cell activation and migration to the relevant lymph nodes. Subsequent research has also demonstrated that *BCGΔsapM* is equally as safe as BCG in severely immunocompromised SCID mice lacking both T- and B-cells, an important hurdle to overcome prior to progression to human clinical trials [56]. Further studies of cytokine excretion and T-cell subtyping are required to characterize the precise effects of *BCGΔsapM* in improving both innate and adaptive immunity, as are human trials demonstrating efficacy. Nonetheless, these findings suggest that an rBCG candidate that performs better than BCG in mice may be produced using only further attenuations to BCG itself.

5.2.2 Alternative Routes of BCG Administration

Calmette and Guérin's early vaccine strains were initially administered orally, although *M.tb* is primarily transmitted via inhaled aerosol droplets invading alveolar sacs in the lungs [57]. Remarkably, the inhaled aerosol route of delivery was tested by Calmette himself as early as the 1920s, using an apparatus of his own construction, and oral routes of delivery were in use well into the 1960s [1]. Intradermal (ID) administration, now the standard route of BCG delivery, was first popularized in Scandinavia in the 1930s [58]. Recently, there has been renewed interest in alternative methods of delivering BCG, as aerosol routes more closely resemble the natural route of infection and pathogenesis of *M.tb*, while oral delivery is more convenient for some groups such as young children and avoids risk of transmission of blood-borne infections such as hepatitis or HIV via needlestick injury, although it may carry a slightly higher risk of cervical lymphadenitis and other systemic complications [59]. Additionally, intravenous (IV)-delivered BCG, although unlikely to be feasible for widespread use across large infant populations, has been described since the 1970s to confer greatly improved efficacy outcomes over conventional BCG in animal models and represents an important model to help identify immune correlates or biomarkers of protection from TB [60].

Two ongoing phase I clinical trials (NCT02709278 and NCT03912207) aim to determine the safety and efficacy of the BCG vaccine administered by the inhaled aerosol route in healthy, BCG naive adults as well as BCG-vaccinated UK adults. These follow several trials that have successfully demonstrated improved immunogenicity in non-human primates (NHPs), with many using novel portable vibrating mesh nebulizers (VMNs) that have the potential to be widely disseminated in future vaccine campaigns worldwide [61, 62]. Notably, pathology measured in extrapulmonary tissues of rhesus macaques following M.tb challenge was significantly reduced in animals that received aerosol BCG compared to animals that received ID BCG. A separate trial recently directly compared IV delivery to aerosol and ID routes, as well as combined aerosol/ID regimens in rhesus macaques, finding that IV delivery strongly outperforms all other alternatives in terms of pathology scores, likely mediated by increased production of antigen-responsive CD4+ T-cells [63]. This follows an earlier study by Sharpe et al. comparing NHPs vaccinated with standard ID BCG compared to those that received ID BCG followed by an intratracheal (IT) boost, or IV BCG [60]. Taken in combination, these trials in NHPs provide strong signals that alternative delivery methods could improve upon standard

ID BCG, but definitive conclusions about the efficacy, safety, and feasibility of such alternatives in common clinical practice remain to be determined and will require further research in larger phase II/III trials.

5.3 Boosting BCG

5.3.1 BCG Revaccination

It is widely accepted that the protection that BCG confers against pulmonary TB generally wanes over time; a large 132-study systematic review and meta-analysis determined that, although often still measurable, a significant degree of protection is likely lost 10–15 years after initial vaccination [64]. What is less clear is whether revaccination with BCG in adolescents and adults could reverse this decline and prolong protection. One large (>100,000 children) cluster-randomized trial of revaccination in Brazilian 7–14-year-olds found no significant improvement in efficacy following BCG revaccination [65]. A separate large (46,000 participants) double-blind, randomized, and placebo-controlled trial in a broader range of age groups (3 months–70 years) in Malawi also found no efficacy of revaccination, although notably in a community for which neonatal BCG itself also seemed to have limited effects [66, 67]. However, neither of these trials measured the *M.tb* or HIV infection status of participants at the outset or tested for previous infections or sensitization events. Similar cohort trials in Hong Kong and Scandinavia have also suggested no benefits to BCG revaccination [68, 69].

However, more recent data have contradicted these results. In a randomized controlled trial of 990 HIV-negative adolescents in a TB-endemic area neonatally vaccinated with BCG who were demonstrably quantiferon-negative, a portion were assigned to receive BCG vaccination or the H4:IC31 subunit vaccine. Those receiving BCG revaccination were significantly less likely to show sustained quantiferon conversion following their second vaccination over the subsequent 2 years [70]. Smaller trials aimed at elucidating the possible immune correlates of protection conferred by revaccination suggest that this effect is likely mediated at least in part by upregulated CD4+ T-cell responses or enhanced trained immunity mechanisms [71, 72]. Looking back toward older community-based trials in India, others have also identified modest revaccination benefits in the data that were not noted at the time [73]. Finally, a recent randomized control trial of 200 healthy adults vaccinated at birth given either BCG revaccination or a control indicated that revaccination improves immunogenicity via enhanced polyfunctional Th1/Th17 and innate effectors, regardless of previous *M.tb* pre-infection status [74]. In the latest trial in QFT–test negative, HIV-negative adolescents, BCG did not provide protection from sustained M.tb infection [75]. Ultimately, further investigations into the possible immunostimulatory effects of BCG revaccination (undertaken with careful consideration of the bias effects generated by previous *M.tb* exposure or local prevalence) will be required across a variety of populations to better understand the conflicting results to date.

5.3.2 Heterologous Prime-Boost

An alternative approach is to continue the administration of BCG at birth and develop a heterologous vaccine to be given at a later time (either in infancy shortly after BCG or in adolescence prior to the rise in TB incidence that occurs in young adulthood) to boost the primed immune response. Such booster vaccines generally comprise one or more *M.tb* antigens combined with either an adjuvant or a recombinant vector delivery system. Importantly, selected antigens must be present in all strains of BCG and show limited variability across circulating M.tb strains if the booster vaccines are to be globally applicable [76].

5.3.2.1 Protein/Adjuvant Vaccine Candidates

Protein subunit vaccines may be a safer and therefore more attractive alternative to live attenuated vaccines. However, a key challenge is induction of sufficient immunogenicity, generally requiring the addition of an adjuvant. Optimal antigen and adjuvant selection are particularly challenging for TB given the lack of validated immune correlates of protection, the multitude of pathogen immune evasion strategies, and the complex clinical manifestations of *M.tb* infection. One approach is the fusion of immunodominant antigens from different stages of infection in the development of multistage subunit vaccines [77].

Leading protein/adjuvant vaccine candidates that are already well-progressed along the clinical pipeline include M72/AS01$_E$ (composed of Mtb32A and Mtb39A immunogenic fusion proteins, with AS01$_E$ as an adjuvant) [78] and ID93 + GLA-SE (composed of Rv2608, Rv2619, Rv3620 and Rv1813 antigens with GLA-SE adjuvant) [79]. H56:IC31 (formed by Ag85B, ESAT-6 and Rv2660c protein fusion antigens with the adjuvant IC31) [71] recently entered a phase IIb double-blind randomized placebo-controlled trial in South Africa and Tanzania, but primary analysis showed that it did not protect against TB recurrence, leading to the discontinuation of development by Statens Serum Institute (SSI), Denmark. GamTBvac, which combines ESAT-6, CFP10, and Ag85A antigens with the novel adjuvant dextran/CpG, is currently in phase III trials to evaluate protective efficacy [80]. AEC/BC02, developed by Anhui Zhifei Longcom, is made from the Ag85B and ESAT-6-CFP-10 proteins and the complex adjuvant system (BC02) composed of cytosine guanine dinucleotide (BCG-cpg-DNA) and aluminum hydroxide of BCG and is currently in phase IIa [81].

H107/CAF01

H107/CAF01 is a recombinant protein subunit candidate vaccine developed by Statens Serum Institut (SSI) in Denmark, designed for co-administration with BCG to complement immunogenicity and efficacy [82]. The earlier construct of H107 consisted of eight *M.tb* proteins: PPE68, ESAT-6, EspI, EspC, EspA, MPT64, MPT70, and MPT83, formulated in a liposome-based Cationic Adjuvant Formulation 1 (CAF01). These proteins are absent or are expressed at very low levels in all BCG vaccine strains. H107/CAF01 replaced its predecessors H64/CAF01 and H74/CAF01. H64/CAF01 consisted of the *M.tb* antigens EsxA, EspD, EspC, EspF,

EspR, and PE35, whereas H74/CAF01 consisted of EspB, EsxA, EspD, EspC, EspA, and EspR, both formulated in CAF01 adjuvant [83].

CB6F1 and B6C3F1 mice vaccinated with three doses of H107 (subcutaneously, intravenously, and intradermally, biweekly) controlled *M.tb* growth following challenge to a similar extent as those vaccinated with BCG alone but significantly better than mice vaccinated with saline (control) [82]. H107 was then assessed for the inhibition of BCG colonization, which could render it unsuitable for co-administration with BCG. Mice vaccinated with H107, followed by BCG had BCG colony-forming unit (CFU) counts similar to mice given saline. However, mice vaccinated with either H4 (composed of Ag85B and TB10.4 antigens present in both *M.tb* and BCG) or H65 (composed of EsxD, EsxC, EsxG, TB10.4, EsxW, and EsxV antigens present in both *M.tb* and BCG), followed by BCG had significantly lower BCG CFU counts than mice vaccinated with H107 or saline [82]. Co-administration of BCG + H107 significantly increased H107-specific CD4+ T-cell and antibody responses and BCG-specific CD4+ T-cell responses. CD4+ T-cells from mice vaccinated with BCG + H107 produced IFN-γ, IL-2, and IL-17, whereas those from mice vaccinated with BCG alone produced mainly IFN-γ and TNF. Additionally, mice vaccinated with BCG + H107 had better control of *M.tb* growth compared to mice vaccinated with BCG alone, H107 alone, or saline [82]. H107 is currently in Phase I clinical trials.

LT70

LT70 is composed of a fusion protein of four *M.tb*-specific proteins, ESAT-6, Ag85B, MPT64, and M.tb8.4, expressed during active replication and growth, as well as two dormancy-related proteins, HSPX and Rv2626c, formulated in a combination of dimethyldioctadecylammonium (DDA) and Poly I:C adjuvant [84]. DDA is a cationic liposome that aids in the delivery of vaccine antigens to the membrane of antigen-presenting cells for uptake, processing, and presentation to T-cells [85]. Poly I:C is a synthetic double-stranded RNA polyriboisosinic:polyribocytidy lic acid which is a potent inducer of Th1 cytokine and CD8+ T-cell responses following recognition by toll-like receptor 3 (TLR3) [86].

LT70 was developed at Lanzhou University, China. When evaluated in C57BL/6 mice, it induced significantly higher IFN-γ responses to ESAT-6, Ag85B, and PPD compared to mice vaccinated with BCG, a fusion protein of ESAT-6-Ag85B-MPT64-Mtb8.4-Mtb10.4-HSPX, or PBS (control) [84]. It also induced significantly higher IgG1 and IgG2c antibody levels to Ag85B and Rv2626c than mice vaccinated with BCG or PBS. Following the challenge of C57BL/6 mice with 50–100 CFU of *M.tb* H37Rv by inhalation, mice prevaccinated with LT70 had a significantly lower bacterial burden in the lung compared to mice prevaccinated with BCG, a fusion protein of ESAT-6-Ag85B-MPT64-Mtb8.4-Mtb10.4-HSPX, or PBS [84]. Priming of C57BL/6 mice with BCG and later boosting with LT70 resulted in significantly higher IFN-γ and IgG1 and IgG2c antibody responses than mice immunized with BCG alone without boosting. Similarly, mice primed with BCG and boosted with LT70 and later challenged with *M.tb* H37Rv by inhalation had a significantly lower bacterial burden in the lungs and spleen and smaller lesions than mice vaccinated with PBS [84].

CysVac2/Advax

CysVac2/Advax, developed at the University of Sydney, Australia, consists of two *M.tb*-specific proteins CysD and Ag85B expressed in *E.coli* as a single fusion protein [87]. CysD (adenylyl transferase) is expressed throughout the course of *M.tb* infection but more strongly during the chronic phase of infection [88]. Both CysD and CysN (GTPase) are core components of a multifunctional enzyme complex ATP sulfurylase which plays significant roles in the assimilation of sulfur from the environment [89]. The resultant sulfur metabolites such as sulfolipids and mycothiol support persistence of *M.tb* in its niches by inhibiting phagosome-lysosome fusion and by shielding from antibiotics and toxic oxidants, respectively [89]. Ag85B on the other hand is a member of the mycolyltransferase Ag85 complex which plays a significant role in the synthesis of mycobacterial cell wall [90]. It is highly expressed during acute stages of *M.tb* infection, but it induces long-lasting memory responses which can be detected during the chronic stages of infection [88].

The initial CysVac2 construct was formulated in an adjuvant comprising monophosphoryl lipid A, TLR4 agonist, and a synthetic surfactant, dimethyl dioctadecyl ammonium bromide (MPL-DDA), a combination that is a potent inducer of Th1 responses [88, 91]. When tested in C57BL/6 mice, CysVac2/MPL-DDA (subcutaneous administration, triple dose) vaccination pre- and post-aerosol *M.tb* challenge induced significantly higher triple functional IFN-γ+ IL2+ TNF+ and dual functional IFN-γ+ TNF+ or IL2+ TNF+ and IL17+ CD4+ T-cell responses compared with BCG Pasteur which mostly induced single positive IFN-γ+ CD4+ T-cells [88]. Subsequently, mice vaccinated with CysVac2/MPL-DDA pre- and post-*M.tb* challenge had better control of bacterial burden in the lungs than mice vaccinated with BCG or unvaccinated mice (control). Protection against *M.tb* in the lungs was significantly improved when CysVac2/MPL-DDA was used as a boost to BCG Pasteur, as these mice had a significantly lower bacterial burden compared to their counterparts vaccinated with BCG + MPL-DDA or MPL-DDA alone (control) [88].

Due to the high reactogenicity and instability associated with the MPL-DDA adjuvant, it was replaced with $\text{Advax}^{\text{CpG}}$ [92]. Intratracheal, and to a lesser extent intramuscular, vaccination with CysVac2/ $\text{Advax}^{\text{CpG}}$ of C57BL/6 mice yielded a similar immunogenicity and efficacy profile as CysVac2/MPL-DDA [87, 92] .

CFMO-DMT

CMFO-DMT, developed at Huazhong University of Science and Technology, China, consists of four recombinant mycobacterial antigens: Rv0577, Rv2875, Rv3044, and Rv2073c expressed as a single protein (designated CMFO) in *E.coli* and formulated in DMT adjuvant [93]. Subcutaneous administration of CMFO-DMT in C57BL/6 mice biweekly conferred superior control of *M.tb* growth in the spleen and lungs and reduced lung pathology compared with mice vaccinated with saline (control), DMT adjuvant or alternative candidate vaccines comprising CTT3H (CFP10-TB10.4-TB8.4-Rv3615c-HBHA), or A1D4 (Rv1813-Rv2660c-Ag85B-Rv2623-HspX) mycobacterial proteins. The protection conferred by CMFO-DMT alone was similar to that conferred by BCG China [93]. In terms of immune responses, CMFO-DMT alone induced significantly higher CMFO-specific antibody responses, Th1, and CD8+ T-cell responses than BCG. Priming mice with BCG, challenging them with *M.tb* H37RV intranasally 4 weeks later, and then boosting with CMFO-DMT achieved sterile immunity in the spleen, and these mice had the lowest bacterial load in the lungs compared to their counterparts boosted with either saline, DMT, BCG or CTT3H, and A1D4 [93].

5.3.2.2 Recombinant Vector Vaccine Candidates

An alternative strategy of delivering antigens to the host is using a vector engineered to express one or more genes from the pathogen of interest. Vectored vaccines usually employ live attenuated replication-deficient viruses such as adenoviruses, poxviruses, herpesviruses, and lentiviruses that express foreign antigen under the control of an exogenous promoter [94]. They offer several advantages over other subunit vaccine approaches, including inducing robust and long-lasting immune responses without the need for an adjuvant. Use of a replicating vector can mimic natural infection, resulting in the induction of cytokines and co-stimulatory molecules that provide a potent adjuvant effect [94].

A number of promising viral-vectored vaccines for TB have been described. Recombinant replication-deficient Modified Vaccinia Ankara (MVA) expressing Ag85A (MVA85A) was the first prophylactic TB vaccine candidate to be evaluated in a phase 2b efficacy trial, but results showed it did not improve upon the efficacy of BCG in South African infants [95]. Another replication-deficient vector, Chimpanzee Adenovirus-vectored Oxford 1 (ChAdOx1), which demonstrated promise as a vector for the AZD1222 (ChAdOx1 nCoV-19) Covid-19 vaccine [96], has since been modified to express Ag85A and used in combination with MVA85A, and a ChAdOx1.85A prime-MVA85A boost regime was well-tolerated and immunogenic in healthy UK adults [97]. Preclinically, ChAdOx1.85A-MVA85A has been shown to be consistently protective, and ChAdOx1.PPE15 (encoding both Ag85A and PPE15 antigens) confers superior protection to BCG alone in mice [98, 99]. Developed by McMaster University and CanSino, Ad5 Ag85A is a human adenovirus type 5 vector expressing Ag85A. It has demonstrated enhanced efficacy over BCG in preclinical studies and demonstrated safety in humans by the intramuscular route with potent stimulation of polyfunctional T-cell responses [100].

ChAdOx1.5Ag/MVA.5Ag

The ChAdOx1.5Ag/MVA.5Ag regime, developed at the University of Oxford UK, consists of recombinant replication-deficient prime-Chimpanzee adenovirus (ChAdOx1) and boost-MVA vectors, both expressing a fusion of Ag85A with four Esx-5a antigens: PE8, PPE-15, EsxI, and EsxJ [101]. Ag85A is a member of the mycolyltransferase Antigen 85 complex also comprising Ag85B and Ag85C. The Ag85 complex plays a significant role in the synthesis of the mycobacterial cell wall, attaching long-chain mycolic acids to arabinogalactan polysaccharides, both core components of the cell wall structure together with peptidoglycans [90]. It also catalyzes the formation of trehalose dimycolate (TDM), cord factor, which is a key virulence factor of *M.tb* [90, 102]. The Esx-5 system plays significant roles in the secretion of *M.tb* proteins (including PE/PPE proteins) and in the activation of the inflammasome [103, 104].

Evaluation of the ChAdOx1.5Ag/MVA.5Ag regime in a murine model (CB6F1 female mice) has been completed [101]. Immunogenicity of both Ag85A and PPE15 is well-established [99]. Therefore, in the murine study for the ChAdOx/MVA.5Ag prime–boost regime, the three new Esx-5a antigens EsxI, EsxJ, and PE8 were assessed for their immunogenicity and efficacy, first individually and then as a fusion protein together with PPE15 and Ag85A. Intradermal and intranasal ChAdOx1.esxI induced the highest IFN-γ ELISpot response and CD4+ and CD8+ T-cell responses, followed by ChAdOx1.PE8. ChAdOx1.esxJ was the least immunogenic construct [101].

Each of the five antigens in the ChAdOx/MVA.5Ag regime was also assessed for its ability to boost BCG-specific immunogenicity and efficacy. Mice vaccinated ID with BCG Pasteur, followed by ChAdOx1 expressing all five antigens (ChAdOx1.5Ag) showed superior control of *M.tb* growth in the lungs and spleen compared to naïve controls or those receiving BCG alone or BCG + ChAdOx1 expressing any of the individual antigens alone [101]. Given the significant boosting of immunogenicity and efficacy observed with intradermal MVA85A following BCG-ChAdOx1.85A [97, 98, 105], boosting of BCG-ChAdOx1.5Ag with MVA expressing all five antigens (MVA.5Ag) was also assessed. Mice vaccinated with BCG, followed by ChAdOx1.5Ag (intranasally) and MVA.5Ag (intradermally) had significantly higher cellular and humoral responses and enhanced control of *M.tb* growth compared with naïve controls or mice vaccinated with BCG alone [101]. Studies evaluating BCG with ChAdOx.5Ag/MVA.5Ag in NHPs are ongoing.

Tri:ChAd:TB

Tri:ChAd:TB, developed at McMaster University, Canada, consists of a chimpanzee adenovirus serotype 68 vector expressing Ag85A, TB10.4, and RpfB as a single transcript. It is a combination of *M.tb* proteins expressed at different stages over the course of infection: Ag85A expressed during acute active infection, TB10.4 expressed throughout infection, and resuscitation-promoting factor B (RpfB) expressed during latency or dormancy [106]. So far, immunogenicity, efficacy, and immunotherapeutic potential of Tri:ChAd:TB have been assessed in *M.tb*-resistant BALB/c mice, *M.tb*-susceptible C3HeB/FeJ mice, and humanized mice.

Regarding immunogenicity, intranasal administration of Tri:ChAd:TB in BALB/c mice induced significantly higher CD8+ T-cell IFN-γ responses than CD4+ T-cell IFN-γ responses to Ag85A, TB10.4, and RpfB in both bronchoalveolar lavage and lung parenchymal tissue assessed 2 weeks post-vaccination. However, both CD8+ and CD4+ T-cell IFN-γ responses were significantly higher in BALB/c mice vaccinated with Tri:ChAd:TB than mice vaccinated with Mono:ChAd:TB consisting of only Ag85A. While the strongest CD8+ T-cell IFN-γ responses observed at 2 weeks post Tri:ChAd:TB vaccination were Ag85A-specific, at 6 weeks post-vaccination, the majority of the CD8+ T-cell IFN-γ responses detected were TB10.4-specific [106].

BALB/c and C3HeB/FeJ mice primed with BCG (subcutaneously) and boosted with Tri:ChAd:TB (intranasally) 4 weeks later had significantly higher BCG-specific and Ag85A-TB10.4-RpfB- specific CD4+ and CD8+ T-cell responses in the bronchoalveolar lavage (BAL) fluid and lung tissue compared to their counterparts boosted with Mono:ChAd:TB or mice given BCG alone. Similarly, BCG-vaccinated BALB/c and C3HeB/FeJ mice boosted with Tri:ChAd:TB had significantly superior control of actively replicating and dormant (persister) *M.tb* and reduced lung immunopathology compared to their counterparts vaccinated with BCG alone, Mono:ChAd:TB alone, Tri:ChAd:TB alone, or BCG + Mono:ChAd:T B. Additionally, superior control of bacterial burden in the lung, protection against weight loss, and reduced lung immunopathology were also observed in humanized mice (irradiated OD-Rag1^{tm1Mom}Il2rg^{tm1Wjl} (NRG) mice reconstituted with CD34+ hematopoietic stem cells from human cord blood) vaccinated with Tri:ChAd:TB alone in comparison to their unvaccinated counterparts [106].

To investigate the immunotherapeutic potential of Tri:ChAd:TB, BALB/c mice were first infected with *M.tb* H37Rv by inhalation, treated with antibiotics orally for 4 weeks, and then immunized with either Tri:ChAd:TB, Mono:ChAd:TB or no vaccination (control). In comparison to controls or BALB/c mice immunized with Mono:ChAd:TB, immunotherapy with Tri:ChAd:TB in addition to the antibiotics significantly reduced bacterial burden in the lungs [106].

RhCMV/TB

RhCMV/TB consists of a replication-competent Rhesus cytomegalovirus (CMV) viral vector expressing a set of nine *M.tb* proteins: ESAT-6, Ag85A, and Ag85B expressed during the active phase of *M.tb* growth; Rv3407, Rv1733, and Rv2626 expressed during latency; and Rpf A, Rpf C, and Rpf D expressed during reactivation [107].

When tested in RhCMV+ rhesus macaques (RM), RhCMV/TB alone (subcutaneous administration) induced significantly higher *M.tb*-specific CD4+ and CD8+ T-cell responses to all the vaccine-insert antigens compared to BCG alone, a combination of BCG (ID) + RhCMV/TB (subcutaneous administration), and no vaccination (control). The CD4+ and CD8+ T-cell responses in RhCMV/TB-vaccinated and BCG + RhCMV/TB-vaccinated RMs were more differentiated, i.e., of the effector memory phenotype producing mostly IFN-γ and TNF and low levels of IL-2. BCG alone induced less differentiated central memory CD4+ T-cell responses producing either TNF or IL-2 and more differentiated effector memory CD8+ T-cell responses producing either TNF or IFN-γ [107]. Surprisingly, following the challenge of these vaccinated animals with *M.tb* Erdman (25 CFUs per animal) intrabronchially, there was no significant difference in the magnitude of T-cell responses to any of the nine vaccine insert antigens between the vaccinated and unvaccinated RMs. However, the extent of pulmonary and extrapulmonary disease in the majority of the RhCMV/TB-vaccinated RMs was mild, characterized by a low lesion volume, low pathology score, and *M.tb* recovery by culture of lung-punch biopsies, lymph nodes, and samples from the trachea [107]. BCG alone, BCG + RhCMV/TB-vaccinated, and unvaccinated RMs developed severe pulmonary and extrapulmonary TB disease. RhCMV/TB prevented *M.tb* infection in >40% of the challenged RMs [107].

Given the nadir of the IgG1 response to all of the vaccine insert antigens following vaccination, the superior control of TB, especially in RhCMV/TB-vaccinated RMs, may have been orchestrated by innate immune mechanisms. Indeed, transcriptional analysis of blood samples from RMs post-vaccination and prior to *M.tb* challenge showed that RhCMV/TB-vaccinated RMs in comparison to BCG + RhCMV/TB-vaccinated or unvaccinated RMs had an increased expression of genes for neutrophil degranulation and innate immune functions, which was associated with enhanced control of TB [107].

Novel Vectors

Due to the potentially derailing impact of pre-existing antivector immunity on the immunogenicity of adenovirus-vectored candidate TB vaccines, several alternative viral and bacterial vectors have been explored. Novel viral vectors include lentivirus-based vectors expressing Ag85A or ESAT-6 singly or in combination (LV-AEG/SVGmu), Sendai virus vector expressing Ag85A and Ag85B, vesicular stomatitis virus vector expressing Rv3615c, M.tb 10.4, and Rv2660c as a single fusion protein, and human parainfluenza virus type 2 and 5 vectors expressing Ag85A or Ag85B [108]. The lentivector expressing nuclear factor-B activator vFLIP and Ag85A (LV vF/85A) induced stronger CD8+ than CD4+ T-cell responses in the lungs and spleens of BALB/c mice, but this construct failed to boost BCG-mediated immunity, and mice vaccinated with BCG had better control of *M.tb* growth compared to their counterparts vaccinated with LV vF/85A. Therefore, this construct was deemed unsuitable for use as a BCG-boosting regimen [109]. On the other hand, foot pad injection of BALB/c mice with the recombinant lentivirus expressing Ag85A and ESAT-6 fused with a dendritic cell target antigen (LV-AEG/SVGmu) induced significantly higher antibody and T-cell responses compared to BCG vaccination, although the capacity of this formulation to boost BCG-mediated immunity was not evaluated [110].

Sendai virus (also known as murine parainfluenza type 1 or murine respirovirus) causes respiratory tract infections in rodents but is not known to cause similar infections in humans. Therefore, its use as a vector for vaccines intended for humans could avoid potential issues around pre-existing antivector immunity. At 8 weeks post-vaccination, mice vaccinated with Sendai virus expressing both Ag85A and Ag85B (SeV85AB, administered intranasally) had significantly higher CD8+ T-cell responses but similar CD4+ T-cell responses and protection from *M.tb* challenge to mice vaccinated with BCG (subcutaneous). Protection was significantly improved when mice were given a prior BCG prime and boosted with SeV85AB: this group had the lowest bacterial burden, reduced pathology, and lung inflammation compared to mice vaccinated with saline (control), BCG alone, and SeV85AB alone [111].

Vesicular stomatitis virus (VSV) is a zoonotic virus that predominantly infects horses, cattle, swine, and deer but can be transmitted to humans following exposure to infected animals. A recombinant VSV expressing Rv3615c,

M.tb 10.4, and Rv2660c as a single fusion protein conferred superior protection against *M.tb* challenge and more sustained CD4+ and CD8+ T-cell responses compared to BCG [112]. Human parainfluenza type 2 (HPIV2) and Parainfluenza type 5 (PIV5) virus-based vectors have also been explored due to their potential to infect a broad range of cell types and their preference for the mucosal system which is a natural route of entry for *M.tb*. Intranasal vaccination of mice with recombinant HPIV2 expressing Ag85B induced formation of inducible bronchus-associated lymphoid tissue (iBALT), which correlated with the enhanced IFN-γ + T-cell responses and IgA responses observed in these mice compared with mice vaccinated with saline. On the other hand, mice vaccinated with a BCG prime and boosted with either PIV5 expressing Ag85A or Ag85B had significantly higher antibody and cellular responses and better control of *M.tb* growth than mice vaccinated with saline [113].

Novel bacteria vectors being explored include the nonpathogenic *Lactobacillus plantarum* and the pathogenic *Listeria monocytogenes*. The *Lactobacillus plantarum* (Lp) formulations have included engineering to carry a plasmid encoding Ag85B and ESAT-6 fused with either a dendritic cell target antigen (Lp_DC construct) or *M.tb* heparin-binding hemagglutinin (Lp_HBHA construct) [114]. Both Lp_DC and Lp_HBHA formulations have been shown to activate human dendritic cells and murine dendritic cells and macrophages, marked by increased expression of the activation markers CD83, CD40, CD80, HLADR, PDL1, and PDL2, MHC molecules I and II, and proinflammatory cytokines IL-1β, IL-6, IL-12, and TNF, following stimulation of cells with the constructs. In terms of adaptive immunity and efficacy, both constructs conferred modest protection and modest T-cell and antibody responses in C57BL/6 mice which were significantly improved (especially for Lp_DC construct) when either constructs were administered as a boost following a prior BCG prime [114].

Given the pathogenic nature of *Listeria monocytogenes (Lm)*, the major virulence genes *actA* and *inlB* have been deleted to permit its safe use as a vector, and this construct further modified by substituting an amino acid in the positive regulatory factor A in order to enhance the vaccine efficacy. Vaccination of mice with recombinant *Lm* expressing a combination of Ag85B, TB10.4, ESAT-6, CFP-10, and MPT-64 significantly boosted BCG immunogenicity and efficacy [115].

5.4 Replacing BCG

5.4.1 Live Attenuated Vaccine Candidates

As noted, live attenuated vaccines such as BCG have a number of advantages over subunit vaccine approaches including the expression of a broader antigenic panel and the ability to replicate and persist, resulting in longer-lived antigenic stimulation. Thus, a range of other live attenuated mycobacterial strains, including *M.tb* itself, have been explored as TB vaccine candidates.

5.4.1.1 Live Attenuated *M.tb*

Vaccine candidates based on *M.tb* may be superior to BCG in their extent of antigenic similarity (given BCG lacks over 100 genes present in *M.tb*) and resemblance to natural infection [108]. However, safety remains a concern with the hypothetical potential for reversion to virulent ancestral phenotypes [116]. Thus, the TB community created the second Geneva consensus which requires at least two stable independent attenuating mutations for the progression of *M.tb* strains into clinical trials [117]. Furthermore, similar to rBCG strains containing ESX-1 or its secreted proteins, attenuated *M.tb* strains may present the challenge of cross-reactivity with IGRAs, leading to positive results and thus inability to distinguish infected from vaccinated individuals. One potential solution is the parallel development of novel diagnostic tools [116].

MTBVAC

MTBVAC is a live attenuated derivative of the clinical *M.tb* isolate Mt103. It was rationally attenuated through two independent stable genetic deletions in the *phoP* and *fadD26* genes which encode major virulence factors [118]. Mutants oversecrete major antigens such as the Ag85 complex and are unable to export the virulence factor ESAT-6, among other properties [119]. A robust safety profile of the doubly attenuated PhoP-/PDIM-deficient prototype SO2 was demonstrated in two SCID mouse models, with superior survival conferred than by BCG vaccination [120]. Further safety studies of MTBVAC were subsequently completed in mice and guinea pigs, as well as biodistribution and formal toxicity studies, with favorable outcomes [119]. Since 2001, there has been rigorous preclinical immunogenicity and efficacy assessment of MTBVAC in mice, guinea pigs, and NHPs. In all cases, MTBVAC has been shown to be comparable or superior to standard BCG vaccination [119]. Notably, in a high-dose challenge long-term survival experiment in guinea pigs, the prototype SO2 conferred 100% survival in guinea pigs compared with 33% survival in the BCG-vaccinated group, as well as a greater reduction in disease severity and lung and spleen bacterial burden [120, 121].

MTBVAC entered clinical trials in 2013, demonstrating safety and immunogenicity in a phase I double-blind randomized controlled dose-escalation trial in HIV-negative volunteers in Switzerland [122] and a phase Ib double-blind randomized dose-escalation trial in a region in South Africa with a high burden of TB [123]. The latter also demonstrated a peak Th1-type CD4+ T-cell response in the group receiving 2.5×10^5 CFU of MTBVAC that was higher than that of the group that received an equivalent dose of BCG. Interestingly dose-related IGRA conversion was noted in several of the MTBVAC-vaccinated infants including 78% of the group vaccinated with a dose of 2.5×10^5 CFU, although reversion occurred in three of the seven infants by day 360 post-vaccination [123]. Two additional clinical trials have also been recently completed in South Africa in adults with and without latent TB and in newborn infants (NCT02933281 and NCT03536117 respectively) and are awaiting results. A phase III trial is currently underway to evaluate efficacy, safety, and immunogenicity in newborn infants with and without HIV exposure at six sites within the TB-endemic regions of sub-Saharan Africa (NCT04975178).

The original MTBVAC is derived from a lineage 4 background, and phoP and fadD26 mutations have recently been generated in lineage 2 and lineage 3 backgrounds (MTBVAC-L2 and MTBVAC-L3, respectively) as comparators. The original MTBVAC demonstrated a superior safety profile in SCID mice with greater attenuation than BCG, while MTBVAC-L2 was less attenuated and MTBVAC-L3 showed an intermediate phenotype [124]. Following challenge with the L4 *M.tb* strain H37Rv, all vaccinated mice had similarly reduced lung bacterial burdens, while MTBVAC and MTBVAC-L2 conferred superior protection compared with BCG against the L2 strain W4-Beijing. MTBVAC and MTBVAC-L3 had the lowest bacterial burdens following challenge with the L3 strain HCU3524 [124]. The superior safety profile and lineage-independent efficacy observed with the original MTBVAC supports the promise of L4 live attenuated vaccines against TB.

Other Live Attenuated *M.tb* Vaccine Candidates

While single mutant vaccine candidates fail to meet the second Geneva consensus requirements [117] and may require further development to meet safety standards, they can be informative in suggesting which mutations could be taken forward into combinations. Mutations are selected based on the ability to attenuate *M.tb* and induce a more potent immune response. A key example is *M.tbΔsigH* based on the deletion of the major *M.tb* stress response factor Sigma H (SigH). This candidate is attenuated for pathology in mice and NHPs [125], and aerosol vaccination with *M.tbΔsigH* in NHPs elicits strong CD4+ and CD8+ central memory T-cell responses together with a robust Th1 response associated with significantly enhanced protection from lethal *M.tb* challenge [126]. Other single-mutant attenuated vaccine candidates showing promise in preclinical challenge studies include *M.tbΔlpqS* (based on deletion of the highly conserved lipoprotein LpqS) [127], *M.tbΔmosR* (based on deletion of the virulence factors and transcriptional repressor *mosR* that is induced during chronic infection) [128], and *M.tbΔechR* (based on deletion of echA7 which encodes a probable enoyl-CoA hydratase and is induced during the early stages of infection) [128]. Plans are underway to combine the latter two deletions in the same *M.tb* strain to reduce the chance of reversion to a virulent wild-type state [129].

In the design of vaccine candidates with multiple attenuating independent mutations, developers must ensure a balance between sufficient attenuation for safety and ability to induce a protective immune response [129]. By way of example, a single bioA mutant strain of *M.tb* was highly attenuated but conferred limited protection against TB in guinea pigs [130], while a triple mutant of mptpA, mptpB, and sapM (*M.tb Δmms*) conferred good levels of protection but caused pathological damage to the spleen [131]. A quadruple gene mutant (*M.tb Δmmsb)* based on the combination of these two strategies was highly attenuated but less protective than BCG [132]. One promising candidate is the unmarked double-mutant *M. tb ΔsigE ΔfadD26* which is significantly more attenuated in SCID mice compared to BCG and confers improved protection against challenge with an *M.tb* Harlem strain (but not a strain of the highly virulent *M.tb* Beijing) [133]. GC1237 Rv1503c::Tn*ΔphoPR* is derived from the *M.tb* Beijing strain G1237 and is inactivated in the Rv1502c gene, which is required for surface glycolipid synthesis, as well as the two-component global regulator *phoP-phoR*. It has demonstrated comparable virulence to BCG in SCID mice, but efficacy may be lineage-dependent with improved protection over BCG following challenge with *M.tb* HN878 but not *M.tb* H37Rv [134].

5.4.1.2 Naturally Attenuated Strains of Other Mycobacteria

Given that BCG likely confers protection to *M.tb* via cross-reactivity to shared antigens, other live avirulent strains of mycobacteria could serve to function in a similar manner. Vaccination of mice with *M. smegmatis*, *M. vaccae*, *M. terrae*, *M. phlei*, *M. trivial*, and *M. tb* H37Ra has been shown to induce differential immune responses, and all groups except *M. phlei* provided protection in the lung against challenge with *M.tb* H37Rv. The most significant protection was conferred by *M.tb* H37Ra and *M. vaccae*, which demonstrated similar efficacy to BCG vaccination [135]. Further study is required to determine the potential for such strains as vaccine candidates. *M. paragordonae* is a naturally temperature-sensitive mycobacterial species that is unable to grow at temperatures greater than 37 °C, thus limiting its ability to infect mammalian hosts. Its potential as a candidate for live vaccination against *M.tb* H37Ra and *M. abscessus* has been explored in mice, with a more protective immune response conferred following vaccination with *M. paragodonae* compared to BCG [136].

Similar to recombinant BCG strategies, naturally attenuated mycobacteria can be genetically modified in an attempt to enhance immunogenicity and efficacy. A recombinant *M. smegmatis* engineered to express a fusion protein of Ag85C, MPT-51, and HspX, known as mc^2-CMX, has been reported to induce an enhanced immune response against *M.tb* compared to BCG vaccination in mice, but lung lesion scores following *M.tb* challenge were similar between mc^2-CMX and BCG-vaccinated groups [137].

5.4.2 Inactivated Vaccine Candidates

Inactivated TB vaccines are composed of whole bacteria that have been killed or otherwise inactivated, or their cleavage fragments. They have several advantages in terms of safety, ease of production, and administration, and thus a number have been developed rapidly with several such vaccines currently in clinical trials and two approved for clinical use [138].

Killed whole cell mycobacteria vaccines include *Mycobacterium indicus pranii* (MIP), *Mycobacterium vaccae* (*M. vaccae*), and DAR-901. MIP is a heat-inactivated mycobacterial strain that has a good safety profile and demonstrated potential to clear *M.tb* in TB patients [139]. The anti-TB properties of *M. vaccae* have long been recognized, and a heat-killed preparation has potential utility as an immunotherapeutic adjunct to drug treatment of active pulmonary TB disease [140], for which it is now licenced for use in China. Results from a placebo-controlled phase III trial of a six-dose vaccination regimen for the prevention of TB disease are awaited

(NCT01979900). DAR-901 is a BCG booster vaccine manufactured from the same seed strain as SRL-172 using a new scalable method. It has demonstrated efficacy as a BCG booster in preclinical studies [141], but in a phase II prevention of infection clinical trial in Tanzania, a three-dose vaccination regime in adolescents previously vaccinated with BCG did not confer efficacy against initial or sustained IGRA conversion [142].

RUTI is composed of cell wall fragments of *M.tb* in a liposome suspension and intended as an immunotherapeutic agent to improve the efficacy and shorten the duration of drug therapy for active TB disease [143]. Both phase I and II trials have been completed, demonstrating safety and immunogenicity in healthy and latent TB-infected (LTBI) volunteers [143, 144], and current trials are focusing on using RUTI as an adjunct to treatment for multidrug-resistant TB (MDR-TB) [129].

5.4.3 Virus-Like Particles

Virus-like particles (VLPs) are nanoscale self-assembled structures of viral proteins that lack viral genetic material. They thus mimic the virus particle but are incapable of infecting host cells. They have several advantages over single protein or peptide subunit vaccines including more similar conformational epitopes to the original pathogen and ability to trigger potent cellular and humoral immune responses [145]. Drawbacks of VLPs include their complex and slow development process, high production cost, and potential for pre-existing antivector antibody responses in humans, although there is little evidence to support any influence on safety and immunogenicity [146]. A range of VLPs based on viruses including hepatitis B virus (HBV), human papilloma virus (HPV), parvovirus, and SV40 have been shown to effectively display foreign peptides and epitopes on their surface [147].

Krammer et al. have described the use of influenza A VLP as a scaffold to display a 20-amino acid sequence from *M.tb* ESAT-6. High serum antibody titers were detected against recombinant ESAT-6 following immunization of mice, demonstrating proof-of-concept for this approach in TB [147]. ESAT-6 has also been used in HBV-based VLPs, with the entire ESAT-6 protein inserted into HBV core (HBc) particles, eliciting a significantly higher ESAT-6-specific antibody and CD4+/CD8+ T-cell response in mice compared to immunization with the recombinant ESAT-6 protein alone [148]. Another HBc VLP bearing *M.tb* CFP-10 has been described, with humoral, cytokine, and splenocyte cell proliferation responses indicating good Th1 immunogenicity [149]. VLPs of HPV have been used as a carrier to insert *M.tb* Ag85B, inducing higher Ag85B-specific antibody responses and T-cell responses compared with recombinant Ag85B immunization in mice [150]. While some advances in the development of VLP-based TB vaccines have been made in recent years, as for subunit vaccines, selection of the optimal antigen(s) remains a major challenge [146].

5.4.4 DNA Vaccines

DNA vaccines consist of nucleic acids encoding antigens of interest that can be designed and optimized directly from pathogen sequences. Genetic material is translocated to the host cell nucleus where the gene(s) are transcribed and translated using the host cellular machinery [151]. DNA vaccines are known to induce strong and sustained cellular responses (which may be of particular relevance for protection against TB), have a high safety margin without any infectious agent, a simple production process, and a robust platform for large-scale production [151]. However, there are a number of drawbacks, including that they are prone to degradation, can have low expression in the human cell nucleus leading to low immunogenicity, have the potential to induce anti-DNA IgG in the host, and could interfere with host DNA [152].

Delivery methods include gene gun, microneedles, electroporation, nanoparticles, and pulmonary or needle-free skin delivery, although viral vectors are the most common method as they can easily infect host cells and exploit cellular molecular machinery to express the target genes and produce native-form antigens. A number of bacteria species have also been used to transfer vaccine plasmids into host cells and generate DNA-containing candidate vaccines, including FnBPA+pValac developed at the Instituto de Ciências Biológicas—Universidade Federal de Minas Gerais, Belo Horizonte, Brazil [153]. Initially, it consisted of *Lactococcus lactis* modified to express fibronectin-binding protein A (FnBPA) genes from *Staphylococcus aureus* and a pValac (vaccination using lactic acid bacteria) plasmid vector [154] carrying *M.tb* H37Rv ESAT-6. Given the nonpathogenic and noninvasive nature of *Lactococcus lactis*, its modification to express the FnBPA invasion genes enhances its invasion of, and internalization by, mammalian host cells [153].

Oral vaccination with FnBPA+pValac:ESAT-6 in BALB/c mice induced significantly higher ESAT-6-specific IFN-γ and secretory IgA responses in colon and fecal extracts compared to mice vaccinated with saline (control), noninvasive *L. lactis* MG1363, noninvasive *L. lactis* MG1363 + pValac:ESAT-6, and invasive *L. lactis* FnBPA (without pValac:ESAT-6). There was no significant difference in the TNF-α, IL-12, IL-10, and IL-4 cytokine responses or IgG, IgG1, and IgG2a antibody responses to recombinant ESAT-6 protein between any of the vaccination groups [153]. Priming of BALB/c mice with subcutaneous BCG, followed by the oral administration of FnBPA+pValac:ESAT-6 resulted in a significant increase in BCG-specific and ESAT-6-specific IFN-γ, IL-6, IL-17, and TNF-α cytokine responses. However, there was no significant boost in the ESAT-6-specific IgG1, IgG2a, and secretory IgA antibody responses [155].

When a construct with the replacement of ESAT-6 with Ag85A from *M.tb* H37Rv (FnBPA+pValac:Ag85A) was administered orally to C57BL/6 mice, there was a significantly higher systemic and mucosal IFN-γ, TNF, and IL-6 cytokine response as well as higher IgG and IgA antibody responses compared to mice vaccinated with saline or FnBPA+pValac not expressing Ag85A [155]. Combining both Ag85A and ESAT-6 in the FnBPA+pValac construct (FnBPA+pValac:e6Ag85A) and evaluating the construct orally in BALB/c mice showed significantly increased

ESAT-6-specific IFN-γ, TNF-α, IL-17, and secretory IgA responses in comparison to saline or FnBPA without pValac:e6Ag85A [156]. Ag85A-specific immune responses following the oral administration of FnBPA+pValac:e6Ag85A were not assessed. BCG-prime FnBPA+pValac:e6Ag85A-boost experiments have also not yet been reported at the time of writing.

A number of DNA vaccines encoding Ag85 complex proteins have been evaluated preclinically [157], as well as a divalent DNA construct encoding Ag85B and MPT64, indicating enhanced protection in mice compared with BCG vaccination or single DNA constructs [158]. A DNA construct encoding ESAT-6 and Ag85A fusion proteins has also been shown to enhance immunogenicity and efficacy in BCG-vaccinated mice [159]. Among other antigens, heat shock proteins including Hsp65 and Hsp70 have shown promise as DNA vaccine candidates in preclinical studies, as well as ESAT-6 and CFP-10 alone or in complex [157]. The only DNA-based TB vaccine to enter clinical trials at the time of writing, GX-70, was a therapeutic vaccine that was terminated due to safety concerns.

5.4.5 RNA Vaccines

The success of mRNA vaccines against COVID-19 has heralded a new era in vaccinology, providing proof-of-concept for this approach that may be widely applicable across disease types. There are two major types of RNA that may be used in vaccines: nonreplicating mRNA which encodes the antigen of interest and contains 5′ and 3’ UTRs and self-amplifying RNA which encodes the antigen of interest together with viral replication genes supporting intracellular RNA amplification and high levels of protein expression [160]. By utilizing the host cell to produce the antigen of interest, the likelihood of correct post-translational modification, folding, and functionality is increased compared with *in vitro* manufacture [161]. Furthermore, mRNA vaccines can be synthesized in a cell-free reaction and are simpler and faster to construct, manufacture, and purify than protein-based subunit vaccines [162]. Other advantages include cost-effectiveness, ability to encode any antigen, multiple antigens on a single mRNA, and avoidance of insertional mutagenesis in the host genome which is a potential risk with DNA vaccines [161].

The application of RNA vaccines in the field of TB is not new. In 2004, Xue et al. described an RNA encoding the *M.tb* MPT83 antigen that was capable of inducing specific humoral and cellular immune responses and conferred modest (less than BCG) but significant protection against *M.tb* challenge in the murine model [163]. Furthermore, an mRNA encoding the Hsp65 protein from *M.leprae* induced protection against *M.tb* challenge in mice following vaccination via the intranasal route [164]. Otherwise, almost two decades passed with little mention of RNA vaccine candidates in the TB literature, perhaps due to issues with stability (due to RNase sensitivity) and potent immunogenicity associated with adverse side-effects *in vivo*. Such obstacles have now been largely overcome [161]. BioNTech (Mainz, Germany) is currently evaluating the safety and immunogenicity of two investigational RNA-based vaccines (BNT164a1 and BNT164b1) in BCG-vaccinated volunteers in the phase I clinical trial (NCT05547464), although no preclinical results have yet been released at the time of writing.

Larsen et al. recently developed a novel VEE virus-based replicating RNA platform (repRNA) as both a homologous TB vaccine and a heterologous strategy to complement protein-adjuvant prophylactic vaccine candidates [165]. The rationale is that the replicating nature will result in longer antigen exposure more similar to replicating BCG than protein-adjuvant approaches, thus enhancing immune responses [166]. RepRNA vaccines have several advantages over mRNA vaccines including the requirement for ~1000-fold lower quantities, ability to induce immune responses after a single immunization, induction of Th1-biased T-cells as well as humoral immunity, and enhanced stability [165]. The second-generation TB vaccine candidate ID91 (encoding a fusion protein of Rv3619, Rv2389, Rv3478, and Rv1886) produced as a repRNA formulated in a nanostructured lipid carrier has been shown to elicit cellular and humoral responses and significantly reduce pulmonary burden in *M.tb*-challenged mice [162, 166].

In 2023, the WHO convened global experts to discuss the feasibility and potential value of mRNA-based TB vaccines [167]. A number of key challenges were raised including lack of consensus around how to rationally select antigens for mRNA vaccines, delays in late-stage clinical development due to the lack of correlates of protection from TB, low manufacturing capabilities in high-burden LMICs, the need for multiple TB vaccines, lack of consensus on vaccine composition, and vaccine acceptability and uptake [167]. Nonetheless, it was agreed that mRNA TB vaccines have a high degree of potential and unique advantages, and recommendations were made for the development of novel mRNA vaccines for TB including strengthening of commitments to address inequalities that may underlie delays in TB mRNA vaccine development, distribution, and access [167]. Notably, the report describes a new TCR-informed TB antigen (TITAN) mRNA vaccine development effort led by the University of Cape Town and University of Witwatersrand, generating mRNA vaccine constructs containing CFP-10, PE13, Wbbl1, and PPE18 and characterizing their immunogenicity and efficacy in mice [167].

5.5 Conclusions

This chapter has discussed the relative pros and cons of current strategies for improving, boosting, or replacing the BCG vaccine, together with study outcomes for the most promising candidates in the preclinical pipeline. Although it is currently unclear which, if any, of these strategies may ultimately progress to clinical use, there is reason to be optimistic that the current status quo of intradermal (ID) BCG, manufactured and delivered in approximately the same way for over a century, will see changes in the near future, despite the many ongoing challenges facing novel TB vaccine development.

Possible improvements to BCG include the development of recombinant BCG strains such as VPM1002 which facilitate enhanced antigen presentation through targeted deletions or additions to the BCG genome [34]. Alternative delivery methods may also improve the immunogenicity of common BCG formulations, particularly via inhaled aerosol droplets which replicate the natural route of *M.tb* infection [168]. BCG could also be improved by facilitating revaccination in specific populations who may benefit, or indeed from boosting BCG with other heterologous subunit vaccines in current development, such as those based on ChAdOx1.5Ag or Rhesus CMV vectors. Finally, traditional BCG could be replaced altogether with more immunogenic alternatives such as MTBVAC, a live attenuated *M.tb* vaccine candidate in phase III trials, or even advanced DNA or RNA vaccines that demonstrated their potential during the COVID-19 pandemic.

Further research, particularly large-scale randomized controlled trials in a variety of TB-endemic populations, will be required before efficacy can be fully demonstrated for any of these strategies and current BCG vaccination regimens replaced. It is also likely that any novel approach will first be implemented in specific population groups/cohorts and geographies for which there is both a demonstrated need and clearly improved efficacy before seeing widespread use. As a result, and rather remarkably, over a hundred years after its invention, Calmette and Guérin's humble BCG vaccine remains our best option for preventing TB in many vulnerable populations.

Competing Interests The author(s) has no competing interests to declare that are relevant to the content of this manuscript.

Ethics Approval The author(s) declares that this manuscript does not include primary research with human participants.

References

1. Gheorgiu M. Antituberculosis BCG vaccine: lessons from the past. In: History of vaccine development. New York: Springer; 2011. p. 47–55.
2. Calmette A. Preventive vaccination against tuberculosis with BCG. Proc R Soc Med. 1931;24:1481–90.
3. Lewis KN, Liao R, Guinn KM, Hickey MJ, Smith S, Behr MA, et al. Deletion of RD1 from Mycobacterium tuberculosis mimics bacille Calmette-Guerin attenuation. J Infect Dis. 2003;187:117–23.
4. Houben D, Demangel C, van Ingen J, Perez J, Baldeon L, Abdallah AM, et al. ESX-1-mediated translocation to the cytosol controls virulence of mycobacteria. Cell Microbiol. 2012;14:1287–98.
5. Brosch R, Gordon SV, Garnier T, Eiglmeier K, Frigui W, Valenti P, et al. Genome plasticity of BCG and impact on vaccine efficacy. Proc Natl Acad Sci USA. 2007;104:5596–601.
6. Favorov M, Ali M, Tursunbayeva A, Aitmagambetova I, Kilgore P, Ismailov S, et al. Comparative tuberculosis (TB) prevention effectiveness in children of Bacillus Calmette-Guerin (BCG) vaccines from different sources, Kazakhstan. PLoS One. 2012;7:e32567.
7. Scriba TJ, Netea MG, Ginsberg AM. Key recent advances in TB vaccine development and understanding of protective immune responses against Mycobacterium tuberculosis. Semin Immunol. 2020;50:101431.
8. Casanova J-L, Jouanguy E, Lamhamedi S, Blanche S, Fischer A. Immunological conditions of children with BCG disseminated infection. Lancet. 1995;346:581.

9. Trunz BB, Fine P, Dye C. Effect of BCG vaccination on childhood tuberculous meningitis and miliary tuberculosis worldwide: a meta-analysis and assessment of cost-effectiveness. Lancet. 2006;367:1173–80.
10. Rodrigues LC, Diwan VK, Wheeler JG. Protective effect of BCG against tuberculous meningitis and miliary tuberculosis: a meta-analysis. Int J Epidemiol. 1993;22:1154–8.
11. Colditz GA, Brewer TF, Berkey CS, Wilson ME, Burdick E, Fineberg HV, et al. Efficacy of BCG vaccine in the prevention of tuberculosis. Meta-analysis of the published literature. JAMA. 1994;271:698–702.
12. Ponnighaus JM, Fine PE, Sterne JA, Wilson RJ, Msosa E, Gruer PJ, et al. Efficacy of BCG vaccine against leprosy and tuberculosis in northern Malawi. Lancet. 1992;339:636–9.
13. Lombardi C, Pedrazzani ES, Pedrazzani JC, Filho PF, Zicker F. Protective efficacy of BCG against leprosy in Sao Paulo. Bull Pan Am Health Organ. 1996;30:24–30.
14. Merle CS, Cunha SS, Rodrigues LC. BCG vaccination and leprosy protection: review of current evidence and status of BCG in leprosy control. Expert Rev Vaccines. 2010;9:209–22.
15. Setia MS, Steinmaus C, Ho CS, Rutherford GW. The role of BCG in prevention of leprosy: a meta-analysis. Lancet Infect Dis. 2006;6:162–70.
16. Smith PG, Revill WD, Lukwago E, Rykushin YP. The protective effect of BCG against Mycobacterium ulcerans disease: a controlled trial in an endemic area of Uganda. Trans R Soc Trop Med Hyg. 1976;70:449–57.
17. Noeske J, Kuaban C, Rondini S, Sorlin P, Ciaffi L, Mbuagbaw J, et al. Buruli ulcer disease in Cameroon rediscovered. Am J Trop Med Hyg. 2004;70:520–6.
18. de Bree LCJ, Koeken VACM, Joosten LAB, Aaby P, Benn CS, van Crevel R, et al. Non-specific effects of vaccines: current evidence and potential implications. Semin Immunol. 2018;39:35–43.
19. Prentice S, Nassanga B, Webb EL, Akello F, Kiwudhu F, Akurut H, et al. BCG-induced non-specific effects on heterologous infectious disease in Ugandan neonates: an investigator-blind randomised controlled trial. Lancet Infect Dis. 2021;21:993.
20. Tverdal A, Funnemark E. Protective effect of BCG vaccination in Norway 1956-73. Tubercle. 1988;69:119–23.
21. Hart PD, Sutherland I. BCG and vole bacillus vaccines in the prevention of tuberculosis in adolescence and early adult life. Br Med J. 1977;2:293–5.
22. Aronson JD. Protective vaccination against tuberculosis, with special reference to BCG vaccine. Minn Med. 1948;31:1336.
23. Hyge TV. The efficacy of BCG-vaccination; epidemic of tuberculosis in a State School, with an observation period of 12 years. Acta Tuberc Scand. 1956;32:89–107.
24. Baily GV. Tuberculosis prevention trial, Madras. Indian J Med Res. 1980;72(Suppl):1–74.
25. Comstock GW, Woolpert SF, Livesay VT. Tuberculosis studies in Muscogee County, Georgia. Twenty-year evaluation of a community trial of BCG vaccination. Public Health Rep. 1976;91:276–80.
26. Shapiro C, Cook N, Evans D, Willett W, Fajardo I, Koch-Weser D, et al. A case-control study of BCG and childhood tuberculosis in Cali, Colombia. Int J Epidemiol. 1985;14:441–6.
27. Sterne JA, Rodrigues LC, Guedes IN. Does the efficacy of BCG decline with time since vaccination? Int J Tuberc Lung Dis. 1998;2:200–7.
28. Miret-Cuadras P, Pina-Gutierrez JM, Juncosa S. Tuberculin reactivity in Bacillus Calmette-Guerin vaccinated subjects. Tuber Lung Dis. 1996;77:52–8.
29. Burl S, Adetifa UJ, Cox M, Touray E, Whittle H, McShane H, et al. The tuberculin skin test (TST) is affected by recent BCG vaccination but not by exposure to non-tuberculosis mycobacteria (NTM) during early life. PLoS One. 2010;5:e12287.
30. Lai R, Ogunsola AF, Rakib T, Behar SM. Key advances in vaccine development for tuberculosis-success and challenges. NPJ Vaccines. 2023;8:158.
31. Scriba TJ, Kaufmann SH, Henri Lambert P, Sanicas M, Martin C, Neyrolles O. Vaccination against tuberculosis with whole-cell mycobacterial vaccines. J Infect Dis. 2016;214:659–64.

32. Schrager LK, Chandrasekaran P, Fritzell BH, Hatherill M, Lambert PH, McShane H, et al. WHO preferred product characteristics for new vaccines against tuberculosis. Lancet Infect Dis. 2018;18:828–9.
33. Portnoy A, Clark RA, Quaife M, Weerasuriya CK, Mukandavire C, Bakker R, et al. The cost and cost-effectiveness of novel tuberculosis vaccines in low- and middle-income countries: a modeling study. PLoS Med. 2023;20:e1004155.
34. Grode L, Ganoza CA, Brohm C, Weiner J 3rd, Eisele B, Kaufmann SH. Safety and immunogenicity of the recombinant BCG vaccine VPM1002 in a phase 1 open-label randomized clinical trial. Vaccine. 2013;31:1340–8.
35. Geoffroy C, Gaillard JL, Alouf JE, Berche P. Purification, characterization, and toxicity of the sulfhydryl-activated hemolysin listeriolysin O from Listeria monocytogenes. Infect Immun. 1987;55:1641–6.
36. Cotton MF, Madhi SA, Luabeya AK, Tameris M, Hesseling AC, Shenje J, et al. Safety and immunogenicity of VPM1002 versus BCG in South African newborn babies: a randomised, phase 2 non-inferiority double-blind controlled trial. Lancet Infect Dis. 2022;22:1472–83.
37. Kaufmann SHE. Vaccination against tuberculosis: revamping BCG by molecular genetics guided by immunology. Front Immunol. 2020;11:316.
38. Nieuwenhuizen NE, Kulkarni PS, Shaligram U, Cotton MF, Rentsch CA, Eisele B, et al. The recombinant Bacille Calmette-Guerin vaccine VPM1002: ready for clinical efficacy testing. Front Immunol. 2017;8:1147.
39. Mazzola TN, da Silva MT, Abramczuk BM, Moreno YM, Lima SC, Zorzeto TQ, et al. Impaired Bacillus Calmette-Guerin cellular immune response in HIV-exposed, uninfected infants. AIDS. 2011;25:2079–87.
40. Hoft DF, Blazevic A, Abate G, Hanekom WA, Kaplan G, Soler JH, et al. A new recombinant bacille Calmette-Guerin vaccine safely induces significantly enhanced tuberculosis-specific immunity in human volunteers. J Infect Dis. 2008;198:1491–501.
41. Ng TW, Saavedra-Avila NA, Kennedy SC, Carreno LJ, Porcelli SA. Current efforts and future prospects in the development of live mycobacteria as vaccines. Expert Rev Vaccines. 2015;14:1493–507.
42. Kaufmann SH, Gengenbacher M. Recombinant live vaccine candidates against tuberculosis. Curr Opin Biotechnol. 2012;23:900–7.
43. Master SS, Rampini SK, Davis AS, Keller C, Ehlers S, Springer B, et al. Mycobacterium tuberculosis prevents inflammasome activation. Cell Host Microbe. 2008;3:224–32.
44. Sander P, Clark S, Petrera A, Vilaplana C, Meuli M, Selchow P, et al. Deletion of zmp1 improves Mycobacterium bovis BCG-mediated protection in a Guinea pig model of tuberculosis. Vaccine. 2015;33:1353–9.
45. Flores-Valdez MA, Kupz A, Subbian S. Recent developments in mycobacteria-based live attenuated vaccine candidates for tuberculosis. Biomedicines. 2022;10:2749.
46. Flores-Valdez MA, Aceves-Sanchez Mde J, Pedroza-Roldan C, Vega-Dominguez PJ, Prado-Montes de Oca E, Bravo-Madrigal J, et al. The cyclic Di-GMP phosphodiesterase gene Rv1357c/BCG1419c affects BCG pellicle production and in vivo maintenance. IUBMB Life. 2015;67:129–38.
47. Flores-Valdez MA, Pedroza-Roldan C, Aceves-Sanchez MJ, Peterson EJR, Baliga NS, Hernandez-Pando R, et al. The BCGDeltaBCG1419c vaccine candidate reduces lung pathology, IL-6, TNF-alpha, and IL-10 during chronic TB infection. Front Microbiol. 2018;9:1281.
48. Sathkumara HD, Pai S, Aceves-Sanchez MJ, Ketheesan N, Flores-Valdez MA, Kupz A. BCG vaccination prevents reactivation of latent lymphatic murine tuberculosis independently of CD4(+) T cells. Front Immunol. 2019;10:532.
49. Aceves-Sanchez MJ, Flores-Valdez MA, Shanley C, Orme I, Bielefeldt-Ohmann H. Vaccination of Guinea pigs with BCGDeltaBCG1419c transiently reduces hematogenous spread of M. tuberculosis to the spleen. Pathog Dis. 2018;76:fty088.
50. Pym AS, Brodin P, Majlessi L, Brosch R, Demangel C, Williams A, et al. Recombinant BCG exporting ESAT-6 confers enhanced protection against tuberculosis. Nat Med. 2003;9:533–9.

51. Muruganandah V, Sathkumara HD, Pai S, Rush CM, Brosch R, Waardenberg AJ, et al. A systematic approach to simultaneously evaluate safety, immunogenicity, and efficacy of novel tuberculosis vaccination strategies. Sci Adv. 2020;6:eaaz1767.
52. Heijmenberg I, Husain A, Sathkumara HD, Muruganandah V, Seifert J, Miranda-Hernandez S, et al. ESX-5-targeted export of ESAT-6 in BCG combines enhanced immunogenicity & efficacy against murine tuberculosis with low virulence and reduced persistence. Vaccine. 2021;39:7265–76.
53. Bottai D, Frigui W, Clark S, Rayner E, Zelmer A, Andreu N, et al. Increased protective efficacy of recombinant BCG strains expressing virulence-neutral proteins of the ESX-1 secretion system. Vaccine. 2015;33:2710–8.
54. Vergne I, Chua J, Lee HH, Lucas M, Belisle J, Deretic V. Mechanism of phagolysosome biogenesis block by viable Mycobacterium tuberculosis. Proc Natl Acad Sci USA. 2005;102:4033–8.
55. Puri RV, Reddy PV, Tyagi AK. Secreted acid phosphatase (SapM) of Mycobacterium tuberculosis is indispensable for arresting phagosomal maturation and growth of the pathogen in Guinea pig tissues. PLoS One. 2013;8:e70514.
56. Festjens N, Vandewalle K, Houthuys E, Plets E, Vanderschaeghe D, Borgers K, et al. SapM mutation to improve the BCG vaccine: genomic, transcriptomic and preclinical safety characterization. Vaccine. 2019;37:3539–51.
57. Hawgood BJ. Albert Calmette (1863-1933) and Camille Guerin (1872-1961): the C and G of BCG vaccine. J Med Biogr. 2007;15:139–46.
58. Edwards PW. Tuberculosis in hospital workers. Br Med J. 1937;2:1261–5.
59. Morrison H, McShane H. BCG: past, present and future direction. In: Vaccines for neglected pathogens: strategies, achievements and challenges. Cham: Springer International Publishing; 2023. p. 171–95.
60. Sharpe S, White A, Sarfas C, Sibley L, Gleeson F, McIntyre A, et al. Alternative BCG delivery strategies improve protection against Mycobacterium tuberculosis in non-human primates: protection associated with mycobacterial antigen-specific CD4 effector memory T-cell populations. Tuberculosis (Edinb). 2016;101:174–90.
61. White AD, Sarfas C, West K, Sibley LS, Wareham AS, Clark S, et al. Evaluation of the immunogenicity of Mycobacterium bovis BCG delivered by aerosol to the lungs of macaques. Clin Vaccine Immunol. 2015;22:992–1003.
62. White AD, Sarfas C, Sibley LS, Gullick J, Clark S, Rayner E, et al. Protective efficacy of inhaled BCG vaccination against ultra-low dose aerosol M. tuberculosis challenge in Rhesus Macaques. Pharmaceutics. 2020;12:12.
63. Darrah PA, Zeppa JJ, Maiello P, Hackney JA, Wadsworth MH 2nd, Hughes TK, et al. Prevention of tuberculosis in macaques after intravenous BCG immunization. Nature. 2020;577:95–102.
64. Abubakar I, Pimpin L, Ariti C, Beynon R, Mangtani P, Sterne JA, et al. Systematic review and meta-analysis of the current evidence on the duration of protection by bacillus Calmette-Guerin vaccination against tuberculosis. Health Technol Assess. 2013;17:1–372, v-vi.
65. Rodrigues LC, Pereira SM, Cunha SS, Genser B, Ichihara MY, de Brito SC, et al. Effect of BCG revaccination on incidence of tuberculosis in school-aged children in Brazil: the BCG-REVAC cluster-randomised trial. Lancet. 2005;366:1290–5.
66. Group KPT. Randomised controlled trial of single BCG, repeated BCG, or combined BCG and killed Mycobacterium leprae vaccine for prevention of leprosy and tuberculosis in Malawi. Karonga Prevention Trial Group. Lancet. 1996;348:17–24.
67. Glynn JR, Fielding K, Mzembe T, Sichali L, Banda L, McLean E, et al. BCG re-vaccination in Malawi: 30-year follow-up of a large, randomised, double-blind, placebo-controlled trial. Lancet Glob Health. 2021;9:e1451–e9.
68. Leung CC, Tam CM, Chan SL, Chan-Yeung M, Chan CK, Chang KC. Efficacy of the BCG revaccination programme in a cohort given BCG vaccination at birth in Hong Kong. Int J Tuberc Lung Dis. 2001;5:717–23.

69. Tala-Heikkila MM, Tuominen JE, Tala EO. Bacillus Calmette-Guerin revaccination questionable with low tuberculosis incidence. Am J Respir Crit Care Med. 1998;157:1324–7.
70. Nemes E, Geldenhuys H, Rozot V, Rutkowski KT, Ratangee F, Bilek N, et al. Prevention of M. tuberculosis infection with H4:IC31 vaccine or BCG revaccination. N Engl J Med. 2018;379:138–49.
71. Bekker LG, Dintwe O, Fiore-Gartland A, Middelkoop K, Hutter J, Williams A, et al. A phase 1b randomized study of the safety and immunological responses to vaccination with H4:IC31, H56:IC31, and BCG revaccination in Mycobacterium tuberculosis-uninfected adolescents in Cape Town, South Africa. EClinicalMedicine. 2020;21:100313.
72. Ahmed A, Tripathi H, van Meijgaarden KE, Kumar NC, Adiga V, Rakshit S, et al. BCG revaccination in adults enhances pro-inflammatory markers of trained immunity along with anti-inflammatory pathways. iScience. 2023;26:107889.
73. Velayutham B, Thiruvengadam K, Kumaran PP, Watson B, Rajendran K, Padmapriyadarsini C. Revisiting the Chingleput BCG vaccination trial for the impact of BCG revaccination on the incidence of tuberculosis disease. Indian J Med Res. 2023;157:152–9.
74. Rakshit S, Ahmed A, Adiga V, Sundararaj BK, Sahoo PN, Kenneth J, et al. BCG revaccination boosts adaptive polyfunctional Th1/Th17 and innate effectors in IGRA+ and IGRA- Indian adults. JCI Insight. 2019;4:e130540.
75. Schmidt AC, Fairlie L, Hellström E, Luabeya Kany Kany A, Middelkoop K, Naidoo K, Hatherill M, et al. BCG Revaccination for the Prevention of Mycobacterium tuberculosis Infection. New England Journal of Medicine. 2025;392(18):1789–1800.
76. Tanner R, McShane H. BCG and other vaccines. In: Friedman LN, Dedicoat M, Davies PD, editors. Cinical Tuberculosis. 6th ed. Boca Raton: CRC Press; 2020.
77. Zhang Y, Xu J-c, Hu Z-d, Fan X-y. Advances in protein subunit vaccines against tuberculosis. Front Immunol. 2023;14:1238586.
78. Tait DR, Hatherill M, Van Der Meeren O, Ginsberg AM, Van Brakel E, Salaun B, et al. Final analysis of a trial of M72/AS01E vaccine to prevent tuberculosis. N Engl J Med. 2019;381:2429–39.
79. Penn-Nicholson A, Tameris M, Smit E, Day TA, Musvosvi M, Jayashankar L, et al. Safety and immunogenicity of the novel tuberculosis vaccine ID93 + GLA-SE in BCG-vaccinated healthy adults in South Africa: a randomised, double-blind, placebo-controlled phase 1 trial. Lancet Respir Med. 6:287–98.
80. Tkachuk AP, Bykonia EN, Popova LI, Kleymenov DA, Semashko MA, Chulanov VP, et al. Safety and immunogenicity of the GamTBvac, the recombinant subunit tuberculosis vaccine candidate: a phase II, multi-center, double-blind, randomized, placebo-controlled study. Vaccine. 2020;8:652.
81. Chen L, Xu M, Wang Z-Y, Chen B-W, Du W-X, Su C, et al. The development and preliminary evaluation of a new Mycobacterium tuberculosis vaccine comprising Ag85b, HspX and CFP-10: ESAT-6 fusion protein with CpG DNA and aluminum hydroxide adjuvants. FEMS Immunol Med Microbiol. 2010;59:42–52.
82. Woodworth JS, Clemmensen HS, Battey H, Dijkman K, Lindenstrøm T, Laureano RS, et al. A Mycobacterium tuberculosis-specific subunit vaccine that provides synergistic immunity upon co-administration with Bacillus Calmette-Guérin. Nat Commun. 2021;12:6658.
83. Aagaard C, Knudsen NPH, Sohn I, Izzo AA, Kim H, Kristiansen EH, et al. Immunization with mycobacterium tuberculosis–specific antigens bypasses T cell differentiation from prior Bacillus Calmette–Guérin vaccination and improves protection in mice. J Immunol. 2020;205:2146–55.
84. Liu X, Peng J, Hu L, Luo Y, Niu H, Bai C, et al. A multistage mycobacterium tuberculosis subunit vaccine LT70 including latency antigen Rv2626c induces long-term protection against tuberculosis. Hum Vaccin Immunother. 2016;12:1670–7.
85. Korsholm KS, Agger EM, Foged C, Christensen D, Dietrich J, Andersen CS, et al. The adjuvant mechanism of cationic dimethyldioctadecylammonium liposomes. Immunology. 2007;121:216–26.

86. Facciolà A, Visalli G, Laganà A, Di Pietro A. An overview of vaccine adjuvants: current evidence and future perspectives. Vaccines (Basel). 2022;10:819.
87. Counoupas C, Ferrell KC, Ashhurst A, Bhattacharyya ND, Nagalingam G, Stewart EL, et al. Mucosal delivery of a multistage subunit vaccine promotes development of lung-resident memory T cells and affords interleukin-17-dependent protection against pulmonary tuberculosis. NPJ Vaccines. 2020;5:105.
88. Counoupas C, Pinto R, Nagalingam G, Hill-Cawthorne GA, Feng CG, Britton WJ, et al. Mycobacterium tuberculosis components expressed during chronic infection of the lung contribute to long-term control of pulmonary tuberculosis in mice. NPJ Vaccines. 2016;1:16012.
89. Pinto R, Tang QX, Britton WJ, Leyh TS, Triccas JA. The Mycobacterium tuberculosis cysD and cysNC genes form a stress-induced operon that encodes a tri-functional sulfate-activating complex. Microbiology. 2004;150:1681–6.
90. Abrahams KA, Besra GS. Mycobacterial cell wall biosynthesis: a multifaceted antibiotic target. Parasitology. 2018;145:116–33.
91. Pedersen GK, Andersen P, Christensen D. Immunocorrelates of CAF family adjuvants. Elsevier. p. 4–13.
92. Counoupas C, Pinto R, Nagalingam G, Britton WJ, Petrovsky N, Triccas JA. Delta inulin-based adjuvants promote the generation of polyfunctional CD4+ T cell responses and protection against Mycobacterium tuberculosis infection. Sci Rep. 2017;7:8582.
93. Ma J, Teng X, Wang X, Fan X, Wu Y, Tian M, et al. A multistage subunit vaccine effectively protects mice against primary progressive tuberculosis, latency and reactivation. EBioMedicine. 2017;22:143–54.
94. Travieso T, Li J, Mahesh S, Mello JDFRE, Blasi M. The use of viral vectors in vaccine development. NPJ Vaccines. 2022;7:75.
95. Tameris MD, Hatherill M, Landry BS, Scriba TJ, Snowden MA, Lockhart S, et al. Safety and efficacy of MVA85A, a new tuberculosis vaccine, in infants previously vaccinated with BCG: a randomised, placebo-controlled phase 2b trial. Lancet. 2013;381:1021–8.
96. Falsey AR, Sobieszczyk ME, Hirsch I, Sproule S, Robb ML, Corey L, et al. Phase 3 safety and efficacy of AZD1222 (ChAdOx1 nCoV-19) Covid-19 vaccine. N Engl J Med. 2021;385:2348–60.
97. Wilkie M, Satti I, Minhinnick A, Harris S, Riste M, Ramon RL, et al. A phase I trial evaluating the safety and immunogenicity of a candidate tuberculosis vaccination regimen, ChAdOx1 85A prime – MVA85A boost in healthy UK adults. Vaccine. 2020;38:779–89.
98. Stylianou E, Griffiths KL, Poyntz HC, Harrington-Kandt R, Dicks MD, Stockdale L, et al. Improvement of BCG protective efficacy with a novel chimpanzee adenovirus and a modified vaccinia Ankara virus both expressing Ag85A. Vaccine. 2015;33:6800–8.
99. Stylianou E, Harrington-Kandt R, Beglov J, Bull N, Pinpathomrat N, Swarbrick GM, et al. Identification and evaluation of novel protective antigens for the development of a candidate tuberculosis subunit vaccine. Infect Immun. 2018;86
100. Smaill F, Jeyanathan M, Smieja M, Medina MF, Thanthrige-Don N, Zganiacz A, et al. A human type 5 adenovirus-based tuberculosis vaccine induces robust T cell responses in humans despite preexisting anti-adenovirus immunity. Sci Transl Med. 2013;5:205ra134.
101. Stylianou E, Pinpathomrat N, Sampson O, Richard A, Korompis M, McShane H. A five-antigen Esx-5a fusion delivered as a prime-boost regimen protects against *M.tb* challenge. Front Immunol. 2023;14:1263457.
102. Ryll R, Kumazawa Y, Yano I. Immunological properties of trehalose dimycolate (cord factor) and other mycolic acid-containing glycolipids – a review. Microbiol Immunol. 2001;45:801–11.
103. Shah S, Cannon JR, Fenselau C, Briken V. A duplicated ESAT-6 region of ESX-5 is involved in protein export and virulence of mycobacteria. Infect Immun. 2015;83:4349–61.
104. Shah S, Briken V. Modular organization of the ESX-5 secretion system in Mycobacterium tuberculosis. Front Cell Infect Microbiol. 2016;6:49.

105. Pinpathomrat N, Bull N, Pasricha J, Harrington-Kandt R, McShane H, Stylianou E. Using an effective TB vaccination regimen to identify immune responses associated with protection in the murine model. Vaccine. 2021;39:1452–62.
106. Afkhami S, D'Agostino MR, Vaseghi-Shanjani M, Lepard M, Yang JX, Lai R, et al. Intranasal multivalent adenoviral-vectored vaccine protects against replicating and dormant M. tb in conventional and humanized mice. NPJ Vaccines. 2023;8:25.
107. Hansen SG, Zak DE, Xu G, Ford JC, Marshall EE, Malouli D, et al. Prevention of tuberculosis in rhesus macaques by a cytomegalovirus-based vaccine. Nat Med. 2018;24:130–43.
108. Watt J, Liu J. Preclinical progress of subunit and live attenuated Mycobacterium tuberculosis vaccines: a review following the first in human efficacy trial. Pharmaceutics. 2020;12:848.
109. Britton G, MacDonald DC, Brown JS, Collins MK, Goodman AL. Using a prime and pull approach, lentivector vaccines expressing Ag85A induce immunogenicity but fail to induce protection against Mycobacterium bovis Bacillus Calmette–Guérin challenge in mice. Immunology. 2015;146:264–70.
110. Shakouri M, Moazzeni SM, Ghanei M, Arashkia A, Etemadzadeh MH, Azadmanesh K. A novel dendritic cell-targeted lentiviral vector, encoding Ag85A-ESAT6 fusion gene of Mycobacterium tuberculosis, could elicit potent cell-mediated immune responses in mice. Mol Immunol. 2016;75:101–11.
111. Hu Z, Wong K-W, Zhao H-M, Wen H-L, Ji P, Ma H, et al. Sendai virus mucosal vaccination establishes lung-resident memory CD8 T cell immunity and boosts BCG-primed protection against TB in mice. Mol Ther. 2017;25:1222–33.
112. Zhang M, Dong C, Xiong S. Vesicular stomatitis virus-vectored multi-antigen tuberculosis vaccine limits bacterial proliferation in mice following a single intranasal dose. Front Cell Infect Microbiol. 2017;7:34.
113. Chen Z, Gupta T, Xu P, Phan S, Pickar A, Yau W, et al. Efficacy of parainfluenza virus 5 (PIV5)-based tuberculosis vaccines in mice. Vaccine. 2015;33:7217–24.
114. Kuczkowska K, Copland A, Øverland L, Mathiesen G, Tran AC, Paul MJ, et al. Inactivated Lactobacillus plantarum carrying a surface-displayed Ag85B-ESAT-6 fusion antigen as a booster vaccine against Mycobacterium tuberculosis infection. Front Immunol. 2019;10:454086.
115. Jia Q, Masleša-Galić S, Nava S, Horwitz MA. Listeria-vectored multiantigenic tuberculosis vaccine enhances protective immunity against aerosol challenge with virulent Mycobacterium tuberculosis in BCG-immunized C57BL/6 and BALB/c mice. MBio. 2022;13:e00687–22.
116. Kupz A. Live attenuated vaccines for tuberculosis. Biochemist. 2021;43:28–32.
117. Walker KB, Brennan MJ, Ho MM, Eskola J, Thiry G, Sadoff J, et al. The second Geneva consensus: recommendations for novel live TB vaccines. Vaccine. 2010;28:2259–70.
118. Arbues A, Aguilo JI, Gonzalo-Asensio J, Marinova D, Uranga S, Puentes E, et al. Construction, characterization and preclinical evaluation of MTBVAC, the first live-attenuated M. tuberculosis-based vaccine to enter clinical trials. Vaccine. 2013;31:4867–73.
119. Marinova D, Gonzalo-Asensio J, Aguilo N, Martin C. MTBVAC from discovery to clinical trials in tuberculosis-endemic countries. Expert Rev Vaccines. 2017;16:565–76.
120. Martin C, Williams A, Hernandez-Pando R, Cardona PJ, Gormley E, Bordat Y, et al. The live Mycobacterium tuberculosis phoP mutant strain is more attenuated than BCG and confers protective immunity against tuberculosis in mice and Guinea pigs. Vaccine. 2006;24:3408–19.
121. Williams A, Hatch GJ, Clark SO, Gooch KE, Hatch KA, Hall GA, et al. Evaluation of vaccines in the EU TB vaccine cluster using a Guinea pig aerosol infection model of tuberculosis. Tuberculosis. 2005;85:29–38.
122. Spertini F, Audran R, Chakour R, Karoui O, Steiner-Monard V, Thierry AC, et al. Safety of human immunisation with a live-attenuated Mycobacterium tuberculosis vaccine: a randomised, double-blind, controlled phase I trial. Lancet Respir Med. 2015;3:953–62.
123. Tameris M, Mearns H, Penn-Nicholson A, Gregg Y, Bilek N, Mabwe S, et al. Live-attenuated Mycobacterium tuberculosis vaccine MTBVAC versus BCG in adults and neonates: a randomised controlled, double-blind dose-escalation trial. Lancet Respir Med. 2019;7:757–70.

124. Pérez I, Uranga S, Sayes F, Frigui W, Samper S, Arbués A, et al. Live attenuated TB vaccines representing the three modern Mycobacterium tuberculosis lineages reveal that the Euro-American genetic background confers optimal vaccine potential. EBioMedicine. 2020;55:102761.
125. Mehra S, Golden NA, Stuckey K, Didier PJ, Doyle LA, Russell-Lodrigue KE, et al. The Mycobacterium tuberculosis stress response factor SigH is required for bacterial burden as well as immunopathology in primate lungs. J Infect Dis. 2012;205:1203–13.
126. Kaushal D, Foreman TW, Gautam US, Alvarez X, Adekambi T, Rangel-Moreno J, et al. Mucosal vaccination with attenuated Mycobacterium tuberculosis induces strong central memory responses and protects against tuberculosis. Nat Commun. 2015;6:8533.
127. Sakthi S, Palaniyandi K, Gupta UD, Gupta P, Narayanan S. Lipoprotein LpqS deficient M. tuberculosis mutant is attenuated for virulence in vivo and shows protective efficacy better than BCG in Guinea pigs. Vaccine. 2016;34:735–43.
128. Marcus SA, Steinberg H, Talaat AM. Protection by novel vaccine candidates, Mycobacterium tuberculosis ΔmosR and ΔechA7, against challenge with a Mycobacterium tuberculosis Beijing strain. Vaccine. 2015;33:5633–9.
129. Schrager LK, Harris RC, Vekemans J. Research and development of new tuberculosis vaccines: a review. F1000Res. 2018;7:1732.
130. Kar R, Nangpal P, Mathur S, Singh S, Tyagi AK. bioA mutant of Mycobacterium tuberculosis shows severe growth defect and imparts protection against tuberculosis in Guinea pigs. PLoS One. 2017;12:e0179513.
131. Chauhan P, Reddy PV, Singh R, Jaisinghani N, Gandotra S, Tyagi AK. Secretory phosphatases deficient mutant of Mycobacterium tuberculosis imparts protection at the primary site of infection in Guinea pigs. PLoS One. 2013;8:e77930.
132. Bahal RK, Mathur S, Chauhan P, Tyagi AK. An attenuated quadruple gene mutant of Mycobacterium tuberculosis imparts protection against tuberculosis in Guinea pigs. Biology Open. 2018;7:bio029546.
133. Hernandez-Pando R, Shin SJ, Clark S, Casonato S, Becerril-Zambrano M, Kim H, et al. Construction and characterization of the Mycobacterium tuberculosis sigE fadD26 unmarked double mutant as a vaccine candidate. Infect Immun. 2019;88:10–1128.
134. Levillain F, Kim H, Kwon KW, Clark S, Cia F, Malaga W, et al. Preclinical assessment of a new live attenuated Mycobacterium tuberculosis Beijing-based vaccine for tuberculosis. Vaccine. 2020;38:1416–23.
135. Liu L, Fu R, Yuan X, Shi C, Wang S, Lu X, et al. Differential immune responses and protective effects in avirulent mycobacterial strains vaccinated BALB/c mice. Curr Microbiol. 2015;71:129–35.
136. Kim B-J, Kim B-R, Kook Y-H, Kim B-J. A temperature sensitive Mycobacterium paragordonae induces enhanced protective immune responses against mycobacterial infections in the mouse model. Sci Rep. 2017;7:15230.
137. Oliveira FM, Trentini MM, Junqueira-Kipnis AP, Kipnis A. The mc 2-CMX vaccine induces an enhanced immune response against Mycobacterium tuberculosis compared to Bacillus Calmette-Guérin but with similar lung inflammatory effects. Mem Inst Oswaldo Cruz. 2016;111:223–31.
138. Gong W, Liang Y, Wu X. The current status, challenges, and future developments of new tuberculosis vaccines. Hum Vaccin Immunother. 2018;14:1697–716.
139. Sharma SK, Katoch K, Sarin R, Balambal R, Kumar Jain N, Patel N, et al. Efficacy and safety of Mycobacterium indicus pranii as an adjunct therapy in category II pulmonary tuberculosis in a randomized trial. Sci Rep. 2017;7:3354.
140. Huang C-Y, Hsieh W-Y. Efficacy of Mycobacterium vaccae immunotherapy for patients with tuberculosis: a systematic review and meta-analysis. Hum Vaccin Immunother. 2017;13:1960–71.
141. Lahey T, Laddy D, Hill K, Schaeffer J, Hogg A, Keeble J, et al. Immunogenicity and protective efficacy of the DAR-901 booster vaccine in a murine model of tuberculosis. PLoS One. 2016;11:e0168521.

142. Munseri P, Said J, Amour M, Magohe A, Matee M, Rees CA, et al. DAR-901 vaccine for the prevention of infection with Mycobacterium tuberculosis among BCG-immunized adolescents in Tanzania: a randomized controlled, double-blind phase 2b trial. Vaccine. 2020;38:7239–45.
143. Nell AS, D'Lom E, Bouic P, Sabate M, Bosser R, Picas J, et al. Safety, tolerability, and immunogenicity of the novel antituberculous vaccine RUTI: randomized, placebo-controlled phase II clinical trial in patients with latent tuberculosis infection. PLoS One. 2014;9:e89612.
144. Vilaplana C, Montané E, Pinto S, Barriocanal AM, Domenech G, Torres F, et al. Double-blind, randomized, placebo-controlled phase I clinical trial of the therapeutical antituberculous vaccine RUTI. Vaccine. 2010;28:1106–16.
145. Nooraei S, Bahrulolum H, Hoseini ZS, Katalani C, Hajizade A, Easton AJ, et al. Virus-like particles: preparation, immunogenicity and their roles as nanovaccines and drug nanocarriers. J Nanobiotechnol. 2021;19:59.
146. Zhou F, Zhang D. Recent advance in the development of tuberculosis vaccines in clinical trials and virus-like particle-based vaccine candidates. Front Immunol. 2023;14:1238649.
147. Krammer F, Schinko T, Messner P, Palmberger D, Ferko B, Grabherr R. Influenza virus-like particles as an antigen-carrier platform for the ESAT-6 epitope of Mycobacterium tuberculosis. J Virol Methods. 2010;167:17–22.
148. Yin Y, Li H, Wu S, Dong D, Zhang J, Fu L, et al. Hepatitis B virus core particles displaying Mycobacterium tuberculosis antigen ESAT-6 enhance ESAT-6-specific immune responses. Vaccine. 2011;29:5645–51.
149. Dhanasooraj D, Kumar RA, Mundayoor S. Vaccine delivery system for tuberculosis based on nano-sized hepatitis B virus core protein particles. Int J Nanomedicine. 2013;8:835–43.
150. Zhou F, Zhang D. Nano-Sized Chimeric Human Papillomavirus-16 L1 Virus-like Particles Displaying Mycobacterium tuberculosis Antigen Ag85B Enhance Ag85B-Specific Immune Responses in Female C57BL/c Mice. Viruses. 2023;15(10):2123. https://doi.org/10.3390/v15102123. PMID: 37896900; PMCID: PMC10612075.
151. Chavda VP, Pandya R, Apostolopoulos V. DNA vaccines for SARS-CoV-2: toward third-generation vaccination era. Expert Rev Vaccines. 2021;20:1549–60.
152. Zhuang L, Ye Z, Li L, Yang L, Gong W. Next-generation TB vaccines: progress, challenges, and prospects. Vaccine. 2023;11:1304.
153. Pereira VB, Saraiva TD, Souza BM, Zurita-Turk M, Azevedo MS, De Castro CP, et al. Development of a new DNA vaccine based on mycobacterial ESAT-6 antigen delivered by recombinant invasive Lactococcus lactis FnBPA+. Appl Microbiol Biotechnol. 2015;99:1817–26.
154. Guimarães V, Innocentin S, Chatel JM, Lefèvre F, Langella P, Azevedo V, et al. A new plasmid vector for DNA delivery using lactococci. Genet Vaccines Ther. 2009;7:4.
155. Pereira VB, da Cunha VP, Preisser TM, Souza BM, Turk MZ, De Castro CP, et al. Lactococcus lactis carrying a DNA vaccine coding for the ESAT-6 antigen increases IL-17 cytokine secretion and boosts the BCG vaccine immune response. J Appl Microbiol. 2017;122:1657–62.
156. de Castro CP, Souza BM, Mancha-Agresti P, Pereira VB, Zurita-Turk M, Preisser TM, et al. Lactococcus lactis FNBPA(+) (pValac:e6ag85a) induces cellular and humoral immune responses after oral immunization of mice. Front Microbiol. 2021;12:676172.
157. Sefidi-Heris Y, Jahangiri A, Mokhtarzadeh A, Shahbazi M-A, Khalili S, Baradaran B, et al. Recent progress in the design of DNA vaccines against tuberculosis. Drug Discov Today. 2020;25:1971–87.
158. Tian X, Cai H, Zhu Y-X. Protection of mice with a divalent tuberculosis DNA vaccine encoding antigens Ag85B and MPT64. Acta Biochim Biophys Sin. 2004;36:269–76.
159. Lu J, Wang C, Zhou Z, Zhang Y, Cao T, Shi C, et al. Immunogenicity and protective efficacy against murine tuberculosis of a prime-boost regimen with BCG and a DNA vaccine expressing ESAT-6 and Ag85A fusion protein. J Immunol Research. 2011;2011:1.
160. Pardi N, Hogan MJ, Porter FW, Weissman D. mRNA vaccines—a new era in vaccinology. Nat Rev Drug Discov. 2018;17:261–79.

161. Zhang G, Tang T, Chen Y, Huang X, Liang T. mRNA vaccines in disease prevention and treatment. Signal Transduct Target Ther. 2023;8:365.
162. Larsen SE, Baldwin SL, Coler RN. Tuberculosis vaccines update: is an RNA-based vaccine feasible for tuberculosis? Int J Infect Dis. 2023;130(Suppl 1):S47–s51.
163. Xue T, Stavropoulos E, Yang M, Ragno S, Vordermeier M, Chambers M, et al. RNA encoding the MPT83 antigen induces protective immune responses against Mycobacterium tuberculosis infection. Infect Immun. 2004;72:6324–9.
164. Lorenzi JC, Trombone AP, Rocha CD, Almeida LP, Lousada RL, Malardo T, et al. Intranasal vaccination with messenger RNA as a new approach in gene therapy: use against tuberculosis. BMC Biotechnol. 2010;10:77.
165. Erasmus JH, Khandhar AP, Guderian J, Granger B, Archer J, Archer M, et al. A nanostructured lipid carrier for delivery of a replicating viral RNA provides single, low-dose protection against Zika. Mol Ther. 2018;26:2507–22.
166. Larsen SE, Erasmus JH, Reese VA, Pecor T, Archer J, Kandahar A, et al. An RNA-based vaccine platform for use against Mycobacterium tuberculosis. Vaccines (Basel). 2023;11:130.
167. Looney MM, Hatherill M, Musvosvi M, Flynn J, Kagina BM, Frick M, et al. Conference report: WHO meeting summary on mRNA-based tuberculosis vaccine development. Vaccine. 2023;41:7060–6.
168. Morrison H, McShane H. BCG: past, present and future direction. Vaccines for neglected pathogens: strategies, achievements and challenges: focus on leprosy, leishmaniasis, melioidosis and tuberculosis. Cham: Springer International Publishing; 2023. p. 171–95.

Pre-clinical Landscape of TB Vaccines: Challenges and Innovations

6

Salem Salman Almujri and Paulo J. G. Bettencourt

6.1 Introduction

Tuberculosis (TB) caused by *Mycobacterium tuberculosis* (*Mtb*) continues to remain a significant global health threat, claiming nearly 4000 lives each day. According to a recent WHO report, in 2024, there were approximately 10.8 million new cases of TB and 1.25 million deaths globally [1]. Among these deaths, 251,000 occurred among individuals who were HIV-positive [2]. The BCG vaccine, the only licensed vaccine available and in use for over a century, has shown inconsistent effectiveness against pulmonary TB, the most prevalent and contagious form of the disease [3]. Clinical trials have also produced inconsistent results, especially in high-prevalence regions, where the vaccine has had little impact on the incidence of pulmonary TB [4]. Furthermore, BCG does not prevent latent TB infection, which can later advance to active TB disease. It also offers only limited protection to adults, who are more likely to develop and transmit the disease [5]. Additionally, BCG does not protect against drug-resistant strains of *Mtb* [6], emphasizing the critical need for new vaccines that provide broader and more reliable protection against all forms and strains of TB. As a result, developing improved vaccines has been a key goal in TB research [7].

To address these challenges, the development of new vaccines against *Mtb* undergoes several pre-clinical stages before advancing to clinical trials. Initially,

S. S. Almujri
Department of Pharmacology, College of Pharmacy, King Khalid University, Asir-Abha, Saudi Arabia

P. J. G. Bettencourt (✉)
Universidade Católica Portuguesa, Center for Interdisciplinary Research in Health, Lisbon, Portugal

Universidade Católica Portuguesa, Faculty of Medicine, Lisbon, Portugal
e-mail: pbettencourt@ucp.pt

P. J. G. Bettencourt (ed.), *Tuberculosis Vaccines*,
https://doi.org/10.1007/978-3-031-94540-3_6

scientists identify specific antigens that can elicit a robust immune response, followed by designing and developing a vaccine candidate based on this information [8]. The pre-clinical phase involves in vitro studies to assess the immune response and animal testing to evaluate safety and efficacy [9]. Researchers obtain regulatory approval from pre-clinical data and then conduct phased clinical trials to assess safety and efficacy. In this context, the chapter addresses various aspects of pre-clinical trials for TB vaccine development. It also explores the challenges encountered in TB vaccine research and future development directions, offering a new perspective on advancing vaccine development.

6.2 Challenges to TB Vaccine Development

Mtb poses significant challenges for vaccine development due to its ability to evade and manipulate the host immune system, making it difficult to target and eliminate [10, 11]. The complexity of the immune response to *Mtb* and the lack of well-defined immunological correlates of protection further complicate the process, as there are no reliable markers to assess immune responses or predict vaccine efficacy [12]. Additionally, replicating human TB in animal models is challenging due to species variations in immune responses and disease progression, which complicates the evaluation of vaccine efficacy [13]. Ensuring that results from animal studies are reproducible and applicable to human disease remains a critical hurdle, making the development of an effective TB vaccine particularly challenging [14].

6.3 Strategies for Antigen Discovery

Antigen discovery is a crucial step in developing effective vaccines and diagnostic tools, particularly for complex diseases like TB. Researchers have employed a variety of strategies for antigen discovery, ranging from traditional empirical screening to advanced techniques like immunopeptidomics. Each approach has its own strengths and limitations, influencing the path toward identifying the most promising antigens for TB vaccine development [15].

6.3.1 Identification of Culture Filtrate Antigens

Tuberculin, a purified protein derivative (PPD) derived from *Mtb*, plays a central role in the diagnosis of TB. It is commonly used in the tuberculin skin test, where a small amount is injected intradermally to detect immune sensitization to TB antigens. Beyond its diagnostic applications, tuberculin has also been instrumental in understanding the antigenic properties of mycobacterial proteins. A key area of research involves the identification of culture filtrate antigens (CFAs), which are proteins secreted by *Mtb* into the culture medium. One of the initial strategies for antigen discovery involves identifying antigens found in the culture filtrates of *Mtb*.

As these proteins are released into the host environment, they are likely to interact with the host's immune system, making them promising candidates for vaccine development.

To identify CFAs, researchers commonly cultivate *Mtb* in liquid culture and subsequently collect the filtrate after eliminating the bacteria. The filtrate contains a blend of secreted proteins, which are analyzed using various biochemical and immunological methods. Proteins that provoke a strong immune response are identified as potential candidates for vaccine development. However, this approach mainly identifies antigens produced during the active growth phase and may overlook those related to latent infection [16]. ESAT-6 was discovered through the analysis of culture filtrates from virulent *Mtb* strains. Researchers observed that this protein is secreted early during infection and is absent in nonvirulent strains, highlighting its potential as a promising candidate for diagnostic and vaccine development. This discovery led to the use of ESAT-6 in interferon-gamma release assays (IGRAs), such as QuantiFERON-TB, which detect TB infections by measuring the immune response to ESAT-6 [17].

6.3.2 Identification of Dormancy Antigens

TB can persist in a dormant state within the host, complicating treatment and control. Identifying antigens linked to this dormant phase is essential for creating vaccines that can address latent TB infections. Dormancy antigens are usually proteins overexpressed by *Mtb* during its nonreplicative or low-metabolic state, enabling the bacterium to survive in harsh conditions within the host.

Researchers often employ dormancy models, like hypoxia or nutrient starvation, to simulate a dormant state in *Mtb* in vitro. Proteins expressed under these conditions are subsequently identified using techniques such as immunoblotting or mass spectrometry (MS). These dormancy-associated antigens could be potential targets for vaccines designed to prevent the reactivation of latent TB or to eradicate dormant bacteria [18]. The Rv1733c antigen was identified through research on the proteomic profile of *Mtb* under hypoxic conditions, which mimic the low-oxygen environments that trigger dormancy. This protein was found to be highly expressed during these dormant states and is believed to contribute to the pathogen's survival in low-oxygen environments within the host [19].

6.3.3 Genome-Wide Approaches

Advances in genomics have transformed the field of antigen discovery through the use of genome-wide approaches. These methods involve systematically screening the entire genome of *Mtb* to identify potential antigens. One approach involves using DNA microarrays or RNA sequencing to examine gene expression profiles under various conditions, helping researchers identify genes that are highly expressed during infection.

Another genome-wide approach is transposon mutagenesis, which entails introducing random mutations across the *Mtb* genome. By determining which mutants are unable to cause disease, researchers can identify critical genes and their corresponding proteins as potential antigens. Furthermore genome-wide association studies (GWAS) can be used to connect specific genetic variations with immune responses, further refining the list of candidate antigens [20]. The M72/AS01E vaccine is currently one of the most promising TB vaccine candidates in development. Its success underscores the value of genome-wide approaches in identifying novel antigens that may not be evident through traditional methods [21].

6.3.4 In Silico Approaches

In silico methods or computational approaches have become increasingly vital in the process of antigen discovery. These methods utilize bioinformatics tools to analyze the *Mtb* genome, proteome, and interactome, allowing for the prediction of proteins that are likely to be immunogenic. By employing algorithms that forecast the protein structure, function, and interactions with the immune system, researchers can identify potential antigens without requiring extensive laboratory experiments.

A widely used in silico method is reverse vaccinology, which involves scanning the entire genome of a pathogen to predict surface-exposed or secreted proteins that could be potential vaccine targets. The predictions are then experimentally validated, making the antigen discovery process more efficient. In silico methods can also integrate data from sources like transcriptomics and proteomics to enhance the precision of antigen prediction [22]. The ID93 antigen is a fusion protein that consists of four *Mtb* proteins: Rv2608, Rv3619, Rv3620, and Rv1813. These proteins were identified through in silico methods, which predicted their immunogenic potential based on sequence conservation, surface localization, and epitope prediction. The ID93/GLA-SE vaccine is currently in further clinical evaluation. Its development demonstrates the effectiveness of in silico approaches in identifying and optimizing TB vaccine candidates, potentially leading to more effective vaccines in the future.

6.3.5 Immunopeptidomics

Immunopeptidomics is an advanced technique that targets the identification of peptides presented by major histocompatibility complex (MHC) molecules on the cell surface. During infection, the MHC-bound peptides, originated from pathogen proteins, are essential for activating T-cells and triggering an immune response. By examining the array of peptides presented by MHC molecules during *Mtb* infection, researchers can identify potential antigens that are naturally processed and detected by the immune system.

This method involves isolating MHC–peptide complexes from infected cells and then using tandem mass spectrometry to identify the peptides bound to these complexes. Immunopeptidomics delivers direct evidence of which pathogen-derived peptides are presented to the immune system, providing strong confidence in their potential as vaccine candidates. Furthermore, this method can uncover variations in antigen presentation among individuals, offering insights into the diversity of immune responses and aiding in the development of personalized vaccines [23].

An earlier study conducted by Flyer et al. employed immunoaffinity chromatography to isolate class I HLA-A*0201-peptide complexes from *Mtb*-infected cells and analyzed the isolated peptides. Three peptides originating from a single *Mtb* protein encoded by the Rv0341 gene were identified. Although no characterized protein has been associated with the Rv0341 gene, it was predicted to encode a 479-amino acid protein with a molecular mass of 43.9 kDa. The three identified peptides, all nested, were shown to be antigenic. They were capable of inducing peptide-specific CD8+ T-cells from healthy blood donors in vitro and demonstrated the ability to recognize and lyse *Mtb* infected dendritic cells. This approach offers a robust tool for identifying *Mtb* proteins that could be explored as potential vaccine candidates [24].

Another study by McMurtey et al. analyzed the ligandome presented by HLA-E during M*tb* infection using a comprehensive mass spectrometry approach. HLA-E is a nonconventional MHC class I molecule recently shown to present pathogen-derived ligands, leading to the TCR-dependent activation of αβ CD8+ T-cells. The study identified 28 *Mtb* ligands originating from 13 distinct source proteins, including members of the Esx protein family. When evaluated for activity with CD8+ T-cells from 16 donors, nine ligands triggered an interferon-gamma (IFN-γ) response in at least one donor, with 14 out of 16 donors responding to the Rv0634A19–29 peptide. Further analysis of the response to this immunodominant peptide confirmed HLA-E restriction and the presence of Rv0634A19–29-reactive CD8+ T-cells in the peripheral blood of human donors. The discovery of an *Mtb* HLA-E ligand commonly recognized could serve as a potential target for a nonconventional vaccine strategy [25].

In a recent study, Bettencourt et al. immunoprecipitated MHC class I and class II complexes from BCG-infected THP-1 macrophages to identify mycobacterial antigens presented by MHC. As a result, 94 mycobacterial peptides presented by MHC-II and 43 by MHC-I, originating from 76 and 41 antigens, respectively, were successfully identified. The identified antigens were predominantly expressed in infected macrophages, with gene ontology analysis revealing their membrane association and roles in lipid biosynthesis and transport. Spectral matching was used to validate the sequences of selected peptides, while their immunogenicity was assessed through IFN-gamma ELISpot assays using peripheral blood mononuclear cells from BCG-vaccinated individuals, latent *Mtb* carriers, and patients with active TB. Three antigens were expressed using viral vectors and assessed as vaccine candidates, either individually or in combination, in a murine aerosol *Mtb* challenge model. When administered together, the candidate vaccines provided significant protection in the lungs and spleen compared to BCG alone, validating this unbiased strategy in identifying novel antigen candidates [26]. Building on this work, the same group identified 64 and 80 unique mycobacterial antigens derived from BCG and *Mtb*, respectively, using the same approach. To ensure broad population coverage, all identified antigens were prioritised based on the density of T-cell epitopes against the most prevalent HLA alleles worldwide using immunoinformatics tools. This yielded a shortlist of promising candidates, among which the metE antigen demonstrated protective efficacy in *in vivo* murine *Mtb* challenge experiments71.

Furthermore, Leddy et al. demonstrated the potential of *Mtb* antigens present on MHC-I that can serve as targets for the TB vaccine. MS analysis of the MHC-I repertoire in *Mtb*-infected primary human macrophages reveals an overrepresentation of *Mtb*-derived peptides from substrates of the type VII secretion systems (T7SS) among those presented on MHC-I. Quantitative, targeted MS demonstrates that ESX-1 activity is essential for the presentation of *Mtb* peptides originating from both ESX-5 and ESX-1 substrates on MHC-I. This supports a model where proteins secreted by multiple type VII secretion systems (T7SSs) access the cytosolic antigen processing pathway through ESX-1-mediated phagosome permeabilization [27].

6.4 Pre-clinical Models

Pre-clinical models are experimental systems utilized to investigate the effects of drugs, treatments, or other interventions before they advance to human clinical trials. These models play a crucial role in biomedical research and drug development, enabling researchers to collect vital data on the safety, efficacy, and mechanisms of action of potential therapies [28].

6.4.1 In Vitro and Ex Vivo Models

In vitro and ex vivo models are valuable tools for studying TB, offering controlled environments to investigate disease mechanisms, assess drug efficacy, and develop vaccines. In vitro models, such as cell culture systems, provide a controlled environment to investigate cellular responses to potential vaccine candidates, utilizing key immune cells like dendritic cells, macrophages, and T-cells. Ex vivo models, on the other hand, involve the examination of tissues or organs from TB-infected or genetically modified organisms outside the body. These models offer a more controlled setting than in vivo studies while retaining some of the complexities of living systems. Additionally, human cells can be employed and infected with the pathogenic strains of *Mtb,* providing a valuable model for studying the disease without the ethical concerns associated with using pathogenic strains in humans [29].

6.4.2 In Vivo Models

Animal models are essential in pre-clinical testing, offering valuable information on the safety, efficacy, and immunogenicity of new vaccines or therapies before human trials. The selection of an animal model depends on factors such as the nature of the disease, the similarity of the animal's immune system to that of humans, and ethical considerations [30]. The different animal models used for TB vaccine development are described in other sections of the book.

6.5 Evaluation of Pre-clinical TB Vaccine Efficacy

6.5.1 Immune Response Assessment Techniques

In the pre-clinical evaluation of TB vaccines, evaluating the immune response is vital to understanding the vaccine's potential efficacy. Several techniques are utilized for this purpose, including

(a) Antibody titers
(b) T-cell responses
(c) Cytokine profiling
(d) Functional assays

(a) *Antibody Titers*

These measurements are used to assess the humoral immune response. Antibodies targeting *Mtb* antigens are quantified through assays such as ELISA (enzyme-linked immunosorbent assay). In this assay, *Mtb* antigens are coated onto a plate, and serum from vaccinated animals is applied. If antibodies against *Mtb* are present in the serum, they will attach to the antigens. Subsequently, a secondary antibody, which targets the animal's antibodies and is coupled with an enzyme, is added. The enzyme's activity, which typically produces a color change, is then measured to determine the quantity of bound antibodies. However, antibodies are not the main line of defence against TB; their presence can still offer valuable insights into the immunity induced by the vaccine [31].

While antibodies play a complementary role to T-cells in TB immunity such as by enhancing bacterial neutralization and phagocytosis, their significance is especially evident in the evaluation of modern vaccine platforms like mRNA and subunit vaccines. Antibody titers also assist in determining the duration of vaccine-induced immunity and guiding the timing of booster doses. In latent TB infections, they may help monitor the immune status and assess the risk of reactivation. However, antibody titers are not definitive markers of protection against TB due to the complex interplay between humoral and cellular immunity. Despite these challenges, their role in TB vaccine research is gaining prominence as part of efforts to optimize immunization strategies and improve outcomes [32].

(b) *T-Cell Responses*

T-cell responses play a critical role in immunity to TB, and understanding these responses is key to the development of effective TB vaccines. Unlike many other infectious diseases, where humoral immunity (antibodies) is the primary defence, TB immunity relies predominantly on the activation of T-cells. These are crucial for effective TB immunity, as they control the infection by activating macrophages and killing infected cells. Unlike antibody-based immunity, TB relies on *CD4+ helper T-cells* and *CD8+ cytotoxic T-cells* to form granulomas and contain the bacteria. Vaccines that stimulate these T-cell responses, especially *memory T-cells*, offer long-term protection and prevent latent TB from reactivating. Enhancing T-cell immunity is essential for overcoming challenges like *T-cell exhaustion* and developing more effective vaccines that can provide lasting protection against TB [10]. The two key techniques that are employed to assess both the magnitude and functionality of these T-cell responses are as follows:

ELISPOT (Enzyme-Linked ImmunoSpot)

This assay determines the frequency of T-cells that produce specific cytokines in response to *Mtb* antigens. PBMCs from vaccinated animals are isolated and cultured with these antigens. The cells are subsequently placed onto a plate coated with an antibody that captures a specific cytokine, such as IFN-γ, as it is released by T-cells. After incubation, the plate is developed, and spots corresponding to individual cytokine-secreting cells are counted, which provide a measure of the number of antigen-specific T cells. ELISPOT assay is highly sensitive and capable of detecting even low-frequency T-cell responses, making it invaluable for early-phase vaccine evaluation [33].

Flow Cytometry Flow cytometry enables detailed characterization of T-cells in response to vaccination. PBMCs are stimulated with *Mtb* antigens and stained with fluorescently labeled antibodies that bind to surface markers to identify T-cell subsets and intracellular cytokines to assess their functionality. The cells are then analyzed using a flow cytometer, which detects the fluorescence and provides information on the quantity and types of T-cells, as well as the cytokines they produce [34].

Flow cytometry offers a comprehensive analysis of the T-cell response, including the proportion of CD4 (helper) and CD8 (cytotoxic) T-cells, their activation status, and the cytokines they produce. This detailed profiling is crucial for understanding the quality of the immune response, such as whether it is predominantly Th1 (proinflammatory and beneficial for TB control) or Th2 (humoral and less effective for TB) [35].

(c) *Cytokine Profiling*

In TB vaccine research, cytokine profiling is essential for identifying the correlates of protection, evaluating vaccine-induced immune responses, and monitoring safety. It helps determine whether a vaccine elicits a robust and appropriate immune response. Various methods are employed for this purpose, including ELISA for quantifying specific cytokines, flow cytometry for single-cell analysis, and multiplex assays that allow simultaneous measurement of multiple cytokines. Transcriptomic approaches provide a broader view by analyzing cytokine mRNA expression profiles [36].

Effective TB vaccines aim to induce a strong Th1-type immune response characterized by IFN-γ, tumor necrosis factor-alpha (TNF-α), and interleukin-2 (IL-2) production. However, a balanced response that includes Th17-associated cytokines like IL-17 is also desirable for sustained immunity and granuloma stability. Conversely, excessive production of Th2 or regulatory cytokines such as IL-4 and IL-10 may indicate an unfavorable shift away from protective immunity. These assays usually employ bead-based platforms, with each bead coated in an antibody specific to a particular cytokine. When a sample containing cytokines is added, the cytokines bind to the corresponding beads. A detection antibody linked to a fluorescent marker is then introduced, and the beads are analyzed using flow cytometry or a similar detection system. This method enables the quantification of a broad range of cytokines, including IFN-γ, IL-2, TNF-α, IL-10, and IL-17 [37].

Despite its potential, cytokine profiling faces challenges such as variability in immune responses across individuals due to genetic and environmental factors, a lack of standardized assays, and the difficulty of identifying reliable biomarkers of protection. Advances in high-throughput multiplex platforms, single-cell technologies, and systems immunology approaches help to address these challenges by providing deeper insights into immune mechanisms and improving the predictive accuracy of vaccine efficacy [38].

(d) *Functional Assays*

Functional assays are essential tools in TB vaccine research, as they provide insights into the quality and efficacy of the immune response induced by candidate vaccines. These assays evaluate the functional capacity of immune cells beyond their activation, shedding light on the mechanisms of protective immunity. These assays test the efficacy of the immune cells from vaccinated animals in preventing the growth of *Mtb* in vitro. For example, PBMCs or macrophages are co-cultured with *Mtb*, and the bacterial load is measured after a specific period, usually by counting colony-forming units (CFUs) or using luminescent reporter strains of *Mtb* [39]. Similarly, micro-CFU assays are typically used to assess whether the vaccine reduces the number of viable bacteria in the lungs or other organs following experimental infection. After vaccination, animals are exposed to TB pathogens, and the bacterial load is measured using micro-CFU techniques, which involve plating diluted samples of tissue homogenates on solid media and counting the microcolonies formed. This approach offers several advantages over traditional CFU assays, including enhanced sensitivity for detecting low levels of viable bacteria, making it especially useful for evaluating vaccines that may not completely eradicate the pathogen but reduce its numbers to a level that the immune system can control [40].

T-cell functional assays are a cornerstone of this research, measuring the production of cytokines like IFN-γ through methods such as IGRAs and polyfunctional T-cell assays, which assess the simultaneous production of multiple cytokines. Proliferation assays evaluate the ability of T-cells to expand upon antigen stimulation, while cytotoxicity assays measure CD8+ T-cells' capacity to kill *Mtb*-infected cells. Macrophage function assays are equally important, as macrophages are the primary host cells for *Mtb*. These assays include phagocytosis tests, mycobacterial growth inhibition assays (MGIA) to assess bacterial killing, and evaluations of antimicrobial mechanisms such as nitric oxide (NO) and reactive oxygen species (ROS) production [41].

Antibody functional assays are gaining attention for their role in TB immunity, measuring processes like opsonophagocytosis, antibody-dependent cellular cytotoxicity (ADCC), and neutralization of *Mtb*. Granuloma-focused assays provide insights into the vaccine's impact on the formation and maintenance of these critical structures that contain infection. In vitro granuloma models and ex vivo analyses allow researchers to study how vaccines influence granuloma integrity and bacterial control. Advances in systems-level approaches, such as single-cell RNA sequencing (scRNA-seq), multiplex cytokine assays, and 3D culture models, further enhance our understanding of vaccine-induced functional immunity. These tools are complemented by high-throughput technologies and organ-on-chip platforms, which aim to replicate physiological conditions more accurately [42].

While functional assays offer valuable insights, challenges such as variability in individual responses, standardization of protocols, and translating findings from in vitro or animal models to humans remain significant. Combining these assays with systems immunology and computational modeling provides a comprehensive framework for optimizing vaccine design [43].

6.5.2 Protective Efficacy Studies in Animal Models

Protective efficacy studies in animal models are crucial for developing TB vaccines. These studies consist of vaccinating animals and then exposing them to virulent strains of *Mtb*. The main objective is to assess whether the vaccine can prevent infection or, at the very least, lessen the severity of the disease [44].

Animal models like guinea pigs, mice, and non-human primates are frequently used because they can mimic various aspects of human TB infection, including the immune response and disease pathology. For example, non-human primates such as rhesus macaques are especially valuable because their immune systems closely resemble those of humans, offering a more accurate prediction of how a vaccine might perform in people. These models enable researchers to assess the vaccine's efficacy in a controlled environment, where factors like dosage, timing, and method of administration can be precisely managed [45].

In TB vaccine studies, candidate vaccines are administered using various routes, such as intramuscular, subcutaneous, or mucosal delivery, often employing a prime–boost strategy. After vaccination, animals are typically challenged with virulent *Mtb* strains via aerosol exposure to mimic natural infection. Control groups, including unvaccinated animals or those receiving the BCG vaccine, provide benchmarks for evaluating efficacy. Protective outcomes are assessed through bacterial load reduction in organs, histopathological examination of granulomas, immune response analysis, and monitoring clinical signs such as weight loss and survival. Cellular immunity, particularly T-cell responses, is a primary focus, as it is critical for TB control [44].

While many candidates demonstrate robust immune responses and reduced bacterial loads in animal models, the translatability of these findings to humans remains a significant challenge. No single model fully replicates human TB, and efficacy in animals does not always predict success in clinical trials. To address these challenges, advancements such as humanized mouse models, standardized protocols, and the identification of immune correlates of protection are being developed. Ethical considerations, including adherence to the principles of Replacement, Reduction, and Refinement (3Rs), are also integral to these studies [46].

6.5.3 Surrogate Immune Markers Between Animal Models and Humans

These biomarkers are used to estimate the presence or intensity of an immune response thought to be linked to protection or disease outcome. In vaccine research, they are frequently employed to forecast a vaccine's effectiveness before conducting human trials [47]. The following are the key considerations for surrogate immune markers when comparing animal models to humans:

Cross-Species Relevance Certain immune markers in animal models, like specific cytokines or antibodies, can reflect similar immune responses in humans. However, not all markers translate seamlessly across species because of differences in immune system physiology and genetics.

Correlation with Human Data Markers such as specific antibody titers or T-cell responses in animal models may sometimes correlate with protective immunity in humans, but the strength and reliability of these correlations can vary.

Validation Validating these markers in both animal models and human studies is essential to ensure their relevance. This process involves verifying that the immune responses observed in animals correspond to similar protection or pathology in humans.

6.5.4 Immunologic Correlates of Protection (ICOPs) in Vaccine Development

Immunologic correlates of protection (ICOPs) are measurable immune responses that are statistically linked to protection against infection or disease. In vaccine development, identifying ICOPs is critical as they serve as benchmarks to predict vaccine efficacy, streamline clinical trials, and guide regulatory approval. These correlates provide insights into the mechanisms of protection, enabling better vaccine design and evaluation [48].

ICOPs can be broadly categorized into *mechanistic correlates* and *nonmechanistic correlates*. Mechanistic correlates are immune responses directly responsible for protection, such as neutralizing antibodies that block viral entry or specific T-cell responses that eliminate infected cells. Nonmechanistic correlates, on the other hand, are immune markers associated with protection but not necessarily causative, like certain cytokine profiles or cell population changes.

In TB, ICOPs are largely focused on cellular immunity, given the pivotal role of T cells in controlling intracellular pathogens like *Mtb*. Key ICOPs under investigation include the production of IFN-γ by antigen-specific CD4+ T-cells, which is crucial for activating macrophages to kill intracellular *Mtb*. Polyfunctional T-cells producing multiple cytokines (e.g., IFN-γ, TNF-α, and IL-2) are considered potential markers of robust and sustained immune responses. Other ICOPs include the frequency and functionality of memory T-cells, cytotoxic CD8+ T-cell responses, and the ability of immune cells to form and maintain granulomas that contain the infection. Emerging research has highlighted the importance of Th17-associated cytokines like IL-17, which contribute to mucosal immunity and granuloma stability, and regulatory cytokines like IL-10, which modulate excessive inflammation but may also suppress protective immunity. Additionally, macrophage activity, such as phagocytosis and mycobacterial growth inhibition, is being explored as a correlate of protection [49].

Defining ICOPs for TB is challenging due to variability in host immune responses, differences in *Mtb* strains, and the lack of a fully protective vaccine for comparison. The BCG vaccine provides partial protection but has inconsistent efficacy, complicating efforts to identify reliable ICOPs. Advanced methodologies, including systems biology, single-cell analyses, and transcriptomic profiling, are increasingly used to uncover novel ICOPs and gain deeper insights into the mechanisms of TB immunity [50].

6.6 Strategies for Pre-clinical TB Vaccine Development

Vaccine development employs several strategies designed to elicit a protective immune response against pathogens [51]. Following are some of the key approaches used in vaccine development.

6.6.1 Live Attenuated Vaccines

These vaccines use a weakened form of the pathogen to provoke immune responses that closely resemble those produced by a natural infection. They generate a broad spectrum of immune responses as they present several antigens, unlike viral or subunit vector vaccines, which typically contain only a few mycobacterial antigens. Live attenuated vaccines might pose a risk to individuals with weakened immune systems, such as those living with HIV/AIDS, as they are at a significantly higher risk of developing active TB disease [52].

A prominent example of a live attenuated vaccine is BCG, which comes from an attenuated form of *Mycobacterium bovis*, a bacterium closely related to *Mtb*. Given the similarity in the cell biology of intracellular infections, both *Mtb* and BCG induce CD4 and CD8 T-cell responses and promote antibody production. During the attenuation process, genomic regions responsible for its major virulence factors are deleted, making BCG safe for use in immunocompetent individuals [53]. The main advantages of live attenuated vaccines are their strong immunogenicity and ability to provide long-lasting protection, due to their capacity to mimic natural infection and persist temporarily in the host. However, they also present challenges, including safety concerns, especially in immunocompromised individuals, and the risk of reversion to virulence. Additionally, these vaccines often require cold-chain storage, which can be a logistical hurdle in resource-limited settings. Despite these challenges, live attenuated vaccines remain a promising avenue for TB prevention, with ongoing research focused on enhancing their safety, stability, and efficacy through genetic modifications and novel delivery methods [54].

6.6.2 Subunit Vaccines

Instead of targeting the whole pathogen, protein subunit vaccines are designed to provoke immune responses against specific antigens derived from the pathogen. Most subunit TB vaccines target particular proteins from *Mtb*, leading to a more limited immune response. In addition, subunit vaccines lack "pathogen-associated microbial patterns" that activate innate immune responses, and they need adjuvants to generate a robust immune response to the target antigen. Therefore, selecting the right adjuvant is a crucial aspect of subunit vaccine design. Examples of such vaccines are H4 and M72/AS01, which have recently completed phase II clinical trials [55]. Despite their promise, subunit vaccines face challenges, including the difficulty of selecting effective antigens, varied immunity across populations due to prior BCG vaccination or *Mtb* exposure, and the need for affordable, scalable production. Additionally, the lack of reliable biomarkers to predict vaccine efficacy complicates their development. Future efforts are focused on optimizing antigens and adjuvants, exploring mucosal delivery for respiratory immunity, and combining subunit vaccines with existing TB vaccines like BCG. These advancements could significantly enhance the global fight against TB [56].

6.6.3 Viral-Vectored Vaccines

Viral-vectored vaccines represent a unique intermediary between live attenuated vaccines and subunit vaccines. Conceptually, they are similar to subunit vaccines in that they focus immune responses on a specific part of the pathogen, rather than targeting the entire pathogen. The viruses, acting as vectors, are engineered to carry genes for *Mtb* proteins. Following immunization with these viral particles, the infected cells begin to produce *Mtb* proteins, leading to a strong immune response without requiring an external adjuvant. This method builds on decades of experience with attenuated virus vaccines (such as those for poliovirus, vaccinia, and measles) and capitalizes on the immune system's robust innate and adaptive responses to viruses [57].

Examples include MVA85A, designed to boost BCG-induced immunity by expressing the Ag85A antigen, and ChAdOx1.85A, an adenovirus-based vaccine targeting the same antigen. While MVA85A demonstrated safety and immunogenicity in early trials, it did not show significant efficacy in preventing TB disease in a Phase IIb trial. Viral-vectored vaccines are particularly effective at inducing both humoral and cellular immunity and can be used as boosters for BCG or other primary vaccines. However, challenges such as pre-existing immunity to some viral vectors, complex manufacturing requirements, and potential safety concerns need to be addressed. Future efforts include developing novel vectors with reduced pre-existing immunity, optimizing prime-boost combinations with other vaccine platforms, and exploring mucosal delivery methods to enhance respiratory immunity [58]. A detailed description of viral-vectored vaccines under clinincal trials can be found on Chap. 11.

6.6.4 DNA Vaccines

DNA vaccines function by delivering a plasmid DNA containing the genetic instructions for a specific pathogen's antigen into the body. The DNA is introduced into cells through various techniques, such as electroporation or gene gun technology. After entering the cells, the plasmid DNA is transported into the nucleus, where it is transcribed into messenger RNA (mRNA). The mRNA then instructs the cell's machinery to produce the pathogen's antigen, which is either displayed on the cell surface or released into the body. This prompts an immune response as the immune system identifies the antigen as foreign. The immune response engages both cellular immunity and humoral immunity (involving B-cells and antibodies), resulting in the formation of immune memory [59].

DNA vaccines, such as those targeting the HSP65 and Ag85A antigens, have shown promise in pre-clinical and early clinical studies, with candidates like the ID93 DNA vaccine aiming to provide broad protection by encoding a fusion of multiple *Mtb* antigens. Key advantages of DNA vaccines include their safety, as they do not involve live pathogens, and their stability, making them suitable for use in resource-limited settings. Additionally, they are cost-effective to produce and can be easily customized to include new antigens. However, challenges remain, including ensuring efficient DNA delivery and expression in host cells, enhancing immune potency, and addressing regulatory concerns regarding long-term safety [60].

6.6.5 Novel Approaches

Novel approaches in pre-clinical vaccine development are focused on improving the efficacy, safety, and broad applicability of vaccines, especially for complex pathogens like *Mtb.* In the development of TB vaccines, innovative strategies such as nanoparticle vaccines, mucosal vaccines, and mRNA vaccines are showing great promise in improving immune responses and vaccine efficacy. Nanoparticle-based vaccines enhance antigen delivery by encapsulating antigens or adjuvants, improving stability and targeted delivery to immune cells like dendritic cells, which strengthen the immune response. These vaccines are particularly useful in TB development, as nanoparticles can deliver *Mtb* antigens, boosting cellular immunity crucial for TB control [61].

Mucosal vaccines, administered orally or intranasally, aim to induce immunity at mucosal surfaces, which are the primary entry points for TB. These vaccines stimulate both local and systemic immune responses, promoting secretory IgA antibodies and cellular immunity, which is important for preventing infection and controlling disease progression in the lungs [24]. While many effective mucosal vaccines are available, the significant advancements achieved with injectable vaccines such as adjuvanted subunit antigens, mRNA, and DNA vaccines have yet to be applied to licensed mucosal vaccines, which are currently limited to live attenuated and inactivated whole-cell formulations.

MRNA vaccines offer rapid production and the flexibility to encode specific *Mtb* antigens, inducing strong humoral and cellular immunity. These vaccines are particularly advantageous in TB research due to their quick scalability and potential to target drug-resistant strains. Furthermore, the in vitro synthesis and purification of mRNA are cell-free, rapid, and easily scalable, unlike the complex and time-consuming production processes required for conventional vaccines [62]. Combining these approaches, nanoparticles for better antigen delivery, mucosal vaccines for localized immune responses, and mRNA vaccines for rapid adaptability, holds great potential in overcoming the challenges of TB, such as latent infection, reinfection, and emerging drug-resistant strains, and could significantly improve TB vaccine development in the future.

6.7 Adjuvants

Adjuvants are substances included in vaccines to enhance or modify the immune response, making vaccines more effective. They work by stimulating the innate immune system, which in turn activates a stronger adaptive immune response. Adjuvants enhance antigen presentation by immune cells like dendritic cells, prolong antigen exposure, and stimulate the production of proinflammatory cytokines, all of which improve the overall immune response. Common types of adjuvants include aluminum salts (e.g., aluminum hydroxide), oil-in-water emulsions (e.g., MF59), TLR agonists (e.g., monophosphoryl lipid A), liposomes, and saponins. These adjuvants work by enhancing immune cell activation, promoting antibody production, or mimicking the structures of pathogens [63].

In the context of TB vaccines, adjuvants are particularly critical for generating strong cellular immunity, which is vital for controlling *Mtb*. Adjuvants like MPL, liposomes, and saponins have been studied for their ability to enhance immune responses in TB vaccine candidates, improving the effectiveness of the vaccine by boosting both the magnitude and duration of immunity. This makes adjuvants an essential component in the development of TB vaccines and other immunotherapies, helping to ensure a balanced immune response that can effectively target the bacteria [64]. The various adjuvants utilized in TB vaccine development are being demonstrated in Table 6.1.

6.8 Conclusions

Pre-clinical TB vaccine research is critically important as it lays the groundwork for creating new and more effective vaccines against TB, a disease that remains a leading cause of death worldwide. At this stage of research, extensive laboratory studies and animal testing are conducted to assess the immune responses triggered by potential vaccines, evaluate their safety, and determine their efficacy before progressing to human trials. Currently, out of the 17 active TB vaccines under clinical development, 8 are subunit vaccines, with 6 of these incorporating or expressing Ag85A or Ag85B proteins [70]. One of the significant challenges in developing TB vaccines is the limited diversity of antigens included and the narrow range of immune responses triggered by the vaccine candidates.

Furthermore, limitations of animal models, such as their inability to accurately mimic human TB pathophysiology and the ethical constraints surrounding their use, further impede vaccine development. A lack of well-defined immune correlates of protection and the genetic diversity of *Mtb* strains add to the difficulty of assessing vaccine efficacy. Additionally, addressing both active and latent TB infection in preclinical studies remains challenging due to limited models for studying latency and reactivation.

Expanding antigen selection and broadening the range of vaccine-induced immune responses are critical steps toward achieving a successful candidate in the coming years. Ongoing research is concentrated on these priorities. The insights

Table 6.1 Adjuvants commonly employed in TB vaccines

No.	Adjuvant type	Composition	Candidate vaccine	Mechanism	Reference
1	Liposome	GLA in a stable oil-in-water SE	ID91 + GLA-SE,ID93 + GLA-SE	Triggers Th1 immune response and generates IL-2, IFN-γ, TNF-α, as well as both IgG3 and IgG1.	[65]
2	Protein	ODN1a, KLK	H1:IC31, H56:IC31	Triggers either Th17 or Th1 immune responses, resulting in the production of IFN-γ, TNF-α, and IL-2.	[66]
3	Nucleic acid	CpG ODN	Ga*MTB*Vac	Induces a Th1 immune response, leading to the production of IFN-γ, IL-6, IL-10, IL-12, TGF-β, and TNF-α. Additionally, it promotes the surface expression of CD40, MHC, and CD86 on peripheral blood cells.	[67]
4	Aluminum salt	CpG DNA, Al(OH)3	BC02/AEC	Trigers both Th1 and Th2 immune responses, leading to the production of IL-4 and stimulating the expression of CD86, CD83, and MHC-II molecules.	[68]
5	Liposome	TDB, DDA	H1:CAF01	It triggers a Th17 immune response, resulting in the production of IL-17 and IgA.	[69]

obtained from pre-clinical research are essential for identifying the most promising vaccine candidates, refining their formulations, and comprehending the mechanisms through which they provide protection. Strengthening the clinical translation pipeline through adaptive trial designs and human challenge models, where ethical, will bridge the gap between pre-clinical and clinical phases. These efforts, combined with global collaboration and technological advancements, will help overcome challenges and pave the way for effective TB vaccines.

Competing Interests The author(s) has no competing interests to declare that are relevant to the content of this manuscript.

Ethics Approval The author(s) declares that this manuscript does not include primary research with human participants.

References

1. Global Tuberculosis Report 2024. https://www.who.int/teams/global-tuberculosis-programme/tb-reports/global-tuberculosis-report-2024.
2. Snow KJ, Sismanidis C, Denholm J, Sawyer SM, Graham SM. The incidence of tuberculosis among adolescents and young adults: a global estimate. Eur Respir J. 2018;51.
3. Walker KB, et al. Novel approaches to preclinical research and TB vaccine development. Tuberculosis (Edinb). 2016;99(Suppl 1):S12–5.
4. Tu HAT, Vu HD, Rozenbaum MH, Woerdenbag HJ, Postma MJ. A review of the literature on the economics of vaccination against TB. Expert Rev Vaccines. 2012;11:303–17.
5. Mangtani P, et al. Protection by BCG vaccine against tuberculosis: a systematic review of randomized controlled trials. Clin Infect Dis. 2014;58:470–80.
6. Orme IM. Beyond BCG: the potential for a more effective TB vaccine. Mol Med Today. 1999;5:487–92.
7. Orme IM. Preclinical testing of new vaccines for tuberculosis: a comprehensive review. Vaccine. 2006;24:2–19.
8. Chugh S, Bahal RK, Dhiman R, Singh R. Antigen identification strategies and preclinical evaluation models for advancing tuberculosis vaccine development. NPJ Vaccines. 2024;9:57.
9. Arroliga AC. Clinics in chest medicine. Clin Chest Med. 1999;20.
10. Balasingam S, et al. Review of current tuberculosis human infection studies for use in accelerating tuberculosis vaccine development: a meeting report. J Infect Dis. 2024;230:e457–64.
11. Krishnan N, et al. A noninvasive BCG skin challenge model for assessing tuberculosis vaccine efficacy. PLoS Biol. 2024;22:e3002766.
12. Wei X, et al. Recent advances and challenges of revolutionizing drug-resistant tuberculosis treatment. Eur J Med Chem. 2024;277:116785.
13. O'Shea MK, McShane H. A review of clinical models for the evaluation of human TB vaccines. Hum Vaccin Immunother. 2016;12:1177–87.
14. Dave S, Patel BM. Preclinical and clinical development for vaccines and formulations. In: Advanced vaccination technologies for infectious and chronic diseases: a guide to vaccinology; 2024. p. 263–78. https://doi.org/10.1016/B978-0-443-18564-9.00016-3.
15. Nguyen TL, Kim H. Discovering peptides and computational investigations of a multiepitope vaccine target Mycobacterium tuberculosis. Synth Syst Biotechnol. 2024;9:391–405.
16. Hu Z, Shi L, Xie J, Fan XY. Editorial: innate and adaptive immunity against tuberculosis infection: diagnostics, vaccines, and therapeutics. Front Immunol. 2024;15:1366976.
17. Larsen SE, Baldwin SL, Coler RN. Tuberculosis vaccines update: is an RNA-based vaccine feasible for tuberculosis? Int J Infect Dis. 2023;130:S47–51.
18. Chen Y, et al. Advancements in the preparation technology of small molecule artificial antigens and their specific antibodies: a comprehensive review. Analyst. 2024; https://doi.org/10.1039/D4AN00501E.
19. Kimuda SG, et al. Humoral responses to Rv1733c, Rv0081, Rv1735c, and Rv1737c DosR regulon-encoded proteins of Mycobacterium tuberculosis in individuals with latent tuberculosis infection. J Immunol Res. 2017;2017:1593143.
20. Xu D, et al. Vaccine design via antigen reorientation. Nat Chem Biol. 2024;20.
21. Simwela NV, et al. Genome-wide screen of Mycobacterium tuberculosis-infected macrophages identified the GID/CTLH complex as a determinant of intracellular bacterial growth. bioRxiv 2024.05.06.592714. 2024. https://doi.org/10.1101/2024.05.06.592714.

22. Sethi G, et al. Immunoinformatics and structural aided approach to develop multi-epitope based subunit vaccine against Mycobacterium tuberculosis. Sci Rep. 2024;14:15923.
23. Abelin JG, Cox AL. Innovations toward immunopeptidomics. Mol Cell Proteomics. 2024;23:100823.
24. Lavelle EC, Ward RW. Mucosal vaccines—fortifying the frontiers. Nat Rev Immunol. 2022;22(4):236–50.
25. McMurtrey C, et al. T cell recognition of Mycobacterium tuberculosis peptides presented by HLA-E derived from infected human cells. PLoS One. 2017;12:1–19.
26. Bettencourt P, et al. Identification of antigens presented by MHC for vaccines against tuberculosis. NPJ Vaccines. 2020;5:2.
27. Leddy O, White FM, Bryson BD. Immunopeptidomics reveals determinants of Mycobacterium tuberculosis antigen presentation on MHC class I. elife. 2023;12:1–24.
28. Hebert JD, Neal JW, Winslow MM. Dissecting metastasis using preclinical models and methods. Nat Rev Cancer. 2023;23:391–407.
29. Alsayed SSR, Gunosewoyo H. Tuberculosis: pathogenesis, current treatment regimens and new drug targets. Int J Mol Sci. 2023;24:5202.
30. Zhuang L, Ye Z, Li L, Yang L, Gong W. Next-generation TB vaccines: progress, challenges, and prospects. Vaccine. 2023;11:1304.
31. Lacámara S, Martin C. MTBVAC: a tuberculosis vaccine candidate advancing towards clinical efficacy trials in TB prevention. Arch Bronconeumol. 2023;59:821–8.
32. Walker KB, et al. Novel approaches to preclinical research and TB vaccine development. Tuberculosis. 2016;99:S12–5.
33. Richeldi L, et al. Using ELISpot technology to improve the diagnosis of tuberculosis infection: from the bench to the T-SPOT.TB assay. Expert Rev Respir Med. 2008;2:253–60.
34. Fuhrmann S, Streitz M, Kern F. How flow cytometry is changing the study of TB immunology and clinical diagnosis. Cytom Part A. 2008;73:1100–6.
35. Parbhoo T, Sampson SL, Mouton JM. Recent developments in the application of flow cytometry to advance our understanding of Mycobacterium tuberculosis physiology and pathogenesis. Cytom Part A. 2020;97:683–93.
36. Painter H, et al. Demonstrating the utility of the ex vivo murine mycobacterial growth inhibition assay (MGIA) for high-throughput screening of tuberculosis vaccine candidates against multiple Mycobacterium tuberculosis complex strains. Tuberculosis. 2024;146:102494.
37. Chen T, et al. Profiling the human immune response to Mycobacterium tuberculosis by human cytokine array. Tuberculosis. 2016;97:108–17.
38. Pandiarajan AN, et al. Distinct TB-antigen stimulated cytokine profiles as predictive biomarkers for unfavorable treatment outcomes in pulmonary tuberculosis. Front Immunol. 2024;15:1392256.
39. Wang H, et al. Enhancing TB vaccine efficacy: current progress on vaccines, adjuvants and immunization strategie. Vaccines. 2023;12:38.
40. Pires D, Bettencourt PJG. Micro-Colony forming unit assay for efficacy evaluation of vaccines against tuberculosis. J Vis Exp. 2023;197:e65447. https://doi.org/10.3791/65447.
41. Painter H, Harriss E, Fletcher HA, McShane H, Tanner R. Development and application of the direct mycobacterial growth inhibition assay: a systematic review. Front Immunol. 2024;15:1355983.
42. Newton S, Martineau A, Kampmann B. A functional whole blood assay to measure viability of mycobacteria, using reporter-gene tagged BCG or M.Tb (BCG lux/M.Tb lux). J Vis Exp. 2011:3332. https://doi.org/10.3791/3332.
43. Tanner R, O'Shea MK, Fletcher HA, McShane H. In vitro mycobacterial growth inhibition assays: a tool for the assessment of protective immunity and evaluation of tuberculosis vaccine efficacy. Vaccine. 2016;34:4656–65.
44. Shim D-H, et al. New animal model of shigellosis in the Guinea pig: its usefulness for protective efficacy studies. J Immunol. 2007;178:2476–82.
45. Hunter L, Ruedas-Torres I, Agulló-Ros I, Rayner E, Salguero FJ. Comparative pathology of experimental pulmonary tuberculosis in animal models. Front Vet Sci. 2023;10:1264833.

46. Gong W, Liang Y, Wu X. Animal models of tuberculosis vaccine research: an important component in the fight against tuberculosis. Biomed Res Int. 2020;2020:4263079.
47. Hölken JM, Teusch N. The monocytic cell line THP-1 as a validated and robust surrogate model for human dendritic cells. Int J Mol Sci. 2023;24:1452.
48. Montoya M, Tchilian E. Principles of vaccinology and vaccine immune response. In: Veterinary vaccines: principles and applications; 2021. p. 11–23. https://doi.org/10.1002/9781119506287.CH2.
49. Scriba TJ, Netea MG, Ginsberg AM. Key recent advances in TB vaccine development and understanding of protective immune responses against Mycobacterium tuberculosis. Semin Immunol. 2020;50:101431.
50. Brazier B, McShane H. Towards new TB vaccines. Semin Immunopathol. 2020;42(3):315–31.
51. Li J, et al. Tuberculosis vaccine development: from classic to clinical candidates. Eur J Clin Microbiol Infect Dis. 2020;39:1405–25.
52. Minor PD. Live attenuated vaccines: historical successes and current challenges. Virology. 2015;479–480:379–92.
53. Belshe RB, Edwards KM, Vesikari T, Black SV, Walker RE, Hultquist M, Kemble G, Connor EM. Live attenuated versus inactivated influenza vaccine in infants and young children. New England Journal of Medicine. 2007;356(7):685–96.
54. Flores-Valdez MA, Kupz A, Subbian S. Recent developments in mycobacteria-based live attenuated vaccine candidates for tuberculosis. Biomedicines. 2022;10:2749.
55. Vartak A, Sucheck SJ. Recent advances in subunit vaccine carriers. Vaccine. 2016;4:1–18.
56. Bellini C, Horváti K. Recent advances in the development of protein- and peptide-based subunit vaccines against tuberculosis. Cells. 2020;9:2673.
57. Ewer KJ, et al. Viral vectors as vaccine platforms: from immunogenicity to impact. Curr Opin Immunol. 2016;41:47–54.
58. Hu Z, Lu SH, Lowrie DB, Fan XY. Research advances for virus-vectored tuberculosis vaccines and latest findings on tuberculosis vaccine development. Front Immunol. 2022;13:895020.
59. Okada M, Kita Y. Tuberculosis vaccine development: the development of a novel (preclinical) DNA vaccine. Hum Vaccin. 2010;6:297–308.
60. Sefidi-Heris Y, et al. Recent progress in the design of DNA vaccines against tuberculosis. Drug Discov Today. 2020;25:1971–87.
61. Gebre MS, et al. Novel approaches for vaccine development. Cell. 2021;184:1589–603.
62. Matarazzo L, Bettencourt PJG. mRNA vaccines: a new opportunity for malaria, tuberculosis and HIV. Front Immunol. 2023;14:1172691.
63. Enriquez AB, et al. Advancing adjuvants for Mycobacterium tuberculosis therapeutics. Front Immunol. 2021;12:740117.
64. Stewart E, Triccas JA, Petrovsky N. Adjuvant strategies for more effective tuberculosis vaccine immunity. Microorganisms. 2019;7:255.
65. Šťastná E, et al. Effects of different immunomodulating liposome-based adjuvants and injection sites on immunogenicity in pigs. Microbes Infect. 2024;26:105346.
66. Cox JC, Coulter AR. Advances in adjuvant technology and application. In: Animal parasite control utilizing biotechnology; 2024. p. 49–112. https://doi.org/10.1201/9781003574880-5.
67. Abbasi S, Uchida S. Multifunctional immunoadjuvants for use in minimalist nucleic acid vaccines. Pharmaceutics. 2021;13:644.
68. Danielsson R, Eriksson H. Aluminium adjuvants in vaccines – a way to modulate the immune response. Semin Cell Dev Biol. 2021;115:3–9.
69. Tretiakova DS, Vodovozova EL. Liposomes as adjuvants and vaccine delivery systems. Biochem (Moscow), Suppl Ser A Membr Cell Biol. 2022;16:1–20.
70. Tait DR, et al. Final analysis of a trial of M72/AS01 E vaccine to prevent tuberculosis. N Engl J Med. 2019;381:2429–39.
71. Almujri SS, Stylianou E, Nicastri A, Satti I, Korompis M, Li S, et al. MetE: a promising protective antigen for tuberculosis vaccine development. Front Immunol. 2025;16:1593263. https://doi.org/10.3389/fimmu.2025.1593263.

7 Pre-clinical Studies and Animal Models

Harindra D. Sathkumara, Ana Maria Valencia-Hernandez, and Andreas Kupz

7.1 In Vitro Assays

The rigorous evaluation of novel vaccine candidates in pre-clinical models is essential in the quest for the development of an effective TB vaccine [1, 2]. Among these models, *in vitro* assays have emerged as indispensable tools, offering insights into vaccine immunogenicity and safety. *In vitro* assays allow the dissection of the intricate interactions between *Mtb* and the host immune system under controlled laboratory conditions. They provide a cost-effective and ethical method for high-throughput screening of vaccine candidates and the evaluation of immune responses at the cellular and molecular levels (Fig. 7.1). These assays not only expedite the identification of promising vaccine candidates but also inform subsequent decisions regarding their advancement to *in vivo* testing [3]. In this part of the chapter, we will delve into the role of *in vitro* assays, including cell lines, primary cells, and organoids in the evaluation of novel anti-TB vaccine candidates. Given the intricate relationship between vaccination and challenge, this part of the chapter will also explore how *in vitro* assays are used to study *Mtb*-host cell interactions.

Authors Harindra D. Sathkumara, Ana Maria Valencia-Hernandez and Andreas Kupz have equally contributed to this chapter.

H. D. Sathkumara · A. M. Valencia-Hernandez · A. Kupz (✉)
Centre for Molecular Therapeutics; Australian Institute of Tropical Health and Medicine, James Cook University, Cairns, QLD, Australia
e-mail: andreas.kupz@jcu.edu.au

P. J. G. Bettencourt (ed.), *Tuberculosis Vaccines*,
https://doi.org/10.1007/978-3-031-94540-3_7

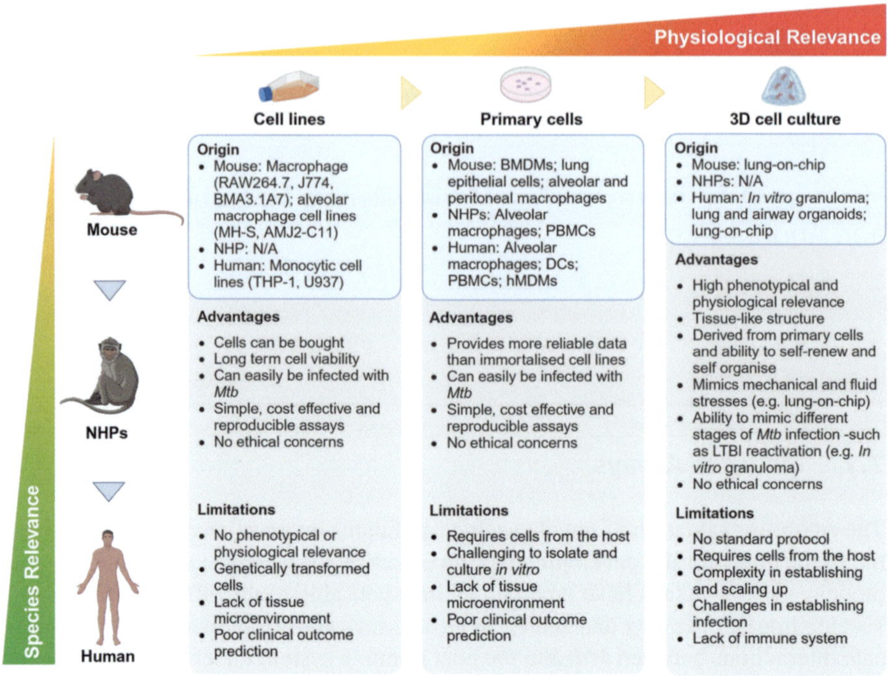

Fig. 7.1 Relevance of *in vitro* assays for the evaluation of TB vaccines. Advantages and limitations of cell lines, primary cells and 3D cell culture systems from various species for the evaluation of TB vaccines. (Figure created with Biorender.com)

7.1.1 Cell Lines

Cell lines offer a versatile platform to dissect the complex interactions between *Mtb,* vaccine candidates and the host immune system. In particular, macrophage-, dendritic cell-, and T cell lines serve as valuable surrogates for primary immune cells, allowing for controlled and reproducible experiments in a laboratory setting. One of the key applications of cell lines is the assessment of vaccine-induced immune responses. Macrophages, specifically alveolar macrophages are among the first responders to *Mtb* infection, and recognition of the bacteria results in phagocytosis and upregulation of proinflammatory responses [4, 5]. In addition to the elimination of bacteria, macrophages can present *Mtb* antigens to T cells to trigger a robust specific adaptive immune response [6].

7.1.1.1 Mouse Cell Lines

RAW264.7 and J774 macrophage cell lines, originating from the BALB/c mouse strain [7, 8] have been used widely. Despite the potential utility of immortalised macrophage cell lines derived from the C57BL/6 background, such as BMA3.1A7, their use has been limited in the past compared to the popular BALB/c-derived cell lines [9]. In addition, MH-S and AMJ2–C11 present two alveolar macrophage cell lines with BALB/c and C57BL/6 backgrounds, respectively [10, 11]. These immortalised macrophage cell lines serve as valuable tools for assessing cytokine production, antimicrobial responses like nitric oxide (NO) production, and the uptake, processing and presentation of antigens from *Mtb,* as well as TB vaccine candidates [12–15].

Generally, intracellular pathogens, including *Mtb*, employ the inhibition of apoptosis as a survival strategy, enabling them to replicate in the infected host cells [16]. RAW264.7 cells have been used to evaluate vaccine-induced apoptosis in *Mycobacterium avium* subsp. paratuberculosis mutant vaccine strains [17]. Similarly, *Mtb*-derived recombinant Rv1654 strain was shown to induce apoptosis through reactive oxygen species (ROS) production via TLR-4-mediated caspase-9/3-dependent manner [18]. Besides the heightened pro-inflammatory cytokine response, RAW264.7 cells have demonstrated elevated expression of surface markers associated with maturation of antigen presenting cells (APCs) upon stimulation with vaccine candidates, including *Mycobacterium smegmatis*-Rv1507A [12]. Furthermore, phagocytosis and antigen presentation abilities of non-genetically enhanced BCG strains were examined within BMA3.1A7 cell lines, utilising both confocal microscopy and flow cytometry [19].

RAW264.7 cells, in conjunction with confocal and transmission electron microscopy, can serve as a valuable tool for assessing autophagy activity and autophagosome formation: properties associated with good vaccine candidates, as demonstrated with the Hsp16.3 gene mutant *Mtb* H37Rv strain Hsp16.3ΔMTB [20]. In addition, these cell lines have been used to investigate the molecular mechanisms and signalling pathways involved in vaccine-induced macrophage activation *in vitro.* For instance, using iTRAQ mass spectrometry, Western blot, and confocal microscopy approaches, it has been identified that the *Mtb* latent antigen Rv2029c from A39 DNA vaccine induced a pro-inflammatory response involving the TLR2/TLR12, MAPKs, NF-κB, and IRF pathways [21]. This approach led to the selective use of knockout mouse strains for downstream *in vivo* validation.

TB research has seen limited utilisation of alveolar macrophage cell lines. However, in a handful of studies, the MH-S cell line was used to evaluate the uptake and antigen presentation of TB vaccine candidates, including the formulated PLGA:H56 [14]. Despite the limited applications, these cells displayed comparable phagocytic activity against *Mtb* to that of resident alveolar macrophages [22]. The use of macrophage cell lines proves invaluable in evaluating the phagocytosis, apoptosis, autophagy, co-stimulation, and antigen presentation abilities of new vaccines.

In a different context, the immunogenic activity of two commercially manufactured BCG formulations (Onco-BCG and ID-BCG) was compared in the J774 macrophage cell line, revealing that the Onco-BCG formulation exhibited a stronger and more sustained proinflammatory response as evident by higher production of TNF-α, IL-6, and NO [23]. These results highlight how different BCG formulations can influence immunogenicity. Another study conducted on RAW264.7 cells revealed a potential link between BCG dosage and macrophage apoptosis [24]. In contrast to conventional practice, where a MOI of 10 is generally considered optimal in *in vitro* mycobacterium infection models, the above study found that a low dose of BCG (MOI of 1) effectively activated macrophages early on [24]. This resulted in a distinctive cytokine profile without inducing cell death or mitochondrial damages typically observed with higher doses, suggesting that BCG infection at a low dose provides an efficient *in vitro* model for studying macrophage/BCG interactions. These studies showcase how *in vitro* methods using cell lines can be utilised to evaluate the safety and ideal dosage of vaccine candidates in the early phases of development.

7.1.1.2 Human Cell Lines

In addition to the mouse-derived macrophage cell lines, human cell lines, such as THP-1 and U937, which can be readily differentiated into macrophage-like cells, have been extensively used in TB vaccine research. THP-1 is a well-characterised human cell line derived from an acute monocytic leukaemia patient [25]. Exposure to PMA differentiates THP-1 cells into adherent macrophages which exhibit phagocytosis [26]. U937 is a human myeloid leukaemia cell line isolated from a histiocytic lymphoma and demonstrate pro-monocytic characteristics [27]. In addition to PMA [28], retinoic acids and 1,25-dihydroxyvitamin D3 (VD3) could also differentiate U937 into macrophages [29]. If needed, these cells can be further differentiated into the classically activated M1 (pro-inflammatory) phenotype or the alternatively activated M2 (anti-inflammatory) phenotype by exposing them to IFN-γ and LPS or IL-4 and IL-13, respectively [30]. While not to the same degree as THP-1 or U937, the human monocytic cell line Mono Mac 6, derived from monoblastic leukaemia [31], has also been employed as an *in vitro* system to assess *Mtb* phagocytosis and intracellular killing in several studies [32, 33].

Prolonged activation through retinoic acids and VD3 led to significant phenotypic alterations in THP-1 cells infected with *Mtb* [34]. This activation resulted in the fusion of these cells with neighbouring THPs, forming multinucleated giant cells containing persistent *Mtb* [34]. This approach showcases a potential *in vitro* framework for investigating the mechanisms involved in latency, a state of dormancy observed in *Mtb* infections.

Similar to the mouse-derived macrophage cell lines described early in this chapter, THP-1 cells have been extensively used to study virulent *Mtb* [35], BCG, and RD1-deleted *Mtb* H37Rv [36]. THP-1 cells have comparable viability, bacterial uptake, intracellular growth, and host immune response to human monocyte-derived macrophages (hMDMs) upon infection with both drug-susceptible and -resistant *Mtb* strains [35]. They were instrumental in revealing the essential role of RD1 in *Mtb* virulence and its critical involvement in BCG attenuation [36]. Interestingly, avirulent *Mtb* H37Ra and BCG were found to induce higher levels of apoptosis in THP-1 cells, akin to human alveolar macrophages [37], which was correlated with elevated TNF-α, IL-1β, and DUSP1 levels [38]. Furthermore, in *in vitro Mtb* infection models, inhibition of TLR8 [39] and targeted pharmacological blockade of NF-κB activation significantly reduced the intracellular survival of bacterium via induction of apoptosis and autophagy in THP-1 cells [40]. The findings in line with hMDMs and human alveolar macrophages showcase the functional similarities between THP-1 cells and primary human cells [35, 40, 41], establishing them as a practical alternative in TB vaccine and infection studies.

In another investigation, U937 cell line has been used to evaluate its ability to phagocytose and present *Mtb* antigens exclusively to human $CD8^+$ cytotoxic T cells [42]. While *Mtb*-infected U937 cells were utilised as an *in vitro* human macrophage model to evaluate HLA class I-restricted CTL function in mycobacterial infections, a comparative study found that U937 cells exhibited notably reduced phagocytic capacity compared to THP-1 and hMDMs despite the comparable production of nitrite, TNF-α and IL-12 [41].

Overall, these findings suggest that cell lines can expedite the assessment of immunogenicity and safety of new vaccine candidates. Nevertheless, owing to inherent limitations, interpretations of the results should be made cautiously. For instance, THP-1 and U937 cells do not possess the mannose receptor (MMR) [43], a crucial macrophage marker in human *Mtb* infection. The bacterium's entry via the MMR plays a significant role in halting phagosome maturation in primary hMDMs [44]. High throughput RNA sequencing data also revealed important transcriptomic differences between bone-marrow-derived mouse macrophages (BMDMs) and J774 cells when infected with live and γ-irradiated *Mtb* [45].

7.1.2 Primary Cells

7.1.2.1 Mouse Primary Cells

While challenging to isolate and culture *in vitro*, primary mouse cells offer distinct advantages by providing more reliable experimental data. BMDMs are the most widely used mouse primary cells in TB vaccine and infection studies. Bone marrow cells are collected from the femurs and tibias, and after differentiation in culture media with macrophage colony-stimulating factor (M-CSF) for approximately 7 days, they mature into macrophages [46]. In comparison to BALB/c, the primary advantage of utilising macrophages from C57BL/6 mice is the accessibility of knockout mutants within this genetic background. For instance, BMDMs have been employed from both wild-type C57BL/6 and TLR2/4 double knockout mice to investigate how *Mtb* alters phagosomal function in a TLR2/4-dependent manner [47]. Similarly, using BMDMs-derived from wild-type and TLR2/4/9 deficient mice, it has been demonstrated that NO-induced apoptosis, not its direct bactericidal action, was responsible for *Mtb* elimination in these macrophages [48]. This enabled other researchers to investigate the specific functions of targeted proteins and pathways in the context of vaccine-induced immune response and/or host-pathogen interactions.

Interestingly, the *ex vivo* usage of BMDMs from BCG vaccinated mice has provided experimental evidence of BCG-induced trained immunity and protection against *Mtb* and other infections [49, 50]. In these experiments, analysis of BMDMs revealed that BCG could imprint a unique transcriptomic profile that promotes myelopoiesis and innate immunity. Gene expression analysis of BMDMs co-cultured with live and γ-irradiated BCG identified IL-17F as a potential requirement for *Mtb* killing in the absence of a T cell response [51]. In a comparative study, factors contributing to the elimination of *Mtb* such as survival kinetics, NO production, and phagosome acidification and maturation were assessed in six different cell types including mouse BMDMs and hMDMs [52]. These BMDMs have also been utilised to evaluate *in vitro* cellular nitrite production induced by BCG and recombinant BCG strains in various comorbid TB models, including those involving type-2 diabetes [53].

In contrast to single biomarker-based assays, the mycobacterial growth inhibition assay (MGIA) offers an unbiased measure of the functional capability of post-vaccination whole blood or cell samples to control mycobacterial growth *in vitro.* In early versions of mouse MGIA, immune splenocytes from vaccinated mice were co-cultured with BMDMs infected with mycobacteria such as *Mtb* Erdman [54]. In this setting, BMDM lysates were plated on solid medium at specific time point to assess the intracellular viability of mycobacteria [54]. The CFU numbers inversely correlated with protection. However, in subsequent research, immune splenocytes from vaccinated mice were directly inoculated with mycobacteria without the requirement for infected macrophages [55–57]. Utilisation of non-virulent BCG or fast-growing *Mycobacterium smegmatis,* along with commercially available liquid medium mycobacterial growth indicator tubes (MGIT) and the BACTEC MGIT automated liquid culture system, not only reduces the assay duration but also simplifies the overall procedure [55, 57]. To this end, immune cells were inoculated with mycobacteria in a tube or plate followed by an incubation at 37 °C for ~3–4 days. The cells were lysed, and the resulting lysates were transferred to MGIT tubes containing PANTA antibiotics and OADC. The time to positivity (TTP) was measured using the BACTEC MGIT detection system. CFU values were calculated using a standard curve of TTP based on the inoculum volume and the CFU [57]. Importantly, findings from MGIA/ MGIT correlate with both *in vivo Mtb* challenge models and *in vitro Mtb* growth inhibition, as well as CFU determinations on solid medium [57, 58]. Furthermore, when integrated with molecular methods like microarray analysis, *ex vivo* stimulated cells utilised in MGIA offered insights into potential mechanisms involved in inhibiting mycobacterial growth [57].

Despite being the more pertinent cell type for *Mtb* infection, the limited yield of alveolar macrophages from mice often deters their utilisation. Instead, peritoneal macrophages are occasionally employed as substitutes for resident macrophages. Alveolar and peritoneal macrophages isolated from bronchoalveolar lavage (BAL) fluid and peritoneal exudate, respectively, have been used to assess bacterial uptake and killing capacity as well as pro-inflammatory cytokine production in *in vitro Mtb* infection models [59, 60]. In addition, primary lung epithelial cells can also be isolated from mouse lungs using commercially available mouse epithelial cell enrichment kits [61]. Using flow cytometry and confocal microscopy, it was demonstrated that primary epithelial cells have the capacity to process and present BCG antigens to sensitised T helper cells akin to peritoneal macrophages [61]. This suggests that these cells play a role in local immune responses, besides their primary function of facilitating gas exchange.

7.1.2.2 NHP Primary Cells

Non-human primates (NHPs) provide a model that closely mimics the progression of human TB, enabling more accurate studies of the disease and vaccination mainly due to their the high-genetic similarity to humans [62]. Despite the wide use of *in vivo* NHP models in TB vaccine research [63–67], NHP-based *in vitro* assays are largely limited to primary alveolar macrophages and peripheral blood mononuclear cells (PBMCs). Alveolar macrophages are the CD14^{+} HLA-DR^{+} adherent cells isolated from BAL fluid [68]. The rapamycin-induced autophagic killing of virulent *Mtb* in alveolar macrophages from rhesus macaques has been assessed using Western blot and immunofluorescence microscopy techniques [68]. With few modifications, this assay can potentially be repurposed to assess the capacity of novel vaccine candidates to induce autophagic killing of *Mtb, in vitro* [69]. In addition, the immunogenicity of vaccines can be assessed *in vitro* by restimulating PBMCs from vaccinated NHPs and measuring antigen-specific cytokine responses using ELISA and intracellular cytokine staining (ICS). In two studies, PBMCs from macaques vaccinated with influenza vector-based TB/FLU-04 L and Ad35-based AERAS-402 vaccines were restimulated with recombinant Ag85A/B, TB10.4, and Ag85B, ESAT-6, respectively [70, 71]. Immunogenicity was evaluated by measuring IFN-γ levels in supernatants and assessing polyfunctional CD4^{+} and CD8^{+} T cells (IFN-γ, IL-2, and TNF) [70, 71].

Interestingly, efforts have been made to modify MGIA for the early evaluation of anti-TB vaccines in NHPs [72]. The assay was performed using whole blood and PBMCs from vaccinated and unvaccinated macaques and inoculating with *Mtb* as a surrogate read-out of vaccine-induced protection [72]. Comparable to some of the small animal MGIAs, *in vitro* growth inhibition directly correlated with the mycobacteria recovered from lymph nodes following *in vivo* challenge of the animals [72]. This approach enables rapid screening of vaccine candidates, accelerating the development of effective TB vaccines and potentially reducing the need for NHPs in efficacy testing.

7.1.2.3 Human Primary Cells

The most common human primary cells being used in TB vaccine research are hMDMs and PBMCs. hMDMs are generated by isolating human monocytes from PBMCs through either CD14 positive/negative selection method or by plastic adherence followed by differentiation with M-CSF and GM-CSF [73]. As described in previous sections, these cells have been widely used to assess the intracellular growth and survival of vaccine and virulent strains, macrophage activation, and the ability to mount an immune response, as well as to investigate the underlying mechanisms [35, 40, 41, 44, 74]. Similar to macrophages, dendritic cells (DCs) play a pivotal role bridging innate and adaptive immune responses through capturing, processing, and presenting *Mtb* antigens to adaptive immune cells [75]. Human DCs have been previously generated by culturing CD14^{+} human monocytes isolated from PBMCs with GM-CSF and IL-4 [76]. Similar to BMDMs and hMDMs, human DCs were used to evaluate the capacity of vaccines including BCG and prototype anti-TB vaccine SO2 to induce cytokine response and promote DC maturation, T cell response, or modulate apoptosis and autophagy [76].

Although it doesn't provide a direct link to clinical efficacy, *in vitro* functional assays like the cytokine secretion assay can be employed to assess the ability of human PBMCs to produce IFN-γ upon *in vitro* stimulation with vaccine antigens [77]. While pro-inflammatory cytokines like IFN-γ, TNFα, IL-1β, IL-6, and IL-12 are recognised as crucial components of anti-TB immunity [78] and are commonly employed as primary immunological indicators in vaccine research, there are numerous instances where they do not align with protective outcomes in both animal models and humans [79, 80]. Thus, MGIA has been widely utilised in human studies involving BCG and other candidates, with human whole blood and PBMCs, serving as commonly used specimens in these assays [81–85]. Although whole blood MGIA offers logistical advantages like using small blood volumes, it might be less suitable for vaccine efficacy testing compared to cellular assays. The limitations of whole blood MGIA include the inability to differentiate between intracellular and extracellular mycobacterial growth, as well as the presence of confounding factors like haemoglobins [86]. Interestingly, MGIA has been adapted to assess physiologically relevant pulmonary immune protection against TB by utilising alveolar macrophages isolated from human BAL fluid [87]. This addresses one of the main criticisms that MGIA often faces, which is not accurately representing the early immune response *in vivo,* involving alveolar macrophages and dendritic cells.

Primary cell-based *in vitro* models are therefore important to evaluate the intracellular persistence of new vaccine candidates, specifically live attenuated strains and their capacity to promote or restrict killing while understanding the underlying molecular mechanisms in a more physiologically relevant context than immortal cell lines.

7.1.3 In Vitro Granulomas, Organoids, and Organ-on-Chips

However advantageous, the outlined *in vitro* methods have a notable drawback. They operate in isolation, lacking the complexity of the body's dynamic interactions, making it challenging to predict real-world outcomes. Formation of granulomas is considered the classic immune response to TB in humans [88]. Thus, advanced three-dimensional (3D) cell culture-based *in vitro* human TB granuloma model systems developed utilising human primary cells, and virulent *Mtb* strains enable exploration of mechanisms and dynamics that may be challenging to investigate in patients and conventional animal models [89, 90]. Furthermore, organs-on-chips and organoids are designed to replicate *in vivo*-like tissue microenvironments, emulating both the structural and biological properties of human organs including lungs [91]. These models aim to enhance our understanding of TB disease, drug responses, and potentially vaccine effectiveness.

7.1.3.1 In Vitro Granulomas

An early human TB granuloma model was established using BCG and PBMCs, exhibiting morphological features akin to a typical epithelioid granuloma. This included fused macrophages forming multinucleated cells, as well as epithelioid macrophages closely connected to surrounding macrophages and lymphocytes [92]. Since then, comparable *in vitro* models of human granulomas have been employed to explore and understand various aspects of granuloma formation. This includes studying the local immune response, functions of crucial cell types, mycobacterial cell wall components, and other virulence factors [93–98]. In a later model, resuscitation of *Mtb* from its dormant state was possible by using anti-TNF-α mAb treatment, as observed during human LTBI reactivation [99]. Therefore, utilising *in vitro* human TB models proves valuable in evaluating the granuloma-inducing potential of new vaccine candidates and assessing the virulence, particularly in live attenuated vaccine strains.

7.1.3.2 Lung Organoids

Organoids are intricate 3D structures formed by a self-organised assembly of diverse cell types such as embryonic stem cells (ESCs), induced pluripotent stem cells (iPSCs), and adult mammalian stem cells, cultivated within gels composed of a complex blend of various extracellular matrix (ECM) proteins [100]. Lung organoids accurately replicate vital aspects of the lung, encompassing various cell types, precise spatial organisation, cells capable of self-renewal and differentiation, and exhibit comparable global transcriptomic profiles [101]. Despite their use in other respiratory infections such as SARS-CoV2 [102, 103], human lung organoids have not been widely explored in TB infection/ vaccine research. However, in a recent investigation, researchers utilised human bronchiolar airway organoids co-cultured with macrophages to study the immune response and infection dynamics during the early stages of *Mtb* infection [104]. Together, these discoveries indicate that human lung organoids offer a promising *in vitro* model for comprehending interactions between the host and *Mtb*. They can also be employed to evaluate the initial immune response in the lungs following mucosal administration of potential vaccine candidates.

7.1.3.3 Lung-on-Chip

Numerous lung-on-chip models have emerged in recent years, incorporating endothelial cells alongside vascular and immune cells from primary sources or iPSC cell lines [105]. Advanced human lung-on-chips, in addition to modelling the tissue microenvironments and vascular perfusion more closely, can also mimic the physiological breathing motion of the lung, representing both solid mechanical and fluid stresses [106, 107]. Although not human, a mouse lung-on-chip has been used to study dynamics of host-*Mtb* interactions and the role of pulmonary surfactants [108]. By employing a novel modular suspended microfluidic coculture platform, a new chip variant was engineered to replicate granuloma-associated immune responses and angiogenesis. This platform provides a prototype for investigating soluble factor signalling within microscale *in vitro* granulomas [109].

7.1.4 Conclusion

Although *in vitro*-based discoveries establish the groundwork for a system to investigate respiratory infections including TB without animal use, these methods must undergo rigorous validation against clinical outcomes, such as protection against natural or experimental mycobacterial infection or disease. Furthermore, as these validated *in vitro* methods evolve, they have the potential not only to streamline effective TB vaccine development but also to cut down on the time and resources required for preclinical evaluation. Moreover, they align with the principles of the 3Rs in the use of animals in biomedical research—Replacing, Reducing, and Refining and promise a deeper understanding of TB immunity. This dual impact positions *in vitro* approaches as critical contributions in the endeavour to combat TB.

7.2 In Vivo Studies

Although experiments conducted with *in vitro* assays can give some insights into immune mechanisms, the complexity of the mammalian immune system cannot be recapitulated by any *in vitro* method. Hence, the safety and efficacy of a vaccine can only be evaluated by conducting vaccination challenge experiments in live animals.

Animal models are not only valuable tools for understanding the pathogenicity and immunology associated with *Mtb* infection but are also essential for the preclinical evaluation of TB vaccine candidates. The choice of animal model largely depends on the intrinsic characteristics of the vaccine candidate, its developmental stage, and the expected readouts. Other reasons that might apply when choosing an animal model include extrinsic constrains, including laboratory conditions, infrastructure, financial resources, and country-specific animal experimentation laws. In general, small animal models are often used for newly developed vaccine strategies or constructs with no pre-existing data from living organisms. Some of these animals include mice, rats, zebrafish, rabbits, and guinea pigs (Fig. 7.2). Encouraging results from small animal models usually trigger the evaluation of the vaccine candidates in large animal models including non-human primates (NHP) or cattle, which resemble more closely the pathogenicity and immune responses of humans. In this part of the chapter, we will discuss the advantages and disadvantages of several vertebrate animal models to evaluate the safety, immunogenicity, and efficacy of TB vaccine candidates.

7.2.1 Mice

7.2.1.1 Inbred-Resistant Mice

The most widely used animal model for the evaluation of TB vaccine candidates are laboratory mice. They are of particular interest given their affordability, the small space required to house them, their rapid reproduction, and importantly, the broad range of immunological assays established for this species. However, there is a

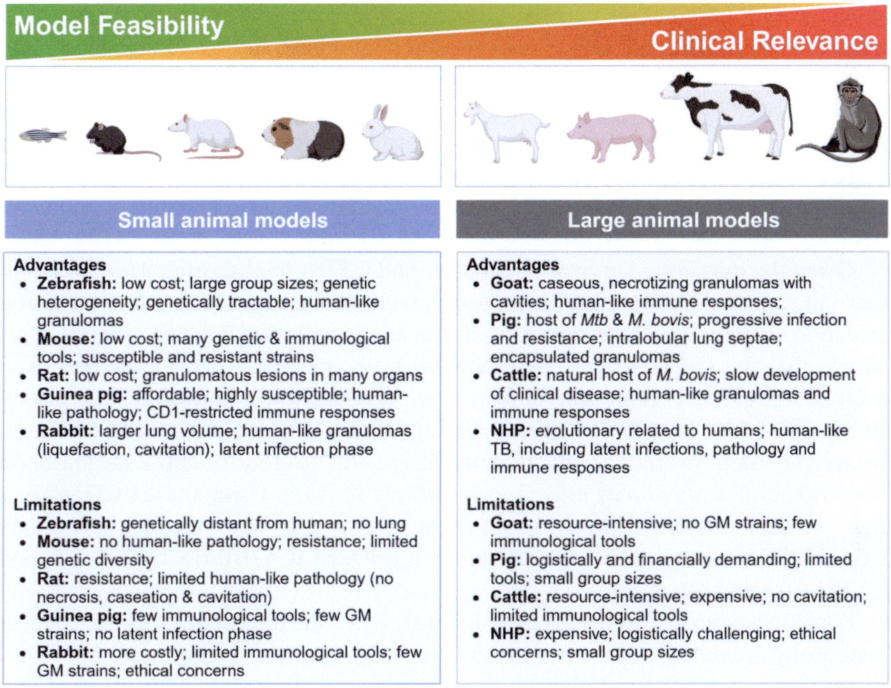

Fig. 7.2 Suitability and clinical relevance of different animal models in TB vaccine research. The advantages and limitations of different vertebrate animal models used in TB vaccine research are summarised. Models have been devided into small and large animals. (Figure created with Biorender.com)

major disadvantage when using mice to evaluate TB vaccines, in most cases they fail to recapitulate the main pathogenic features of the disease. Mice don't develop typical defined granulomas nor cavitations like humans do when infected with *Mtb* [110–112]. In fact, the most commonly used mouse strains C57BL/6 and BALB/c mice are considered resistant to *Mtb* infection, as they survive for long periods of time without developing symptoms of disease [113]. However, *Mtb* is capable of colonising, spreading, and growing in several organs in mice. For that reason, bacterial burden after infection is one of the readouts when assessing vaccine efficacy in mice.

Immune responses to BCG in mice depend on several factors, including the route of administration, the mouse strain, and the vaccination dose. Early reports indicated that after BCG vaccination, C57BL/6 mice exhibit a strong Th1 response characterised by elevated expression of IL-12 and TNF-α, leading to IFN-γ production and enhanced *Mtb* protection. Conversely, BCG-vaccinated BALB/c mice present lower levels of Th1 cytokines and substantial production of IL-4 with higher bacterial burden after challenge [114–116]. Importantly, the differences between C57BL/6 and BALB/c mice reported in these early studies came as a result of administering BCG intravenously, and more recent publications confirm that subcutaneous vaccination with BCG and recombinant BCG (rBCG) strains also induce strong Th1-type immune responses in both mouse strains. In fact, a growing number of reports show that subcutaneous and intradermal administration of most BCG and rBCG vaccines promote high levels of IL-2, TNF-α, and IFN-γ accompanied by enhanced IgG2/IgG1 ratios and equivalent protective efficacy in C57BL/6 or BALB/c mouse models [117–128]. Moreover, intradermal administration with other vaccine types, including DNA-based vaccines are also capable of inducing strong humoral and Th1-type responses in BALB/c and C57BL/6 mice [129, 130].

Given the long-term survival of BALB/c and C57BL/6 mice after *Mtb* infection, these mouse strains have also been used to recreate chronic and latent/reactivation infection models where therapeutic vaccines can be tested. In fact, studies have shown that the rBCG strains, BCGΔBCG1419c, and BCGΔ*ureC::hly* improved protection against chronic *Mtb* infection in BALB/c mice, compared to parental BCG strain [126, 131]. In two models of latent infection, reactivation and increased bacterial burden was induced by administering corticosterone or anti-CD4 antibody to resistant mice previously infected with *Mtb* [132, 133]. Using these two reactivation models, studies have shown that BCG and the vaccine candidate BCGΔBCG1419c can prevent reactivation in B6D2F1 (C57BL/6 × DBA/2, F1) and C57BL/6 mice [126, 134].

For TB vaccine research, C57BL/6 mice are often the preferred strain, since most genetically modified mice were generated in this genetic background. However, these mice come with limitations as they are not only resistant to *Mtb* infection, but they also lack certain class-I and a class-II MHC genes compared to BALB/c mice. Moreover, identifying effective vaccine strategies that increase disease immunity and immunological correlates of protection can be a challenging task when using C57BL/6 mice. For instance, contradictory findings for the role of T cell-mediated cytokine responses, which are both essential for control of TB infection and not correlated with vaccine efficacy, highlights the difficulty in finding surrogates of protection. For example, IFN-γ deficient mice were unable to contain and control a sublethal dose of *Mtb* and BCG [135, 136], while other studies show that *Mtb*-specific IFN-γ T cell responses alone after vaccination do not correlate with protection [79, 137]. Another aspect that interferes with the pre-clinical value of C57BL/6 mice is whether the promising vaccine candidates tested using this model will be effective in genetically diverse hosts like humans. To allow for more diversity in MHC restriction, some investigators have recently used F1 hybrids of inbred laboratory mouse strains including CB6F1 ($H2^{b,d}$) and B6C3F1 ($H2^{b,k}$). In these studies, hybrid mice are initially immunised with BCG and then boosted with a modified viral vector or a fusion protein, allowing the identification of immunodominant epitopes and antigen-specific T cells using tetramers raised for C57BL/6 and BALB/c mice [138–141].

7.2.1.2 Genetically Diverse DO and CC Mice

Classic inbred mouse strains typically show consistent immune responses to the same infection because their genomes are largely functionally identical. However, it's now understood that human and NHP responses to similar *Mtb* exposures vary significantly, likely due to genetic disparities amongst the population. This variability is observed in human *Mtb* infection outcomes and is often reflected in the diverse efficacy levels of BCG vaccination [142–145]. To address this challenge, mouse populations with highly diverse genetic backgrounds were generated through a selective breeding process involving eight distinct founder strains (C57BL/6 J, 129S1/SvImJ, A/J, NOD/ShiLtJ, NZO/HiLtJ, CAST/EiJ, PWK/PhJ, and WSB/EiJ). This process resulted in a random assortment of genetic traits amongst the offspring [146, 147]. The resultant highly diverse reproducible inbred strains became known as the collaborative cross (CC) mice. The diversity outbred (DO) mice originate from further breeding of an initial group of CC strains, creating an outbred population through random crossings [148].

A panel of CC mice have shown heterogeneity of disease progression following aerosol *Mtb* infection, with organ CFU burdens in lungs and spleens varying from 1000- to 10,000-fold [149, 150]. Interestingly, BCG vaccination failed to conferred long-term protection against *Mtb*, mirroring the absence of BCG-induced protection in a human population [149]. In a recent investigation involving mice vaccinated with BCG across 24 CC strains, it was discovered that the effectiveness of BCG is not directly linked to the inherent susceptibility to *Mtb* [151]. Variability in vaccine-induced protection primarily stemmed from host genetics rather than the specific T cell composition or functionality elicited by BCG [151]. Moreover, several of the CC strains that were protected exhibited distinct forms of immunity, suggesting multiple routes to protection [151].

The DO mice are highly susceptible to aerosol *Mtb* infection [152]. While subcutaneous BCG vaccination enhanced the survival rates of vaccinated animals, lung CFU counts did not show significant reduction when compared to naive DO mice exhibiting heterogenous bacterial burdens [152]. Most disease parameters, including *Mtb* burden, weight loss, and lung pathology, had weak or no correlations with each other nor with protection [152]. Although the survival was higher in mice that received intravenous vaccination compared to subcutaneous BCG administration, it did not significantly alter organ bacterial loads or lung inflammation in DO mice [153]. Low dose aerosol *Mtb* infection in these mice revealed lung necrosis and neutrophil influx as correlates of TB disease susceptibility [154]. Additionally, diagnostic-quality serum protein biomarkers of human TB, such as CXCL1 were identified [155], indicating the relevance of this model to human disease. Alongside the observed inverse correlation between IFN-γ and protection, recent single-cell RNA sequencing analysis in a group of new wild-derived inbred mice from the *Mus musculus domesticus* subspecies identified a unique neutrophil signature linked to the inability to control the infection [156]. Given the wide range of disease presentations after *Mtb* infection in vaccinated or un-vaccinated DO mice, large number of mice are usually required to find significant differences, and in-depth transcriptomic analysis are needed to identify correlates of protection due to the diverse TB disease progression observed in vaccinated DO mice [152, 153, 157].

Collectively, findings from recent human and animal studies suggest that tailoring a vaccine for a specific standard laboratory mouse strain might not ultimately guarantee broad efficacy in a genetically diverse population. The varied responses seen in genetically diverse mice during both vaccination and infection contribute to the understanding of general immunity to *Mtb* and the genetics influencing of the vaccination outcomes. Therefore, genetically diverse strains such as CC and DO offer a reliable *in vivo* platform to facilitate the development of vaccines that protect a diverse range of genotypes against *Mtb* infection.

7.2.1.3 "Dirty" and Wild Mice

Humans are constantly exposed to pathogenic and non-pathogenic microbes which modulate the internal immunological landscape from birth to death. On the other hand, laboratory mice are usually housed and bred under specific pathogen-free (SPF) conditions and therefore possess minimal immunological memory. Wild mice or mice from pet stores, which have been exposed to multiple pathogens and commensal microbes have a mature immune system that resembles more closely the one from adult humans [158, 159]. Consequently, dirty mice are now considered an important model for preclinical studies and a critical tool in the path to translation. There are several methods to generate dirty mice, including co-housing SPF mice with pet store mice, infection with a panel of known experimental pathogens, exposure to fomites from dirty bedding or transfer of natural microbiota ("re-wilding"). Microbial exposure has profound consequences for the immune system; in fact, the reconstitution of germ-free laboratory mice with microbiota from wild mice promoted survival and reduced inflammatory responses to a lethal dose of influenza A virus and colorectal cancer [159]. Dirty mice also harbour an increased number of phenotypically diverse memory cells, including tissue resident memory T cells [158, 160], important for local immunosurveillance at barrier tissues, including the lung. Recent vaccination studies have shown that dirty mice have a different transcriptional signature compared to SPF mice after immunisation and similar to the signature observed in humans [161, 162]. Interestingly, humoral and cellular responses after influenza vaccination were reduced in dirty mice, resulting in poor control of viral load after challenge [161]. Another important aspect of having increased numbers of antigen experienced immune cells is that these cells can promote antigen-independent responses, important for early pathogen detection and clearance [163–165]. These recent findings suggest that dirty mice represent a more relevant animal model for testing vaccines designed to generate immune responses at barrier tissues, critical for diseases caused by pathogens like *Mtb*, HIV, and respiratory viruses. To our knowledge, minimal research has been performed using dirty mice in the context of *Mtb* infection or for testing TB vaccine candidates. We urge the scientific community to include this model in their preclinical studies, especially for vaccine candidates that performed well in SPF mice.

7.2.1.4 Inbred Susceptible Mice

To overcome some of the shortcomings of using resistant inbred mice, different genetically modified and knock-out inbred mice lacking immune cell populations have been used to study specific aspects of the immune responses to mycobacterial infections and live attenuated vaccines. These mice succumb to *Mtb* infection, and some can recapitulate traits of human *Mtb* infection and TB disease, including the generation of caseous granulomas and necrosis.

While C3HeB/FeJ mice possess an intact and functional immune system, they are highly susceptible to *Mtb* infection and develop multiple lung micro-lesions which progress to highly organised encapsulated granulomas with liquefactive necrosis [166–168]. The ability of C3HeB/FeJ mice to recapitulate the human hallmark of TB infection (e.g., pulmonary necrotic granulomas) makes them an important model for the evaluation of drugs and new vaccines. Interestingly, a vaccination study showed that susceptible C3HeB/FeJ mice but not their resistant counterpart C3H/HeOuJ mice were protected by BCG at later time points [169]. The authors of this study proposed that BCG could survive longer in C3Heb/FeJ mice, inducing a better memory T cell response compared to the resistant C3H/HeOuJ mice, which translated to reduced bacterial burden and enhanced protection of susceptible mice. These results contradict previous reports, indicating that susceptible and resistant murine strains from this lineage generate similar adaptive T cell responses after BCG vaccination [170]. Once again, these conflicting findings can be explained by the route of immunisation, while BCG was administered intravenously for the early study, for the more recent study mice were vaccinated by the subcutaneous route. Further investigation into the immune responses of vaccine candidates in C3HeB/FeJ mice are required to understand underlying molecular mechanisms and to make informed decisions for the design of new TB vaccines.

Two other mouse strains that are classified as highly susceptible to *Mtb* are the 129Sv and DBA/2 mice [113]. While these mice fail to generate necrotic granulomas such as C3HeB/FeJ do, they develop lung lesions characterised by the accumulation of foamy macrophages that in turn support the spread and progression of *Mtb* replication [171, 172]. There are several publications using 129Sv and DBA/2 transgenic mice lacking cytokines (e.g., TNF-α, IFN-γ, IL-6) or TLR genes to investigate molecular mechanisms involved in the granuloma formation upon *Mtb* infection. Only few studies used these susceptible mouse strains to investigate vaccine efficacy. Some reports suggest that vaccination of 129Sv mice with BCG had limited protection against *Mtb* challenge [149, 173]; however, a more recent study proposed that BCG can confer better protection in female than in male 129Sv mice [174]. On the contrary, subcutaneous immunisation with BCG or with Ag85 antigen plus adjuvant protect susceptible DBA/2 mice from *Mtb* infection [173, 175]; and the protective efficacy of BCG is increased when administered intranasally [176]. Immunogenicity studies on DBA/2 mice revealed that the ratio of monocyte to lymphocyte and the proportion of IFN-γ and IL-17 by memory T cells might play a role on the protective efficacy of BCG [173, 175, 176].

After *Mtb* infection, moderately susceptible CBA/J mice develop an increased lung bacterial load and die earlier compared to C57BL/6 mice. Disease progression in these mice has been linked to IL-10 production in the lung [177] and IL-10 deficient CBA/J mice control *Mtb* infection by forming mature lung granulomas [178]. Furthermore, vaccination studies have shown that blockade of IL-10 signalling during BCG immunisation increased Th1 and Th17 responses leading to enhance protection in CBA/J mice [179]. In the same study, authors demonstrated that in absence of IL-10, BCG vaccination increases IFN-γ and IL-17 production and protection against *Mtb* challenge in C57BL/6 mice [179].

Highly immunocompromised SCID mice, lacking T- and B lymphocytes, are a reference model for safety profiling of live attenuated vaccines including recombinant BCG and attenuated *Mtb* strains in preclinical studies [180, 181]. Conventional BCG grows progressively in SCID mice when delivered intravenously, and all mice succumb by 6–8 weeks with enlarged spleens and lymph nodes and high bacterial burdens [182]. In fact, there are several reports of auxotrophic and other rBCG strains with enhanced safety compared to conventional BCG [182–184]. Similar safety studies can be performed in $Rag^{-/-}$ or $Rag^{-/-}IL2rg^{-/-}$ double knockout mice [185], a more stringent model of immunosuppression that does not sustain "leaky" T and B cell responses as reported in SCID mice [186]. However, $Rag^{-/-}$ mice survive between 17 and 25 weeks post-BCG infection (twice as long as SCID mice), thus, safety studies of live attenuated vaccines using these mice required much longer monitoring times [187, 188].

7.2.1.5 Humanised Mice

Humanised mouse models for TB research use extremely immunodeficient mice deficient in B, T, and NK cells, allowing the engraftment with human hematopoietic stem cells and foetal tissues, which in turn populate the host tissues with human immune cells. Since 2013, humanised mouse models have been used to study lung pathology caused by *Mtb* infection, demonstrating the formation of organised granulomas with necrosis formed by human T cells and macrophages in mice [189–191]. More recent studies have also compared immune responses to BCG and vaccine candidates including subunit and viral-vector-based strategies. Results indicate that BCG and other vaccine candidates are indeed able to induce human T cells responses specific to *Mtb* antigens in those mice [192, 193]. Although the use of humanised animal models faces major limitations such as the inability to support the development of major human cell populations (e.g., erythrocytes), as well as logistic limitations related to the high cost of production, these models play an important role for pre-clinical studies of TB vaccines.

In summary, a large body of TB research has been performed in mice with several immune cells and host components described as essential for disease protection and progression. Likewise, mice are commonly used to assess TB vaccine candidates to understand the immunological mechanisms underlying vaccine-mediated immunity. However, several of the best performing vaccine candidates tested in mice don't show promising results in large animals nor in humans. These contrasting results might be a consequence of the intrinsic limitations of using mouse models, which include (i) failure to recapitulate human-like lung pathology; (ii) inherent resistance; and (iii) lack of genetic diversity. Under such circumstances, the identification of immunological correlates of protection and the discovery of vaccine candidates effective in genetically diverse hosts (e.g., humans) is a difficult goal to achieve. Although animal studies are useful to determine factors essential for TB protection, their vaccine efficacy predictive value is uncertain [194, 195]. Despite these shortcomings, mouse models that resemble more closely human pathology and immune responses have been developed and therefore are more relevant for the investigation of novel vaccine candidates.

7.2.2 Other Animal Models

While mice, with their genetic tractability and cost-effectiveness, are excellent models for early screening and mechanistic studies of experimental TB vaccines, their differences in TB pathology from humans limits their relevance for some aspects of TB vaccine research. Selecting an appropriate alternative animal model depends on the specific research goals and available resources. In the section below, we will highlight the advantages and disadvantages of other vertebrate animal species that have been used for TB vaccine research.

7.2.3 Rats

Rats, once considered insensitive to *Mtb* infection, have emerged as valuable models in TB research due to several advantages they offer, including ease of experimentation, affordability, robust resistance, and convenient blood collection methods [196]. Contrary to earlier beliefs [197, 198], some studies have demonstrated that rats exhibit sensitivity to *Mtb* [199, 200]. While rats are predominantly used for TB drug testing, they have also contributed to assess the efficacy of TB vaccines, including BCG [201, 202]. *Mtb*-infected rats of various species (American cotton, Lewis, Wistar, and Sprague-Dawley) show granulomatous lesions in the spleen, liver, lung, and lymph nodes. However, these lesions lack central necrosis and fail to fully mimic human lung pathology, such as caseation, fibrosis, calcification, and cavitation [200, 203, 204]. Wistar rats are commonly used in vaccination studies due to their widespread availability, ease of handling, well-defined physiology, and the potential to obtain larger sample sizes compared to mice [205]. Interestingly, the rats' dietary microelement status, particularly zinc deficiency, has been shown to impact their immune responses to BCG and ESAT-6/CFP-10 vaccination [206]. A rat model of type I diabetes has also demonstrated increased susceptibility to TB [207]; however, no vaccine efficacy tests have been performed in this model.

7.2.4 Guinea Pigs

Compared to mice and rats, guinea pigs present several advantages for TB vaccine research and provide a balance between cost-effectiveness and similarity to human TB pathology [196, 205]. Their ease of handling and maintenance makes them a practical choice for medium-sized vaccine studies. They are often the preferred small animal model for further efficacy and safety testing of TB vaccine candidates that have shown promising results in mice and are particularly useful for early vaccine screening. Due to their remarkable susceptibility to *Mtb* infection via the airways, guinea pigs have been extensively utilised for various aspects of TB studies, including lymphocyte proliferation assays, dermal reactivity evaluations, and assessing the transmission of multidrug-resistant *Mtb* strains [208–212].

One of the key areas of research involving guinea pigs is the study of pathological lesions caused by *Mtb* infection. Granulomas in their lungs closely resemble those found in humans and include Langerhans giant cells and epithelioid cells. These lesions, both inside and outside the lungs, have provided essential insights into vaccine-mediated protection against pulmonary TB [213–215]. Moreover, guinea pigs exhibit distinct pathological tubercles in their spleens following *Mtb* infection, a phenomenon not observed in mice. This feature makes guinea pigs an invaluable model for understanding the impact of vaccination on pathophysiology [216–221]. However, it's essential to note that guinea pigs are not suitable for studying vaccines against latent TB reactivation due to the absence of a latent phase in their infection [211, 222, 223]. Instead, they are excellent models for progressive and fatal TB infections. Because guinea pigs are highly responsive to anti-TB drugs [224], they are also an excellent choice for assessing the efficacy of experimental anti-TB compounds against drug-resistant *Mtb* strains. Immune responses to TB vaccine candidates in guinea pigs have been probed by utilising antibody-mediated blocking of immune cells and pathways, flow cytometry, and transcriptomics. These investigations have unveiled the intricate dynamics of the immune system's response to *Mtb* infection. Initially, responding T cells, primarily $CD4^+$ T cells, are activated following infection. However, T cell numbers decline significantly by approximately one month after infection. In contrast, B cells and granulocytes gradually increase during that period [225]. This nuanced understanding of immune responses in guinea pigs is important for assessing the immunogenicity of novel vaccine candidates. Another intriguing aspect of guinea pig immunology is the induction of a CD1-restricted immune response following immunisation with mycobacterial lipid antigens. This CD1-restricted response is unique and distinguishes guinea pigs from murine rodents, aligning them more closely with human immune responses. The CD1-T cell axis, due to its interaction with mycobacterial lipids, has been a significant focus of TB vaccine research in guinea pigs [226–232].

Despite their strong impact on TB vaccine research, guinea pigs have limitations due to the lack of many immunological tools and the absence of genetically modified animals. Recent advancements have addressed some of these limitations. The development of guinea pig-specific immunological reagents, including cloned guinea pig IL-17A, IL-10 IL-4, and IFN-γ, has significantly enhanced the potential of guinea pigs as a model organism [233, 234]. Moreover, molecular screening techniques, such as qRT-PCR, gene arrays, and cell stimulation assays, have allowed more comprehensive investigations into guinea pig immunology [235–238]. It is also important to note that guinea pigs display considerable inter-animal variability in terms of disease progression, which can introduce complexities in data interpretation, particularly when assessing vaccine efficacy. This variability must be considered and controlled for experimental design and data analysis to ensure reliable and reproducible results.

7.2.5 Rabbits

Compared to mice and guinea pigs, rabbits have played a relatively modest role in evaluating TB vaccine candidates. Their notably larger lung volumes, when compared to rodents, make rabbits an ideal choice for investigating various aspects of pulmonary TB. Furthermore, rabbits can be infected via aerosol exposure, closely mimicking the natural infection route seen in humans. They also offer a compromise between cost and pathology relevance.

Rabbit models were initially very prevalent in TB research, particularly in the first half of the twentieth century [239–244]. Over time, they have been partially replaced by rodent models, particularly mice. However, rabbits remain an useful model for studying TB, primarily due to the similarity in lesion manifestations, such as granulomas, liquefaction, and cavitation, [245–248]. These similarities have made rabbits valuable for screening and evaluating TB vaccine candidates, including BCG, *M. vaccae*, *M. microti*, and multiple subunit and other live-attenuated vaccines [249–254]. Rabbits have also been instrumental in investigating the pathogenesis of cavities induced by different *Mtb* strains. It is now well established that infections with *Mtb* Erdman, *Mtb* H37Rv, and *Mtb* CDC1551 result in varying pulmonary pathologies in New Zealand white rabbits [255]. For example, large confluent granulomas with extensive central necrosis can be seen in rabbit lungs infected with the *Mtb* HN878 strain [256]. This variability underscores the importance of the virulence of *Mtb* strains in determining lesion severity in rabbit models and can be used to evaluate how vaccination impacts lung histopathology.

Overall, rabbits are not highly susceptible to *Mtb*, and they can contain the infection in a latent form, which can be reactivated with corticosteroids to model LTBI reactivation [257–259]. This unique feature allows to explore the dynamics of TB latency and reactivation in the context of vaccination and has revealed the crucial role of rapid innate immunity, particularly early activation of NK cells, in controlling bacterial growth. Once bacterial growth is controlled, T cell activation is often reduced, which leads to spontaneous latency [260]. Additionally, the rabbit BCG challenge skin model has also been used to evaluate the effectiveness of experimental TB vaccines [261], and rabbits have also been useful in investigating rare forms of TB, such as cutaneous TB and TB meningitis [262]. When infected with *M. bovis*, rabbits experience extended lung tissue damage that ultimately leads to the formation of cavities, a feature similar to post-primary TB in humans. This model has helped elucidate the role of matrix-metallo-proteases in the formation of TB cavities [260, 263]. However, the capacity to cause cavities depends on the *Mtb* strain used, with strong cavity induction seen with hypervirulent *Mtb* W-Beijing, while less virulent strains like CDC1551 tend to trigger LTBI. While currently understudied, all those disease manifestations should be used for the pre-clinical evaluation of TB vaccine candidates.

Like guinea pigs, a limitation in rabbit TB research is the scarcity of immunological reagents, which constraints the depth of mechanistic studies and hinders more sophisticated vaccinology studies [196, 205, 208]. Conducting rabbit studies can be financially demanding, and ethical concerns may arise due to their larger size and the requirement for more extensive care. Like with guinea pigs, inter-animal variability in response to vaccination and *Mtb* infection impacts experimental consistency and can confound data interpretation.

7.2.6 Non-human Primates

NHPs have played a pivotal role in TB vaccine research, owing to their natural susceptibility to *Mtb* and their close evolutionary relationship with humans [216, 264]. This unique similarity has made NHPs one of the most relevant animal models for studying TB, with their disease pathology, and clinical manifestations closely mirroring those of humans, including the development of latent TB infections [264]. One of the distinguishing features of NHP models is their ability to replicate the entire spectrum of human TB, ranging from active disease to latent infection and TB reactivation [196, 205, 208]. This comprehensive representation of the disease allows insights into different stages of TB, including the complexities of granuloma formation and the varying individual outcomes. Notably, NHPs, particularly macaques, exhibit immune responses that closely parallel those of humans, rendering them invaluable for assessing vaccine immunogenicity. Moreover, NHPs permit in-depth clinical monitoring, including advanced imaging studies to provide insights into vaccine efficacy and disease dynamics over time [66, 265].

Their use in vaccine research is particularly valuable for screening improved TB vaccines that do not interfere with TB diagnosis methods like the tuberculin skin test and interferon-gamma release assay. NHP models have been used to assess the efficacy of various vaccines, including those delivered through respiratory mucosal routes [265, 266]. Of particular importance is the fact that intravenous vaccination of NHPs with BCG can lead to sterile immunity, a feature not observed in any other animal model of TB [66, 67, 267]. This unique feature has recently allowed closer insights into the potential correlates of protection induced by intravenous vaccination [267–269]. Although NHPs closely resemble humans in genetic background, immune responses, clinical symptoms, and pathogenesis, their use in TB vaccine research is limited due to ethical concerns, high costs, variability amongst individuals, and space requirements. Furthermore, variations in responses after BCG vaccination in different NHP species make it somewhat difficult to compare results across species [63]. Rhesus macaques and cynomolgus macaques have been the primary NHP species used in TB research [270, 271]. Depending on factors such as the *Mtb* strain, infection route, and dose, macaques can accurately replicate various forms of TB, including acute, latent, and reactivated TB, complete with human-like granuloma structures [205]. These granulomas, characterised by necrotic cores surrounded by macrophages and lymphocyte zones, closely resemble those observed in humans and provide a valuable platform for studying the impact of vaccination on TB pathophysiology [264, 272]. In addition to disease progression monitoring through MRI and PET-CT scans, NHPs have allowed to identify correlates of protection and susceptibility [267, 272]. Factors like $CD4^+$ T cells, tertiary lymphoid structures, and *Mtb*-specific B cells have all been implicated in influencing disease outcomes [273, 274]. Intradermal BCG vaccination in NHPs has provided insights into its variable protection against human pulmonary TB [275–277], and NHPs have also been instrumental in evaluating the safety and efficacy of preclinical and clinical TB vaccine candidates, including M72/AS01E [278] and MTBVAC [279].

NHP models in TB vaccine research come with inherent disadvantages, as their use is costly, demanding specialised facilities, equipment, and trained personnel. NHPs' genetic relatedness to humans raises ethical concerns about their use in research more broadly. Additionally, the limited availability of NHPs, especially specific pathogen-free macaques, poses a significant challenge for conducting large-scale and long-term vaccination studies [205, 208]. Balancing these advantages and limitations is crucial in determining the appropriateness of NHP models for TB vaccine evaluation. Despite their high cost and ethical concerns, NHPs are still widely considered essential for assessing vaccine immunogenicity, especially for candidates transitioning to clinical trials.

7.2.7 Livestock Animals

7.2.7.1 Cattle

Cattle serve as natural hosts for *M. bovis* infections, a significant source of economic losses, animal welfare issues, and zoonotic risks, particularly in developing countries [280]. Cattle models offer a unique opportunity to assess TB vaccine candidates with potential applications in both human and veterinary medicine. BCG-vaccinated cattle exhibit increased IFN-γ responses, fewer lesions, and reduced bacteria per lesion in comparison to non-vaccinated cattle [281, 282]. Additionally, key immune cells associated with infection, such as macrophages and IFN-γ^+ T cells, were significantly diminished in lymph node granulomas of BCG-vaccinated cattle [283, 284]. Moreover, 2,3-dioxygenase, a molecule implicated in immunoregulation during *Mtb* infection, was reduced within granulomas of BCG-vaccinated cattle [285]. While protection of BCG in cattle initially wanes [286], revaccination with BCG can restore protection, suggesting potential effectiveness in populations with a negative response to the tuberculin skin test (TST) in humans [286, 287]. The cattle model is suited for follow-up screening of advanced TB vaccine candidates and, more broadly, for assessing immune responses against mycobacteria [288]. This model's advantages include the slow development of clinical disease, similarities in granuloma formation and immune responses to human TB, and the feasibility of neonatal calf vaccination [289].

Major drawbacks of the cattle model are the requirement for long-term, resource-intensive studies due to the slower disease progression, high costs, and the absence of cavitations seen in infected humans. Additionally, cattle, like some other animal models, have limited access to immunological tools and reagents compared to more commonly used models like mice, limiting in-depth of mechanistic studies. Lastly, ethical and space constraints pose challenges in maintaining cattle in research facilities, as they require substantial space and adherence to strict animal welfare standards, further complicating logistical aspects of the research.

7.2.7.2 Goats

Goats can naturally contract *M. caprae* or *M. bovis* infections and can be used to evaluate TB vaccine efficacy. Vaccinated goats show differences in body weight, pathology, and bacterial burden, when compared to unvaccinated goats [290]. The goat model infected with *M. caprae* demonstrates caseous necrotising granulomas with liquefactive necrosis and cavities, akin to active TB in humans [196]. Recent investigations have shown that BCG vaccination provides some protection against experimental *M. bovis* or *M. caprae* challenge in goats [291], by reducing the number of lung lesions and bacterial burden in pulmonary lymph nodes and by increased weight [291, 292]. Interestingly, a number of studies from groups in Spain have shown that the route of TB vaccination may influence the resulting immune response in goats [196]. While subcutaneous, intranasal, and intramuscular vaccination with heat inactivated *Mycobacterium bovis,* BCG, or *Mtb* SO_2 led to a detectable immune responses measured by the single intradermal test and/or interferon gamma assays [291, 293, 294], this was not observed in orally vaccinated goats [295]. Goats were also used to evaluate the advanced clinical TB vaccine candidate VPM1002 and its next-generation derivatives [296, 297]. Goats offer advantages over cattle and NHPs due to their smaller size, lower cost, and the presence of human-like caseous and cavitary granulomatous lesions [292, 298].

7.2.7.3 Pigs

Mtb and *M. bovis* can also infect pigs and mini pigs [205, 208]. While an infection with *M. bovis* often leads to progressive disease, pigs sometimes can clear an infection with *Mtb* making them suitable models for investigating pathology and correlates of protection against *Mtb* [299]. The anatomy of the pig lung is related to human lungs with the presence of intralobular septae [208], and natural *Mtb* complex infections generate granulomas in various stages, including contained fibrotic encapsulated granulomas and necrotic lesions with extracellular mycobacteria [299, 300]. The immune response in pigs mirrors human TB, with significant increase in IFN-γ-producing $CD4^+$ T cells and *M. bovis*-specific B cells. However, $CD8^+$ T cell activation appears lower compared to $CD4^+$ T cells. In pigs, bacilli transmission from infected to naïve animals is possible due to cavity formation. Notably, BCG vaccination of pigs showed only marginal protection against *Mtb* challenge [301]. However, in more recent studies, it was demonstrated that BCG-vaccinated piglets develop effector and memory T cells that persist over time [302]. Given the logistical and financial implications associated with breeding, maintaining, and infecting pigs, this model has not been more widely used for TB vaccination studies. However, if taken up more widely by the TB research community, vaccination studies in piglets could offer unique insights into immune responses in neonatal hosts.

7.2.8 Zebrafish

Zebrafish are used as an animal model for TB due to their natural susceptibility to *Mycobacterium marinum*, a non-tuberculous relative of *Mtb*. Zebrafish offer several advantages, including their small size, ease of reproduction, and cost-effectiveness [303, 304]. When infected with *M. marinum*, adult zebrafish and their larval stages develop granulomas that closely resemble those found in humans. The immune responses (innate and adaptive) mounted against *M. mariunum* in zebrafish share key components with those in humans [304–306]. Additionally, the transparency of zebrafish larvae makes them amenable to fluorescence imaging. Studies using zebrafish have demonstrated that both BCG and DNA vaccination can protect adult fish from *M. marinum*-induced disease [306, 307]. These vaccinations reduce mortality and bacterial counts, mainly driven by adaptive immune response and increased production of IFN-γ. Zebrafish models have not only been employed for preclinical vaccine screening but have also contributed to our understanding of the mechanisms underlying granuloma formation and the reactivation of latent mycobacterial infections [308]. While significant anatomical and physiological differences to humans are evident, a *M. marinum* infection in zebrafish mirrors the continuum of human TB, enabling cost-efficient pre-clinical testing of vaccines against both primary and latent TB infections.

Zebrafish can be vaccinated via intraperitoneal or intramuscular injections, but mucosal immunisation is also possible [307, 309]. Biomarkers and reagents for assessing antigen immunogenicity in zebrafish are limited, and hence, survival rates, bacterial and granulomatous burden, and the involvement of other organs are predominantly assessed when evaluating vaccine efficacy. BCG has served as the standard vaccination control in zebrafish models against acute or chronic *M. marinum* infections [310, 311]. Like in humans, BCG does not prevent *M. marinum* infection in zebrafish but does provide limited and variable protection against disease. This limited protection is likely due to the poor replication of BCG in zebrafish [312]. Furthermore, BCG vaccination enhances survival in zebrafish with acute *M. marinum* infections and reduces bacilli numbers in chronic infections. Notably, this protective effect is amplified when a booster DNA vaccination, encoding antigens such as Ag85B, ESAT-6, and RpfE, is administered [312]. While the precise immunological mechanisms responsible for this protection in zebrafish are not fully understood, it is known that BCG induces Th1 and Th17-dependent immune responses, both in humans and multiple animal models [313]. Similarly, BCG administration to zebrafish triggers the expression of genes encoding proteins involved in innate and adaptive immune responses, including IL17 and its receptor [312]. Additionally, the reduced disease in vaccinated zebrafish is linked to a restrained pro-inflammatory response mediated by TNF [312]. While zebrafish are genetically the most distant vertebrate animal model from human, they exhibit genetic heterogeneity, similar to the natural diversity in the human population and large group sizes can be used in experimental settings.

7.2.9 Conclusion

In conclusion, choosing the right animal model for TB vaccine research is a crucial decision that impacts the validity and relevance of the results. Each model offers distinct advantages and disadvantages, and the choice should align with the specific research goals, budget, and ethical considerations. In addition to the vertebrate models described above, non-vertebrate fruit flies and amoeba can also be infected with mycobacteria [196] but are not particularly useful for TB vaccine research due to the absence of adaptive immune responses. Ultimately, a combination of animal models, alongside *in vitro* and computational approaches, may be the most effective strategy for advancing TB vaccine research towards the goal of TB eradication.

7.3 Routes of Vaccine Administration and Challenge Dose

While we have tried to cover the impact of different vaccination routes on TB disease in different animal models in the section above, we would like to end this chapter by discussing the advantages and disadvantages of various alternative vaccination routes, including aerosol, oral, intranasal, intratracheal, transdermal, and intravenous delivery more broadly (Fig. 7.3). Traditional routes of TB vaccine delivery, such as intradermal or subcutaneous injections, have shown limited success in achieving the desired level of protection. In recent years, many groups have explored some of those alternative routes of vaccine administration to enhance TB vaccine efficacy.

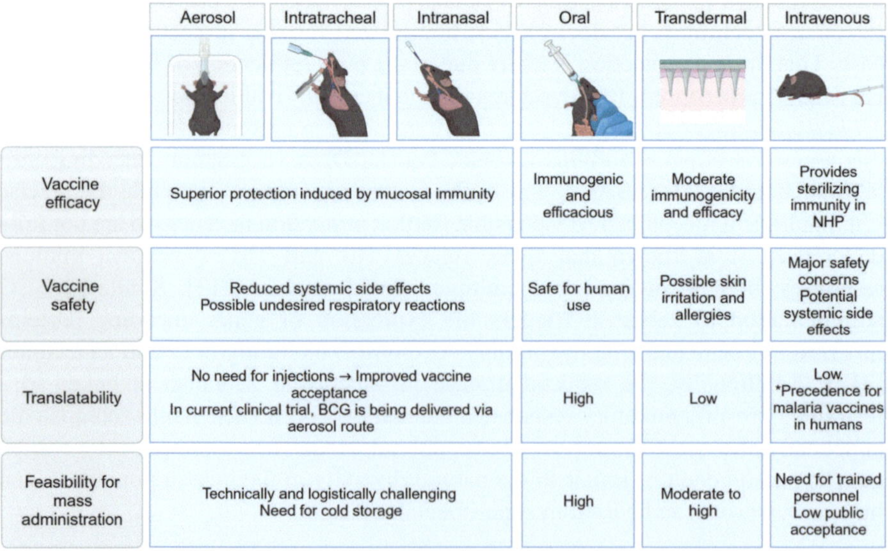

Fig. 7.3 Vaccine delivery routes. A summary of alternative TB vaccine delivery routes and their impact on vaccine efficacy, safety, and translatability as well as their potential for mass administration in a human population. (Figure created with Biorender.com)

7.3.1 Aerosol Delivery

Aerosol delivery involves the administration of vaccines in the form of droplets or particles suspended in air, targeting the respiratory mucosa [314]. This method aims to mimic the natural route of infection for *Mtb*. Compared to intradermal vaccine delivery, aerosolised vaccination more strongly induces mucosal immunity, including the generation of lung-resident memory T cells, which have been shown to offer significant protection against *Mtb* infection [315]. It also targets and leads to transcriptional changes in alveolar macrophages which are contained in the respiratory mucosa [316]. Compared to systemic injection, aerosol delivery often results in lower systemic exposure, reducing the risk of systemic side effects. Aerosol delivery also eliminates the need for needles, potentially improving vaccine acceptance and reducing the risk of needlestick injuries. Multiple TB vaccine candidates have been tested via aerosol (or intranasal/ intratracheal) delivery in animal models, with often superior protection compared to parental vaccine delivery [265, 268, 317–319]. It is important to note that aerosol vaccination with BCG of human volunteers is currently being trialled at the University of Oxford [320]. While these studies are predominantly geared towards the development of a human *Mtb* challenge model [321], they will undoubtedly also provide important safety data on aerosol BCG vaccination.

However, achieving consistent and precise aerosol delivery can be technically challenging, especially in resource-limited settings. Furthermore, concerns regarding the impact on lung gas exchange function and the potential for unintended aerosol exposure during administration require careful consideration. Hence, further studies are needed to evaluate these concerns and to assess whether existing mucosal delivery devices can be repurposed for the delivery of TB vaccines [322].

7.3.2 Oral Delivery

Oral vaccine delivery involves administering the vaccine through the mouth, typically in the form of capsules, tablets, or liquid formulations [323]. Oral vaccines are relatively easy to administer and do not require trained medical personnel, making them suitable for mass vaccination campaigns. The cost of oral vaccine administration is generally lower than injectable methods, as it does not require needles or syringes [323]. Oral vaccines can stimulate gut-associated lymphoid tissue, potentially providing systemic and mucosal immunity. Oral vaccines can be more stable than injectable formulations, reducing the need for cold storage and transportation. Importantly, when BCG was first introduced in 1921 it was administered orally for several decades, including the first dose ever given to a French infant [324]. The early success of BCG in reducing TB around the world clearly indicates that oral BCG vaccination is immunogenic and efficacious. Hence, it is interesting that few experimental human and animal TB vaccine candidates have been tested as oral formulations [79, 325–327]. However, some vaccine types, especially protein-based ones, may not induce robust immune responses when administered orally, the digestive environment can degrade them, and the absorption in the gut can be inconsistent, leading to variability in immune responses. Some orally delivered vaccines also require booster doses to maintain long-term protection [323]. Nevertheless, it appears logical that new TB vaccine candidates should also be tested as oral formulations in the future [328].

7.3.3 Intranasal and Intratracheal Delivery

Intranasal vaccine delivery involves administering vaccines through the nasal mucosa, and intratracheal vaccination through the oropharynx, collectively targeting the respiratory tract's local immune system [329]. Just like aerosol delivery, intranasal delivery stimulates mucosal immune responses, which may be critical for TB protection, given the respiratory route of infection [315]. Intranasal vaccines can induce rapid immune responses at the site of infection, potentially providing immediate protection [330]. This method is non-invasive, easy to administer, and does not require needles. Similar to aerosol delivery, intranasal vaccines often result in reduced systemic exposure, minimising systemic side effects [315]. As mentioned above, multiple TB vaccine candidates have shown superior protective efficacy and immunogenicity when administered intranasally or intratracheally in animal models [70, 331–333]. Compared to aerosol delivery, intranasal vaccine administration may also be more feasible for mass administration, particularly in resource poor settings [330]. It is, however, important to note that nasal congestion or blockage can hinder vaccine delivery and absorption and immune responses induced by intranasal vaccines may have a shorter duration compared to other delivery routes. In particular, compared to aerosol delivery, intranasal delivery in humans will predominantly target the upper airways with consequences for the resulting immune responses and vaccine efficacy. Intranasal vaccines may also have limited stability, requiring cold storage and careful handling, and concerns about the potential for respiratory infections or adverse reactions must be addressed.

7.3.4 Transdermal Delivery

Transdermal delivery involves administering vaccines through the skin, often using patches, microneedles, or other delivery systems [334]. Transdermal delivery is generally painless and does not involve needles, making it well-tolerated [335]. Controlled release systems can provide precise dosing, enhancing vaccine efficacy. The risk of infection or contamination is lower with transdermal delivery compared to injections. Some transdermal systems allow for self-administration, improving vaccine accessibility [335]. Not all vaccines are suitable for transdermal delivery, as they may not penetrate the skin effectively. Transdermal delivery may also result in slower immune responses compared to mucosal or systemic routes, and some individuals may experience skin irritation or allergic reactions to transdermal patches. Vaccine stability and shelf-life can be a concern with transdermal delivery systems.

To our knowledge, only very few TB vaccine candidates have been tested via transdermal delivery with modest success [336]. At this stage, it appears unlikely that a successful BCG replacement vaccine may be delivered via the transdermal route.

7.3.5 Intravenous Delivery

Intravenous vaccination for TB has recently re-emerged as a promising approach for TB vaccine delivery [66]. Based on seminal studies performed in NHPs, one of the primary advantages of intravenous BCG vaccination appears to be its ability to elicit a robust induction of airway T cells [267], mycobacteria-specific antibodies and NK cell activation [269, 337]. Intravenous BCG even prevented TB in simian immunodeficiency virus (SIV)—infected macaques—a high bar to cross [67]. While intravenous testing of TB vaccine candidates is not new [338, 339], access to modern high dimensional immune readouts and sophisticated imaging techniques allowed the more recent studies to gain mechanistic insights into the protective effects of intravenous BCG vaccination. TB often manifests as a latent infection, and intravenous vaccination may be more effective at targeting LTBI, as it can activate systemic immune responses as well as tissue-specific responses. While these findings are encouraging, intravenous TB vaccination is still in the experimental phase, and extensive research, including clinical trials, is needed to validate its safety and efficacy in humans. There is precedence for safe intravenous delivery for malaria vaccines, however the injected malaria sporozoites were irradiated and could not replicate within the human body [340–342]. Currently, the TB research community appears to be divided about the feasibility of intravenous BCG vaccination in humans. On the one hand, BCG has a proven safety record, is licensed for human use and billions of doses have been administered. On the other hand, intravenous injection with a live microorganism (although attenuated) will likely face stiff resistance from some groups, including parents and doctors. One promising strategy to overcome the safety considerations appears to be either the inclusion of "kill-switches" into BCG or other live-attenuated TB vaccines to limit their replication and induce controlled death of the bacterium [343, 344] or the development of auxotrophic strain [345, 346]. Regardless, it is essential to proceed with caution, conduct rigorous clinical trials, and address safety concerns before intravenous delivery can be widely implemented as part of global TB vaccination strategies. However, if successful, intravenous BCG vaccination could significantly contribute to the goal of TB eradication.

7.3.6 Effects of *Mtb* Challenge Dose

The initial *Mtb* infectious dose can shape disease progression and severity as well as the immune responses and the formation of defined lung granulomas. In resistant mouse models, animals infected with high doses of aerosolised *Mtb* (>1000 CFUs) die more rapidly than those infected with lower doses (50–100 CFUs). In early studies, susceptible mice lacking pro-inflammatory cytokines (IFN-γ, IL-12, IL-1) infected with 10^{5-6} CFU of *Mtb* succumbed earlier than resistant mice but survived for up to 100 days [347, 348]. A previous study had calculated that an initial dose of 10^{5-6} CFU ensured an uptake of approximately 200–500 viable bacilli [349], and it is possible that these early studies aimed for a safe approach to ensure infection. However, different results were observed after the same mouse strains were exposed to lower *Mtb* doses, ranging from 50 to 300 CFU, as these mice succumbed after 40 days of infection [350–353]. These contra-intuitive results suggest that choosing a more physiological initial *Mtb* inoculum is not a trivial task and can influence not only the disease outcomes but also the immune responses induced by vaccination.

Immunisation studies in macaques have shown that lower *Mtb* doses (<20 CFU), not only allowed better discrimination of vaccine efficacies between different immunisation protocols but also enabled the observation of vaccine-mediated sterilising immunity [66, 265, 354]. Although most of the NHP vaccination studies use very low *Mtb* doses for challenge experiments, this is not the standard approach in mice, which are usually infected with the so-called "conventional dose" (100–300 CFU). However, as mentioned before, NHP studies are expensive and testing all novel vaccine candidates in NHPs is not feasible. Importantly, promising results from a model of ultra-low dose (1–3 CFU) infection in mice, indicate that this method can recapitulate the formation of well-defined granulomas and that a mouse blood RNA signature can predict *Mtb* infection outcomes across species, including NHP and humans [355]. Altogether, these findings support the idea that using different animal models in conjunction with more physiological very low doses of *Mtb* for challenge experiments offer several advantages for pre-clinical testing of vaccine candidates.

7.3.7 Conclusion

Alternative routes of TB vaccine delivery offer the potential to improve vaccine efficacy and accessibility. Each route has its advantages and limitations, and the choice should align with the specific goals of TB vaccine development, as well as logistical and safety considerations. Aerosol and intranasal delivery hold promise for mimicking the natural route of infection and inducing mucosal immunity. Oral delivery is cost-effective and suitable for mass vaccination campaigns, while transdermal delivery provides a painless and controlled dosing option. Intravenous delivery appears to be most protective and capable of inducing sterile immunity. The selection of the most appropriate delivery route should be made based on careful consideration and may be specific for different types of vaccine modalities. Similarly, the choice of *Mtb* challenge dose should align with the animal model and aim to mimic the human infectious dose. Overall, it appears that low and ultra-low infectious doses more closely model human-like granulomas, TB disease progression, and the variable efficacy of BCG observed in different human populations.

Competing Interests The author(s) has no competing interests to declare that are relevant to the content of this manuscript.

Ethics Approval The author(s) declares that this manuscript does not include primary research with human participants.

References

1. Ottenhoff TH, Kaufmann SH. Vaccines against tuberculosis: where are we and where do we need to go? PLoS Pathog. 2012;8(5):e1002607. https://doi.org/10.1371/journal.ppat.1002607.
2. Flores-Valdez MA, Segura-Cerda CA. Preclinical evaluation of tuberculosis vaccine candidates: is it time to harmonize study design and readouts for prioritizing their development? Vaccine. 2021;39(2):173–5. https://doi.org/10.1016/j.vaccine.2020.11.073.
3. Zhang X, Wu X, He Q, Wang J, Mao Q, Liang Z, et al. Research progress on substitution of in vivo method(s) by in vitro method(s) for human vaccine potency assays. Expert Rev Vaccines. 2023;22(1):270–7. https://doi.org/10.1080/14760584.2023.2178421.
4. Pieters J. Mycobacterium tuberculosis and the macrophage: maintaining a balance. Cell Host Microbe. 2008;3(6):399–407. https://doi.org/10.1016/j.chom.2008.05.006.
5. Giacomini E, Iona E, Ferroni L, Miettinen M, Fattorini L, Orefici G, et al. Infection of human macrophages and dendritic cells with Mycobacterium tuberculosis induces a differential cytokine gene expression that modulates T cell response. J Immunol. 2001;166(12):7033–41. https://doi.org/10.4049/jimmunol.166.12.7033.
6. Harding CV, Boom WH. Regulation of antigen presentation by Mycobacterium tuberculosis: a role for Toll-like receptors. Nat Rev Microbiol. 2010;8(4):296–307. https://doi.org/10.1038/nrmicro2321.
7. Raschke WC, Baird S, Ralph P, Nakoinz I. Functional macrophage cell lines transformed by Abelson leukemia virus. Cell. 1978;15(1):261–7. https://doi.org/10.1016/0092-8674(78)90101-0.
8. Ralph P, Nakoinz I. Phagocytosis and cytolysis by a macrophage tumour and its cloned cell line. Nature. 1975;257(5525):393–4. https://doi.org/10.1038/257393a0.
9. Radzioch D, Hudson T, Boule M, Barrera L, Urbance JW, Varesio L, et al. Genetic resistance/susceptibility to mycobacteria: phenotypic expression in bone marrow derived macrophage lines. J Leukoc Biol. 1991;50(3):263–72. https://doi.org/10.1002/jlb.50.3.263.
10. Mbawuike IN, Herscowitz HB. MH-S, a murine alveolar macrophage cell line: morphological, cytochemical, and functional characteristics. J Leukoc Biol. 1989;46(2):119–27. https://doi.org/10.1002/jlb.46.2.119.
11. Palleroni AV, Varesio L, Wright RB, Brunda MJ. Tumoricidal alveolar macrophage and tumor infiltrating macrophage cell lines. Int J Cancer. 1991;49(2):296–302. https://doi.org/10.1002/ijc.2910490226.
12. Arora SK, Alam A, Naqvi N, Ahmad J, Sheikh JA, Rahman SA, et al. Immunodominant Mycobacterium tuberculosis protein Rv1507A elicits Th1 response and modulates host macrophage effector functions. Front Immunol. 2020;11:1199. https://doi.org/10.3389/fimmu.2020.01199.
13. Miller BH, Fratti RA, Poschet JF, Timmins GS, Master SS, Burgos M, et al. Mycobacteria inhibit nitric oxide synthase recruitment to phagosomes during macrophage infection. Infect Immun. 2004;72(5):2872–8. https://doi.org/10.1128/IAI.72.5.2872-2878.2004.
14. Roces CB, Hussain MT, Schmidt ST, Christensen D, Perrie Y. Investigating prime-pull vaccination through a combination of parenteral vaccination and intranasal boosting. Vaccines (Basel). 2019;8(1). https://doi.org/10.3390/vaccines8010010

15. Liu S, Jia H, Hou S, Zhang G, Xin T, Li H, et al. Recombinant TB10.4 of Mycobacterium bovis induces cytokine production in RAW264.7 macrophages through activation of the MAPK and NF-kappaB pathways via TLR2. Mol Immunol. 2014;62(1):227–34. https://doi.org/10.1016/j.molimm.2014.06.026.
16. Briken V, Miller JL. Living on the edge: inhibition of host cell apoptosis by Mycobacterium tuberculosis. Future Microbiol. 2008;3(4):415–22. https://doi.org/10.2217/17460913.3.4.415.
17. Barletta RG, Bannantine JP, Stabel JR, Muthukrishnan E, Anderson DK, Dutta E, et al. Mycobacterium avium subsp. paratuberculosis candidate vaccine strains are pro-apoptotic in RAW 264.7 murine macrophages. Vaccines (Basel). 2023;11(6). https://doi.org/10.3390/vaccines11061085.
18. Lee KI, Choi S, Choi HG, Gurmessa SK, Dang TB, Back YW, et al. Recombinant Rv1654 protein of Mycobacterium tuberculosis induces mitochondria-mediated apoptosis in macrophage. Microbiol Immunol. 2021;65(4):178–88. https://doi.org/10.1111/1348-0421.12880.
19. Liao TY, Lau A, Joseph S, Hytonen V, Hmama Z. Improving the immunogenicity of the Mycobacterium bovis BCG vaccine by non-genetic bacterial surface decoration using the Avidin-Biotin system. PLoS One. 2015;10(12):e0145833. https://doi.org/10.1371/journal.pone.0145833.
20. Yang L, Zhang C, Zhao Y, Zhao N, Wu P, Zhang H, et al. Effects of Mycobacterium tuberculosis mutant strain Hsp16.3 gene on murine RAW 264.7 macrophage autophagy. DNA Cell Biol. 2018;37(1):7–14. https://doi.org/10.1089/dna.2016.3599.
21. Su H, Zhu S, Zhu L, Kong C, Huang Q, Zhang Z, et al. Mycobacterium tuberculosis latent antigen Rv2029c from the multistage DNA vaccine A39 drives TH1 responses via TLR-mediated macrophage activation. Front Microbiol. 2017;8:2266. https://doi.org/10.3389/fmicb.2017.02266.
22. Melo MD, Stokes RW. Interaction of Mycobacterium tuberculosis with MH-S, an immortalized murine alveolar macrophage cell line: a comparison with primary murine macrophages. Tuber Lung Dis. 2000;80(1):35–46. https://doi.org/10.1054/tuld.1999.0228.
23. Darieva ZA, Lasunskaia EB, Kipnis TL, Dias Da Silva W. Two BCG vaccine formulations prepared from the same strain with different J774 macrophage activation capacities and patterns of NF-kappaB induction. Int J Mol Med. 2000;6(5):575–80. https://doi.org/10.3892/ijmm.6.5.575.
24. Chavez-Galan L, Vesin D, Martinvalet D, Garcia I. Low dose BCG infection as a model for macrophage activation maintaining cell viability. J Immunol Res. 2016;2016:4048235. https://doi.org/10.1155/2016/4048235.
25. Tsuchiya S, Yamabe M, Yamaguchi Y, Kobayashi Y, Konno T, Tada K. Establishment and characterization of a human acute monocytic leukemia cell line (THP-1). Int J Cancer. 1980;26(2):171–6. https://doi.org/10.1002/ijc.2910260208.
26. Tsuchiya S, Kobayashi Y, Goto Y, Okumura H, Nakae S, Konno T, et al. Induction of maturation in cultured human monocytic leukemia cells by a phorbol diester. Cancer Res. 1982;42(4):1530–6.
27. Sundstrom C, Nilsson K. Establishment and characterization of a human histiocytic lymphoma cell line (U-937). Int J Cancer. 1976;17(5):565–77. https://doi.org/10.1002/ijc.2910170504.
28. Chun EM, Park YJ, Kang HS, Cho HM, Jun DY, Kim YH. Expression of the apolipoprotein C-II gene during myelomonocytic differentiation of human leukemic cells. J Leukoc Biol. 2001;69(4):645–50.
29. Rots NY, Iavarone A, Bromleigh V, Freedman LP. Induced differentiation of U937 cells by 1,25-dihydroxyvitamin D3 involves cell cycle arrest in G1 that is preceded by a transient proliferative burst and an increase in cyclin expression. Blood. 1999;93(8):2721–9.
30. Chanput W, Mes JJ, Wichers HJ. THP-1 cell line: an in vitro cell model for immune modulation approach. Int Immunopharmacol. 2014;23(1):37–45. https://doi.org/10.1016/j.intimp.2014.08.002.
31. Ziegler-Heitbrock HW, Thiel E, Futterer A, Herzog V, Wirtz A, Riethmuller G. Establishment of a human cell line (Mono Mac 6) with characteristics of mature monocytes. Int J Cancer. 1988;41(3):456–61. https://doi.org/10.1002/ijc.2910410324.

32. Shattock RJ, Friedland JS, Griffin GE. Phagocytosis of Mycobacterium tuberculosis modulates human immunodeficiency virus replication in human monocytic cells. J Gen Virol. 1994;75(Pt 4):849–56. https://doi.org/10.1099/0022-1317-75-4-849.
33. Horvati K, Fodor K, Palyi B, Henczko J, Balka G, Gyulai G, et al. Novel assay platform to evaluate intracellular killing of Mycobacterium tuberculosis: in vitro and in vivo validation. Front Immunol. 2021;12:750496. https://doi.org/10.3389/fimmu.2021.750496.
34. Estrella JL, Kan-Sutton C, Gong X, Rajagopalan M, Lewis DE, Hunter RL, et al. A novel in vitro human macrophage model to study the persistence of Mycobacterium tuberculosis using vitamin D(3) and retinoic acid activated THP-1 macrophages. Front Microbiol. 2011;2:67. https://doi.org/10.3389/fmicb.2011.00067.
35. Madhvi A, Mishra H, Leisching GR, Mahlobo PZ, Baker B. Comparison of human monocyte derived macrophages and THP1-like macrophages as in vitro models for M. tuberculosis infection. Comp Immunol Microbiol Infect Dis. 2019;67:101355. https://doi.org/10.1016/j.cimid.2019.101355.
36. Lewis KN, Liao R, Guinn KM, Hickey MJ, Smith S, Behr MA, et al. Deletion of RD1 from Mycobacterium tuberculosis mimics bacille Calmette-Guerin attenuation. J Infect Dis. 2003;187(1):117–23. https://doi.org/10.1086/345862.
37. Riendeau CJ, Kornfeld H. THP-1 cell apoptosis in response to Mycobacterial infection. Infect Immun. 2003;71(1):254–9. https://doi.org/10.1128/IAI.71.1.254-259.2003.
38. Liu Z, Wang J, Dai F, Zhang D, Li W. DUSP1 mediates BCG induced apoptosis and inflammatory response in THP-1 cells via MAPKs/NF-kappaB signaling pathway. Sci Rep. 2023;13(1):2606. https://doi.org/10.1038/s41598-023-29900-6.
39. Tang J, Zhan L, Qin C. Inhibition of TLR8 mediated signaling promotes BCG induced apoptosis in THP-1 cells. Microb Pathog. 2016;93:78–82. https://doi.org/10.1016/j.micpath.2015.11.028.
40. Bai X, Feldman NE, Chmura K, Ovrutsky AR, Su WL, Griffin L, et al. Inhibition of nuclear factor-kappa B activation decreases survival of Mycobacterium tuberculosis in human macrophages. PLoS One. 2013;8(4):e61925. https://doi.org/10.1371/journal.pone.0061925.
41. Mendoza-Coronel E, Castanon-Arreola M. Comparative evaluation of in vitro human macrophage models for mycobacterial infection study. Pathog Dis. 2016;74(6):ftw052. https://doi.org/10.1093/femspd/ftw052.
42. Passmore JS, Lukey PT, Ress SR. The human macrophage cell line U937 as an in vitro model for selective evaluation of mycobacterial antigen-specific cytotoxic T-cell function. Immunology. 2001;102(2):146–56. https://doi.org/10.1046/j.1365-2567.2001.01164.x.
43. Vigerust DJ, Vick S, Shepherd VL. Characterization of functional mannose receptor in a continuous hybridoma cell line. BMC Immunol. 2012;13:51. https://doi.org/10.1186/1471-2172-13-51.
44. Schlesinger LS. Macrophage phagocytosis of virulent but not attenuated strains of Mycobacterium tuberculosis is mediated by mannose receptors in addition to complement receptors. J Immunol. 1993;150(7):2920–30.
45. Andreu N, Phelan J, de Sessions PF, Cliff JM, Clark TG, Hibberd ML. Primary macrophages and J774 cells respond differently to infection with Mycobacterium tuberculosis. Sci Rep. 2017;7:42225. https://doi.org/10.1038/srep42225.
46. Francke A, Herold J, Weinert S, Strasser RH, Braun-Dullaeus RC. Generation of mature murine monocytes from heterogeneous bone marrow and description of their properties. J Histochem Cytochem. 2011;59(9):813–25. https://doi.org/10.1369/0022155411416007.
47. Podinovskaia M, Lee W, Caldwell S, Russell DG. Infection of macrophages with Mycobacterium tuberculosis induces global modifications to phagosomal function. Cell Microbiol. 2013;15(6):843–59. https://doi.org/10.1111/cmi.12092.
48. Herbst S, Schaible UE, Schneider BE. Interferon gamma activated macrophages kill mycobacteria by nitric oxide induced apoptosis. PLoS One. 2011;6(5):e19105. https://doi.org/10.1371/journal.pone.0019105.

49. Kaufmann E, Sanz J, Dunn JL, Khan N, Mendonca LE, Pacis A, et al. BCG educates hematopoietic stem cells to generate protective innate immunity against tuberculosis. Cell. 2018;172(1–2):176–90 e19. https://doi.org/10.1016/j.cell.2017.12.031.
50. Khan N, Downey J, Sanz J, Kaufmann E, Blankenhaus B, Pacis A, et al. M. tuberculosis reprograms hematopoietic stem cells to limit Myelopoiesis and impair trained immunity. Cell. 2020;183(3):752–70 e22. https://doi.org/10.1016/j.cell.2020.09.062.
51. Bickett TE, McLean J, Creissen E, Izzo L, Hagan C, Izzo AJ, et al. Characterizing the BCG induced macrophage and neutrophil mechanisms for defense against Mycobacterium tuberculosis. Front Immunol. 2020;11:1202. https://doi.org/10.3389/fimmu.2020.01202.
52. Jordao L, Bleck CK, Mayorga L, Griffiths G, Anes E. On the killing of mycobacteria by macrophages. Cell Microbiol. 2008;10(2):529–48. https://doi.org/10.1111/j.1462-5822.2007.01067.x.
53. Sathkumara HD, Muruganandah V, Cooper MM, Field MA, Alim MA, Brosch R, et al. Mucosal delivery of ESX-1-expressing BCG strains provides superior immunity against tuberculosis in murine type 2 diabetes. Proc Natl Acad Sci USA. 2020;117(34):20848–59. https://doi.org/10.1073/pnas.2003235117.
54. Parra M, Yang AL, Lim J, Kolibab K, Derrick S, Cadieux N, et al. Development of a murine mycobacterial growth inhibition assay for evaluating vaccines against Mycobacterium tuberculosis. Clin Vaccine Immunol. 2009;16(7):1025–32. https://doi.org/10.1128/CVI.00067-09.
55. Zelmer A, Tanner R, Stylianou E, Damelang T, Morris S, Izzo A, et al. A new tool for tuberculosis vaccine screening: ex vivo mycobacterial growth inhibition assay indicates BCG-mediated protection in a murine model of tuberculosis. BMC Infect Dis. 2016;16:412. https://doi.org/10.1186/s12879-016-1751-4.
56. Yang AL, Schmidt TE, Stibitz S, Derrick SC, Morris SL, Parra M. A simplified mycobacterial growth inhibition assay (MGIA) using direct infection of mouse splenocytes and the MGIT system. J Microbiol Methods. 2016;131:7–9. https://doi.org/10.1016/j.mimet.2016.09.010.
57. Marsay L, Matsumiya M, Tanner R, Poyntz H, Griffiths KL, Stylianou E, et al. Mycobacterial growth inhibition in murine splenocytes as a surrogate for protection against Mycobacterium tuberculosis (M. tb). Tuberculosis (Edinb). 2013;93(5):551–7. https://doi.org/10.1016/j.tube.2013.04.007.
58. Kolibab K, Parra M, Yang AL, Perera LP, Derrick SC, Morris SL. A practical in vitro growth inhibition assay for the evaluation of TB vaccines. Vaccine. 2009;28(2):317–22. https://doi.org/10.1016/j.vaccine.2009.10.047.
59. Alim MA, Kupz A, Sikder S, Rush C, Govan B, Ketheesan N. Increased susceptibility to Mycobacterium tuberculosis infection in a diet-induced murine model of type 2 diabetes. Microbes Infect/Institut Pasteur. 2020;22(8):303–11. https://doi.org/10.1016/j.micinf.2020.03.004.
60. Alim MA, Sikder S, Sathkumara H, Kupz A, Rush CM, Govan BL, et al. Dysregulation of key cytokines may contribute to increased susceptibility of diabetic mice to Mycobacterium bovis BCG infection. Tuberculosis (Edinb). 2019;115:113–20. https://doi.org/10.1016/j.tube.2019.02.005.
61. Kumari M, Saxena RK. Relative efficacy of uptake and presentation of Mycobacterium bovis BCG antigens by type I mouse lung epithelial cells and peritoneal macrophages. Infect Immun. 2011;79(8):3159–67. https://doi.org/10.1128/IAI.05406-11.
62. Foreman TW, Mehra S, Lackner AA, Kaushal D. Translational research in the nonhuman primate model of tuberculosis. ILAR J. 2017;58(2):151–9. https://doi.org/10.1093/ilar/ilx015.
63. Harris SA, White A, Stockdale L, Tanner R, Sibley L, Sarfas C, et al. Development of a nonhuman primate BCG infection model for the evaluation of candidate tuberculosis vaccines. Tuberculosis (Edinb). 2018;108:99–105. https://doi.org/10.1016/j.tube.2017.11.006.
64. Joslyn LR, Pienaar E, DiFazio RM, Suliman S, Kagina BM, Flynn JL, et al. Integrating non-human primate, human, and mathematical studies to determine the influence of BCG timing on H56 vaccine outcomes. Front Microbiol. 2018;9:1734. https://doi.org/10.3389/fmicb.2018.01734.

65. Pena JC, Ho WZ. Non-human primate models of tuberculosis. Microbiol Spectr. 2016;4(4) https://doi.org/10.1128/microbiolspec.TBTB2-0007-2016.
66. Darrah PA, Zeppa JJ, Maiello P, Hackney JA, Wadsworth MH 2nd, Hughes TK, et al. Prevention of tuberculosis in macaques after intravenous BCG immunization. Nature. 2020;577(7788):95–102. https://doi.org/10.1038/s41586-019-1817-8.
67. Larson EC, Ellis-Connell AL, Rodgers MA, Gubernat AK, Gleim JL, Moriarty RV, et al. Intravenous Bacille Calmette-Guerin vaccination protects simian immunodeficiency virus-infected macaques from tuberculosis. Nat Microbiol. 2023;8:2080. https://doi.org/10.1038/s41564-023-01503-x.
68. Pacheco SA, Powers KM, Engelmann F, Messaoudi I, Purdy GE. Autophagic killing effects against Mycobacterium tuberculosis by alveolar macrophages from young and aged rhesus macaques. PLoS One. 2013;8(6):e66985. https://doi.org/10.1371/journal.pone.0066985.
69. Khan A, Bakhru P, Saikolappan S, Das K, Soudani E, Singh CR, et al. An autophagy-inducing and TLR-2 activating BCG vaccine induces a robust protection against tuberculosis in mice. NPJ Vaccines. 2019;4:34. https://doi.org/10.1038/s41541-019-0122-8.
70. Shurygina AP, Zabolotnykh N, Vinogradova T, Khairullin B, Kassenov M, Nurpeisova A, et al. Preclinical evaluation of TB/FLU-04L-an intranasal influenza vector-based boost vaccine against tuberculosis. Int J Mol Sci. 2023;24(8). https://doi.org/10.3390/ijms24087439.
71. Hokey DA, Wachholder R, Darrah PA, Bolton DL, Barouch DH, Hill K, et al. A nonhuman primate toxicology and immunogenicity study evaluating aerosol delivery of AERAS-402/Ad35 vaccine: evidence for transient t cell responses in peripheral blood and robust sustained responses in the lungs. Hum Vaccin Immunother. 2014;10(8):2199–210. https://doi.org/10.4161/hv.29108.
72. Tanner R, White AD, Boot C, Sombroek CC, O'Shea MK, Wright D, et al. A non-human primate in vitro functional assay for the early evaluation of TB vaccine candidates. NPJ Vaccines. 2021;6(1):3. https://doi.org/10.1038/s41541-020-00263-7.
73. Nielsen MC, Andersen MN, Moller HJ. Monocyte isolation techniques significantly impact the phenotype of both isolated monocytes and derived macrophages in vitro. Immunology. 2020;159(1):63–74. https://doi.org/10.1111/imm.13125.
74. Madhvi A, Mishra H, Chegou NN, Mkhonza MN, Ndou S, Tromp G, et al. Comparison of cytokines expression from human monocyte-derived macrophages infected with different species of mycobacteria. J Interferon Cytokine Res. 2022;42(4):141–52. https://doi.org/10.1089/jir.2021.0216.
75. Mihret A. The role of dendritic cells in Mycobacterium tuberculosis infection. Virulence. 2012;3(7):654–9. https://doi.org/10.4161/viru.22586.
76. Etna MP, Giacomini E, Severa M, Pardini M, Aguilo N, Martin C, et al. A human dendritic cell-based in vitro model to assess Mycobacterium tuberculosis SO2 vaccine immunogenicity. ALTEX. 2014;31(4):397–406. https://doi.org/10.14573/altex.1311041.
77. Ming M, Bernardo L, Williams K, Kolattukudy P, Kapoor N, Chan LG, et al. An in vitro functional assay to measure the biological activity of TB vaccine candidate H4-IC31. Vaccine. 2019;37(22):2960–6. https://doi.org/10.1016/j.vaccine.2019.04.035.
78. Domingo-Gonzalez R, Prince O, Cooper A, Khader SA. Cytokines and chemokines in Mycobacterium tuberculosis infection. Microbiol Spectr. 2016;4(5). https://doi.org/10.1128/microbiolspec.TBTB2-0018-2016.
79. Mittrücker HW, Steinhoff U, Köhler A, Krause M, Lazar D, Mex P, et al. Poor correlation between BCG vaccination-induced T cell responses and protection against tuberculosis. Proc Natl Acad Sci USA. 2007;104(30):12434–9. https://doi.org/10.1073/pnas.0703510104.
80. Kagina BM, Abel B, Scriba TJ, Hughes EJ, Keyser A, Soares A, et al. Specific T cell frequency and cytokine expression profile do not correlate with protection against tuberculosis after bacillus Calmette-Guerin vaccination of newborns. Am J Respir Crit Care Med. 2010;182(8):1073–9. https://doi.org/10.1164/rccm.201003-0334OC.
81. Tanner R, Smith SG, van Meijgaarden KE, Giannoni F, Wilkie M, Gabriele L, et al. Optimisation, harmonisation and standardisation of the direct mycobacterial growth inhi-

bition assay using cryopreserved human peripheral blood mononuclear cells. J Immunol Methods. 2019;469:1–10. https://doi.org/10.1016/j.jim.2019.01.006.
82. Worku S, Hoft DF. In vitro measurement of protective mycobacterial immunity: antigen-specific expansion of T cells capable of inhibiting intracellular growth of bacille Calmette-Guerin. Clin Infect Dis. 2000;30(Suppl 3):S257–61. https://doi.org/10.1086/313887.
83. Fletcher HA, Tanner R, Wallis RS, Meyer J, Manjaly ZR, Harris S, et al. Inhibition of mycobacterial growth in vitro following primary but not secondary vaccination with Mycobacterium bovis BCG. Clin Vaccine Immunol. 2013;20(11):1683–9. https://doi.org/10.1128/CVI.00427-13.
84. Bobadilla-Del-Valle M, Leal-Vega F, Torres-Gonzalez P, Ordaz-Vazquez A, Garcia-Garcia ML, Tovar-Vargas MLA, et al. Mycobacterial growth inhibition assay (MGIA) as a host directed diagnostic tool for the evaluation of the immune response in subjects living with type 2 diabetes mellitus. Front Cell Infect Microbiol. 2021;11:640707. https://doi.org/10.3389/fcimb.2021.640707.
85. Harris SA, Meyer J, Satti I, Marsay L, Poulton ID, Tanner R, et al. Evaluation of a human BCG challenge model to assess antimycobacterial immunity induced by BCG and a candidate tuberculosis vaccine, MVA85A, alone and in combination. J Infect Dis. 2014;209(8):1259–68. https://doi.org/10.1093/infdis/jit647.
86. Tanner R, O'Shea MK, Fletcher HA, McShane H. In vitro mycobacterial growth inhibition assays: a tool for the assessment of protective immunity and evaluation of tuberculosis vaccine efficacy. Vaccine. 2016;34(39):4656–65. https://doi.org/10.1016/j.vaccine.2016.07.058.
87. Radloff J, Heyckendorf J, van der Merwe L, Sanchez Carballo P, Reiling N, Richter E, et al. Mycobacterium growth inhibition assay of human alveolar macrophages as a correlate of immune protection following Mycobacterium bovis Bacille Calmette-Guerin vaccination. Front Immunol. 2018;9:1708. https://doi.org/10.3389/fimmu.2018.01708.
88. Silva Miranda M, Breiman A, Allain S, Deknuydt F, Altare F. The tuberculous granuloma: an unsuccessful host defence mechanism providing a safety shelter for the bacteria? Clin Dev Immunol. 2012;2012:139127. https://doi.org/10.1155/2012/139127.
89. Elkington P, Lerm M, Kapoor N, Mahon R, Pienaar E, Huh D, et al. In vitro granuloma models of tuberculosis: potential and challenges. J Infect Dis. 2019;219(12):1858–66. https://doi.org/10.1093/infdis/jiz020.
90. Fitzgerald LE, Abendano N, Juste RA, Alonso-Hearn M. Three-dimensional in vitro models of granuloma to study bacteria-host interactions, drug-susceptibility, and resuscitation of dormant mycobacteria. Biomed Res Int. 2014;2014:623856. https://doi.org/10.1155/2014/623856.
91. Gkatzis K, Taghizadeh S, Huh D, Stainier DYR, Bellusci S. Use of three-dimensional organoids and lung-on-a-chip methods to study lung development, regeneration and disease. Eur Respir J. 2018;52(5):1800876. https://doi.org/10.1183/13993003.00876-2018.
92. Puissegur MP, Botanch C, Duteyrat JL, Delsol G, Caratero C, Altare F. An in vitro dual model of mycobacterial granulomas to investigate the molecular interactions between mycobacteria and human host cells. Cell Microbiol. 2004;6(5):423–33. https://doi.org/10.1111/j.1462-5822.2004.00371.x.
93. Taflin C, Miyara M, Nochy D, Valeyre D, Naccache JM, Altare F, et al. FoxP3+ regulatory T cells suppress early stages of granuloma formation but have little impact on sarcoidosis lesions. Am J Pathol. 2009;174(2):497–508. https://doi.org/10.2353/ajpath.2009.080580.
94. Lay G, Poquet Y, Salek-Peyron P, Puissegur MP, Botanch C, Bon H, et al. Langhans giant cells from M. tuberculosis-induced human granulomas cannot mediate mycobacterial uptake. J Pathol. 2007;211(1):76–85. https://doi.org/10.1002/path.2092.
95. Puissegur MP, Lay G, Gilleron M, Botella L, Nigou J, Marrakchi H, et al. Mycobacterial lipomannan induces granuloma macrophage fusion via a TLR2-dependent, ADAM9- and beta1 integrin-mediated pathway. J Immunol. 2007;178(5):3161–9. https://doi.org/10.4049/jimmunol.178.5.3161.

96. Wang C, Peyron P, Mestre O, Kaplan G, van Soolingen D, Gao Q, et al. Innate immune response to Mycobacterium tuberculosis Beijing and other genotypes. PLoS One. 2010;5(10):e13594. https://doi.org/10.1371/journal.pone.0013594.
97. Crouser ED, White P, Caceres EG, Julian MW, Papp AC, Locke LW, et al. A novel in vitro human granuloma model of sarcoidosis and latent tuberculosis infection. Am J Respir Cell Mol Biol. 2017;57(4):487–98. https://doi.org/10.1165/rcmb.2016-0321OC.
98. Guirado E, Mbawuike U, Keiser TL, Arcos J, Azad AK, Wang SH, et al. Characterization of host and microbial determinants in individuals with latent tuberculosis infection using a human granuloma model. MBio. 2015;6(1):e02537–14. https://doi.org/10.1128/mBio.02537-14.
99. Kapoor N, Pawar S, Sirakova TD, Deb C, Warren WL, Kolattukudy PE. Human granuloma in vitro model, for TB dormancy and resuscitation. PLoS One. 2013;8(1):e53657. https://doi.org/10.1371/journal.pone.0053657.
100. Clevers H. Modeling development and disease with organoids. Cell. 2016;165(7):1586–97. https://doi.org/10.1016/j.cell.2016.05.082.
101. Dye BR, Hill DR, Ferguson MA, Tsai YH, Nagy MS, Dyal R, et al. In vitro generation of human pluripotent stem cell derived lung organoids. elife. 2015;4:e05098. https://doi.org/10.7554/eLife.05098.
102. Katsura H, Sontake V, Tata A, Kobayashi Y, Edwards CE, Heaton BE, et al. Human lung stem cell-based alveolospheres provide insights into SARS-CoV-2-mediated interferon responses and pneumocyte dysfunction. Cell Stem Cell. 2020;27(6):890–904 e8. https://doi.org/10.1016/j.stem.2020.10.005.
103. Salahudeen AA, Choi SS, Rustagi A, Zhu J, van Unen V, de la OS, et al. Progenitor identification and SARS-CoV-2 infection in human distal lung organoids. Nature. 2020;588(7839):670–5. https://doi.org/10.1038/s41586-020-3014-1.
104. Iakobachvili N, Leon-Icaza SA, Knoops K, Sachs N, Mazeres S, Simeone R, et al. Mycobacteria-host interactions in human bronchiolar airway organoids. Mol Microbiol. 2022;117(3):682–92. https://doi.org/10.1111/mmi.14824.
105. Francis I, Shrestha J, Paudel KR, Hansbro PM, Warkiani ME, Saha SC. Recent advances in lung-on-a-chip models. Drug Discov Today. 2022;27(9):2593–602. https://doi.org/10.1016/j.drudis.2022.06.004.
106. Huh D, Matthews BD, Mammoto A, Montoya-Zavala M, Hsin HY, Ingber DE. Reconstituting organ-level lung functions on a chip. Science. 2010;328(5986):1662–8. https://doi.org/10.1126/science.1188302.
107. Zamprogno P, Wuthrich S, Achenbach S, Thoma G, Stucki JD, Hobi N, et al. Second-generation lung-on-a-chip with an array of stretchable alveoli made with a biological membrane. Commun Biol. 2021;4(1):168. https://doi.org/10.1038/s42003-021-01695-0.
108. Thacker VV, Dhar N, Sharma K, Barrile R, Karalis K, McKinney JD. A lung-on-chip model of early Mycobacterium tuberculosis infection reveals an essential role for alveolar epithelial cells in controlling bacterial growth. elife. 2020;9:e59961. https://doi.org/10.7554/eLife.59961.
109. Berry SB, Gower MS, Su X, Seshadri C, Theberge AB. A modular microscale granuloma model for immune-microenvironment signaling studies in vitro. Front Bioeng Biotechnol. 2020;8:931. https://doi.org/10.3389/fbioe.2020.00931.
110. Gupta UD, Katoch VM. Animal models of tuberculosis for vaccine development. Indian J Med Res. 2009;1(129):11–8.
111. Kaplan G, Post FA, Moreira AL, Wainwright H, Kreiswirth BN, Tanverdi M, et al. Mycobacterium tuberculosis growth at the cavity surface: a microenvironment with failed immunity. Infect Immun. 2003;71(12):7099–108. https://doi.org/10.1128/IAI.71.12.7099-7108.2003.
112. Ulrichs T, Kaufmann SH. New insights into the function of granulomas in human tuberculosis. J Pathol. 2006;208(2):261–9. https://doi.org/10.1002/path.1906.

113. Medina E, North RJ. Resistance ranking of some common inbred mouse strains to Mycobacterium tuberculosis and relationship to major histocompatibility complex haplotype and Nramp1 genotype. Immunology. 1998;93(2):270–4. https://doi.org/10.1046/j.1365-2567.1998.00419.x.
114. Huygen K, Abramowicz D, Vandenbussche P, Jacobs F, Bruyn JDE, Kentos A, et al. Spleen cell cytokine secretion in Mycobacterium bovis BCG-infected mice. In: Infection and Immunity; 1992. p. 2880–6.
115. Yoshida A, Koide Y, Uchijima M, Yoshida T. Dissection of strain difference in acquired protective immunity against Mycobacterium bovis Calmette-Gu6rin Bacillus (BCC) macrophages regulate the susceptibility through cytokine network and the induction of nitric oxide synthase. J Immunol. 1995:2057–66.
116. Flynn JL, Coldstein MM, Triebold KJ, Sypek J, Wolf S, Bloom BR. IL-12 increases resistance of BALB/c mice to Mycobacterium tuberculosis infection. J Immunol. 1995;155:2515.
117. Garcia-Pelayo MC, Bachy VS, Kaveh DA, Hogarth PJ. BALB/c mice display more enhanced BCG vaccine induced Th1 and Th17 response than C57BL/6 mice but have equivalent protection. Tuberculosis (Edinb). 2015;95(1):48–53. https://doi.org/10.1016/j.tube.2014.10.012.
118. Yang E, Lu Y, Xu Y, Liang Q, Wang C, Wang H, et al. Recombinant BCG coexpressing Ag85B, ESAT-6 and Rv3620c elicits specific Th1 immune responses in C57BL/6 mice. Microb Pathog. 2014;69-70:53–9. https://doi.org/10.1016/j.micpath.2014.03.011.
119. Lu Y, Xu Y, Yang E, Wang C, Wang H, Shen H. Novel recombinant BCG coexpressing Ag85B, ESAT-6 and Rv2608 elicits significantly enhanced cellular immune and antibody responses in C57BL/6 mice. Scand J Immunol. 2012;76(3):271–7. https://doi.org/10.1111/j.1365-3083.2012.02726.x.
120. Christy AJ, Dharman K, Dhandapaani G, Palaniyandi K, Gupta UD, Gupta P, et al. Epitope based recombinant BCG vaccine elicits specific Th1 polarized immune responses in BALB/c mice. Vaccine. 2012;30(7):1364–70. https://doi.org/10.1016/j.vaccine.2011.12.059.
121. Yuan X, Teng X, Jing Y, Ma J, Tian M, Yu Q, et al. A live attenuated BCG vaccine overexpressing multistage antigens Ag85B and HspX provides superior protection against Mycobacterium tuberculosis infection. Appl Microbiol Biotechnol. 2015;99(24):10587–95. https://doi.org/10.1007/s00253-015-6962-x.
122. Shen H, Wang C, Yang E, Xu Y, Liu W, Yan J, et al. Novel recombinant BCG coexpressing Ag85B, ESAT-6 and mouse TNF-alpha induces significantly enhanced cellular immune and antibody responses in C57BL/6 mice. Microbiol Immunol. 2010;54(8):435–41. https://doi.org/10.1111/j.1348-0421.2010.00232.x.
123. Dobakhti F, Naghibi T, Taghikhani M, Ajdary S, Rafinejad A, Bayati K, et al. Adjuvanticity effect of sodium alginate on subcutaneously injected BCG in BALB/c mice. Microbes Infect. 2009;11(2):296–301. https://doi.org/10.1016/j.micinf.2008.12.003.
124. Lu M, Xia ZY, Bao L. A Mycobacterium bovis BCG-naked DNA prime-boost vaccination strategy induced CD4(+) and CD8(+) T-cell response against Mycobacterium tuberculosis immunogens. J Immunol Res. 2014;2014:395626. https://doi.org/10.1155/2014/395626.
125. Sander P, Clark S, Petrera A, Vilaplana C, Meuli M, Selchow P, et al. Deletion of zmp1 improves Mycobacterium bovis BCG-mediated protection in a Guinea pig model of tuberculosis. Vaccine. 2015;33(11):1353–9. https://doi.org/10.1016/j.vaccine.2015.01.058.
126. Pedroza-Roldan C, Guapillo C, Barrios-Payan J, Mata-Espinosa D, Aceves-Sanchez Mde J, Marquina-Castillo B, et al. The BCGDeltaBCG1419c strain, which produces more pellicle in vitro, improves control of chronic tuberculosis in vivo. Vaccine. 2016;34(40):4763–70. https://doi.org/10.1016/j.vaccine.2016.08.035.
127. Counoupas C, Pinto R, Nagalingam G, Britton WJ, Triccas JA. Protective efficacy of recombinant BCG over-expressing protective, stage-specific antigens of Mycobacterium tuberculosis. Vaccine. 2018;36(19):2619–29. https://doi.org/10.1016/j.vaccine.2018.03.066.
128. Da Costa AC, Costa ADO, De Oliveira FM, Nogueira SV, Rosa JD, Resende DP, et al. A new recombinant BCG vaccine induces specific Th17 and Th1 effector cells with higher protective efficacy against tuberculosis. PLoS One. 2014;9(11):e112848. https://doi.org/10.1371/journal.pone.0112848.

129. Roupie V, Romano M, Zhang L, Korf H, Lin MY, Franken KL, et al. Immunogenicity of eight dormancy regulon-encoded proteins of Mycobacterium tuberculosis in DNA-vaccinated and tuberculosis-infected mice. Infect Immun. 2007;75(2):941–9. https://doi.org/10.1128/IAI.01137-06.
130. Tang J, Cai Y, Liang J, Tan Z, Tang X, Zhang C, et al. In vivo electroporation of a codon-optimized BER(opt) DNA vaccine protects mice from pathogenic Mycobacterium tuberculosis aerosol challenge. Tuberculosis (Edinb). 2018;113:65–75. https://doi.org/10.1016/j.tube.2018.07.003.
131. Gengenbacher M, Kaiser P, Schuerer S, Lazar D, Kaufmann SH. Post-exposure vaccination with the vaccine candidate Bacillus Calmette-Guerin DeltaureC::hly induces superior protection in a mouse model of subclinical tuberculosis. Microbes Infect. 2016;18(5):364–8. https://doi.org/10.1016/j.micinf.2016.03.005.
132. Phyu S, Mustafa T, Hofstad T, Nilsen R, Fosse R, Bjune G, et al. A mouse model for latent tuberculosis. Scand J Infect Dis. 1998:59–68.
133. Kupz A, Zedler U, Staber M, Kaufmann SH. A mouse model of latent tuberculosis infection to study intervention strategies to prevent reactivation. PLoS One. 2016;11(7):e0158849. https://doi.org/10.1371/journal.pone.0158849.
134. Sathkumara HD, Pai S, Aceves-Sanchez MJ, Ketheesan N, Flores-Valdez MA, Kupz A. BCG vaccination prevents reactivation of latent lymphatic murine tuberculosis independently of CD4(+) T cells. Front Immunol. 2019;10:532. https://doi.org/10.3389/fimmu.2019.00532.
135. Cooper AM, Dalton DK, Stewart TA, Griffin JP, Russell DG, Orme IM. Disseminated tuberculosis in interferon gamma gene-disrupted mice. J Exp Med. 1993;178(6):2243–7. https://doi.org/10.1084/jem.178.6.2243.
136. Dalton DK, Pitts-Meek S, Keshav S, Figari IS, Bradley A, Stewart TA. Multiple defects of immune cell function in mice with disrupted interferon-gamma genes. Science. 1993;259(5102):1739–42. https://doi.org/10.1126/science.8456300.
137. Kamath AT, Feng CG, Macdonald M, Briscoe H, Britton WJ. Differential protective efficacy of DNA vaccines expressing secreted proteins of Mycobacterium tuberculosis. Infect Immun. 1999;67(4):1702–7. https://doi.org/10.1128/iai.67.4.1702-1707.1999.
138. Bettencourt P, Müller J, Nicastri A, Cantillon D, Madhavan M, Charles PD, et al. Identification of antigens presented by MHC for vaccines against tuberculosis. NPJ Vaccines. 2020;5(1):2. https://doi.org/10.1038/s41541-019-0148-y.
139. Stylianou E, Harrington-Kandt R, Beglov J, Bull N, Pinpathomrat N, Swarbrick GM, et al. Identification and evaluation of novel protective antigens for the development of a candidate tuberculosis subunit vaccine. Infect Immun. 2018;86(7). https://doi.org/10.1128/IAI.00014-18.
140. Aagaard C, Knudsen NPH, Sohn I, Izzo AA, Kim H, Kristiansen EH, et al. Immunization with Mycobacterium tuberculosis-specific antigens bypasses T cell differentiation from prior Bacillus Calmette-Guerin vaccination and improves protection in mice. J Immunol. 2020;205(8):2146–55. https://doi.org/10.4049/jimmunol.2000563.
141. Woodworth JS, Clemmensen HS, Battey H, Dijkman K, Lindenstrom T, Laureano RS, et al. A Mycobacterium tuberculosis-specific subunit vaccine that provides synergistic immunity upon co-administration with Bacillus Calmette-Guerin. Nat Commun. 2021;12(1):6658. https://doi.org/10.1038/s41467-021-26934-0.
142. Zumla A, Raviglione M, Hafner R, von Reyn CF. Tuberculosis. N Engl J Med. 2013;368(8):745–55. https://doi.org/10.1056/NEJMra1200894.
143. Andersen P, Doherty TM. The success and failure of BCG - implications for a novel tuberculosis vaccine. Nat Rev Microbiol. 2005;3(8):656–62. https://doi.org/10.1038/nrmicro1211.
144. Martinez L, Cords O, Liu Q, Acuna-Villaorduna C, Bonnet M, Fox GJ, et al. Infant BCG vaccination and risk of pulmonary and extrapulmonary tuberculosis throughout the life course: a systematic review and individual participant data meta-analysis. Lancet Glob Health. 2022;10(9):e1307–e16. https://doi.org/10.1016/S2214-109X(22)00283-2.

145. Mangtani P, Abubakar I, Ariti C, Beynon R, Pimpin L, Fine PE, et al. Protection by BCG vaccine against tuberculosis: a systematic review of randomized controlled trials. Clin Infect Dis. 2014;58(4):470–80. https://doi.org/10.1093/cid/cit790.
146. Churchill GA, Airey DC, Allayee H, Angel JM, Attie AD, Beatty J, et al. The collaborative cross, a community resource for the genetic analysis of complex traits. Nat Genet. 2004;36(11):1133–7. https://doi.org/10.1038/ng1104-1133.
147. Noll KE, Ferris MT, Heise MT. The collaborative cross: a systems genetics resource for studying host-pathogen interactions. Cell Host Microbe. 2019;25(4):484–98. https://doi.org/10.1016/j.chom.2019.03.009.
148. Churchill GA, Gatti DM, Munger SC, Svenson KL. The diversity outbred mouse population. Mammalian Genome. 2012;23(9–10):713–8. https://doi.org/10.1007/s00335-012-9414-2.
149. Smith CM, Proulx MK, Olive AJ, Laddy D, Mishra BB, Moss C, et al. Tuberculosis susceptibility and vaccine protection are independently controlled by host genotype. MBio. 2016;7(5). https://doi.org/10.1128/mBio.01516-16.
150. Smith CM, Baker RE, Proulx MK, Mishra BB, Long JE, Park SW, et al. Host-pathogen genetic interactions underlie tuberculosis susceptibility in genetically diverse mice. elife. 2022;11:11. https://doi.org/10.7554/eLife.74419.
151. Lai R, Gong DN, Williams T, Ogunsola AF, Cavallo K, Lindestam Arlehamn CS, et al. Host genetic background is a barrier to broadly effective vaccine-mediated protection against tuberculosis. J Clin Invest. 2023;133(13). https://doi.org/10.1172/JCI167762.
152. Kurtz SL, Rossi AP, Beamer GL, Gatti DM, Kramnik I, Elkins KL. The diversity outbred mouse population is an improved animal model of vaccination against tuberculosis that reflects heterogeneity of protection. mSphere. 2020;5(2). https://doi.org/10.1128/mSphere.00097-20.
153. Kurtz SL, Mittereder LR, Lehman CC, Khan H, Gould VA, Elkins KL. Intravenous BCG vaccination of diversity outbred mice results in moderately enhanced protection against challenge with Mycobacterium tuberculosis compared to intradermal vaccination. Infect Immun. 2023;91(7):e0016823. https://doi.org/10.1128/iai.00168-23.
154. Niazi MK, Dhulekar N, Schmidt D, Major S, Cooper R, Abeijon C, et al. Lung necrosis and neutrophils reflect common pathways of susceptibility to Mycobacterium tuberculosis in genetically diverse, immune-competent mice. Dis Model Mech. 2015;8(9):1141–53. https://doi.org/10.1242/dmm.020867.
155. Koyuncu D, Niazi MKK, Tavolara T, Abeijon C, Ginese ML, Liao Y, et al. CXCL1: a new diagnostic biomarker for human tuberculosis discovered using diversity outbred mice. PLoS Pathog. 2021;17(8):e1009773. https://doi.org/10.1371/journal.ppat.1009773.
156. Mariëtta MR-C, Erik Van D, Douglas F, Xammy HN, Sagar LR, Mallory AB, et al. Tuberculosis susceptibility in genetically diverse mice reveals functional diversity of neutrophils. bioRxiv. 2023:2023.06.29.547125. https://doi.org/10.1101/2023.06.29.547125.
157. Kurtz SL, Ryden P, Elkins KL. Transcriptional signatures measured in whole blood correlate with protection against tuberculosis in inbred and outbred mice. PLoS One. 2023;18(8):e0289358. https://doi.org/10.1371/journal.pone.0289358.
158. Beura LK, Hamilton SE, Bi K, Schenkel JM, Odumade OA, Casey KA, et al. Normalizing the environment recapitulates adult human immune traits in laboratory mice. Nature. 2016;532(7600):512–6. https://doi.org/10.1038/nature17655.
159. Rosshart SP, Vassallo BG, Angeletti D, Hutchinson DS, Morgan AP, Takeda K, et al. Wild mouse gut microbiota promotes host fitness and improves disease resistance. Cell. 2017;171(5):1015–28 e13. https://doi.org/10.1016/j.cell.2017.09.016.
160. Beura LK, Wijeyesinghe S, Thompson EA, Macchietto MG, Rosato PC, Pierson MJ, et al. T cells in nonlymphoid tissues give rise to lymph-node-resident memory T cells. Immunity. 2018;48(2):327–38.e5. https://doi.org/10.1016/j.immuni.2018.01.015.
161. Fiege JK, Block KE, Pierson MJ, Nanda H, Shepherd FK, Mickelson CK, et al. Mice with diverse microbial exposure histories as a model for preclinical vaccine testing. Cell Host Microbe. 2021;29(12):1815–27 e6. https://doi.org/10.1016/j.chom.2021.10.001.

162. Reese TA, Bi K, Kambal A, Filali-Mouhim A, Beura LK, Burger MC, et al. Sequential infection with common pathogens promotes human-like immune gene expression and altered vaccine response. Cell Host Microbe. 2016;19(5):713–9. https://doi.org/10.1016/j.chom.2016.04.003.
163. Chu T, Tyznik AJ, Roepke S, Berkley AM, Woodward-Davis A, Pattacini L, et al. Bystander-activated memory CD8 T cells control early pathogen load in an innate-like, NKG2D-dependent manner. Cell Rep. 2013;3(3):701–8. https://doi.org/10.1016/j.celrep.2013.02.020.
164. Schenkel JM, Fraser KA, Vezys V, Masopust D. Sensing and alarm function of resident memory CD8 + T cells. Nat Immunol. 2013;14(5):509–13. https://doi.org/10.1038/ni.2568.
165. Kastenmuller W, Torabi-Parizi P, Subramanian N, Lammermann T, Germain RN. A spatially-organized multicellular innate immune response in lymph nodes limits systemic pathogen spread. Cell. 2012;150(6):1235–48. https://doi.org/10.1016/j.cell.2012.07.021.
166. Kramnik I, Dietrich WF, Demant P, Bloom BR. Genetic control of resistance to experimental infection with virulent Mycobacterium tuberculosis. 2000;97:8560.
167. Driver ER, Ryan GJ, Hoff DR, Irwin SM, Basaraba RJ, Kramnik I, et al. Evaluation of a mouse model of necrotic granuloma formation using C3HeB/FeJ mice for testing of drugs against Mycobacterium tuberculosis. Antimicrob Agents Chemother. 2012;56(6):3181–95. https://doi.org/10.1128/AAC.00217-12.
168. Harper J, Skerry C, Davis SL, Tasneen R, Weir M, Kramnik I, et al. Mouse model of necrotic tuberculosis granulomas develops hypoxic lesions. J Infect Dis. 2012;205(4):595–602. https://doi.org/10.1093/infdis/jir786.
169. Henao-Tamayo M, Obregon-Henao A, Creissen E, Shanley C, Orme I, Ordway DJ. Differential Mycobacterium bovis BCG vaccine-derived efficacy in C3Heb/FeJ and C3H/HeOuJ mice exposed to a clinical strain of Mycobacterium tuberculosis. Clin Vaccine Immunol. 2015;22(1):91–8. https://doi.org/10.1128/CVI.00466-14.
170. Yan B-S, Pichugin AV, Jobe O, Helming L, Eruslanov EB, Gutiérrez-Pabello JA, et al. Progression of pulmonary tuberculosis and efficiency of Bacillus Calmette-Guérin vaccination are genetically controlled via a common sst1-mediated mechanism of innate immunity 1. J Immunol. 2007:6919–32.
171. Cardona PJ, Gordillo S, Diaz J, Tapia G, Amat I, Pallares A, et al. Widespread bronchogenic dissemination makes DBA/2 mice more susceptible than C57BL/6 mice to experimental aerosol infection with Mycobacterium tuberculosis. Infect Immun. 2003;71(10):5845–54. https://doi.org/10.1128/IAI.71.10.5845-5854.2003.
172. Brandenburg J, Marwitz S, Tazoll SC, Waldow F, Kalsdorf B, Vierbuchen T, et al. WNT6/ACC2-induced storage of triacylglycerols in macrophages is exploited by Mycobacterium tuberculosis. J Clin Invest. 2021;131(16). https://doi.org/10.1172/JCI141833.
173. Zelmer A, Stockdale L, Prabowo SA, Cia F, Spink N, Gibb M, et al. High monocyte to lymphocyte ratio is associated with impaired protection after subcutaneous administration of BCG in a mouse model of tuberculosis. F1000Res. 2018;7:296. https://doi.org/10.12688/f1000research.14239.2.
174. Nieuwenhuizen NE, Zyla J, Zedler U, Bandermann S, Abu Abed U, Brinkmann V, et al. Weaker protection against tuberculosis in BCG-vaccinated male 129 S2 mice compared to females. Vaccine. 2021;39(50):7253–64. https://doi.org/10.1016/j.vaccine.2021.09.039.
175. Beamer GL, Cyktor J, Flaherty DK, Stromberg PC, Carruthers B, Turner J. CBA/J mice generate protective immunity to soluble Ag85 but fail to respond efficiently to Ag85 during natural Mycobacterium tuberculosis infection. Eur J Immunol. 2012;42(4):870–9. https://doi.org/10.1002/eji.201142054.
176. Aguilo N, Alvarez-Arguedas S, Uranga S, Marinova D, Monzón M, Badiola J, et al. Pulmonary but not subcutaneous delivery of BCG vaccine confers protection to tuberculosis-susceptible mice by an interleukin 17-dependent mechanism. J Infect Dis. 2015;212(11):831–9. https://doi.org/10.1093/infdis/jiv503.
177. Beamer GL, Flaherty DK, Assogba BD, Stromberg P, Gonzalez-Juarrero M, De R, et al. Interleukin-10 promotes Mycobacterium tuberculosis disease progression in CBA/J mice 1. J Immunol. 2008:5545–50.

178. Cyktor JC, Carruthers B, Kominsky RA, Beamer GL, Stromberg P, Turner J. IL-10 inhibits mature fibrotic granuloma formation during mycobacterium tuberculosis infection. J Immunol. 2013;190(6):2778–90. https://doi.org/10.4049/jimmunol.1202722.
179. Pitt JM, Stavropoulos E, Redford PS, Beebe AM, Bancroft GJ, Young DB, et al. Blockade of IL-10 signaling during bacillus Calmette-Guerin vaccination enhances and sustains Th1, Th17, and innate lymphoid IFN-gamma and IL-17 responses and increases protection to Mycobacterium tuberculosis infection. J Immunol. 2012;189(8):4079–87. https://doi.org/10.4049/jimmunol.1201061.
180. Zhang L, Ru HW, Chen FZ, Jin CY, Sun RF, Fan XY, et al. Variable virulence and efficacy of BCG vaccine strains in mice and correlation with genome polymorphisms. Mol Ther. 2016;24(2):398–405. https://doi.org/10.1038/mt.2015.216.
181. Walker KB, Brennan MJ, Ho MM, Eskola J, Thiry G, Sadoff J, et al. The second Geneva consensus: recommendations for novel live TB vaccines. Vaccine. 2010;28(11):2259–70. https://doi.org/10.1016/j.vaccine.2009.12.083.
182. Guleria I, Teitelbaum R, McAdam RA, Kalpana G, Jacobs WR Jr, Bloom BR. Auxotrophic vaccines for tuberculosis. Nat Med. 1996;2(3):334–7.
183. Gengenbacher M, Nieuwenhuizen N, Vogelzang A, Liu H, Kaiser P, Schuerer S, et al. Deletion of nuoG from the vaccine candidate Mycobacterium bovis BCG DeltaureC::hly improves protection against tuberculosis. MBio. 2016;7(3). https://doi.org/10.1128/mBio.00679-16.
184. Aceves-Sanchez MJ, Flores-Valdez MA, Pedroza-Roldan C, Creissen E, Izzo L, Silva-Angulo F, et al. Vaccination with BCGDeltaBCG1419c protects against pulmonary and extrapulmonary TB and is safer than BCG. Sci Rep. 2021;11(1):12417. https://doi.org/10.1038/s41598-021-91993-8.
185. Shinkai Y, Rathbun G, Lam K-P, Oltz EM, Stewart V, Mendelsohn M, et al. RAG-2-deficient mice lack mature lymphocytes owing to inability to initiate V(D)J rearrangement. Cell. 1992:855–67.
186. Bosma GC, Fried M, Custer RP, Carroll A, Gibson DM, Bosma MJ. Evidence of functional lymphocytes in some (leaky) SCID mice. J Exp Med. 1988;167:1016.
187. Triccas JA, Shklovskaya E, Spratt J, Ryan AA, Palendira U, Barbara BF, et al. Effects of DNA- and Mycobacterium bovis BCG-based delivery of the Flt3 ligand on protective immunity to Mycobacterium tuberculosis. Infect Immun. 2007;75(11):5368–75. https://doi.org/10.1128/IAI.00322-07.
188. Spratt JM, Britton WJ, Triccas JA. In vivo persistence and protective efficacy of the bacille Calmette Guerin vaccine overexpressing the Hspx latency antigen. Bioengineered Bugs. 2010;1(1):61–5.
189. Heuts F, Gavier-Widen D, Carow B, Juarez J, Wigzell H, Rottenberg ME. CD4+ cell-dependent granuloma formation in humanized mice infected with mycobacteria. Proc Natl Acad Sci USA. 2013;110(16):6482–7. https://doi.org/10.1073/pnas.1219985110.
190. Calderon VE, Valbuena G, Goez Y, Judy BM, Huante MB, Sutjita P, et al. A humanized mouse model of tuberculosis. PLoS One. 2013;8(5):e63331. https://doi.org/10.1371/journal.pone.0063331.
191. Arrey F, Lowe D, Kuhlmann S, Kaiser P, Moura-Alves P, Krishnamoorthy G, et al. Humanized mouse model mimicking pathology of human tuberculosis for in vivo evaluation of drug regimens. Front Immunol. 2019;10:89. https://doi.org/10.3389/fimmu.2019.00089.
192. Yao Y, Lai R, Afkhami S, Haddadi S, Zganiacz A, Vahedi F, et al. Enhancement of antituberculosis immunity in a humanized model system by a novel virus-vectored respiratory mucosal vaccine. J Infect Dis. 2017;216(1):135–45. https://doi.org/10.1093/infdis/jix252.
193. Grover A, Troy A, Rowe J, Troudt JLM, Creissen E, McLean J, et al. Humanized NOG mice as a model for tuberculosis vaccine-induced immunity: a comparative analysis with the mouse and Guinea pig models of tuberculosis. Immunology. 2017;152(1):150–62. https://doi.org/10.1111/imm.12756.
194. Counoupas C, Triccas JA, Britton WJ. Deciphering protective immunity against tuberculosis: implications for vaccine development. Expert Rev Vaccines. 2019;18(4):353–64. https://doi.org/10.1080/14760584.2019.1585246.

195. Satti I, McShane H. Current approaches toward identifying a correlate of immune protection from tuberculosis. Expert Rev Vaccines. 2019;18(1):43–59. https://doi.org/10.1080/14760584.2019.1552140.
196. Gong W, Liang Y, Wu X. Animal models of tuberculosis vaccine research: an important component in the fight against tuberculosis. Biomed Res Int. 2020;2020:4263079. https://doi.org/10.1155/2020/4263079.
197. Bodkin GE. A case of tuberculosis in a rat. J Hyg (Lond). 1918;17(1):10–2. https://doi.org/10.1017/s0022172400007038.
198. Gabler E, Pendl O. Inborn resistance to tubercle bacilli (H 37 Rv) in albino rats. Med Thorac. 1966;23(1):36–51.
199. Gray DF. The relative natural resistance of rats and mice to experimental pulmonary tuberculosis. J Hyg (Lond). 1961;59(4):471–7. https://doi.org/10.1017/s0022172400039164.
200. Singhal A, Aliouat el M, Hervé M, Mathys V, Kiass M, Creusy C, et al. Experimental tuberculosis in the Wistar rat: a model for protective immunity and control of infection. PLoS One. 2011;6(4):e18632. https://doi.org/10.1371/journal.pone.0018632.
201. McFarland CT, Ly L, Jeevan A, Yamamoto T, Weeks B, Izzo A, et al. BCG vaccination in the cotton rat (Sigmodon hispidus) infected by the pulmonary route with virulent Mycobacterium tuberculosis. Tuberculosis (Edinb). 2010;90(4):262–7. https://doi.org/10.1016/j.tube.2010.03.014.
202. Singhal A, Mathys V, Kiass M, Creusy C, Delaire B, Aliouat el M, et al. BCG induces protection against Mycobacterium tuberculosis infection in the Wistar rat model. PLoS One. 2011;6(12):e28082. https://doi.org/10.1371/journal.pone.0028082.
203. Elwood RL, Wilson S, Blanco JC, Yim K, Pletneva L, Nikonenko B, et al. The American cotton rat: a novel model for pulmonary tuberculosis. Tuberculosis (Edinb). 2007;87(2):145–54. https://doi.org/10.1016/j.tube.2006.07.001.
204. Sugawara I, Yamada H, Mizuno S. Pathological and immunological profiles of rat tuberculosis. Int J Exp Pathol. 2004;85(3):125–34. https://doi.org/10.1111/j.0959-9673.2004.00379.x.
205. Corleis B, Bastian M, Hoffmann D, Beer M, Dorhoi A. Animal models for COVID-19 and tuberculosis. Front Immunol. 2023;14:1223260. https://doi.org/10.3389/fimmu.2023.1223260.
206. Shi L, Zhang L, Li C, Hu X, Wang X, Huang Q, et al. Dietary zinc deficiency impairs humoral and cellular immune responses to BCG and ESAT-6/CFP-10 vaccination in offspring and adult rats. Tuberculosis (Edinb). 2016;97:86–96. https://doi.org/10.1016/j.tube.2016.01.002.
207. Sugawara I, Mizuno S. Higher susceptibility of type 1 diabetic rats to Mycobacterium tuberculosis infection. Tohoku J Exp Med. 2008;216(4):363–70. https://doi.org/10.1620/tjem.216.363.
208. Williams A, Orme IM. Animal models of tuberculosis: an overview. Microbiol Spectr. 2016;4(4). https://doi.org/10.1128/microbiolspec.TBTB2-0004-2015.
209. Hasløv K, Closs O, Møller S, Bentzon MW. Studies on the development of tuberculin sensitivity in immunized Guinea pigs with demonstration of a close relationship between results of skin tests and the lymphocyte transformation technique. Int Arch Allergy Appl Immunol. 1984;73(2):114–22. https://doi.org/10.1159/000233450.
210. Dharmadhikari AS, Basaraba RJ, Van Der Walt ML, Weyer K, Mphahlele M, Venter K, et al. Natural infection of Guinea pigs exposed to patients with highly drug-resistant tuberculosis. Tuberculosis (Edinb). 2011;91(4):329–38. https://doi.org/10.1016/j.tube.2011.03.002.
211. Clark S, Hall Y, Williams A. Animal models of tuberculosis: Guinea pigs. Cold Spring Harb Perspect Med. 2014;5(5):a018572. https://doi.org/10.1101/cshperspect.a018572.
212. Hasløv K, Andersen A, Nagai S, Gottschau A, Sørensen T, Andersen P. Guinea pig cellular immune responses to proteins secreted by Mycobacterium tuberculosis. Infect Immun. 1995;63(3):804–10. https://doi.org/10.1128/iai.63.3.804-810.1995.
213. Palanisamy GS, Smith EE, Shanley CA, Ordway DJ, Orme IM, Basaraba RJ. Disseminated disease severity as a measure of virulence of Mycobacterium tuberculosis in the Guinea pig model. Tuberculosis (Edinb). 2008;88(4):295–306. https://doi.org/10.1016/j.tube.2007.12.003.

214. Basaraba RJ. Experimental tuberculosis: the role of comparative pathology in the discovery of improved tuberculosis treatment strategies. Tuberculosis (Edinb). 2008;88(Suppl 1):S35–47. https://doi.org/10.1016/s1472-9792(08)70035-0.
215. Basaraba RJ, Dailey DD, McFarland CT, Shanley CA, Smith EE, McMurray DN, et al. Lymphadenitis as a major element of disease in the Guinea pig model of tuberculosis. Tuberculosis (Edinb). 2006;86(5):386–94. https://doi.org/10.1016/j.tube.2005.11.003.
216. Cardona PJ, Williams A. Experimental animal modelling for TB vaccine development. Int J Infect Dis. 2017;56:268–73. https://doi.org/10.1016/j.ijid.2017.01.030.
217. Commandeur S, van den Eeden SJ, Dijkman K, Clark SO, van Meijgaarden KE, Wilson L, et al. The in vivo expressed Mycobacterium tuberculosis (IVE-TB) antigen Rv2034 induces $CD4^+$ T-cells that protect against pulmonary infection in HLA-DR transgenic mice and Guinea pigs. Vaccine. 2014;32(29):3580–8. https://doi.org/10.1016/j.vaccine.2014.05.005.
218. Skeiky YA, Dietrich J, Lasco TM, Stagliano K, Dheenadhayalan V, Goetz MA, et al. Non-clinical efficacy and safety of HyVac4:IC31 vaccine administered in a BCG prime-boost regimen. Vaccine. 2010;28(4):1084–93. https://doi.org/10.1016/j.vaccine.2009.10.114.
219. Aagaard C, Hoang TT, Izzo A, Billeskov R, Troudt J, Arnett K, et al. Protection and polyfunctional T cells induced by Ag85B-TB10.4/IC31 against Mycobacterium tuberculosis is highly dependent on the antigen dose. PLoS One. 2009;4(6):e5930. https://doi.org/10.1371/journal.pone.0005930.
220. Clark S, Cross ML, Nadian A, Vipond J, Court P, Williams A, et al. Oral vaccination of Guinea pigs with a Mycobacterium bovis bacillus Calmette-Guerin vaccine in a lipid matrix protects against aerosol infection with virulent M. bovis. Infect Immun. 2008;76(8):3771–6. https://doi.org/10.1128/iai.00052-08.
221. Watanabe Y, Watari E, Matsunaga I, Hiromatsu K, Dascher CC, Kawashima T, et al. BCG vaccine elicits both T-cell mediated and humoral immune responses directed against mycobacterial lipid components. Vaccine. 2006;24(29–30):5700–7. https://doi.org/10.1016/j.vaccine.2006.04.049.
222. Grover A, Troudt J, Arnett K, Izzo L, Lucas M, Strain K, et al. Assessment of vaccine testing at three laboratories using the Guinea pig model of tuberculosis. Tuberculosis (Edinb). 2012;92(1):105–11. https://doi.org/10.1016/j.tube.2011.09.003.
223. Williams A, Hall Y, Orme IM. Evaluation of new vaccines for tuberculosis in the Guinea pig model. Tuberculosis (Edinb). 2009;89(6):389–97. https://doi.org/10.1016/j.tube.2009.08.004.
224. Ordway DJ, Shanley CA, Caraway ML, Orme EA, Bucy DS, Hascall-Dove L, et al. Evaluation of standard chemotherapy in the Guinea pig model of tuberculosis. Antimicrob Agents Chemother. 2010;54(5):1820–33. https://doi.org/10.1128/aac.01521-09.
225. Turner OC, Basaraba RJ, Orme IM. Immunopathogenesis of pulmonary granulomas in the Guinea pig after infection with Mycobacterium tuberculosis. Infect Immun. 2003;71(2):864–71. https://doi.org/10.1128/IAI.71.2.864-871.2003.
226. Larrouy-Maumus G, Layre E, Clark S, Prandi J, Rayner E, Lepore M, et al. Protective efficacy of a lipid antigen vaccine in a Guinea pig model of tuberculosis. Vaccine. 2017;35(10):1395–402. https://doi.org/10.1016/j.vaccine.2017.01.079.
227. Dascher CC, Hiromatsu K, Naylor JW, Brauer PP, Brown KA, Storey JR, et al. Conservation of a CD1 multigene family in the Guinea pig. J Immunol. 1999;163(10):5478–88.
228. Dascher CC, Hiromatsu K, Xiong X, Sugita M, Buhlmann JE, Dodge IL, et al. Conservation of CD1 intracellular trafficking patterns between mammalian species. J Immunol. 2002;169(12):6951–8. https://doi.org/10.4049/jimmunol.169.12.6951.
229. Hiromatsu K, Dascher CC, Sugita M, Gingrich-Baker C, Behar SM, LeClair KP, et al. Characterization of Guinea-pig group 1 CD1 proteins. Immunology. 2002;106(2):159–72. https://doi.org/10.1046/j.1365-2567.2002.01422.x.
230. Van Rhijn I, Godfrey DI, Rossjohn J, Moody DB. Lipid and small-molecule display by CD1 and MR1. Nat Rev Immunol. 2015;15(10):643–54. https://doi.org/10.1038/nri3889.
231. Minnikin DE, Kremer L, Dover LG, Besra GS. The methyl-branched fortifications of Mycobacterium tuberculosis. Chem Biol. 2002;9(5):545–53. https://doi.org/10.1016/s1074-5521(02)00142-4.

232. Hiromatsu K, Dascher CC, LeClair KP, Sugita M, Furlong ST, Brenner MB, et al. Induction of CD1-restricted immune responses in Guinea pigs by immunization with mycobacterial lipid antigens. J Immunol. 2002;169(1):330–9. https://doi.org/10.4049/jimmunol.169.1.330.
233. Schäfer H, Burger R. Tools for cellular immunology and vaccine research the in the Guinea pig: monoclonal antibodies to cell surface antigens and cell lines. Vaccine. 2012;30(40):5804–11. https://doi.org/10.1016/j.vaccine.2012.07.012.
234. Schäfer H, Kliem G, Kropp B, Burger R. Monoclonal antibodies to Guinea pig interferon-gamma: tools for cytokine detection and neutralization. J Immunol Methods. 2007;328(1–2):106–17. https://doi.org/10.1016/j.jim.2007.08.012.
235. McMurray DN, Allen SS, Jeevan A, Lasco T, Cho H, Skwor T, et al. Vaccine-induced cytokine responses in a Guinea pig model of pulmonary tuberculosis. Tuberculosis (Edinb). 2005;85(5–6):295–301. https://doi.org/10.1016/j.tube.2005.08.012.
236. Allen SS, McMurray DN. Coordinate cytokine gene expression in vivo following induction of tuberculous pleurisy in Guinea pigs. Infect Immun. 2003;71(8):4271–7. https://doi.org/10.1128/iai.71.8.4271-4277.2003.
237. Spohr C, Kaufmann E, Battenfeld S, Duchow K, Cussler K, Balks E, et al. A new lymphocyte proliferation assay for potency determination of bovine tuberculin PPDs. ALTEX. 2015;32(3):201–10. https://doi.org/10.14573/altex.1502101.
238. Ordway D, Palanisamy G, Henao-Tamayo M, Smith EE, Shanley C, Orme IM, et al. The cellular immune response to Mycobacterium tuberculosis infection in the Guinea pig. J Immunol. 2007;179(4):2532–41. https://doi.org/10.4049/jimmunol.179.4.2532.
239. Lurie MB. Studies on the mechanism of immunity in tuberculosis : the mobilization of mononuclear phagocytes in normal and immunized animals and their relative capacities for division and phagocytosis. J Exp Med. 1939;69(4):579–99. https://doi.org/10.1084/jem.69.4.579.
240. Lurie MB. Studies on the mechanism of immunity in tuberculosis : the RÔLE of extracellular factors and local immunity in the fixation and inhibition of growth of tubercle bacilli. J Exp Med. 1939;69(4):555–78. https://doi.org/10.1084/jem.69.4.555.
241. Lurie MB, Zappasodi P, Cardona-Lynch E, Dannenberg AM Jr. The response to the intracutaneous inoculation of BCG as an index of native resistance to tuberculosis. J Immunol. 1952;68(4):369–87.
242. Dannenberg AM Jr. Cellular hypersensitivity and cellular immunity in the pathogensis of tuberculosis: specificity, systemic and local nature, and associated macrophage enzymes. Bacteriol Rev. 1968;32(2):85–102. https://doi.org/10.1128/br.32.2.85-102.1968.
243. Dannenberg AM Jr. Pathogenesis of tuberculosis: local and systemic immunity and cellular hypersensitivity. Bull Int Union Tuberc. 1970;43:177–8.
244. Dannenberg AM. Delayed-type hypersensitivity and cell-mediated immunity in the pathogenesis of tuberculosis. Immunol Today. 1991;12(7):228–33. https://doi.org/10.1016/0167-5699(91)90035-R.
245. O'Brien P, Vinnard C, Subbian S. An improved protocol to establish experimental tuberculous meningitis in the rabbit. MethodsX. 2020;7:100832. https://doi.org/10.1016/j.mex.2020.100832.
246. Tsenova L, Fallows D, Kolloli A, Singh P, O'Brien P, Kushner N, et al. Inoculum size and traits of the infecting clinical strain define the protection level against Mycobacterium tuberculosis infection in a rabbit model. Eur J Immunol. 2020;50(6):858–72. https://doi.org/10.1002/eji.201948448.
247. Dehnad A, Ravindran R, Subbian S, Khan IH. Development of immune-biomarkers of pulmonary tuberculosis in a rabbit model. Tuberculosis (Edinb). 2016;101:1–7. https://doi.org/10.1016/j.tube.2016.07.008.
248. Nedeltchev GG, Raghunand TR, Jassal MS, Lun S, Cheng Q-J, Bishai WR. Extrapulmonary dissemination of <i>Mycobacterium bovis</i> but not <i>Mycobacterium tuberculosis</i> in a Bronchoscopic rabbit model of cavitary tuberculosis. Infect Immun. 2009;77(2):598–603. https://doi.org/10.1128/iai.01132-08.

249. Dannenberg AM Jr. Liquefaction and cavity formation in pulmonary TB: a simple method in rabbit skin to test inhibitors. Tuberculosis (Edinb). 2009;89(4):243–7. https://doi.org/10.1016/j.tube.2009.05.006.
250. Bishai WR, Dannenberg AM Jr, Parrish N, Ruiz R, Chen P, Zook BC, et al. Virulence of Mycobacterium tuberculosis CDC1551 and H37Rv in rabbits evaluated by Lurie's pulmonary tubercle count method. Infect Immun. 1999;67(9):4931–4. https://doi.org/10.1128/iai.67.9.4931-4934.1999.
251. Tsenova L, Sokol K, Freedman VH, Kaplan G. A combination of thalidomide plus antibiotics protects rabbits from mycobacterial meningitis-associated death. J Infect Dis. 1998;177(6):1563–72. https://doi.org/10.1086/515327.
252. Dorman SE, Hatem CL, Tyagi S, Aird K, Lopez-Molina J, Pitt ML, et al. Susceptibility to tuberculosis: clues from studies with inbred and outbred New Zealand White rabbits. Infect Immun. 2004;72(3):1700–5. https://doi.org/10.1128/iai.72.3.1700-1705.2004.
253. Sun H, Ma X, Zhang G, Luo Y, Tang K, Lin X, et al. Effects of immunomodulators on liquefaction and ulceration in the rabbit skin model of tuberculosis. Tuberculosis (Edinb). 2012;92(4):345–50. https://doi.org/10.1016/j.tube.2012.03.005.
254. Dannenberg AM Jr, Collins FM. Progressive pulmonary tuberculosis is not due to increasing numbers of viable bacilli in rabbits, mice and Guinea pigs, but is due to a continuous host response to mycobacterial products. Tuberculosis (Edinb). 2001;81(3):229–42. https://doi.org/10.1054/tube.2001.0287.
255. Mantilla Galindo A, Ocampo M, Patarroyo MA. Experimental models used in evaluating anti-tuberculosis vaccines: the latest advances in the field. Expert Rev Vaccines. 2019;18(4):365–77. https://doi.org/10.1080/14760584.2019.1583558.
256. Tsenova L, Harbacheuski R, Sung N, Ellison E, Fallows D, Kaplan G. BCG vaccination confers poor protection against M. Tuberculosis HN878-induced central nervous system disease. Vaccine. 2007;25(28):5126–32. https://doi.org/10.1016/j.vaccine.2006.11.024.
257. Kesavan AK, Brooks M, Tufariello J, Chan J, Manabe YC. Tuberculosis genes expressed during persistence and reactivation in the resistant rabbit model. Tuberculosis (Edinb). 2009;89(1):17–21. https://doi.org/10.1016/j.tube.2008.08.004.
258. Manabe YC, Dannenberg AM Jr, Tyagi SK, Hatem CL, Yoder M, Woolwine SC, et al. Different strains of Mycobacterium tuberculosis cause various spectrums of disease in the rabbit model of tuberculosis. Infect Immun. 2003;71(10):6004–11. https://doi.org/10.1128/iai.71.10.6004-6011.2003.
259. Manabe YC, Kesavan AK, Lopez-Molina J, Hatem CL, Brooks M, Fujiwara R, et al. The aerosol rabbit model of TB latency, reactivation and immune reconstitution inflammatory syndrome. Tuberculosis (Edinb). 2008;88(3):187–96. https://doi.org/10.1016/j.tube.2007.10.006.
260. Subbian S, Tsenova L, O'Brien P, Yang G, Kushner NL, Parsons S, et al. Spontaneous latency in a rabbit model of pulmonary tuberculosis. Am J Pathol. 2012;181(5):1711–24. https://doi.org/10.1016/j.ajpath.2012.07.019.
261. Chen H, Liu X, Ma X, Wang Q, Yang G, Niu H, et al. A new rabbit-skin model to evaluate protective efficacy of tuberculosis vaccines. Front Microbiol. 2017;8:842. https://doi.org/10.3389/fmicb.2017.00842.
262. Peng X, Knouse JA, Hernon KM. Rabbit models for studying human infectious diseases. Comp Med. 2015;65(6):499–507.
263. Subbian S, Bandyopadhyay N, Tsenova L, O'Brien P, Khetani V, Kushner NL, et al. Early innate immunity determines outcome of Mycobacterium tuberculosis pulmonary infection in rabbits. Cell Commun Signal. 2013;11:60. https://doi.org/10.1186/1478-811X-11-60.
264. Flynn JL, Capuano SV, Croix D, Pawar S, Myers A, Zinovik A, et al. Non-human primates: a model for tuberculosis research. Tuberculosis (Edinb). 2003;83(1–3):116–8. https://doi.org/10.1016/s1472-9792(02)00059-8.
265. Dijkman K, Sombroek CC, Vervenne RAW, Hofman SO, Boot C, Remarque EJ, et al. Prevention of tuberculosis infection and disease by local BCG in repeatedly exposed rhesus macaques. Nat Med. 2019;25(2):255–62. https://doi.org/10.1038/s41591-018-0319-9.

266. Aguilo N, Uranga S, Mata E, Tarancon R, Gómez AB, Marinova D, et al. Respiratory immunization with a whole cell inactivated vaccine induces functional mucosal immunoglobulins against tuberculosis in mice and non-human primates. Front Microbiol. 2020;11:1339. https://doi.org/10.3389/fmicb.2020.01339.
267. Darrah PA, Zeppa JJ, Wang C, Irvine EB, Bucsan AN, Rodgers MA, et al. Airway T cells are a correlate of i.v. Bacille Calmette-Guerin-mediated protection against tuberculosis in rhesus macaques. Cell Host Microbe. 2023;31(6):962–77.e8. https://doi.org/10.1016/j.chom.2023.05.006.
268. Vierboom MPM, Dijkman K, Sombroek CC, Hofman SO, Boot C, Vervenne RAW, et al. Stronger induction of trained immunity by mucosal BCG or MTBVAC vaccination compared to standard intradermal vaccination. Cell Rep Med. 2021;2(1):100185. https://doi.org/10.1016/j.xcrm.2020.100185.
269. Irvine EB, Darrah PA, Wang S, Wang C, McNamara RP, Roederer M, et al. Humoral correlates of protection against Mycobacterium tuberculosis following intravenous Bacille Calmette-Guérin vaccination in rhesus macaques. bioRxiv 2023. https://doi.org/10.1101/2023.07.31.551245.
270. Lin PL, Rodgers M, Smith L, Bigbee M, Myers A, Bigbee C, et al. Quantitative comparison of active and latent tuberculosis in the cynomolgus macaque model. Infect Immun. 2009;77(10):4631–42. https://doi.org/10.1128/iai.00592-09.
271. Maiello P, DiFazio RM, Cadena AM, Rodgers MA, Lin PL, Scanga CA, et al. Rhesus macaques are more susceptible to progressive tuberculosis than Cynomolgus macaques: a quantitative comparison. Infect Immun. 2018;86(2). https://doi.org/10.1128/iai.00505-17.
272. Gideon HP, Hughes TK, Tzouanas CN, Wadsworth MH 2nd, Tu AA, Gierahn TM, et al. Multimodal profiling of lung granulomas in macaques reveals cellular correlates of tuberculosis control. Immunity. 2022;55(5):827–46.e10. https://doi.org/10.1016/j.immuni.2022.04.004.
273. Lin PL, Rutledge T, Green AM, Bigbee M, Fuhrman C, Klein E, et al. CD4 T cell depletion exacerbates acute Mycobacterium tuberculosis while reactivation of latent infection is dependent on severity of tissue depletion in cynomolgus macaques. AIDS Res Hum Retrovir. 2012;28(12):1693–702. https://doi.org/10.1089/aid.2012.0028.
274. Yao S, Huang D, Chen CY, Halliday L, Wang RC, Chen ZW. CD4+ T cells contain early extrapulmonary tuberculosis (TB) dissemination and rapid TB progression and sustain multieffector functions of CD8+ T and CD3- lymphocytes: mechanisms of CD4+ T cell immunity. J Immunol. 2014;192(5):2120–32. https://doi.org/10.4049/jimmunol.1301373.
275. Verreck FAW, Tchilian EZ, Vervenne RAW, Sombroek CC, Kondova I, Eissen OA, et al. Variable BCG efficacy in rhesus populations: pulmonary BCG provides protection where standard intra-dermal vaccination fails. Tuberculosis (Edinb). 2017;104:46–57. https://doi.org/10.1016/j.tube.2017.02.003.
276. Langermans JA, Andersen P, van Soolingen D, Vervenne RA, Frost PA, van der Laan T, et al. Divergent effect of bacillus Calmette-Guérin (BCG) vaccination on Mycobacterium tuberculosis infection in highly related macaque species: implications for primate models in tuberculosis vaccine research. Proc Natl Acad Sci USA. 2001;98(20):11497–502. https://doi.org/10.1073/pnas.201404898.
277. Scanga CA, Flynn JL. Modeling tuberculosis in nonhuman primates. Cold Spring Harb Perspect Med. 2014;4(12):a018564. https://doi.org/10.1101/cshperspect.a018564.
278. Darrah PA, DiFazio RM, Maiello P, Gideon HP, Myers AJ, Rodgers MA, et al. Boosting BCG with proteins or rAd5 does not enhance protection against tuberculosis in rhesus macaques. NPJ Vaccines. 2019;4(1):21. https://doi.org/10.1038/s41541-019-0113-9.
279. White AD, Sibley L, Sarfas C, Morrison A, Gullick J, Clark S, et al. MTBVAC vaccination protects rhesus macaques against aerosol challenge with M. Tuberculosis and induces immune signatures analogous to those observed in clinical studies. NPJ Vaccines. 2021;6(1):4. https://doi.org/10.1038/s41541-020-00262-8.
280. Palmer MV. Mycobacterium bovis: characteristics of wildlife reservoir hosts. Transbound Emerg Dis. 2013;60(Suppl 1):1–13. https://doi.org/10.1111/tbed.12115.

281. Canto Alarcon GJ, Rubio Venegas Y, Bojorquez Narvaez L, Pizano Martínez OE, García Casanova L, Sosa Gallegos S, et al. Efficacy of a vaccine formula against tuberculosis in cattle. PLoS One. 2013;8(10):e76418. https://doi.org/10.1371/journal.pone.0076418.
282. Villarreal-Ramos B, Berg S, Chamberlain L, McShane H, Hewinson RG, Clifford D, et al. Development of a BCG challenge model for the testing of vaccine candidates against tuberculosis in cattle. Vaccine. 2014;32(43):5645–9. https://doi.org/10.1016/j.vaccine.2014.08.009.
283. Salguero FJ, Gibson S, Garcia-Jimenez W, Gough J, Strickland TS, Vordermeier HM, et al. Differential cell composition and cytokine expression within lymph node granulomas from BCG-vaccinated and non-vaccinated cattle experimentally infected with Mycobacterium bovis. Transbound Emerg Dis. 2017;64(6):1734–49. https://doi.org/10.1111/tbed.12561.
284. Maggioli MF, Palmer MV, Thacker TC, Vordermeier HM, Waters WR. Characterization of effector and memory T cell subsets in the immune response to bovine tuberculosis in cattle. PLoS One. 2015;10(4):e0122571. https://doi.org/10.1371/journal.pone.0122571.
285. Garcia-Jimenez WL, Villarreal-Ramos B, Grainger D, Hewisnon RG, Vordermeier HM, Salguero FJ. The expression of Indoleamine 2, 3-dioxygenase (IDO) is reduced in granulomas from BCG vaccinated cattle compared to granulomas from unvaccinated controls after experimental challenge with Mycobacterium bovis. Vet Immunol Immunopathol. 2018;203:52–6. https://doi.org/10.1016/j.vetimm.2018.08.002.
286. Thom ML, McAulay M, Vordermeier HM, Clifford D, Hewinson RG, Villarreal-Ramos B, et al. Duration of immunity against Mycobacterium bovis following neonatal vaccination with bacillus Calmette-Guérin Danish: significant protection against infection at 12, but not 24, months. Clin Vaccine Immunol. 2012;19(8):1254–60. https://doi.org/10.1128/cvi.00301-12.
287. Parlane NA, Shu D, Subharat S, Wedlock DN, Rehm BH, de Lisle GW, et al. Revaccination of cattle with bacille Calmette-Guérin two years after first vaccination when immunity has waned, boosted protection against challenge with Mycobacterium bovis. PLoS One. 2014;9(9):e106519. https://doi.org/10.1371/journal.pone.0106519.
288. Buddle BM, Skinner MA, Wedlock DN, de Lisle GW, Vordermeier HM, Glyn HR. Cattle as a model for development of vaccines against human tuberculosis. Tuberculosis (Edinb). 2005;85(1–2):19–24. https://doi.org/10.1016/j.tube.2004.09.003.
289. Siddiqui N, Price S, Hope J. BCG vaccination of neonatal calves: potential roles for innate immune cells in the induction of protective immunity. Comp Immunol Microbiol Infect Dis. 2012;35(3):219–26. https://doi.org/10.1016/j.cimid.2011.11.003.
290. de Val PB, López-Soria S, Nofrarías M, Martín M, Vordermeier HM, Villarreal-Ramos B, et al. Experimental model of tuberculosis in the domestic goat after endobronchial infection with Mycobacterium caprae. Clin Vaccine Immunol. 2011;18(11):1872–81. https://doi.org/10.1128/cvi.05323-11.
291. Pérez de Val B, Villarreal-Ramos B, Nofrarías M, López-Soria S, Romera N, Singh M, et al. Goats primed with Mycobacterium bovis BCG and boosted with a recombinant adenovirus expressing Ag85A show enhanced protection against tuberculosis. Clin Vaccine Immunol. 2012;19(9):1339–47. https://doi.org/10.1128/cvi.00275-12.
292. Vidal E, Arrieta-Villegas C, Grasa M, Mercader I, Domingo M, Pérez de Val B. Field evaluation of the efficacy of Mycobacterium bovis BCG vaccine against tuberculosis in goats. BMC Vet Res. 2017;13(1):252. https://doi.org/10.1186/s12917-017-1182-5.
293. Arrieta-Villegas C, Perálvarez T, Vidal E, Puighibet Z, Moll X, Canturri A, et al. Efficacy of parenteral vaccination against tuberculosis with heat-inactivated Mycobacterium bovis in experimentally challenged goats. PLoS One. 2018;13(5):e0196948. https://doi.org/10.1371/journal.pone.0196948.
294. Bezos J, Casal C, Puentes E, Díez-Guerrier A, Romero B, Aguiló N, et al. Evaluation of the immunogenicity and diagnostic interference caused by M. tuberculosis SO2 vaccination against tuberculosis in goats. Res Vet Sci. 2015;103:73–9. https://doi.org/10.1016/j.rvsc.2015.09.017.
295. Roy A, Risalde MA, Casal C, Romero B, de Juan L, Menshawy AM, et al. Oral vaccination with heat-inactivated Mycobacterium bovis does not interfere with the antemortem diagnos-

tic techniques for tuberculosis in goats. Front Vet Sci. 2017;4:124. https://doi.org/10.3389/fvets.2017.00124.
296. Figl J, Köhler H, Wedlich N, Liebler-Tenorio EM, Grode L, Parzmair G, et al. Safety and immunogenicity of recombinant Bacille Calmette-Guérin Strain VPM1002 and its derivatives in a Goat model. Int J Mol Sci. 2023;24(6). https://doi.org/10.3390/ijms24065509.
297. Liebler-Tenorio EM, Heyl J, Wedlich N, Figl J, Köhler H, Krishnamoorthy G, et al. Vaccine-induced subcutaneous granulomas in goats reflect differences in host-Mycobacterium interactions between BCG- and recombinant BCG-derivative vaccines. Int J Mol Sci. 2022;23(19). https://doi.org/10.3390/ijms231910992.
298. Sanchez J, Tomás L, Ortega N, Buendía AJ, del Rio L, Salinas J, et al. Microscopical and immunological features of tuberculoid granulomata and cavitary pulmonary tuberculosis in naturally infected goats. J Comp Pathol. 2011;145(2–3):107–17. https://doi.org/10.1016/j.jcpa.2010.12.006.
299. Niroula N, Lim ZL, Walker S, Huang Y, Gerdts V, Zriba S, et al. Domestic pigs experimentally infected with Mycobacterium bovis and Mycobacterium tuberculosis exhibit different disease outcomes. Tuberculosis (Edinb). 2022;133:102167. https://doi.org/10.1016/j.tube.2022.102167.
300. Gil O, Díaz I, Vilaplana C, Tapia G, Díaz J, Fort M, et al. Granuloma encapsulation is a key factor for containing tuberculosis infection in Minipigs. PLoS One. 2010;5(4):e10030. https://doi.org/10.1371/journal.pone.0010030.
301. Hayes FHC, Traum J. Vaccination of swine against tuberculosis with Calmette-Guérin culture. BCG Hilgardia. 1932;7(6):235–61. https://doi.org/10.3733/hilg.v07n06p235.
302. Ramos L, Obregon-Henao A, Henao-Tamayo M, Bowen R, Izzo A, Lunney JK, et al. Minipigs as a neonatal animal model for tuberculosis vaccine efficacy testing. Vet Immunol Immunopathol. 2019;215:109884. https://doi.org/10.1016/j.vetimm.2019.109884.
303. Swaim LE, Connolly LE, Volkman HE, Humbert O, Born DE, Ramakrishnan L. Mycobacterium marinum infection of adult zebrafish causes caseating granulomatous tuberculosis and is moderated by adaptive immunity. Infect Immun. 2006;74(11):6108–17. https://doi.org/10.1128/iai.00887-06.
304. Saralahti AK, Uusi-Mäkelä MIE, Niskanen MT, Rämet M. Integrating fish models in tuberculosis vaccine development. Dis Model Mech. 2020;13(8). https://doi.org/10.1242/dmm.045716.
305. Traver D, Herbomel P, Patton EE, Murphey RD, Yoder JA, Litman GW, et al. The zebrafish as a model organism to study development of the immune system. Adv Immunol. 2003;81:253–330.
306. Myllymäki H, Niskanen M, Oksanen KE, Sherwood E, Ahava M, Parikka M, et al. Identification of novel antigen candidates for a tuberculosis vaccine in the adult zebrafish (Danio rerio). PLoS One. 2017;12(7):e0181942. https://doi.org/10.1371/journal.pone.0181942.
307. Oksanen KE, Halfpenny NJ, Sherwood E, Harjula SK, Hammarén MM, Ahava MJ, et al. An adult zebrafish model for preclinical tuberculosis vaccine development. Vaccine. 2013;31(45):5202–9. https://doi.org/10.1016/j.vaccine.2013.08.093.
308. Lugo-Villarino G, Balla KM, Stachura DL, Bañuelos K, Werneck MB, Traver D. Identification of dendritic antigen-presenting cells in the zebrafish. Proc Natl Acad Sci USA. 2010;107(36):15850–5. https://doi.org/10.1073/pnas.1000494107.
309. Risalde MA, López V, Contreras M, Mateos-Hernández L, Gortázar C, de la Fuente J. Control of mycobacteriosis in zebrafish (Danio rerio) mucosally vaccinated with heat-inactivated Mycobacterium bovis. Vaccine. 2018;36(30):4447–53. https://doi.org/10.1016/j.vaccine.2018.06.042.
310. Su H, Peng B, Zhang Z, Liu Z, Zhang Z. The Mycobacterium tuberculosis glycoprotein Rv1016c protein inhibits dendritic cell maturation, and impairs Th1 /Th17 responses during mycobacteria infection. Mol Immunol. 2019;109:58–70. https://doi.org/10.1016/j.molimm.2019.02.021.

311. Ru H, Liu X, Lin C, Yang J, Chen F, Sun R, et al. The impact of genome region of difference 4 (RD4) on mycobacterial virulence and BCG efficacy. Front Cell Infect Microbiol. 2017;7:239. https://doi.org/10.3389/fcimb.2017.00239.
312. Oksanen KE, Myllymäki H, Ahava MJ, Mäkinen L, Parikka M, Rämet M. DNA vaccination boosts bacillus Calmette-Guérin protection against mycobacterial infection in zebrafish. Dev Comp Immunol. 2016;54(1):89–96. https://doi.org/10.1016/j.dci.2015.09.001.
313. Gopal R, Lin Y, Obermajer N, Slight S, Nuthalapati N, Ahmed M, et al. IL-23-dependent IL-17 drives Th1-cell responses following Mycobacterium bovis BCG vaccination. Eur J Immunol. 2012;42(2):364–73. https://doi.org/10.1002/eji.201141569.
314. Kanojia G, Have RT, Soema PC, Frijlink H, Amorij JP, Kersten G. Developments in the formulation and delivery of spray dried vaccines. Hum Vaccin Immunother. 2017;13(10):2364–78. https://doi.org/10.1080/21645515.2017.1356952.
315. Stylianou E, Paul MJ, Reljic R, McShane H. Mucosal delivery of tuberculosis vaccines: a review of current approaches and challenges. Expert Rev Vaccines. 2019;18(12):1271–84. https://doi.org/10.1080/14760584.2019.1692657.
316. Jeyanathan M, Fritz DK, Afkhami S, Aguirre E, Howie KJ, Zganiacz A, et al. Aerosol delivery, but not intramuscular injection, of adenovirus-vectored tuberculosis vaccine induces respiratory-mucosal immunity in humans. JCI Insight. 2022;7(3). https://doi.org/10.1172/jci.insight.155655.
317. Kaushal D, Foreman TW, Gautam US, Alvarez X, Adekambi T, Rangel-Moreno J, et al. Mucosal vaccination with attenuated Mycobacterium tuberculosis induces strong central memory responses and protects against tuberculosis. Nat Commun. 2015;6:8533. https://doi.org/10.1038/ncomms9533.
318. Heijmenberg I, Husain A, Sathkumara HD, Muruganandah V, Seifert J, Miranda-Hernandez S, et al. ESX-5-targeted export of ESAT-6 in BCG combines enhanced immunogenicity & efficacy against murine tuberculosis with low virulence and reduced persistence. Vaccine. 2021;39:7265. https://doi.org/10.1016/j.vaccine.2021.08.030.
319. White AD, Sibley L, Sarfas C, Morrison AL, Bewley K, Churchward C, et al. Influence of aerosol delivered BCG vaccination on immunological and disease parameters following SARS-CoV-2 challenge in rhesus macaques. Front Immunol. 2021;12:801799. https://doi.org/10.3389/fimmu.2021.801799.
320. Oxford Uo. Aerosol-based TB vaccine begins human trials.: Available at: https://www.ox.ac.uk/news/2022-07-06-aerosol-based-tb-vaccine-beginshuman-trial.; 2022.
321. Gordon SB, Sichone S, Chirwa AE, Hazenberg P, Kafuko Z, Ferreira DM, et al. Practical considerations for a TB controlled human infection model (TB-CHIM); the case for TB-CHIM in Africa, a systematic review of the literature and report of 2 workshop discussions in UK and Malawi. Wellcome Open Res. 2023;8:71. https://doi.org/10.12688/wellcomeopenres.18767.2.
322. Puri M, Miranda-Hernandez S, Subbian S, Kupz A. Repurposing mucosal delivery devices for live attenuated tuberculosis vaccines. Front Immunol. 2023;14:1159084. https://doi.org/10.3389/fimmu.2023.1159084.
323. Kwong KW, Xin Y, Lai NC, Sung JC, Wu KC, Hamied YK, et al. Oral vaccines: a better future of immunization. Vaccines (Basel). 2023;11(7). https://doi.org/10.3390/vaccines11071232.
324. Luca S, Mihaescu T. History of BCG vaccine. Maedica (Bucur). 2013;8(1):53–8.
325. Juste RA, Blanco-Vázquez C, Barral M, Prieto JM, Varela-Castro L, Lesellier S, et al. Efficacy of heat-inactivated Mycobacterium bovis vaccine delivered to European badgers (Meles meles) through edible bait. Heliyon. 2023;9(9):e19349. https://doi.org/10.1016/j.heliyon.2023.e19349.
326. Aldwell FE, Tucker IG, de Lisle GW, Buddle BM. Oral delivery of Mycobacterium bovis BCG in a lipid formulation induces resistance to pulmonary tuberculosis in mice. Infect Immun. 2003;71(1):101–8. https://doi.org/10.1128/iai.71.1.101-108.2003.
327. Rigano MM, Dreitz S, Kipnis AP, Izzo AA, Walmsley AM. Oral immunogenicity of a plant-made, subunit, tuberculosis vaccine. Vaccine. 2006;24(5):691–5. https://doi.org/10.1016/j.vaccine.2005.08.009.

328. Monteiro-Maia R, Pinho RT. Oral bacillus Calmette-Guérin vaccine against tuberculosis: why not? Memorias do Instituto Oswaldo Cruz. 2014;109(6):838–45. https://doi.org/10.1590/0074-0276140091.
329. Shrewsbury SB. The upper nasal space: option for systemic drug delivery, mucosal vaccines and "nose-to-brain". Pharmaceutics. 2023;15(6). https://doi.org/10.3390/pharmaceutics15061720.
330. Sonvico F, Colombo G, Quarta E, Guareschi F, Banella S, Buttini F, et al. Nasal delivery as a strategy for the prevention and treatment of COVID-19. Expert Opin Drug Deliv. 2023;20(8):1115–30. https://doi.org/10.1080/17425247.2023.2263363.
331. Perdomo C, Zedler U, Kühl AA, Lozza L, Saikali P, Sander LE, et al. Mucosal BCG vaccination induces protective lung-resident memory T cell populations against tuberculosis. MBio. 2016;7(6). https://doi.org/10.1128/mBio.01686-16.
332. Afkhami S, D'Agostino MR, Vaseghi-Shanjani M, Lepard M, Yang JX, Lai R, et al. Intranasal multivalent adenoviral-vectored vaccine protects against replicating and dormant M.tb in conventional and humanized mice. NPJ Vaccines. 2023;8(1):25. https://doi.org/10.1038/s41541-023-00623-z.
333. Gomez M, Ahmed M, Das S, McCollum J, Mellett L, Swanson R, et al. Development and testing of a spray-dried tuberculosis vaccine candidate in a mouse model. Front Pharmacol. 2021;12:799034. https://doi.org/10.3389/fphar.2021.799034.
334. Malek-Khatabi A, Sadat Razavi M, Abdollahi A, Rahimzadeghan M, Moammeri F, Sheikhi M, et al. Recent progress in PLGA-based microneedle-mediated transdermal drug and vaccine delivery. Biomater Sci. 2023;11(16):5390–409. https://doi.org/10.1039/d3bm00795b.
335. McNamee M, Wong S, Guy O, Sharma S. Microneedle technology for potential SARS-CoV-2 vaccine delivery. Expert Opin Drug Deliv. 2023;20(6):799–814. https://doi.org/10.1080/17425247.2023.2209718.
336. Platteel ACM, Nieuwenhuizen NE, Domaszewska T, Schürer S, Zedler U, Brinkmann V, et al. Efficacy testing of H56 cDNA tattoo immunization against tuberculosis in a mouse model. Front Immunol. 2017;8:1744. https://doi.org/10.3389/fimmu.2017.01744.
337. Irvine EB, O'Neil A, Darrah PA, Shin S, Choudhary A, Li W, et al. Robust IgM responses following intravenous vaccination with Bacille Calmette-Guérin associate with prevention of Mycobacterium tuberculosis infection in macaques. Nat Immunol. 2021;22(12):1515–23. https://doi.org/10.1038/s41590-021-01066-1.
338. Barclay WR, Anacker RL, Brehmer W, Leif W, Ribi E. Aerosol-induced tuberculosis in subhuman primates and the course of the disease after intravenous BCG vaccination. Infect Immun. 1970;2(5):574–82. https://doi.org/10.1128/iai.2.5.574-582.1970.
339. Anacker RL, Brehmer W, Barclay WR, Leif WR, Ribi E, Simmons JH, et al. Superiority of intravenously administered BCG and BCG cell walls in protecting rhesus monkeys (Macaca mulatta) against airborne tuberculosis. Z Immunitatsforsch Exp Klin Immunol. 1972;143(4):363–76.
340. Oneko M, Cherop YR, Sang T, Gutman JR, Wiegand R, Nyang'au EM, et al. Feasibility of direct venous inoculation of the radiation-attenuated plasmodium falciparum whole sporozoite vaccine in children and infants in Siaya, western Kenya. Vaccine. 2020;38(29):4592–600. https://doi.org/10.1016/j.vaccine.2020.05.008.
341. Steinhardt LC, Richie TL, Yego R, Akach D, Hamel MJ, Gutman JR, et al. Safety, tolerability, and immunogenicity of plasmodium falciparum Sporozoite vaccine administered by direct venous inoculation to infants and Young children: findings from an age de-escalation, dose-escalation, double-blind, randomized controlled study in Western Kenya. Clin Infect Dis. 2020;71(4):1063–71. https://doi.org/10.1093/cid/ciz925.
342. Seder RA, Chang LJ, Enama ME, Zephir KL, Sarwar UN, Gordon IJ, et al. Protection against malaria by intravenous immunization with a nonreplicating sporozoite vaccine. Science. 2013;341(6152):1359–65. https://doi.org/10.1126/science.1241800.
343. Rottinghaus AG, Ferreiro A, Fishbein SRS, Dantas G, Moon TS. Genetically stable CRISPR-based kill switches for engineered microbes. Nat Commun. 2022;13(1):672. https://doi.org/10.1038/s41467-022-28163-5.

344. Stirling F, Bitzan L, O'Keefe S, Redfield E, Oliver JWK, Way J, et al. Rational design of evolutionarily stable microbial kill switches. Mol Cell. 2017;68(4):686–97.e3. https://doi.org/10.1016/j.molcel.2017.10.033.
345. Dellagostin OA, Borsuk S, Oliveira TL, Seixas FK. Auxotrophic Mycobacterium bovis BCG: updates and perspectives. Vaccines (Basel). 2022;10(5). https://doi.org/10.3390/vaccines10050802.
346. Tiwari S, van Tonder AJ, Vilcheze C, Mendes V, Thomas SE, Malek A, et al. Arginine-deprivation-induced oxidative damage sterilizes Mycobacterium tuberculosis. Proc Natl Acad Sci USA. 2018;115(39):9779–84. https://doi.org/10.1073/pnas.1808874115.
347. Yamada H, Mizumo S, Horai R, Iwakura Y, Sugawara I. Protective role of interleukin-1 in mycobacterial infection in IL-1 alpha/beta double-knockout mice. Lab Investig. 2000;80(5):759–67. https://doi.org/10.1038/labinvest.3780079.
348. Juffermans NP, Florquin S, Camoglio L, Verbon A, Kolk AH, Speelman P, et al. Interleukin-1 signaling is essential for host defense during murine pulmonary tuberculosis. J Infect Dis. 2000;182(3):902–8.
349. Sugawara I, Yamada H, Kaneko H, Mizuno S, Takeda K, Akira S. Role of Interleukin-18 (IL-18) in mycobacterial infection in IL-18-gene-disrupted mice. Infect Immun. 1999;67(5):2585–9.
350. Fremond CM, Togbe D, Doz E, Rose S, Vasseur V, Maillet I, et al. IL-1 receptor-mediated signal is an essential component of MyD88-dependent innate response to Mycobacterium tuberculosis infection. J Immunol. 2007;179(2):1178–89. https://doi.org/10.4049/jimmunol.179.2.1178.
351. Scanga CA, Bafica A, Feng CG, Cheever AW, Hieny S, Sher A. MyD88-deficient mice display a profound loss in resistance to Mycobacterium tuberculosis associated with partially impaired Th1 cytokine and nitric oxide synthase 2 expression. Infect Immun. 2004;72(4):2400–4. https://doi.org/10.1128/IAI.72.4.2400-2404.2004.
352. Mayer-Barber KD, Andrade BB, Barber DL, Hieny S, Feng CG, Caspar P, et al. Innate and adaptive interferons suppress IL-1alpha and IL-1beta production by distinct pulmonary myeloid subsets during Mycobacterium tuberculosis infection. Immunity. 2011;35(6):1023–34. https://doi.org/10.1016/j.immuni.2011.12.002.
353. Maglione PJ, Xu J, Chan J. B cells moderate inflammatory progression and enhance bacterial containment upon pulmonary challenge with Mycobacterium tuberculosis. J Immunol. 2007;178(11):7222–34. https://doi.org/10.4049/jimmunol.178.11.7222.
354. Hansen SG, Zak DE, Xu G, Ford JC, Marshall EE, Malouli D, et al. Prevention of tuberculosis in rhesus macaques by a cytomegalovirus-based vaccine. Nat Med. 2018;24(2):130–43. https://doi.org/10.1038/nm.4473.
355. Plumlee CR, Duffy FJ, Gern BH, Delahaye JL, Cohen SB, Stoltzfus CR, et al. Ultra-low dose aerosol infection of mice with Mycobacterium tuberculosis more closely models human tuberculosis. Cell Host Microbe. 2021;29(1):68–82 e5. https://doi.org/10.1016/j.chom.2020.10.003.

Pre-clinical Tuberculosis Vaccine Development: Understanding Immune Response to Infection to Inform Next-Generation Vaccine Development

8

Dylan Kain, David Lewinsohn, and Deborah Lewinsohn

8.1 Beating BCG: Need for a Better Vaccine

8.1.1 Introduction

First administered in 1921 [1], *Mycobacterium bovis* bacilli Calmette-Guérin (BCG) remains the only licensed vaccine for prevention of Tuberculosis (TB). Discovered through ~230 serial passages of virulent *Mycobacterium bovis*, by Calmette and Guérin, BCG lacks several important genomic regions including the region of difference 1 (RD1), a nine gene locus encoding for ESAT-6, CFP-10, PE35, PPE68, Rv3871, Rv3876, Rv3877, Rv3878, and Rv3879c [2]. Loss of this region has been shown to impair the virulence of the *Mycobacterium* [3]. Given to over 88% of children worldwide in the first year of life in 2019, BCG is one of the most widely used vaccines in history [3].

Despite its widespread use, many questions about BCG's efficacy and mechanism of action remain. BCG provides more than 70% protection in children against severe and disseminated TB disease, including TB meningitis, especially in the first year of life, however, consistent benefit in adults has not been demonstrated [4]. Reasons for this difference in response based on age remain unknown. Beyond protection against TB, BCG has also been well described to provide heterologous protection against other communicable and non-communicable diseases and improved survival [5–7]. Recent work is only just beginning to disentangle the specific and heterologous mechanisms of protection from BCG, mediated by both the adaptive

Permission: Biorender purchase receipt uploaded. No other permissions.

D. Kain · D. Lewinsohn · D. Lewinsohn (✉)
Department of Medicine, Oregon Health and Sciences University, Portland, OR, USA
e-mail: kain@ohsu.edu; lewinsod@ohsu.edu; lewinsde@ohsu.edu

P. J. G. Bettencourt (ed.), *Tuberculosis Vaccines*,
https://doi.org/10.1007/978-3-031-94540-3_8

immune system, but also the innate immune system through trained immunity [8–10].

With the exclusion of a few newly developed vaccines (e.g., the COVID mRNA vaccine), all licensed vaccines have been developed empirically, that is, without requiring understanding of immune mechanisms of protection. Moreover, typically, correlates of protective immunity, such as antibody titers, can be empirically defined and used as a surrogate for protection in clinical trials of candidate vaccines. Of these empirically developed vaccines, the vast majority are significantly more effective than BCG. One only has to compare the number of TB cases worldwide (7.5 million in 2022, including 1.3 million children), the vast majority of which occur in BCG-vaccinated individuals [11], with the eradication of smallpox and near eradication of polio worldwide, as well as the rarity of diphtheria, tetanus, or disease, due to hepatitis B virus, or *H. influenzae* among vaccinated individuals. Therefore, a designer approach to vaccine development will likely be required to improve upon BCG. This approach first requires developing an understanding of the mechanisms of immune protection, followed by the design of vaccine candidates that target these protective components, and ultimately definition of mechanistic correlates of protection (COP) to be used as surrogates of efficacy in clinical trials. Having surrogate efficacy endpoints is especially useful in trials of TB vaccines given the prolonged time course from Mtb exposure to symptom onset compared to many other pathogens. A summary of the components of TB host defense as defined in animal TB models and in humans, and as relevant to vaccine development, follows. In Sect. 8.7, COP are discussed.

8.1.2 Cellular Immunity: Innate Immune Cells

Early studies in the murine TB model de-emphasized a potential for antibody-mediated immunity in TB host defense, which led to the subsequent, and almost exclusive study of cellular immunity rather than antibody-mediated immunity [12]. Among innate immune cells, macrophages, dendritic cells (DC), NK cells, as well as innate-like T cells (discussed below), all initiate the host immune response to Mtb infection [13]. Following inhalation of Mtb bacilli, lung macrophages represent both the primary host cell for infection but also the first line of defense, as infection activates multiple effector mechanisms. These effector mechanisms promote both containment of intracellular infection and attraction of additional innate immune cells to the site of infection. Among these innate immune cells are immature DC, which are activated upon infection, signaling maturation and trafficking to regional lymph nodes. In the lymph node, DC are the predominant cell type that prime naïve T cells. With relevance to vaccines, innate cells may serve as targets of adjuvants. For example, adjuvants that promote the secretion of IL-12 by DC and macrophages in turn promote the development of naïve T cells into Th1 $CD4^+$ and $CD8^+$ T cells, which are essential for TB host defense. Furthermore, increasing evidence supports that live attenuated TB vaccines (e.g., BCG, MTBVAC) induce trained immunity in macrophages, which in turn may provide heterologous protection from pathogens unrelated to Mtb [14].

8.1.3 Cellular Immunity: $CD4^+$ T Cells

Adaptively acquired (conventional) $CD4^+$ T cells recognize short peptides presented within the context of Major Histocompatibility Complex (MHC) Class II molecules (HLA DR, DQ, and DP in humans). MHC Class II molecules are expressed by professional antigen presenting cells (APC), including macrophages, as well as additional activated cell types. Evidence from the murine TB model suggest an essential role for $CD4^+$ T cells in TB host defense [15]. Moreover, individuals with HIV/AIDS and marked $CD4^+$ T cell depletion are exquisitely susceptible to TB [16]. $CD4^+$ T cells subsets express pro-inflammatory cytokines, including IFN-γ, TNF, and IL-17. Murine TB studies and characterization of individuals with Mendelian Susceptibility to Mycobacterial Disease (MSMD) support a critical role for IFN-γ, and hence the $CD4^+$ T cell subset which produces IFN-γ, Th1 $CD4^+$ T cells [17, 18]. Murine TB studies also demonstrate an adjunctive role for IL-17, and therefore the $CD4^+$ T cell subset which produce IL-17, Th17 $CD4^+$ T cells [18]. Thus, Th1 $CD4^+$ T cells, and more recently Th17 $CD4^+$ T cells represent important targets for TB vaccine candidates and have been extensively evaluated as a COP in pre-clinical and human TB vaccine studies.

8.1.4 Cellular Immunity: $CD8^+$ T Cells

Conventional $CD8^+$ T cells recognize short peptides presented within the context of MHC Class I molecules (HLA A, B, & C in humans). MHC Class I molecules are expressed by all nucleated cells and therefore are expressed more broadly than MHC Class II molecules. Murine TB studies demonstrate an important role for $CD8^+$ T cells, especially within the setting of heavy bacillary burden [19]. In humans, pro-inflammatory Mtb-specific $CD8^+$ T cells have been identified in individuals with latent TB infection (LTBI) and TB disease [20]. $CD8^+$ have redundant effector function to $CD4^+$ T cells, such as production of IFN-γ and TNF but also have enhanced cytolytic function and can recognize and destroy heavily infected macrophages, eliminate infected MHC class II-negative cells such as epithelial cells, endothelial cells and fibroblasts, inhibit mycobacterial growth, and induce apoptosis in infected cells. Moreover, in humans, $CD8^+$ T cells also produce mycobactericidal proteins, such as granulysin and IL-26, a molecule that directly kills intracellular Mtb [21]. Therefore, $CD8^+$ T cells represent a target for novel TB vaccines, and the presence of $CD8^+$ T cells have more recently started to be evaluated as a COP.

8.1.5 Cellular Immunity: Donor-Unrestricted T Cells (DURTs)

Several T cell subsets comprise the category of Donor Unrestricted T cells (DURTs), which are characterized by restriction by non-polymorphic molecules and recognition of predominantly non-peptide ligands (lipids, glycolipids, metabolites, and phospholipids) [22]. DURTs include: (1) MR1T cells that are MR1-restricted T cells and include the predominant subset, Mucosal-Associated Invariant T (MAIT) cells. MR1T cells recognize microbial-derived riboflavin biosynthesis intermediate derivatives, such as 5-OP-RU (5-(2- oxopropylideneamino)-6-d-ribitylaminouracil), and a broad spectrum of microbes that synthesize riboflavin, including Mtb [22]; (2) γδ T cells, named according to the TCR variable (V) segments, recognize small phosphorylated non-peptide antigens through a mechanism involving butyrophilin 3A1 [22, 23]. γδ T cells are implicated in host defense to TB and the Vγ9Vδ2 subset, which constitute the predominant subset in humans, recognize Mtb-infected cells (3). CD1-restricted T cells can be categorized as belonging to Group 1 (CD1a,b,c-restricted) or Group 2 (CD1d-restricted, iNKT). CD1-restricted T cells recognize lipids including Mtb components (lipids, glycolipids, galactoceramides) [24]; (4) HLA-E-restricted T cells also recognize Mtb-infected cells and recognize both peptide and glycopeptide antigens.

As relevant to vaccine targets, in addition to recognizing Mtb, DURT cells produce pro-inflammatory cytokines (e.g., IFN-γ, TNF) and are cytotoxic [25]. DURTs have been primarily characterized as innate T cells yet have features of adaptive immunity, including attributes of memory T cells [26–28]. Therefore, innate properties of DURT cells could be targeted by a vaccine to augment the adjuvant activity of a vaccine, promoting the development of adaptively acquired, conventional $CD4^+$ and $CD8^+$ T cells [29]. More specifically, as pre-armed effector T cells, IFN-γ-producing DURTs could provide an early source of this cytokine at the site of infection to promote the maturation of DC to those that efficiently elicit Th1 $CD4^+$ T cells and cytotoxic $CD8^+$ T cells. Furthermore, there is evidence from non-human primate (NHP) models that the microbial antigen HMBPP is needed for the expansion and effector functions of the Vγ9Vδ2 subset of γδ T cells during infection and that these cells can increase immune resistance to Mtb infection in macaques [30, 31]. On the other hand, the adaptive immunity features of DURTs could be targeted by a vaccine to elicit a memory T cell population with attributes of immunologic recall with re-exposure to antigen, which is the hallmark of vaccine-elicited immunity.

8.1.6 Revisiting a Role for Antibody-Mediated Immunity: B Cells

Early literature demonstrated limited efficacy of immune sera for protection against Mtb infection [32]. Due to these initial studies and dogma in the field that antibodies were unlikely to play a role in intracellular infections in general, a role for B cell immunity in TB host defense was largely ignored in the TB vaccine field [12, 33]. However, more recently, a role for B cells to complement T cell immunity, both through the production of antibodies and through the provision of T cell help is being revisited [12, 33]. These studies include murine TB studies more extensively evaluating the route and dose of Mtb challenge in B-cell deficient mice, as well as studies of TB vaccine candidates that target B cell immunity. In humans, also supportive of a role for antibody-mediated immunity are observational studies comparing antibody responses in individuals with LTBI to those with TB disease with regard to antibody subtype and glycosylation patterns of the antibody Fc region. This could suggest that certain Fc glycosylation patterns are associated with protection. Finally, a recent NHP vaccine study demonstrating that the dramatic efficacy of intravenous (IV) BCG correlated with antibody titers in the bronchoalveolar lavage of protected animals [34] has engendered enthusiasm as well. Therefore, interest in targeting B cell immunity in preclinical vaccine studies is gaining momentum. Moreover, these more detailed studies of antibodies in animal models and humans have engendered increased interest in studying antibody titers as COP as well.

8.2 New Strategies to Improve, Replace, or Boost BCG

Given its long track-record of safety, coupled with its efficacy in preventing severe and disseminated TB in young children, much effort has been put into altering or improving BCG. This can be done through changes in BCG vaccination schedule (e.g., re-vaccination), changes in route of administration (e.g., aerosol delivery), using heterologous vaccines (e.g., viral-vectored vaccines) in a prime-boost strategy, or alternatively through changes directly to BCG, altering the immune response to the vaccination. Finally, alternative live attenuated mycobacterial vaccines are also in development, with the aim of replacing BCG with another option that may have improved efficacy, safety, or durability.

8.2.1 Boosting BCG: Revaccination

The simplest strategy for attempting to boost the efficacy or durability of BCG is re-vaccination. However, studies to date have not shown clear benefit from revaccination [35], and as a result, the WHO does not currently recommend revaccination [36]. Studying BCG revaccination is complex, and many variables including BCG strain, timing of revaccination, exposure to environmental mycobacterium, and many others could influence the results [4, 37, 38]. Because of this, BCG revaccination is very much still an ongoing area of research, and as of January 2024 there are 12 ongoing studies registered on clinicaltrials.gov investigating BCG revaccination to improve its efficacy, durability, or response in adults [39]. Furthermore, given the rising evidence of heterologous protection against a host of both communicable and non-communicable diseases, BCG revaccination strategies are also an active area of study for diseases beyond TB [40–47].

One major challenge in determining the efficacy of BCG revaccination strategies is that current methods for determining asymptomatic Mtb infection cannot be measured directly, only indirectly through tuberculin skin test (TST) or interferon gamma release assay (IGRA) responses. This makes it extremely challenging to determine the efficacy of BCG revaccination on prevention of infection, or for that matter, any future prevention of infection vaccine. Nonetheless, in a study from 2018, Nemes et al. addressed this challenge by following adolescents who were vaccinated with BCG at birth, in a high risk setting for 6 months following BCG revaccination, vaccination with H4:IC31 (a candidate Mtb subunit vaccine) or placebo [48]. They found that neither H4:IC31 nor BCG vaccination was successful in prevention of the primary study endpoint of initial QuantiFERON-TB Gold conversion (QFT), however, sustained QFT conversion over the duration of the study was significantly reduced by 45.4% ($p = 0.03$) in the BCG revaccination group [48]. Despite these promising results, two recent larger studies in Africa did not show clear benefit of BCG revaccination in prevention of infection [49, 50]. In an earlier study, BCG did lead to a 49% reduction in the diagnosis of another mycobacterial infection; leprosy [51]. Further work is needed to determine if there is potential utility of BCG revaccination in prevention of Mtb.

8.2.2 Boosting BCG: Alternative Delivery Routes

BCG is classically given intradermally, and while this method creates a robust systemic immune response, it often does not create a robust mucosal immune response. Mtb's initial interaction with the immune system is, however, predominantly at the mucosal surface of the lungs, and alternative routes of BCG delivery have been proposed as a strategy to boost the vaccine's efficacy [52]. This strategy garnered increased attention following a landmark study in 2020 by Darrah et al. showing complete protection against Mtb following IV BCG vaccination in an NHP model [34]. IV BCG was found to elicit increased antigen-responsive $CD4^+$ and $CD8^+$ T cells including in the bronchoalveolar lavage and lung lymph nodes, suggesting there was increased production of lung mucosal immunity derived from IV BCG [34].

While possible, IV delivery of BCG in humans is unlikely to be seriously pursued both due to safety concerns about IV delivery of a live vaccine, especially in neonates or those who are immunocompromised, but also due to feasibility and practicality issues of IV delivery for the majority of those living in endemic areas, where medical resources are limited. While IV delivery in humans may not be feasible, it does provide a proof of concept that alternative routes of delivery of BCG could provide increased protection. Moreover, given the sterilizing protection provided by IV BCG in the NHP TB model [34], IV BCG may suggest mechanistic COPs to be pursued.

One alternative route that is actively being investigated is intrapulmonary delivery of BCG. This could potentially improve the mucosal immunity derived from BCG, while reducing the safety and feasibility issues of IV BCG delivery. Studies in mice have shown that mucosal BCG vaccination led to induction of more lung tissue cells with a protective phenotype compared to intradermal vaccination [53].

Another study also showed that intratracheal BCG vaccination led to reduced bacterial counts after subsequent Mtb challenge [54]. In rhesus macaques, endobronchial BCG delivery led to increased lung-resident memory T cells and improved protection compared to intradermal or subcutaneous delivery [53, 55, 56]. Aerosol delivery of BCG has also been shown to produce higher protection in NHP models [57, 58] and is currently in early phase clinical trials (NCT02709278) [59].

Intranasal delivery of BCG also aims to deliver vaccination into the airways, the first contact point for Mtb in human infection, and may provide an easier and more reliable way to delivery vaccination compared to intrapulmonary methods. Pre-clinical work in mouse models shows that compared to intradermal BCG, intranasal BCG led to increased antigen-specific IFN-γ-producing cells, and that this was associated with reduced bacterial burden in the lungs [60–65].

Alternative routes including oral administration and intralymphatic administration have also been investigated. Oral administration actually was the initial means by which BCG was administered after its creation in the 1920s. There is evidence from mouse models that there is an increased response of multifunctional $CD4^+$ T cells in the lungs compared to alternative routes [66]. Later studies, however, have shown that this response is likely significantly blunted in the presence of helminthic or *H. pylori* infection [67, 68]. Given that the majority of BCG vaccination occurs in areas with high prevalence of helminthic or *H. pylori* infection, justification for trials of oral BCG would be hard to justify. Intralymphatic administration has been shown in mice to produce stronger BCG-specific immune responses, however, practicality of this delivery method will make development challenging [69].

8.2.3 Recombinant BCG

Despite over 100 years of experience with the BCG vaccine, our understanding of the immune mechanisms of protection it provides is limited. It is clear, however, that there are potentially important ways in which BCG poorly stimulates critical components of the immune system. Modified BCG, or recombinant BCG (rBCG), is one strategy to try and improve the immune response to BCG, and thus the efficacy and/or durability of protection. rBCG has several advantages over other strategies. First, it benefits from the safety profile of BCG, with over 100 years of clinical experience. Second, it takes advantage of the efficacy BCG has already demonstrated in neonates and young children. Finally, it has the potential to utilize the established infrastructure of the current BCG vaccine production, storage, and delivery, meaning costs are likely to be lower than an independently developed novel vaccine [70]. There are many ways in which BCG had been modified to try and improve its efficacy and durability, and these have recently been reviewed by Kowalewicz-Kulbat and Locht [71]. Major strategies utilized in rBCG include strains producing cytokines, modification of strains to increase expression of immunodominant antigens, strains expressing bacterial effector proteins and toxins, strains producing non-bacterial proteins or non-protein molecules that modify the immune system response, and deletion of components of BCG strains with immunosuppressive effects.

O'Donnell et al. were the first to develop recombinant BCG (rBCG) that produced IL-2 and showed that it led to increased IFN-γ by splenocytes [72]. Since then, there have been many other BCG strains engineered to produce a host of cytokines including IFN-γ [73–77], IFN-α [78–83], IL-7 [84], IL-12 [85–89], IL-15 [90–93], IL-18 [91, 94–98], IL-21 [99], IL-35 [100], GM-CSF [89, 101–105], TNF [106], and other IL-2 producing strains [107–114]. These rBCG strains have been tested mainly in mouse models with most leading to an increased inflammatory response compared to BCG. However, while some have shown lower bacterial burden or improved outcomes against Mtb infection [83, 86, 98, 108], others have shown no significant difference [73, 84, 88, 112]. rBCG-producing cytokines have not been tested in other animal model systems or in humans to date, and more work is needed to ensure their safety and efficacy outside of murine models. In particular, a safety response outside of mice is needed to ensure rBCG vaccines do not trigger an overly robust immune response.

Modifications to improve immunodominant antigen responses can be accomplished through over expression of immunodominant antigens found in BCG or addition of *M. bovis* or Mtb-specific antigens that are not present in BCG. Genomic analysis has revealed that compared to Mtb, BCG has lost 16 genomic regions of differentiation (RD1-RD16 plus nRD18) [115, 116]. RD1 is of particular interest, as this region encodes for critical Mtb virulence factors including ESAT-6, CFP-10, and PPE protein [117], and restoration of RD1 genes to BCG leads to increased protection from Mtb infection in mouse and guinea pig models [118]. Ag85A, Ag85B, and Ag85C have also been targets for rBCG, as these proteins are major fractions of Mtb-secreted proteins and represent immunodominant antigens to infection [119, 120]. A phase I human trial of rBCG-30 over-expressing Ag85B showed increased Ag85B-specific T cells that were able to inhibit intracellular mycobacteria [121], however, clinical trials have not advanced to date [70].

Bacterial effector proteins and toxins are well known for their ability to modify immune responses and for their adjuvant properties. Taking advantage of this, rBCG that produce bacterial proteins or toxins is a strategy to improve the immune response to BCG. The concept behind this strategy is that these effector proteins or toxins may act directly as adjuvants or indirectly as adjuvants by leading to increased damage and inflammation. Multiple bacterial toxins are currently being investigated in this regard and include *E. coli* labile toxin A or B subunit [122–124], Cholera toxin B subunit [125, 126], pertussis toxin A subunit [127–131], *C. perfringens* toxin perfringolysin O [132–134], and *L. monocytogenes* toxin listeriolysin O [135–144]. rBCG expressing Ag85A, Ag85B, and Rv3407 along with mutant perfringolysin entered phase I clinical trials, however, has not progressed due to increased development of varicella zoster infection in those vaccinated [145]. rBCG expressing listeriolysin O toxin with *ureC* gene removed to decrease phagosomal pH for optimal toxin activity was created with the purpose of increasing cytosolic mycobacterial antigens to improved $CD8^+$ T cell responses [146]. This vaccine has now entered phase III clinical trials under the name VPM1002 [147].

While bacterial toxins are one of the methods for immune manipulation, many other protein and non-protein molecules have been shown to be able to manipulate the immune system and have been exploited in the development of rBCG strains. Proteins that activate the innate immune system are one mechanism by which this can be accomplished and include Fms-like tyrosine kinase 3 ligand (Ftl3L) that functions as a ligand that increases the development of APC [148], monocyte chemotactic protein 3 (MCP-3) that functions as a chemokine receptor for innate and adaptive immune cells [149], and BAX which functions as a pro-apoptotic protein triggering apoptosis of macrophages to enhance the immune response [150]. rBCG overexpressing Ftl3L or MCP-3 led to increased IFN-γ production in a mouse model, however, in neither case did this result in protection from Mtb challenge [148, 149]. rBCG over-expressing BAX also led to an enhanced Th1 T cell response, but has not been evaluated for its efficacy against Mtb challenge [150]. BCG has also been engineered to counteract immunosuppressive components of the immune system to improve the response to vaccination, and one important example of this is through rBCG strains that produce a suppressor of cytokine signaling 1 (SOCS1) antagonist (rBCG::SOCS1DN) [151]. Mycobacterial infection normally triggers SOCS1 production and this dampens IFN-γ production and negatively affects mycobacterial control [152]. Thus, rBCG::SOCS1DN was able to increase effector memory $CD8^+$ T cells and protect against Mtb in mice [151]. Cathepsin S is a protease involved in MHC II antigen presentation and is repressed by BCG, thus limiting MHC II antigen presentation [153]. rBCG-producing cathepsin S was developed to overcome this and has been shown to improve MHC II antigen presentation and in vitro Mtb killing although this has not yet been tested in vivo [154].

Non-protein immunomodulatory molecules can also be utilized in the development of rBCG. One example of this is rBCG:PGL-1, a BCG strain that synthesizes phenolic glycolipid 1 (PGL-1), a glycolipid found by *M. leprae* [155]. rBCG:PGL-1 has been shown to increase the efficiency by which BCG invaded and grew within macrophages and dendritic cells, which could theoretically improve the efficacy of BCG through a prolonged and more robust reponse [155]. However, effects on critical cytokines including TNF and IL-12 have been conflicting, with some studies showing reduced levels of inflammatory cytokines [155] and others showing increased levels [156]. Another rBCG strategy utilizing non-protein immunomodulatory molecules is re-engineered BCG over-expressing the STING agonist, cyclic di-AMP. This has been shown to augment trained immunity in response to rBCG and improved outcomes in a bladder cancer model [157].

As with other mycobacterial infection, BCG produces immunosuppressive molecules. Modifications of BCG to remove genes associated with immunosuppression is another strategy to increase the immune response to BCG. Some important genes associated with immunosuppression that have been targeted to date are extracytoplasmic sigma factor SigH (rBCGΔ*sigH*) [158], secreted acid phosphatase (rBCG*sapM*::Tn) [159, 160], aminoglycoside acetyltransferase (rBCGΔ*2432c*) [161], and zinc metalloprotease (rBCGΔ*zmp1*) [162, 163]. SigH is one of the factors responsible for antioxidant production, and this suppresses the immune response. rBCGΔ*sigH*, missing the gene for SigH, has been shown to increase polyfunctional CD8⁺ T cells in mice, leading to improved response to Mtb challenge [164]. SapM has been shown to dephosphorylate phosphatidylinositol 3-phosphate (PI3P), and this leads to reduction in phagolysosomal fusion and prevention of mycobacterial clearance. Deletion of *sapM* in BCG vaccination has been shown to be protective in BALB/c mice challenged with Mtb [160]. Deletion of *BCG_2432c* also leads to more robust immune responses to BCG due to increased autophagy, and this has been shown to improve bacterial burden in mouse models [161]. Zmp1 produced from BCG and other mycobacteria interferes with inflammasome activation and phagosome maturation [162], and deletion of the *zmp1* gene from BCG has been shown to be beneficial in protection against Mtb challenge [163]. rBCGΔ*zmp1* has now entered phase I human clinical trials [147].

8.2.4 Heterologous BCG Prime Boost Strategies

One method to further boost the humoral and cellular immunity derived from BCG is through heterologous prime boost strategies. This strategy relies on priming the immune system against specific antigens, followed by a later boosting with the original antigens combined with an immunogen to increase the response [165, 166]. Heterologous BCG boosting can be accomplished in three major ways following BCG prime: boosting with viral vector regimens, boosting with DNA vaccines, or boosting with mycobacterial antigens.

Recombinant adenoviruses (Ad) and modified vaccinia virus Ankara strain (MVA) have both been extensively studied as viral vectors for TB vaccine development and as boosting regimens following BCG prime. This was first shown in 2003, where mice initially primed with BCG were boosted with recombinant MVA expressing Ag85A (M.85A) leading to increased Ag85A-specific $CD4^+$ and $CD8^+$ T cell responses [167]. Studies using Ad-based viral vector vaccines expressing Mtb antigens for BCG boosting have shown similar results in mice with increased IFN-γ^+ $CD8^+$ T cells with viral-vector boosting [168, 169]. Human phase I studies using AERAS-402 (recombinant Ad expressing Ag85A, Ag85B, and TB10.4), as a boosting regimen following BCG priming, have shown similarly increased immune response with increased polyfunctional $CD4^+$ and $CD8^+$ T cells [170, 171]. DNA vaccines expressing Mtb antigens have also been studied as boosting regimes following priming with BCG. Studies have shown reduced bacterial burden and lung pathology in BCG-primed mice boosted with a DNA vaccine-expressing ESAT-6 and Ag85A [172], or Ag85A alone [173].

Mycobacterial antigens have been used as boosting regimens following BCG-prime as well. Heparin-binding hemagglutin adhesion (HBHA) alone provides similar protection to BCG, but when used as a boosting regimen has been shown to increase protection against Mtb [174], and is also associated with generation of HBHA-induced IFN-γ, IL-12, and TGFβ [175]. Combining HBHA with cholera toxin as a boosting regimen has been shown to lead to IFN-γ but also IL-17 production by HBHA-specific T cells in the lungs [176]. Given that the vast majority of those infected with Mtb worldwide have latent infection, vaccines specifically designed to target dormant Mtb, potentially eradicating or controlling infection at this point are potentially very powerful. Alpha-crystalline protein 1 (Acr1) or HspX is one such antigen that is expressed during latency [177], and when liposomized and given as a booster to BCG-primed mice, it has been shown to increase IFN-γ/TNF-producing $CD4^+$ and $CD8^+$ T cells [178]. Similar results were also seen in a guinea pig model of Mtb, and this also led to lower bacilli burden and reduced lung pathology [179]. Recombinant protein, H56 (containing Ag85B, ESAT-6 and Rv2660c) with the IC31 adjuvant has been shown in NHP models to effectively boost BCG, with reduced clinical disease, but also reduced latent disease [180]. H56 is currently in phase 2b clinical trials in remotely BCG-vaccinated individuals [147].

8.2.5 Conclusions: New Strategies to Improve, Replace, or Boost BCG

BCG remains the oldest vaccine still in use today and with over 100 years of safety and efficacy it remains one of the most powerful tools in the arsenal for TB prevention. However, despite its widespread use [3], TB remains the leading infectious disease killer globally. This highlights the urgent need for improved vaccine options to prevent Mtb. Given the benefits derived in prevention of severe and disseminated disease in infants and young children, along with its long safety record, making modifications to improve or boost BCG are highly attractive. We are only just beginning to discover the mechanisms of protection afforded by BCG, and this sheds new hope for next-generation TB vaccines.

8.3 Vaccine Design and Development

8.3.1 Introduction: Spectrum of TB Disease and Vaccine Efficacy Points

Following exposure to aerosolized Mtb, there is a wide spectrum of possible outcomes from complete clearance of infection to progressive active disease in the lungs or disseminating to other sites of the body (Fig. 8.1) [181]. In particular, many who have a significant exposure will contain the infection, but not be able to eliminate Mtb entirely, often referred to as latent TB infection (LTBI), as defined by a positive IGRA or TST. Individuals who convert their TST/IGRA from negative to positive are at high risk over the subsequent 1–2 years to progress to active disease, but also may develop active disease remotely even decades later [182–185]. Even with availability of effective antibiotics, many with active TB disease will fail treatment and can develop recurrent disease [186]. There are many reasons for this, including toxicity to treatment, lack of compliance, and drug-resistant TB without appropriate therapy among other possibilities [187]. This is particularly problematic as those with recurrent TB are at high risk for developing drug resistant disease

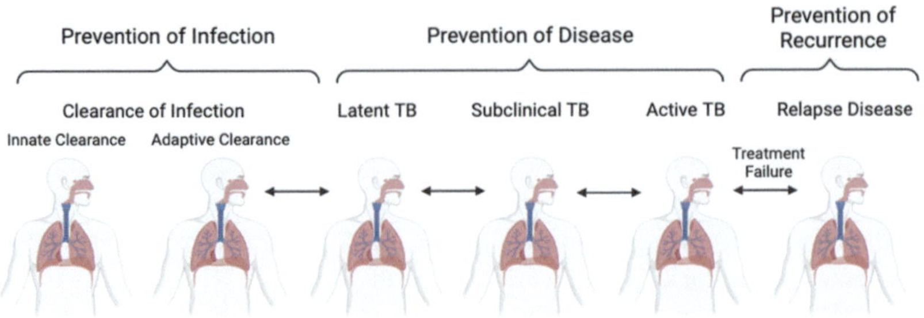

	Innate Clearance	Adaptive Clearance	Latent TB	Subclinical TB	Active TB	Relapse Disease
TST/IGRA	Negative	Positive	Positive	Positive	Usually Positive	Usually Positive
Culture	Negative	Negative	Negative	Intermittent	Positive	Positive
Imaging	None	None	None	Positive	Positive	Positive
Symptomatic	None	None	None	None	Yes	Yes

Fig. 8.1 Spectrum of tuberculosis disease and opportunities for vaccine prevention. (Adapted from Pai et al. [181] TST = TB skin test. IGRA = interferon gamma release assay. Imaging refers to chest x-ray, Computed Tomography (CT) scan or Positron Emission Tomography (PET)/CT scan)

[188]. This spectrum of disease provides several different points at which a TB vaccine can potentially work and include prevention of infection, prevention of disease and prevention of recurrence, also called therapeutic vaccines (Fig. 8.1). Prevention of infection vaccines aim to prevent the development of any signs of infection, including evidence of LTBI, as reflected by TST/IGRA conversion, whereas prevention of disease vaccines aims to control progression from LTBI to symptomatic or active TB disease. Prevention of recurrence or therapeutic vaccines meanwhile aim to improve the treatment for TB by reducing the duration of treatment, reducing the toxicity of therapy, or preventing recurrence following completion of therapy. These vaccines would be particularly useful for multi-drug resistant (MDR) or extensive drug-resistant (XDR) TB, where treatments can be prolonged with significant drug toxicity [189].

8.3.2 Types of Vaccines in Development of TB

Broadly speaking, there are 11 different types of vaccine platforms in clinical use or in experimental development which include: live attenuated, killed whole organisms, toxoid, subunit, virus-like particle, outer membrane vesicles, protein-polysaccharide conjugate, viral vectored, nucleic acid (e.g., mRNA), bacterial vectored, and APC vaccines [190]. TB vaccines in current pre-clinical and clinical development generally fall into five of these categories: whole cell live attenuated vaccines, inactivated whole cell vaccines or lysates, subunit vaccines, viral-vectored vaccines, and nucleic acid vaccines [191].

Live attenuated vaccine strategies utilize a closely related, but less virulent organism, or the organism of interest is attenuated to be less virulent. This strategy dates back to the origins of vaccination with the observation of Edward Jenner in 1798 that milkmaids were protected from smallpox due to acquisition of the less virulent cowpox [192]. He subsequently demonstrated that scratching cowpox lesions into the skin of an 8-year-old boy protected him from smallpox [192]. The only currently licensed TB vaccine and oldest vaccine still in use, BCG (attenuated *M. bovis*), is an example of a live attenuated whole cell vaccine. The mechanisms of protection induced by BCG are only just beginning to be understood. It likely induces some protection through generation of memory T cell responses against shared antigens with Mtb. However, there is also growing evidence that it also induces protection through a variety of other mechanisms, including direct effects on innate cells, a process referred to as trained immunity [193, 194]. BCG along with rBCG vaccines in development are reviewed above. There is one live attenuated TB vaccine in development, MTBVAC, which is being tested in phase III clinical trials [147]. MTBVAC is attenuated via genetic mutations to delete the virulence factors phoP and fadD26 [195]. This sufficiently reduces the virulence of Mtb to prevent clinical disease but allows induction of protection through generation of immune response to Mtb antigens [196–199].

Killed or inactivated whole organism vaccines function through a very similar premise to live attenuated vaccines, in that the whole organism is used to generate a broad immune response. The main advantage of this strategy is that since the organism is no longer viable, it is generally safer to be given to immunocompromised hosts, whereas live vaccines such as BCG are usually not given, due to the risk of infection progressing to disease. This however comes at the loss of antigens only produced during live infection. There are several killed or inactivated whole organism TB vaccines currently in development, and these include DAR-901, RUTI, and oral V7 vaccine. DAR-901 is inactivated *M. obuense*, and despite being protective in a murine model of TB [200], in a phase 2b clinical trial in Tanzania it did not prevent initial or persistent interferon gamma release assay (IGRA) conversion [201]. Two other inactivated whole cell vaccines, RUTI and oral V7, are being tested as therapeutic vaccines. RUTI is derived from purified and liposomal fragments of Mtb and had been shown to be protective in murine models with reduction of bacterial burden [202]. It is currently being tested in phase 2b clinical trials [147]. Oral V7 is derived from inactivated *M. vaccae*, and in 2019, was shown to be effective as a therapeutic vaccine in reducing hepatoxicity as a result of side effects from TB treatment [203].

Subunit vaccines employ specific antigens from the organism, rather than the whole organism. This has the major advantage of increased safety, especially in those with compromised immune systems, as there is no danger of causing an infection. This is particularly important given the high prevalence of HIV infection in those at highest TB risk. However, since they provide only specific antigens, rather than the whole organism, their efficacy is dependent on understanding antigens that activate a protective immune response. This is a challenging determination for Mtb given the breath of possible antigens produced by the organism and current lack of understanding which of these will induce a protective immune response [204]. This is discussed further below. Subunit vaccines typically induce robust Th1 $CD4^+$ T cell responses and antibody responses but are poorly immunogenic for $CD8^+$ T cell responses. There are several subunit vaccines currently in clinical trials for TB prevention along with different adjuvants. H4:IC31 is a subunit vaccine containing Mtb antigens Ag85B and TB10.4, paired with an adjuvant [205]. The adjuvant, IC31, is composed of the immunostimulatory oligonucleotide (ODN1a), which acts as a TLR9 agonist, and a synthetic antimicrobial peptide (KLK) that stabilizes the delivery of ODN1a that signals through TLR9 [206]. It was successful in decreasing bacillary burden in preclinical models [205, 207–208], however when tested in a phase IIb trial in South Africa, it failed to provide protection from Mtb infection (IGRA conversion, LTBI) [48]. M72/$AS01_E$ is another TB subunit vaccine that is comprised of a recombinant fusion protein of two Mtb antigens (Mtb32A and Mtb39A) along with the adjuvant $AS01_E$. $AS01_E$ is made up of MPL and QS-21, which activate the innate immune system through TLR4 signaling pathways, but also enhance antigen uptake and presentation [209]. After success in preclinical studies [210–212], M72/$AS01_E$ was recently tested for prevention of disease in a phase IIb trial in those with LTBI in South Africa. It was found to reduce developing active disease by 49.7% in these participants over the trial period [213]. Two other prominent subunit candidates, H56:IC31 (containing Mtb antigens Ag85B, ESAT-6 and Rv2660c) [214] and ID93/GLA-SE (containing Mtb antigens Rv1813c, Rv2608, Rv3619c, and Rv3620c) [215, 216] have also entered early phase clinical trials [217, 218]. GLA-SE (glucopyranosyl lipid adjuvant-stable emulsion), similar to $AS01_E$ works through TLR4 activation and increasing antigen presentation [219].

Viral-vectored vaccines also rely on understanding critical antigens for inducing immune protection. They utilize a virus as the vector to deliver the Mtb antigens to the immune system, but also the viral-vector itself functions as an adjuvant, activating a more robust immune response. Furthermore, viral-vectored vaccines deliver Mtb antigens intracellularly and therefore induce $CD8^+$ T cell responses in addition to Th1 $CD4^+$ and $CD8^+$ T cell responses. There are many viral-vectored platforms currently in development using different human-attenuated viruses including adenoviruses (Ad), modified vaccinia virus Ankara (MVA, which is an attenuated vaccinia virus), and cytomegaloviruses (CMV). Undergoing a single round of replication, Ad vectors and MVA provide short-term expression of Mtb antigens. As a persistent virus, CMV vectors provide longer term expression of Mtb antigens. Examples studied in human clinical trials include AdHu85A [220], AdHu35 [221], and MVA85A. AdHu85A and AdHu35, utilize an adenoviral platform, has been evaluated in a phase I clinical trial. MVA85, recombinant MVA expressing Ag85, has been evaluated in both phase I as well a phase 2b clinical trial [222, 223]. RhCMV/TB is a CMV-viral-vectored vaccine that has shown significant preclinical trial promise, with a 68% reduction in Mtb infection or disease in a rhesus macaque model of TB [224]. The use of CMV as a platform has several exciting advantages including its ability to induce strong T cell responses and as CMV persists in human host, it has the ability to continue to eliciting sustained Mtb-specific immune responses [225]. However, the persistence of CMV in humans means additional work is still needed to ensure safety of this platform. At present, it is being engineered to be suitable for human trials, with phase I trials ongoing with the focus on safety of this novel platform. One of the major problems with utilizing attenuated human viruses as viral-vectored vaccine platforms is that there can pre-existing immunity to the viral-vector, and due to pre-existing neutralizing antibodies, this can result in the viral-vector being eliminated prior to inducing an effective immune response to the Mtb antigens. To combat this problem, researchers have used rare human serotypes (e.g. AdHu85A) [221] or non-human viruses for their viral vectors (e.g., ChAd68Ag85A and ChAdOx1.85A) [226–229].

mRNA vaccine platforms have garnered an unprecedented amount of attention over recent years given incredible success during the SARS-CoV-2 pandemic [230]. There are several key advantages of mRNA vaccines including their speed and flexibility, induction of both robust Th1 $CD4^+$ and $CD8^+$ T cell responses, as well as their lack of need for additional adjuvant [231]. Recent work by Larsen et al. have demonstrated feasibility of mRNA-based platforms for TB vaccine development with adaption of the TB vaccine candidate ID91 (containing Mtb antigens esxV, RpfD, PPE60, and Ag85B) to an mRNA vaccine platform and modest efficacy in reducing bacterial burden in murine models of disease [232]. As with subunit vaccines and viral-vectored vaccines, success of mRNA vaccines against a complex pathogen with over 4000 genes [204], is selection of the correct genes for producing antigens that will lead to a protective immune response. This is currently still severely limited by our lack of understanding of protective immune responses against Mtb and the antigens that may be important in eliciting those responses, and this is further explored in the next section.

8.4 Safety

8.4.1 Vaccine Safety

Given that vaccines are predominantly given to healthy individuals for prevention of disease, their safety is imperative. A lack of safety can have profound impacts beyond even the direct costs to individuals. This was recently demonstrated in the Philippines with the surge of increased measles cases fueled by vaccine hesitance in the wake of the scandal surrounding the rollout of Sanofi's Dengvaxia [233]. Further complicating the development of a safe TB vaccine is the intimate relationship of TB and HIV, as with 167,000 deaths, TB is the leading cause of death in those living with HIV [234]. Development of a vaccine that is safe in those with HIV or other immunocompromising disease states is imperative in protecting these individuals in high-risk areas.

The pipeline for novel TB vaccine development traditionally progresses in a similar manner to other novel drug or vaccine development, first establishing proof of concept, safety data, and dosing regimen in preclinical and animal models before progressing into traditional human clinical trials. Prior to entering animal trials, safety must first be established in vitro, to ensure the candidate is suitable for animal studies. This must consider all components of the future vaccine, including ensuring that there is no evidence of toxicity from adjuvants that will accompany the vaccine [235]. Following this, candidate vaccines can generally progress into animal models with mice often being used first given their availability and relative cost.

Different vaccine types in development carry inherently different risks. Live attenuated vaccines have a long track record of use and safety, with BCG being the oldest vaccine still in clinical use. Despite this long safety issue, they remain theoretically dangerous for those with defects in their immune system, and BCG is not recommended by the WHO for those living with HIV [236]. Live attenuated vaccines also carry the risk of mutations allowing them to become virulent again. This has been well established with the oral polio vaccine, which was able to genetically reverse the attenuation to become virulent again and lead to vaccine-induced polio [237]. While this is theoretically possible with live attenuated mycobacterial vaccines, the lower rates of spontaneous mutations in Mtb [238] compared to viruses make it considerably less likely. Guidelines for testing novel live attenuated vaccines have been well established and are extensively outlined elsewhere [239]. Generally, they consist of ensuring absence of excessive signs of inflammation at the injection site, and also repeated dosing to ensure there is no evidence of anaphylaxis [240]. For live attenuated vaccines, there is also concurrent testing in immunocompromised mice, including $RAG1^{-/-}$ and severe combined immunodeficient (SCID) mice, to ensure candidate vaccines are as safe or safer than BCG [235].

Whole cell inactivated vaccines are safer in this regard, however, without proper oversight failures of inactivation can have disastrous consequences. This was the case in 1955, when at Cutter Laboratories batches of live polio was given to the public having failed inactivation despite passing safety testing [241]. Overall this led to an estimated 220,000 infections, 164 severe cases of paralysis, and 10 deaths [242]. Even before the Cutter incident, another tragic incident occurred with early BCG vaccine administration in Lübeck, Germany [243]. In 1929, 251 neonates were accidentally administered BCG vaccination contaminated with Mtb, resulting in the deaths of 72 infants [243]. Since the time of those tragic incidents, regulations for vaccines have improved substantially, but theoretical risk remains. Other vaccine types, including subunit vaccines, viral-vectored vaccines, and mRNA vaccines, do not carry the risk of infection, however, other risks remain. For viral-vectored vaccines, risks in particular stem from the virus used as the vector, however, there is already a huge body of safety literature on these platforms, and further guidance is provided in the guidance document: WHO guidelines on non-clinical evaluation of vaccines [244]. For protein or subunit vaccines, idiosyncratic vaccine reactions have been reported but remain extremely rare [241].

8.5 Identification of Antigens for Inclusion in TB Vaccines

8.5.1 Identification of Immunodominant T Cell Antigens

Vaccine discovery, including TB vaccines, have been mainly driven by empiric trial and error of various attenuated versions or critical components of the organisms. Only over recent decades have there been an increase in the involvement of immunologists and a more nuanced approach taken to vaccine design. This is particularly important in the development of TB vaccines for several reasons. As previously alluded to, Mtb has over 4000 genes [204] and coupled with the genetic diversity seen among different Mtb strains [245] which means there is an overwhelming number of potential antigens generated by Mtb that makes it essentially impossible to empirically test all of them. This problem is further compounded by challenges with animal models accurately capitulating human disease (discussed below in preclinical studies and animal models). Therefore, efforts have been directed toward selection of Mtb proteins that can be shown to represent immunodominant antigens, which as defined in humans are antigens that are commonly and strongly recognized by Mtb-specific T cells. The concept of utilizing immunodominant antigens in vaccine design is straight forward, in that antigens that produce stronger responses in preclinical or early phase human clinical trials are intuitively more likely to be antigens that activate protective immune responses. In this regard, there are two general strategies for antigen discovery: targeted screening of a protein or interest or whole proteome screening approaches. In either case, proteins are typically screened for recognition by $CD4^+$ or $CD8^+$ T cells isolated from cohorts of individuals infected with Mtb (LTBI or active TB disease) or vaccinated with BCG. As discussed above, it has long been understood that IFN-γ, produced by Th1 $CD4^+$ T cells and $CD8^+$ T cells along with other cell types, is extremely important in Mtb control in murine TB models [246, 247]. Given this importance, IFN-γ is the main method for screening for immunodominant CD4 and CD8 antigens [248].

8.5.2 CD4 Antigen Discovery

Dating back to the early 1990s, efforts were taken to dissect the secreted Mtb proteome and discover immunodominant antigens [249–252]. The secreted Mtb proteome was targeted initially because of the importance that many of these proteins play in Mtb's survival and its virulence. In particular, this early work focused on secreted protein-derived antigens that were able to induce a $CD4^+$ T cell protective effect in mice and guinea pigs [253–255]. The first step in this antigen discovery process was the isolation of secreted proteins, which was frequently done through the use of two-dimensional gel electrophoresis. These proteins were then purified and examined for immunodominant $CD4^+$ T cell responses. This early work identified many important Mtb proteins that continue to be used in TB vaccine development, including Ag85A, part of a complex of proteins (Ag85A, Ag85B, and Ag85C) [252], CFP-10 and ESAT-6 among others [256, 257].

Although initial work was focused on secreted Mtb proteins, these may not be the only proteins that play a role in protection from disease. One of the complexities of Mtb as a pathogen is its ability to change its metabolic state from active replication to slow or non-replicative states. These shifts from replicated to non-replicative states, or vice versa, result in dramatically different protein production that can be disease-stage specific [258–260]. Identification of latency-associated proteins can, however, be challenging [261]. Granuloma conditions include hypoxia, low pH, NO, nutrient deprivation, and along with increased host immune pressure, induce alternate gene expression from Mtb. Replicating these conditions in the lab is one method to determine the proteins expressed within this context [262–264]. Proteins expressed during latency can then be screened for T cell recognition, including by humans with LTBI. Evaluation of latency proteins, and the antigens derived from them, can be challenging given the lack of high-quality animal models that recapitulate LTBI in humans. This will be discussed further below in the section on animal models of TB disease.

Inclusion of immunodominant CD4 antigens discovered using a targeted approach have yielded some successes. In particular, the M72/AS01$_E$ vaccine, a recombinant fusion protein of the immunodominant Mtb antigen (Mtb39A) delivered with the AS01$_E$ adjuvant, demonstrated a 49.7% reduction in progression to active TB in those with LTBI [213]. Yet, there are also examples of failures. Most notably, while the MVA85A vaccine, encoding immunodominant CD4 antigen Ag85, was able to induce a modest Th1 CD4$^+$ T cell response, it did not provide protection from TB disease in infants, when provided as a boost to neonatal BCG [223]. In addition to the modest CD4$^+$ T cell response, the MVA85A vaccine did not induce CD8$^+$ T cell responses in these infants, possibly providing at least a partial explanation for its lack of efficacy. As discussed below, more recent work has attempted to better define CD8 immunodominant antigens, which have been far less explored, and found many CD8 immunodominant antigens from Mtb-proteins that had not been previously described [265].

Conventional targeted antigen discovery is inherently biased in the selection of proteins to study, and this can be problematic. For example, it has been suggested that since many secreted proteins are not essential for the survival of Mtb [266], these could be secreted by the bacteria as a decoy to prevent the immune system from recognition of more critical antigens [267]. However, following the publishing of the genomic sequencing of Mtb in 1998 [268], and advances in high-throughput peptide synthesis methods and computational methods, whole proteome discovery approaches to immunodominant CD4 antigen discovery became possible. One notable example has been the work by Lindestam Arlehamn et al. [269] They first used protein sequences from several Mtb genomes and predicted binding capacity of all 15-mer peptides for the most common human HLA alleles. Then they screened all of these 15-mers using ex-vivo ELISPOT analysis in individuals with LTBI [269]. This work demonstrated the utility of unbiased whole-genome approaches to antigen discovery, as they found not just secreted proteins being immunodominant but also the proteins that comprise these secretion systems inducing immunodominant responses [269]. This work was then used to develop a pool of 300 15-mer peptides of immunodominant CD4 epitopes recognized by South African and US populations named the MTB300 pool [269, 270]. This pool remains a powerful tool for studying CD4+ T cell responses to Mtb in multiple populations [271–274].

8.5.3 CD8 Antigen Discovery

As discussed above, several studies in mice and NHP models have shown that CD8+ T cells are also important in Mtb protection [275–278]. Thus, using both targeted and proteome-wide approaches, immunodominant CD8 antigens have been identified for inclusion in TB vaccine candidates. For example, using a targeted approach, several well-known immunodominant CD4 antigens, such as CFP-10 were demonstrated to represent immunodominant CD8 antigens as well [279]. In addition, a proteome-wide HLA allele independent approach greatly expanded the known repertoire of immunodominant antigens [265]. Using an integrated computational and proteomic approach, Lewinsohn et al. created a synthetic peptide library representing 10% of the Mtb proteome, selected to be enriched for Mtb antigens, and then screened this library utilizing CD8+ T cells isolated from individuals with LTBI or TB [265]. A set of immunodominant CD8 antigens including part or all of 74, Mtb proteins, only 16 of which are previously known CD8 antigens, were defined.

To contribute to vaccine efficacy, CD8 antigens must be processed and presented by Mtb-infected cells, yet not all Mtb epitopes are effectively displayed on infected macrophages [280]. For the studies discussed above, the CD8+ T cells used for antigen discovery were isolated from Mtb-infected individuals and therefore were necessarily primed by Mtb-infected cells in vivo. "Immunopeptidomics" represents another approach that ensures that antigens are effectively processed and presented by Mtb-infected cells. This approach identifies peptides bound to MHC Class I molecules using mass spectrometry at a whole-proteome scale [281]. This has been employed in Mtb antigen discovery in several recent papers by Leddy et al. and Bettencourt et al. to use mass spectrometry to analyze the entire repertoire of MHC-I antigens in Mtb-infected macrophages [282, 283]. Using this method, they were able to identify several candidate antigens from Mtb proteins that are accessible for presentation on MHC-I and represent candidate antigens for future CD8+ activating TB vaccine development.

8.5.4 Moving Beyond Immunodominant Antigens: Definition of Antigens Associated with Protection

The major limitation of all of the previously described work is that although many immunodominant antigens can be discovered, it is unclear the degree to which T cell responses to these antigens correlate with protection. It has also even been proposed that some immunodominant antigens may actually be evolutionarily advantageous to Mtb [284]. For example, a more robust immune response could lead to increased phagocytosis assisting Mtb to reach its intracellular nice within macrophages, or increase cavitation within the lung, a feature that increases transmission [285].

One novel approach to address this shortcoming was exemplified in a recent paper by Musvosvi et al. [286] In this paper, they utilized human samples from large cohort studies of individuals with LTBI who either progressed to develop active disease or who controlled infection. T cells from these individuals were stimulated with Mtb lysate, flow sorted for activated T cells, and single-cell TCR sequencing performed. Using a novel bioinformatics tool, GLIPH2 [287], which clusters TCRs predicted to bind to similar antigens to define TCR similarity groups, they were able to find 17 TCR similarity sequences that were associated with control of infection and 7 that were associated with progression to disease. They then expressed these TCR sequences in a reporter cell line and using genome-wide Mtb-antigen screening were able to resolve the antigens these TCRs recognized in three cases. Of note, there was significant enrichment of TCR similarity groups that recognized Mtb antigens PE13 and CFP-10 in those that controlled infection. This would suggest that these antigens are potentially more important in a protective response to infection and could be prioritized for future vaccine development.

Despite these promising results, there were limitations to this study. This approach is labor-intensive and only 3/24 enriched TCR similarity groups were able to be resolved to the antigen they recognize. In addition, as Mtb lysate was used to activate the T cells, only activated $CD4^+$ T cells would be identified. Nonetheless, this is a critical step in the process of determining antigens that show biological signs of being important in TB control, rather than just immunodominant ones. As bioinformatic and machine- learning approaches continue to improve, and likely being to incorporate more sophisticated artificial intelligent systems, this approach is likely to be extremely fruitful.

8.6 Preclinical Studies and Animal Models

8.6.1 Introduction and Overview of Model Systems

As with vaccine development for other diseases, preclinical and animal models are essential for testing both efficacy and also safety of candidate vaccines for TB. As with the use of animal models for the study of any disease, ethical considerations must be taken to ensure suffering is minimized. This has led to the concept of "replacement, reduction and refinement" first proposed in 1959 [288]. Animals used for TB vaccine development can be broadly divided into small mammal models (mice, guinea pigs, rabbits, and rats), large mammal models (cattle, goats, and NHP), and invertebrate models (zebrafish, and fruit flies). Each different animal model has distinct benefits and draw backs, and ongoing work continues to modify these models to improve their utility. However, despite improvements, none of these model systems fully captures the complexity of human disease, and it is therefore imperative to understand the unique benefits and limitations of each model system in order to best use them in the pursuit of better TB vaccine development. The majority of animal models are reviewed in other sections of the manuscript, but given their importance in TB vaccine testing, non-human primate (NHP) models are reviewed below.

8.6.2 Non-Human Primates (NHP)

Of all animal models for TB vaccine development, NHP are evolutionarily the closest to humans and as a result it is not surprising that they closely replicate human disease, both with respect to immune response but also the clinical spectrum seen in humans [289]. The existence of simian immunodeficiency virus (SIV) that closely resembled HIV means that NHPs are also an ideal model for TB/HIV co-infection studies. Therefore, NHP models are the most informative of all animal models for candidate vaccine testing; however, there are significant ethical and economic restrictions on their use that prevent their widespread use [290]. There are two commonly use NHP models for TB research, and these are the cynomolgus macaques (*Macaca fascicularis*) and the rhesus macaques (*Macaca mulatta*). Although very similar, there are significant differences between species which have implication for TB vaccine research [291]. Cynomolgus macaques are relatively resistant to Mtb infections and have been used to study LTBI and chronic persistent TB, whereas rhesus macaques are more susceptible and can be used to study progressive disease [292]. Despite these differences in susceptibility, both cynomolgus and rhesus macaques can develop close to the full range of human disease following aerosolized Mtb exposure, albeit not identical to human disease.

Another significant difference between cynomolgus and rhesus macaques is the protection afforded to them by BCG vaccination. In a study by Langermans et al., intradermal BCG vaccination provided an almost complete protection against pathology in cynomolgus macaques, and this was coupled with a 2-log reduction in bacillary load in the lungs [293]. Rhesus macaques meanwhile were not protected by intradermal BCG vaccination. A more recent landmark study by Darrah et al. showed that IV BCG vaccination, unlike intradermal vaccination, provided complete sterilizing immunity in rhesus macaques against subsequent Mtb challenge [34]. IV BCG induced airway T cells that correlated with the protection, suggesting that IV BCG induced protective mucosal T cell immunity [294]. Although IV BCG vaccination poses both logistical and safety concerns that limit its ability to be translated into humans, this work highlights the potential importance of route of vaccine delivery in providing protection. Several other studies have shown increased protection through alternative routes of BCG delivery [295–297]. The discovery that IV BCG provides sterilizing immunity in rhesus macaques has also allowed researchers to explore mechanistic COP to attempt to tease apart how protection is derived. Follow-up work by Liu et al. has shown that early innate immune responses including type I interferon, DC activation, and RIG-I-like receptor were correlated with both the adaptive immune response in the lungs at 4–8 weeks and protection from Mtb infection [298].

In another landmark study, Hansen et al. showed that a novel CMV viral-vectored TB vaccine candidate, RhCMV/TB, was able to reduce TB by 68% ~1 year after initial vaccination [224]. Compared to intradermal BCG, RhCMV/TB was able to produce increased circulating and tissue-resident Mtb-specific CD4$^+$ and CD8$^+$ memory T cells, and these were correlated with protection [224]. Further work exploring other COP and comparisons with protection induced by IV BCG holds promise for eliciting further potential mechanisms of protection in humans. Using NHP models, many important studies have been conducted examining SIV/TB co-infection, which is of critical importance given the high rates of HIV in individuals at risk of TB. Work by Larsen et al. has shown that IV BCG also provided protection for rhesus macaques co-infected with SIV, providing promise that protection derived from IV BCG will also provide protection in those living with HIV [299].

DURTs possess features of both the innate and adaptive immunity and represent a potential bridge between the two. Their enrichment in mucosal surfaces including the lung, ability to respond quickly and robustly to mycobacterial infection, and lack of significant polymorphism in the human population of the restriction alleles required for antigen presentation make DURTs attractive candidates for future TB vaccine development. Unlike other animal models, NHP DURTs much more accurately represent human DURTs in both their frequencies and function and allows researchers to directly examine the role these cells play in the Mtb immune response. In a recent study by Winchell et al., cynomolgus macaques were depleted of CD8β expressing cells, depleting only conventional CD8$^+$ T cells that express CD8αβ or depleted of CD8α expressing cells, depleting conventional CD8$^+$ T cells and CD8αα expressing DURTs [278]. They showed that CD8α depletion led to significantly worse outcomes with increased lung granulomas, increased thoracic bacillary load, associated with disseminated Mtb, and extrapulmonary disease [278]. Meanwhile, CD8β depletion only influenced the Mtb bacillary load in draining lymph nodes, suggesting that DURTs play a critical role in early protection against TB [278].

8.6.3 Animal Models: Fit for Purpose

Many animal models for TB exist, each with unique advantages and drawbacks and none fully recapitulating human disease. Human TB disease is a wide spectrum (Fig. 8.1), and careful consideration must be taken as animal models generally only mimic small sections of this spectrum during any experimental design. The use of animal models to replicate different human disease states is summarized in Fig. 8.2.

Animal models generally best recapitulate primary TB and active disease, and all animal models can be used for this purpose. Some animals will, however, more accurately represent different components of active disease. For example, although mice will develop active progressive TB disease, other models such as guinea pigs, rabbits, and NHPs develop granulomas that much more accurately reflect human granulomas. As previously discussed, modifications to traditional animal models can be used to better match the granulomas seen in humans, including using C3HeB/FeJ mice or ultra-low dose infection models. Despite all animal models being able

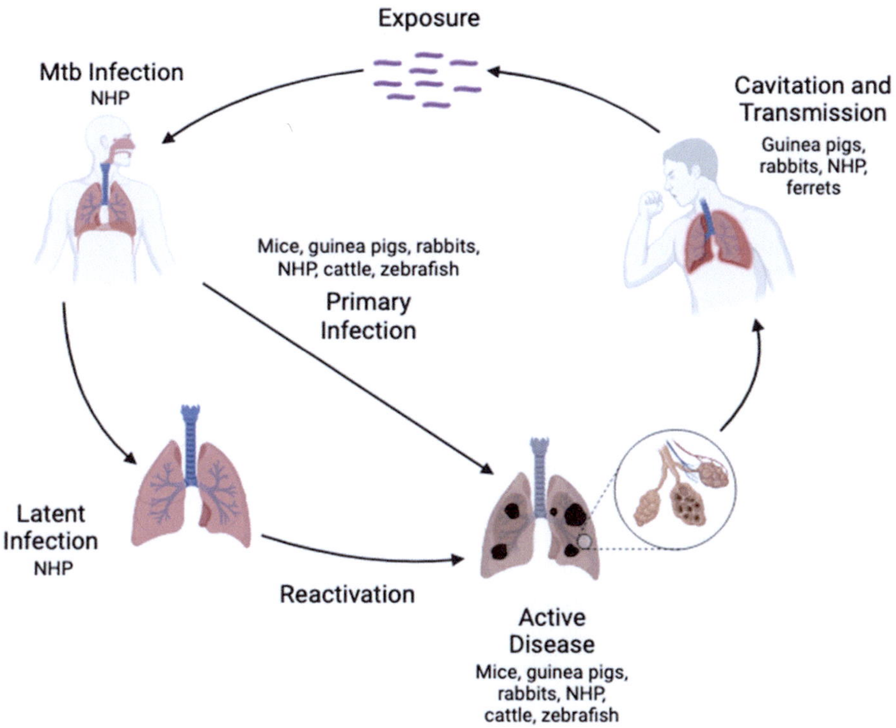

Fig. 8.2 Fit for purpose of different animal models

to develop active progressive TB disease, few animal models are able to accurately capture extrapulmonary disease, especially TB meningitis.

In humans, the majority of those infected with Mtb will contain the infection, resulting in LTBI. Animal models are generally much less adept at modelling this, as most will progress to active disease after infection. In particular, more available and less expensive smaller mammal model do not traditionally represent LTBI well. Older models in mice and guinea pigs used shorter courses of chemotherapy to prevent development of active disease in an attempt to mimic LTBI [300, 301]. This, however, represents a very different pathophysiology compared to humans who are mainly able to contain infection without the need for antibiotics, and therefore it is unclear how representative these models are to human disease. More recently, the CMTB model was developed in mice and is a better representation of LTBI in humans [302, 303]. Further work using this model to evaluate prevention of disease vaccine candidates holds promise for better translation of findings from the TB murine model to humans.

Transmission is an extremely important component of TB disease that is much less well studied. In particular, with respect to vaccine development, it is possible that vaccines could protect an individual from disease, but not prevent transmission. Conversely, vaccines could be insufficient to prevent infection or disease in an individual but could still be beneficial from a public health perspective, if they reduce transmission. This is especially important in consideration of prevention of recurrence vaccines, where shortening the period of transmissibility could have large implications on cost of treatment and quality of life of those needing prolonged therapy for MDR or XDR TB. Although rarely utilized, some animal models are useful for transmission modelling. In particular, guinea pig models of natural infection have potential utility in evaluating vaccine efficacy in prevention of transmission, although logistically could be difficult to implement.

8.6.4 Summary and Conclusions

Animal models are and will for the foreseeable future remain a crucial component of candidate vaccine testing. Even though there are multiple well-developed animal models for TB that are very valuable in candidate vaccine testing, there remain gaps in these models. In particular, animal models of latent Mtb infection poorly mimic human disease and continue to represent a major barrier to TB vaccine development. Furthermore, traditionally candidate vaccine testing is often thought of in a linear fashion, with new candidates first evaluated in mouse models before moving into guinea pig models and the NHP models and if successful entering human clinical trials [304]. This linear model, however, leads to significant bottlenecks and misses opportunities to better understand Mtb immunity. In particular, there are very few primate centers around the world, with only seven centers in North America and nine in Europe. This makes NHP studies a particularly scarce resource, and correctly determining the most promising candidates is extremely important. To better understand which candidates should move forward in testing, we must first better understand COPs across species and also in humans. To do this, we must use information on COPs garnered from humans or other animal models and evaluate their applicability for other species in a circular fashion (Fig. 8.3). This is particularly important as more candidate TB vaccines move through clinical trials, as COP may be relatively unique to individual vaccine platforms.

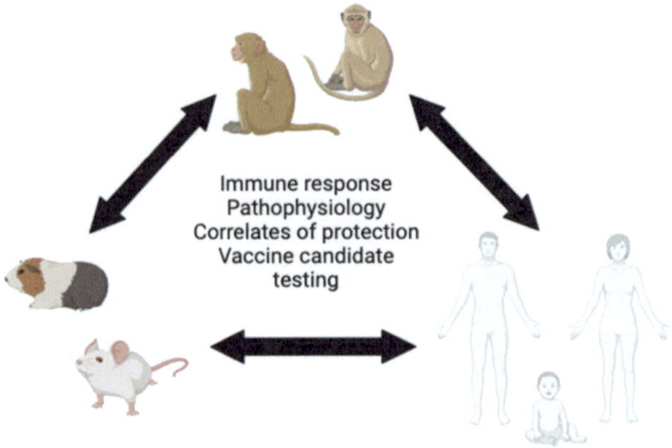

Fig. 8.3 Circular model for utilizing animal models in TB vaccine development and understand TB immunology

8.7 Concluding Remarks

The recent initiation of a Phase 3 trial to assess the efficacy of the Bill & Melinda Gates Medical Research Institute (Gates MRI) M72/AS01E tuberculosis (TB) vaccine candidate highlights both the excitement of the first vaccine in over 100 years to enter last stage testing and the inherent challenges to the evaluation of TB vaccines [305]. As opposed to exposure to and infection with SARS-COV2, the likelihood of developing TB following exposure Mtb is low, such that the Phase 3 trial will require as many as 20,000 participants and is estimated to cost an estimated $550 million dollars (USD) [306].

To allow the more rapid and cost-effective development of novel vaccines, COP are urgently needed. In this regard, it seems likely that these correlates will vary based both on the vaccine composition and on the clinical indication. For example, the M72/AS01E vaccine has been shown to be a potent inducer of poly-functional $CD4^+$ T cells [307], while whole cell vaccines such as TBVAC would be expected to elicit a more diverse immune response including DURTs. Additionally, it seems likely that immune correlates for infants might not be the same as those for adults or adolescents or in the elderly. The gold standard for a COP is a vaccine-induced immune marker that is associated with protection after vaccination. Importantly, these markers are necessarily predictive, but not necessarily mechanistic. As a result, it is imperative to use successful vaccination studies in humans to determine true COP [308]. In parallel, having animal models that reflect the full spectrum of infection and control of infection with Mtb will facilitate the development of these markers. While the mouse model is necessarily used as a means to establish vaccine efficacy, this model does not reflect resistance to infection (IGRA negative in household contacts) and resistance to disease once infected (IGRA positive). As a result, the development and standardization of animal models that reflect these endpoints will allow for more rapid vaccine development and licensure.

References

1. Calmette A, Guérin C, Boquet A, Négre L. La vaccination preventive contre la tuberculose par le “BCG.” Masson, Paris. 1927.
2. Mahairas GG, Sabo PJ, Hickey MJ, et al. Molecular analysis of genetic differences between Mycobacterium bovis BCG and virulent M. Bovis. J Bacteriol. 1996;178:1274–82.
3. Lange C, Aaby P, Behr M, et al. 100 years of *Mycobacterium bovis* bacilli Calmette-Guérin. Lancet Infectious Disease. 2022;22(1):e2–e12.
4. Mangtani P, Abubaka I, Ariti C, et al. Protection by BCG vaccination against tuberculosis: a systematic review of randomized controlled trials. Clin Infect Dis. 2014;58(4):470–80.
5. Benn CS, Roth A, Garly ML, et al. BCG scarring and improved child survival: a combined analysis of studies of BCG scarring. J Intern Med. 2020;288:614–24.
6. Garly ML, Martins CL, Balé C, et al. BCG scar and positive tuberculin reaction associated with reduced child mortality in West Africa. A non-specific beneficial effect of BCG? Vaccine. 2003;21:2782–90.
7. Ahmed A, Rakshit S, Adiga V, et al. A century of BCG: impact on tuberculosis control and beyond. Immunol Rev. 2021;301:98–121.

8. Netea MG, Giamarellos-Bourboulis EJ, Domínguez-Andrés J, et al. Trained immunity: a tool for reducing susceptibility to and the severity of SARS-CoV-2 infection. Cell. 2020;181:969–77.
9. O'Neill LAJ, Netea MG. BCG-induced trained immunity: can it offer protection against COVID-19? Nat Rev Immunol. 2020;20:335–7.
10. Netea MG, Joosten LA, Latz E, et al. Trained immunity: a program of innate immune memory in health and disease. Science. 2016;352:aaf1098.
11. Global Tuberculosis Report 2023. Geneva: World Health Organization; 2023.
12. Rijnink WF, Ottenhoff THM, Joosten SA. B-cells and antibodies as contributors to effector immune responses in tuberculosis. Front Immunol. 2021;12:640168.
13. Sia JK, Rengarajan J. Immunology of *mycobacterium tuberculosis* infections. Microbiol Spectr. 2019;7(4):10.1128.
14. Ferluga J, Yasmin H, Al-Ahdal MN, et al. Natural and trained innate immunity against mycobacterium tuberculosis. Immunobiology. 2020;225(3):151951.
15. Lindestam Arlehamn CS, Lewinsohn DM, Sette A, et al. Antigens for CD4 and CD8 T cells in tuberculosis. Cold Spring Harb Perspect Med. 2014a;4(7):a018465.
16. Scriba TJ, Coussens AK, Fletcher HA. Human immunology of tuberculosis. Microbiol Spectr. 2017a;5(1):TBTB2-0016-2016.
17. Bustamante J, Boisson-Dupuis S, Abel L, Casanova JL. Mendelian susceptibility to mycobacterial disease: genetic, immunological, and clinical features of inborn errors of IFN-γ immunity. Semin Immunol. 2014;26(6):454–70. https://doi.org/10.1016/j.smim.2014.09.008. Epub 2014 Oct 26. PMID: 25453225
18. Lyadova IV, Panteleev AV. Th1 and Th17 cells in tuberculosis: protection, pathology and biomarkers. Mediators Inflamm. 2015;2015:854507.
19. Behar SM. Antigen-specific CD8(+) T cells and protective immunity to tuberculosis. Adv Exp Med Biol. 2013;783:141–63.
20. Lin PL, Flynn JL. CD8 T cells and mycobacterium tuberculosis infection. Semin Immunopathol. 2015;37(3):239–49.
21. Ernst WA, Thoma-Uszynski S, Teitelbaum R, et al. Granulysin, a T cell product, kills bacteria by altering membrane permeability. J Immunol. 2000;165(12):7102–8.
22. Godfrey DI, Uldrich AP, McCluskey J, et al. The burgeoning family of unconventional T cells. Nat Immunol. 2015;16(11):1114–23.
23. Sandstrom A, Peigne CM, Leger A, et al. The intracellular B30.2 domain of butyrophilin 3A1 binds phosphoantigens to mediate activation of human Vgamma9Vdelta2 T cells. Immunity. 2014;40(4):490–500.
24. Van Rhijn I, Moody DB. CD1 and mycobacterial lipids activate human T cells. Immunol Rev. 2015;264(1):138–53.
25. Kim SJ, Karamooz E. MR1- and HLA-E-dependent antigen presentation of *mycobacterial tuberculosis*. Int J Mol Sci. 2022;23(22):14412.
26. James CA, Seshadri C. T cell responses to mycobacterial glycolipids: on the spectrum of "innateness". Front Immunol. 2020;11:170.
27. Gold MC, Eid T, Smyk-Pearson S, et al. Human thymic MR1-restricted MAIT cells are innate pathogen-reactive effectors that adapt following thymic egress. Mucosal Immunol. 2013;6(1):35–44.
28. Swarbrick GM, Gela A, Cansler ME, et al. Postnatal expansion, maturation, and functionality of MR1T cells in humans. Front Immunol. 2020;11:556695.
29. Joosten SA, Ottenhoff THM, Lewinsohn DM, et al. Harnessing donor unrestricted T-cells for new vaccines against tuberculosis. Vaccine. 2019;37(23):3022–30.
30. Spencer CT, Abate G, Blazevic A, Hoft DF. Only a subset of Phosphoantigen-responsive $\gamma_9\delta_2$ T cells mediate protective tuberculosis immunity. J Immunol. 2008;181(7):4471–84.
31. Chen ZW. Protective immune responses of major Vγ2Vδ2 T-cell subset in *M. tuberculosis* infection. Curr Opin Immunol. 2016;42:105–12.

32. Glatman-Freedman A, Casadevall A. Serum therapy for tuberculosis revisited: reappraisal of the role of antibody-mediated immunity against mycobacterium tuberculosis. Clin Microbiol Rev. 1998;11:514–32.
33. Larsen SE, Williams BD, Rais M, et al. It takes a village: the multifaceted immune response to *mycobacterium tuberculosis* infection and Vaccine-induced immunity. Front Immunol. 2022;10(13):840225.
34. Darrah PA, Zeppa JJ, Maiello P, et al. Prevention of tuberculosis in macaques after intravenous BCG immunization. Nature. 2020;577:95–102.
35. Rodrigues LC, Pereira SM, Cunha SS, et al. Effect of BCG revaccination on incidence of tuberculosis in school-aged children in Brazil: the BCG-REVAC cluster-randomised trial. Lancet. 2005;366:1290–5.
36. WHO Report. BCG vaccine: WHO position paper, February 2018—Recommendations.
37. Zhang L, Ru HW, Chen FZ, et al. Variable virulence and efficacy of BCG vaccination strains in mice and correlation with genome polymorphisms. Mol Ther. 2016;24(2):398–405.
38. Poyntz HC, Stylianou E, Griffiths KL, et al. Non-tuberculosis mycobacteria have diverse effects on BCG efficacy against *Mycobacterium tuberculosis*. Tuberculosis. 2014;94(3):226–37.
39. National Library of Medicine. Clinicaltrials.gov. Accessed on 11 Jan 2024.
40. Aaby P, et al. Randomized trial of BCG vaccination at birth to low-birth-weight children: beneficial nonspecific effects in the neonatal period? J Infect Dis. 2011;204(2):245–52.
41. Williams SK, et al. Intravesical therapy for bladder cancer. Expert Opin Pharmacother. 2010;11(6):947–58.
42. Stewart JHT, Levine EA. Role of bacillus Calmette-Guerin in the treatment of advanced melanoma. Expert Rev Anticancer Ther. 2011;11(11):1671–6.
43. Biering-Sorensen S, et al. Small randomized trial among low-birth-weight children receiving bacillus Calmette-Guerin vaccination at first health center contact. Pediatr Infect Dis J. 2012;31(3):306–8.
44. Higgins JP, et al. Association of BCG, DTP, and measles containing vaccines with childhood mortality: systematic review. BMJ. 2016;355:i5170.
45. Pollard AJ, Finn A, Curtis N. Non-specific effects of vaccines: plausible and potentially important, but implications uncertain. Arch Dis Child. 2017;
46. Faustman DL, et al. Proof-of-concept, randomized, controlled clinical trial of Bacillus-Calmette-Guerin for treatment of long-term type 1 diabetes. PLoS One. 2012;7(8):e41756.
47. Ristori G, et al. Effects of Bacille Calmette-Guerin after the first demyelinating event in the CNS. Neurology. 2014;82(1):41–8.
48. Nemes E, Geldenhuys H, Rozot V, et al. Prevention of *M. tuberculosis* Infection with H4:IC31 Vaccine or BCG Revaccination. NEJM. 2018;379:138–49.
49. Glynn JR, Fielding K, Mzembe K, et al. BCG revaccination in Malawi: 30-year follow-up of a large, randomized, double-blind, placebo-controlled trial. Lancet Global Health. 2021a;9(10):e1451–e9.
50. Glynn JR, Dube A, Fielding K, et al. The effect of BCG revaccination on all-cause mortality beyond infancy: 30-year follow-up of a population-based, double-blind, randomized placebo-controlled trial in Malawi. Lancet Infect Dis. 2021b;21(11):1590–7.
51. Karonga Prevention Trial Group. Randomised controlled trial of single BCG, repeated BCG, or combined BCG and killed *Mycobacterium leprae* vaccine for prevention of leprosy and tuberculosis in Malawi. Lancet. 1996;348:17–24.
52. Kallenius G, Pawlowshi A, Brandtzaeg P, Stevenson S. Should a new tuberculosis vaccine be administered intranasally? Tuberculosis. 2007;87(4):257–66.
53. Perdomo C, Zedler U, Kuhl AA, et al. Mucosal BCG vaccination induces protective lung-resident memory T cell populations against tuberculosis. MBio. 2016;7(6):1–11.
54. Aguilo N, Toledo AM, Lopez-Roman EM, et al. Pulmonary mycobacterium bovis BCG vaccination confers dose-dependent superior protection compared to that of subcutaneous vaccination. Clin Vaccine Immunol. 2014;21(4):594–7.

55. Verreck FAW, Tchilian EZ, Vervenne RAW, et al. Variable BCG efficacy in rhesus populations: pulmonary BCG provides protection where standard intra-dermal vaccination fails. Tuberculosis. 2017a;104:46–57.
56. Sharpe S, White A, Sarfas C, et al. Alternative BCG delivery strategies improve protection against mycobacrterium tuberculosis in non-human primates: protection associated with mycobacterial antigen-specific CD4 effector memory T-cell populations. Tuberculosis. 2016a;202:274–90.
57. Vierboom MPM, Dijkman K, Sombroek CC, et al. Stronger induction of trained immunity by mucosal BCG or MTBVAC vaccination compared to standard intradermal vaccination. Cell Rep Med. 2021;2(1):100185.
58. Barclay WR, Busey WM, Dalgard DW, et al. Protection of monkeys against airborne tuberculosis by aerosol vaccination with bacillus calmette-guerin. Am Rev Respir Dis. 1973;107(3):351–8.
59. McShane H, Moss P. Aerosol BCG Challenge Trial in Healthy UK Adults. ClinicalTrials.gov identifier: NCT02709278. Updated November 18th, 2023. Accessed 12 Jan 2024. https://clinicaltrials.gov/study/NCT02709278
60. Uranga S, Marinova D, Martin C, Aguilo N. Protective efficacy and pulmonary immune response following subcutaneous and intranasal BCG administration in mice. J Visual Experiment. 2016;115:1–8.
61. Chen L, Wang J, Zganiacz A, Xing Z. Single intranasal mucosal mycobacterium bovis BCG vaccination confers improved protection compared to subcutaneous vaccination against pulmonary tuberculosis. Infection Immun. 2004;72(1):238–46.
62. Giri PK, Verma I, Khuller GK. Protective efficacy of intranasal vaccination with mycobacterium bovis BCG against airway mycobacterium tuberculosis challenge in mice. J infection. 2006;53(5):350–6.
63. Derrick SC, Kolibab K, Yang A, Morris SL. Intranasal administration of mycobacterium bovis BCG induces superior protection against aerosol infection with mycobacterium tuberculosis in mice. Clin Vaccine Immunol. 2014;21(10):1443–51.
64. Aguilo N, Alvarez-Arguedas S, Uranga S, Marinova D, Monzon M, Badiola J, et al. Pulmonary but not subcutaneous delivery of BCG vaccine confers protection to tuberculosis-susceptible mice by an interleukin 17-dependent mechanism. J Infect Dis. 2016;213(5):831–9.
65. Bull NC, Stylianou E, Kaveh DA, Pinpathomrat N, Pasricha J, HarringtonKandt R, et al. Enhanced protection conferred by mucosal BCG vaccination associates with presence of antigen-specific lung tissue-resident PD-1(+) KLRG1 (−) CD4(+) T cells. Mucosal Immunol. 2019;12(2):555–64.
66. Ancelet LR, Aldwell FE, Rich FJ, Kirman JR. Oral vaccination with lipid-formulated BCG induces a long-lived, multifunctional CD4(+) T cell memory immune response. PLoS One. 2012;7(9):e45888.
67. Abolhassani M, Lagranderie M, Chavarot P, Balazuc AM, Marchal G. Mycobacterium bovis BCG induces similar immune responses and protection by rectal and parenteral immunization routes. Infection Immun. 2000;68(10):5657–62.
68. Lagranderie M, Chavarot P, Balazuc AM, Marchal G. Immunogenicity and protective capacity of mycobacterium bovis BCG after oral or intragastric administration in mice. Vaccine. 2000;18(13):1186–95.
69. Waeckerle-Men Y, Bruffaerts N, Liang Y, Jurion F, Sander P, Kundig TM, et al. Lymph node targeting of BCG vaccines amplifies CD4 and CD8 T-cell responses and protection against mycobacterium tuberculosis. Vaccine. 2013;31(7):1057–64.
70. Singh S, Saavedra-Avila NA, Tiwari S, Porcelli SA. A century of BCG vaccination: immune mechanisms, animal models, non-traditional routes and implications for COVID-19. Front Immunol. 2022a;13:1–22.
71. Kowalewicz-Kulbat M, Locht C. Recombinant BCG to enhance its immunomodulatory activities. MDPI. 2022;10(5):827.

72. O'Donnell MA, Aldovini A, Duda RB, et al. Recombinant *Mycobacterium bovis* BCG secreting functional interleukin-2 enhances gamma interferon production by splenocytes. Infect Immun. 1994;62(6):2508–14.
73. Moreira AL, Tsenova L, Murray PJ, et al. Aerosol infection of mice with recombinant BCG secreting murine IFN-g partially reconstitutes local protective immunity. Microb Pathog. 2000;29:175–85.
74. Wangoo A, Brown IN, Marshall BG, et al. Bacille Calmette-Guérin (BCG)-associated inflammation and fibrosis: modulation by recombinant BCG expressing interferon-gamma (IFN-g). Clin Exp Immunol. 2000;119:92–8.
75. Xu U, Zhu B, Wang Q, et al. Recombinant BCG overexpressing Ag85A, ESAT-6 and mouse IFN-g confers effective protection against *Mycobacterium tuberculosis* in C57BL/6 mice. FEMS Immunol Med Microbiol. 2007;51:480–7.
76. Liu W, Xu Y, Shen H, et al. Recombinant Bacille Calmette-Guérin coexpressing Ag85B-IFN-g enhances the cell-mediated immunity in C57BL/6 mice. Exp Ther Med. 2017;13:2339–47.
77. Arnold J, de Boer EC, O'Donnell MA, et al. Immunotherapy of experimental bladder cancer with recombinant BCG expressing interferon-gamma. J Immunother. 2004;27:116–23.
78. Gan YH, Zhang Y, Khoo HE, Esuvaranathan K. Antitumor immunity of Bacillus Calette-Guérin and interferon alpha in murine bladder cancer. Eur J Cancer. 1999;35:1123–9.
79. Luo Y, Chen R, Han M, O'Donnell M. Recombinant bacille Calmette-Guérin (BCG) expressing human interferon-alpha 2B demonstrates enhanced immunogenicity. Clin Exp Immunol. 2001;123:264–70.
80. Fan X, Han R. Study of recombinant human IFN-a-2b bacilli Calmette-Guérin activated killer cells against bladder cancer cells in vitro. Front Med China. 2007;1:377–80.
81. Ding G, Yu Y, Shen Z, et al. Antitumor effects of human interferon-alpha 2b secreted by recombinant bacillus Calmette-Guérin vaccine on bladder cancer cells. J Zhejiang Univ Sci B. 2012;13:335–41.
82. Sun E, Nian X, Liu C, et al. Construction of recombinant human IFN-a-2b BCG and its antitumor effects on bladder cancer cells in vitro. Genet Mol Res. 2015a;14:3436–49.
83. Sun E, Fan X, Wang L, et al. Recombinant hIFN-a2b-BCG inhibits tumor growth in a mouse model of bladder cancer. Onc Rep. 2015b;34:183–94.
84. Hatano S, Tamura T, Umemura M, et al. Recombinant *Mycobacterium bovis* bacillus Calmette-Guérin expressing Ag85B-IL-7 fusion protein enhances IL-17A-producing innate gd T cells. Vaccine. 2016;34:2490–5.
85. Lin CW, Su IJ, Chang JR, et al. Recombinant BCG coexpressing Ag85B, CFP10, and interleukin-12 induces multifunctional Th1 and memory T cells in mice. Ampis. 2012a;120:72–80.
86. Chen YY, Lin CW, Huang WF, et al. Recombinant bacille Calmette-Guérin coexpressing Ag85b, CFP10, and interleukin-12 elicits effective protection against *Mycobacterium tuberculosis*. J Microbiol Immunol Infect. 2017;50:90–6.
87. Deng Y, Bao L, Yang X. Evaluation of immunogenicity and protective efficacy against *Mycobacterium tuberculosis* infection elicited by recombinant *Mycobacterium bovis* BCG expressing human interleukin-12p70 and early secretory antigen target-6 fusion protein. Microbiol Immunol. 2011;55:798–808.
88. Deng YH, He HY, Zhang FJ. Immunogenicity and protective efficacy conferred by a novel recombinant *Mycobacterium bovis* bacillus Calmette-Guérin strain expressing interleukin-12p70 of human cytokine and Ag85A of *Mycobacterium tuberculosis* fusion protein. Scan J Immunol. 2013;76:497–506.
89. Dai FY, Wang JF, Gong XL, et al. Immunogenicity and protective efficacy of recombinant bacille Calmette-Guérin strains expressing mycobacterium antigens Ag85A, CFP10, ESAT-6, GM-CSF and IL-12p70. Hum Vaccin Immunother. 2017;13:1425–32.
90. Perera LP, Goldman CK, Waldmann TA. IL-15 induces the expression of chemokines and their receptors in T lymphocytes. J Immunol. 1999;162:2606–12.
91. Chapdelaine Y, Smith DK, Pedras-Vasconcelos JA, et al. Increased $CD8^+$ T cell memory to concurrent infection at the expense of increased erosion of pre-existing memory: the paradoxical role of IL-15. J Immunol. 2003;171:5454–60.

92. Takeuchi A, Eto M, Tatsugami K, et al. Antitumor activity of recombinant Bacille Calmette-Guérin secreting interleukin-15-Ag85B fusion protein against bladder cancer. Int Immunopharmacol. 2016;35:327–31.
93. Tang C, Yamada H, Shibata K, et al. Efficacy of recombinant Bacille Calmette-Guérin vaccine secreting interleukin-15/antigen 85B fusion protein in providing protection against *Mycobacterium tuberculosis*. J Infect Dis. 2008;197:1263–74.
94. Biet F, Kremer L, Wolowczuk I, et al. *Mycobacterium bovis* BCG producing interleukin-18 increases antigen-specific gamma interferon production in mice. Infect Immun. 2002;70:5649–6557.
95. Luo Y, Yamada H, Chen X, et al. Recombinant *Mycobacterium bovis* bacillus Calmette-Guérin (BCG) expressing mouse IL-18 augments Th1 immunity and macrophage cytotoxicity. Clin Exp Immunol. 2004;137:24–34.
96. Biet F, Duez C, Kremer L, et al. Recombinant *Mycobacterium bovis* BCG producing IL-18 reduces IL-5 production and bronchoalveolar eosinophilia induced by an allergic reaction. Allergy. 2005;60:1065–72.
97. Szpakowshi P, Biet B, Locht C, et al. Dendritic cell activity driven by recombinant *Mycobacterium bovis* BCG producing human IL-18 in healthy BCG vaccinated adults. J Immunol. 2015;2015:359153.
98. Kowalewicz-Kulbat M, Szpakowski P, Krawczyk KT, et al. Decrease of IL-5 production by naïve T cells cocultured with IL-18-producing BCG-pulsed dendritic cells from patients allergic to house dust mite. Vaccine. 2021;9:277.
99. Huang Y, Matsumura Y, Hatano S, et al. IL-21 inhibits IL-17A-producing gd T-cell response after infection with bacillus Calmette-Guérin via induction of apoptosis. Innate Immun. 2016;22:588–97.
100. Peng W, Wang L, Zhang G, et al. Effects of recombinant IL-35-BCG on Treg/Th17 cell imbalance and inflammatory response in asthmatic newborn mice induced by RSV. Inflammation. 2021;44:2476–85.
101. Ryan AA, Wozniak TM, Shklovskaya E, et al. Improved protection against disseminated tuberculosis by *Mycobacterium bovis* bacillus Calmette-Guérin secreting murine GM-CSF is associated with expansion and activation of APCs. J Immunol. 2007a;179:8414–24.
102. Xang X, Bao L, Deng Y. A novel recombinant *Mycobacterium bovis* bacillus Calmette-Guérin strain expressing human granulocyte macrophage colony-stimulating factor and *Mycobacterium tuberculosis* early secretory antigenic target 6 complex augments Th1 immunity. Acta Biochim Biophys Sin. 2011;43:511–81.
103. Yuan S, Shi C, Ling R, et al. Immunization with two recombinant bacillus Calmette-Guérin vaccines that combine the expression of multiple tandem repeats of mucin-1 and colony stimulating-facto suppress breast tumor growth in mice. J Cancer Res Clin Oncol. 2010;136:1359–67.
104. Xue QJ, Li YQ, Yang CQ, et al. Anti-tumor research of recombinant BCG using BZLF1 and hGM-CSF fusion genes. Vaccine. 2017;35:1599–607.
105. Yan Y, Xue OJ, Liu A, et al. EB virus-positive tumors are inhibited by rBCG expressing hGM-CSF and LMP2A. Hum Vaccin Immunother. 2020;16:654–63.
106. Shen H, Wang C, Yang E, et al. Novel recombinant BCG co-expressing Ag85B, ESAT-6 and mouse TNF-a induces significantly enhanced cellular immune and antibody responses in C57BL/6 mice. Microbiol Immunol. 2010;54:435–41.
107. Kong D, Kunimoto DY. Secretion of human interleukin 2 by recombinant *Mycobacterium bovis* BCG. Infect Immun. 1995;63:799–803.
108. Luo Y, Chen X, Szilvasi A, O'Donnell MA. Co-expression of interleukin-2 and green fluorescent protein reporter in mycobacteria: in vivo application for monitoring antimycobacterial immunity. Mol Immunol. 2000;37:527–36.
109. Murray PJ, Aldovini A, Young RA. Manipulation and potentiation of antimycobacterial immunity using recombinant bacille Calmette-Guérin strains that secrete cytokines. Proc Natl Acad Sci USA. 1996;93:934–9.

110. Slobbe L, Lockhart E, O'Donnell MA, et al. An in vivo comparison of bacillus Calmette-Guérin (BCG) and cytokine-secreting BCG vaccines. Immunology. 1999;96:517–23.
111. Young S, O'Donnell M, Lockhart E, et al. Manipulation of immune responses to *Mycobacterium bovis* by vaccination with IL-2- and IL-18-secreting recombinant bacillus Calmette Guérin. Immunol Cell Biol. 2002a;80:209–15.
112. Young SL, O'Donnell MA, Buchan GS. IL-2-secreting recombinant bacillus Calmette Guérin can overcome a type 2 immune response and corticosteroid-induced immunosuppression to elicit a type 1 immune response. Int Immunol. 2002b;14:793–800.
113. Fan XL, Yu TH, Gao Q, Yao W. Immunological properties of recombinant *Mycobacterium bovis* Bacillus Calmette-Guérin strain expressing fusion protein IL-2-ESAT-6. Acta Biochim Biophys Sin. 2006;38:683–90.
114. Duda RB, Yang H, Dooley DD, Abu-Jawdeh G. Recombinant BCG therapy suppresses melanoma tumor growth. Ann Surg Oncol. 1995;2:542–9.
115. Brosch R, Gordon SV, Pym A, et al. Comparative genomics of the mycobacteria. Int J Med Microbiol. 2000;290:143–52.
116. Joung SM, Ryoo S. BCG vaccine in Korea. Clin Exp Vaccine Res. 2014;2:83–91.
117. Cole ST, Brosch R, Parkhill J, et al. Deciphering the biology of *Mycobacterium tuberculosis* from the complete genomic sequence. Nature. 1998a;393:537–44.
118. Pym AS, Brodin P, Majlessi L, et al. Recombinant BCG exporting ESAT-6 confers enhanced protection against tuberculosis. Nat Med. 2003;9:533–9.
119. Wiker HG, Harboe M. The antigen 85 complex: a major secretion product of mycobacterium tuberculosis. Microbiological Rev. 1992;56(4):648–61.
120. Belisle JT, Vissa VD, Sievert T, et al. Role of the major antigen of mycobacterium tuberculosis in cell wall biogenesis. Science. 1997;276(5317):1420–2.
121. Hoft DF, Blazevic A, Abate G, et al. A new recombinant Bacille Calmette-Guérin vaccine safely induces significantly enhanced tuberculosis-specific immunity in human volunteers. J Infect Dis. 2008;198(10):1491–501.
122. Hayward CMM, O'Gaora P, Young DB. Construction and murine immunogenicity of recombinant Bacille Calmette Guerin vaccines expressing the B subunit of *E. coli* heat labile enterotoxin. Vaccine. 1999;17:272–1281.
123. Nascimento IP, Rodriguez D, Issamu AK, et al. Recombinant BCG expressing LTAK63 adjuvant induces superior protection against Mycobacterium tuberculosis. Sci Rep. 2017;7:2109.
124. Dos Santos CC, Rodriguez D, Issamu AK, et al. Recombinant BCG expressing the LTAK63 adjuvant induces increased early and long-term immune responses against mycobacteria. Hum Vaccin Immunother. 2020;16:673–83.
125. Biet F, Kremer L, Wolowczuk I, et al. Immune response induced by recombinant Mycobacterium bovis BCG producing the cholera toxin B subunit. Infect Immun. 2003;71:2933–7.
126. Kim PH, Eckmann L, Lee WJ, et al. Cholera toxin and cholera toxin B subunit induce IgA switching through the action of TGF-beta. J Immunol. 1998;160:1198–203.
127. Rodriguez D, Goulart C, Pagliarone AC, et al. In vitro evidence of human immune responsiveness shows the improved potential of a recombinant BCG strain for bladder cancer treatment. Front Immunol. 2019;10:1460.
128. Chade DC, Borra RC, Nascimento IP, et al. Immunomodulatory effects of recombinant BCG expressing pertussis toxin on TNF-alpha and IL-10 in a bladder cancer model. J Exp Clin Cancer Res. 2008;27:78.
129. Andrade PM, Chade DC, Borra RC, et al. The therapeutic potential of recombinant BCG expressing the antigen S1PT in the intravesical treatment of bladder cancer. Urol Oncol. 2010;28:520–5.
130. Kanno AI, Boraschi D, Leite LCC, Rodriguez D. Recombinant BCG expressing the subunit 1 of pertussis toxin induces innate immune memory and confers protection against non-related pathogens. Vaccine. 2022;10:234.

131. Christ AP, Rodriguez D, Bortolatto J, et al. Enhancement of Th1 lung immunity induced by recombinant *Mycobacterium bovis* bacillus Calmette-Guérin attenuates airway allergic disease. Am J Respir Cell Mol Biol. 2010;43:243–52.
132. Sun R, Skeiky YA, Izzo A, et al. Novel recombinant BCG expressing perfringolysin O and the over-expression of key immunodominant antigens: pre-clinical characterization, safety and protection against challenge with *Mycobacterium tuberculosis*. Vaccine. 2009;27:4412–23.
133. Henao-Tamayo M, Shanley CA, Verma D, et al. The efficacy of the BCG vaccine against newly emerging clinical strains of *Mycobacterium tuberculosis*. PLoS One. 2015;10:e0136500.
134. Magalhaes I, Sizemore DR, Ahmed RK, et al. rBCG induces strong antigen-specific T cell responses in rhesus macaques in a prime-boost setting with an adenovirus 35 tuberculosis vaccine vector. PLoS One. 2008;3:e3790.
135. Hess J, Miko D, Catic A, et al. *Mycobacterium bovis* bacilli Calmette-Guérin strains secreting listeriolysin of *listeria monocytogenes*. Proc Natl Acad Sci USA. 1998;95:5299–304.
136. Conradt P, Hess J, Kaufmann SHE. Cytotoxic T-cell responses to human dendritic cells and macrophages infected with *Mycobacterium bovis* BCG and recombinant BCG secreting listeriolysin. Microbes Infect. 1999;1:753–64.
137. Grode L, Seiler P, Baumann S, et al. Increased vaccine efficacy against tuberculosis of recombinant *Mycobacterium bovis* bacille Calmette-Guérin mutants that secrete listeriolysin. J Clin Infest. 2005;115:2472–9.
138. Vogelzang A, Perdomo C, Zedler U, et al. Central memory $CD4^+$ T cells are responsible for the recombinant Bacillus Calmette-Guérin Δ*ureC::hly* vaccine's superior protection against tuberculosis. J Infect Dis. 2014;210:1928–37.
139. Desel C, Dorhoi A, Bandermann S, et al. Recombinant BCGΔ*ureChly*$^+$ induces superior protection over parental BCG by stimulating a balanced combination of type 1 and type 17 cytokine responses. J Infect Dis. 2011;204:1573–84.
140. Saiga H, Nieuwenhuizen N, Gengenbacher M, et al. The recombinant BCGΔ*ureC::hly* vaccine targets the AIM2 inflammasome to induce autophagy and inflammation. J Infect Dis. 2015;211:1831–41.
141. Grode L, Ganoza CA, Brohm C, et al. Safety and immunogenicity of the recombinant BCG vaccine VPM1002 in a phase I open-label randomized clinical trial. Vaccine. 2013;31:1340–8.
142. Loxton AG, Knaul JK, Grode L, et al. Safety and immunogenicity of the recombinant *Mycobacterium bovis* BCG vaccine VPM1002 in HIV-unexposed newborn infants in South Africa. Clin Vaccine Immunol. 2017;2:e00439–16.
143. Gengenbacher M, Nieuwenhuizen N, Vogelzang A, et al. Deletion of *nuoG* from the vaccine candidate *Mycobacterium bovis* BCGΔ*ureC::hly* improves protection against tuberculosis. MBio. 2016;7:e00679–16.
144. Rentsch CA, Bosshard P, Mayor G, et al. Results of the phase I open label clinical trial SAKK 06/14 assessing safety of intravesical instillation of VPM1002BC, a recombinant *mycobacterium* bacillus Calmette Guérin (BCG), in patients with non-muscle invasive bladder cancer and previous failure of conventional BCG therapy. Onco Targets Ther. 2020;9:e1748981.
145. Hoft DF, Blazevic A, Selimovic A, et al. Safety and immunogenicity of the recombinant BCG Vaccine AERAS-422 in healthy BCG-naïve adults: a randomized, active-controlled, first-in-human phase 1 trial. EBioMedicine. 2016;7:278–86.
146. Nieuwenhuizen NE, Kulkarni PS, Shaligram U, et al. The recombinant Bacille Calmette–Guérin vaccine VPM1002: ready for clinical efficacy testing. Front Immunol. 2017;8:1147.
147. StopTBPartnership. TB Vaccine Clinical Pipeline. Accessed 20 Jan 2024. https://newtbvaccines.org/tb-vaccine-pipeline/clinical-phase/
148. Triccas JA, Shklovskaya E, Spratt J, et al. Effects of DNA- and *Mycobacterium bovis* BCG-based delivery of the Flt3 ligand on protective immunity to *Mycobacterium tuberculosis*. Infect Immun. 2007;75:5368–75.
149. Ryan AA, Spratt JM, Britton WJ, Triccas JA. Secretion of functional monocyte chemotactic protein 3 by recombinant *Mycobacterium bovis* BCG attenuates vaccine virulence and maintains protective efficacy against *M. tuberculosis* infection. Infect Immun. 2007b;75:523–6.

150. Li G, Liu G, Song N, et al. A novel recombinant BCG-expressing pro-apoptotic potein BAX enhances Th1 protective immune responses in mice. Mol Immunol. 2015;66:346–56.
151. Mizuno S, Soma S, Inada H, et al. SOCS1 antagonist-expressing Calmette-Guérin enhances antituberculosis protection in a mouse model. J Immunol. 2019;203:188–97.
152. Carow B, Ye X, Gaver-Widen D, Bhuju S, et al. Silencing suppressor of cytokine signaling-1 (SOCS1) in macrophages improves *Mycobacterium tuberculosis* control in an interferon-gamma (IFN-gamma)-dependent manner. J Biol Chem. 2011;286:26873–87.
153. Sendide K, Deghmane AE, Pechkovsky D, et al. *Mycobacterium bovis* BCG attenuates surface expression of mature class II molecules through IL-10-dependent inhibition of cathepsin S. J Immunol. 2005;175:5324–32.
154. Soualhine H, Deghmane AE, Sun J, et al. Mycobacterium bovis bacilli Calmette-Guérin secreting active cathepsin S stimulates expression of mature MHC class II molecules and antigen presentation in human macrophages. J Immunol. 2007;179:5137–45.
155. Tabouret G, Astarie-Dequeker C, Demangel C, et al. *Mycobacterium leprae* phenolglycolipid-1 expressed by engineered *M. bovis* BCG modulates early interaction with human phagocytes. PLoS One. 2010;6:e1001159.
156. Manca C, Peixoto B, Malaga W, et al. Modulation of the cytokine response in human monocytes by *Mycobacterium leprae* phenolic glycolipod-1. J Interf Cytokine Res. 2012;32:27–33.
157. Singh AK, Praharaj M, Lombardo KA, et al. Re-engineered BCG overexpressing cyclic di-AMP augments trained immunity and exhibits improved efficacy against bladder cancer. Nat Comms. 2022b;13:878.
158. Sadagopal S, Braunstein M, Hager CC, et al. Reducing the activity and secretion of microbial antioxidants enhances the immunogenicity of BCG. PLoS One. 2009;4:e5531.
159. Festjens N, Bogaert P, Batni A, et al. Disruption of the SapM locus of *Mycobacterium bovis* BCG improves its protective efficacy as a vaccine against *M. tuberculosis*. EMBO Mol Med. 2011;3:222–34.
160. Festjens N, Vandewalle K, Houthuys E, et al. SapM mutation to improve the BCG vaccine: genomic, transcriptomic and preclinical safety characterization. Vaccine. 2019;37:3539–51.
161. Wu Y, Zhang Y, Peng H, et al. Deletion of *BCG_2432c* from the bacillus Calmette-Guérin vaccine enhances autophagy-mediated immunity against tuberculosis. Allergy. 2022;77:619–32.
162. Johansen P, Fettelschoss A, Amstutz B, et al. Relief from Zmp1-mediated arrest of phagosome maturation is associated with facilitated presentation and enhanced immunogenicity of mycobacterial antigens. Clin Vaccine Immunol. 2011;18:907–13.
163. Sander P, Clark S, Petrera A, et al. Deletion of *zmp1* improves *Mycobacterium bovis* BCG-mediated protection in a Guinea pig model of tuberculosis. Vaccine. 2015;33:1353–9.
164. Shoen CM, DeStefano MS, Hager CC, et al. A modified Bacillus Calmette-Guérin (BCG) vaccine with reduced activity of antioxidants and glutamine synthetase exhibits enhanced protection of mice despite diminished in vivo persistence. Vaccine. 2013;1:34–57.
165. Woodland DL. Jump-starting the immune system: prime-boosting comes of age. Trends Immunol. 2004;25(2):98–104.
166. Estcourt MH, Ramsay AJ, Brooks A, et al. Prime-boost immunization generates a high frequency, high-avidity CD8(+) cytotoxic T lymphocyte population. Int Immunol. 2002;14(1):31–7.
167. Goonetilleke NP, McShane H, Hannan CM, et al. Enhanced immunogenicity and protective efficacy against mycobacterium tuberculosis of bacille calmette-guerin vaccine using mucosal administration and boosting with a recombinant modified vaccinia virus Ankara. J Immunol. 2003;171(3):1602–9.
168. Kaveh DA, Garcia-Pelayo MC, Webb PR, et al. Parenteral adenoviral boost enhances BCG induced protection, but not long-term survival in a murine model of bovine TB. Vaccine. 2016;34(34):4003–11.
169. Santosuosso M, McCormick S, Zhang X, et al. Intranasal boosting with an adenovirus-vectored vaccine markedly enhances protection by parenteral mycobacterium bovis BCG immunization against pulmonary tuberculosis. Infect Immun. 2006;74(8):4634–43.

170. Abel B, Tameris M, Mansoor N, et al. The novel tuberculosis vaccine, AERAS-402, induces robust and polyfunctional CD4+ and CD8+ T cells in adults. Am J Respir Crit Care Med. 2010;181(12):1407–17.
171. Hoft DF, Blazevic A, Stanley J, et al. A recombinant adenovirus expressing immunodominant TB antigens can significantly enhance BCG-induced human immunity. Vaccine. 2012;30(12):2098–108.
172. Lu J, Wang C, Zhou Z, et al. Immunogenicity and protective efficacy against murine tuberculosis of a prime-boost regimen with BCG and a DNA vaccine expressing ESAT-6 and Ag85A fusion protein. Clin Dev Immunol. 2011;2011:617892.
173. Kang H, Yuan Q, Ma H, et al. Enhanced protective efficacy against mycobacterium tuberculosis afforded by BCG prime-DNA boost regimen in an early challenge mouse model is associated with increased splenic interleukin-2-producing CD4 T-cell frequency post-vaccination. Immunology. 2014;143(4):661–9.
174. Rahman MJ, Fernandez C. Neonatal vaccination with mycobacterium bovis BCG: potential effects as a priming agent shown in a heterologous prime boost immunization protocol. Vaccine. 2009;27(30):4038–46.
175. Guerrero GG, Debrie AS, Locht C. Boosting with mycobacterial heparin binding haemagglutinin enhances protection of mycobacterium bovis BCG vaccinated newborn mice against *M. Tuberculosis*. Vaccine. 2010;28(27):4340–7.
176. Fukui M, Shinjo K, Umemura M, et al. Enhanced effect of BCG vaccine against pulmonary mycobacterium tuberculosis infection in mice with lung Th17 response to mycobacterial heparin-binding hemagglutinin adhesin antigen. Microbiol Immunol. 2015;59(12):735–43.
177. Demissie A, Leyten EM, Abebe M, et al. Recognition of stage-specific mycobacterial antigens differentiates between acute and latent infections with mycobacterium tuberculosis. Clin Vaccine Immunol. 2006;13(2):179–86.
178. Siddiqui KF, Amir M, Khan N, et al. Prime-boost vaccination strategy with bacillus calmette-guerin (BCG) and liposomized alpha-crystalline protein 1 reinvigorates BCG potency. Clin Exp Immunol. 2015;181(2):286–96.
179. Dey B, Jain R, Gupta UD, et al. A booster vaccine expressing a latency-associated antigen augments BCG induced immunity and confers enhanced protection against tuberculosis. PLoS One. 2011;6(8):e23360.
180. Lin PL, Dietrich J, Tan E, et al. The multistage vaccine H56 boosts the effects of BCG to protect cynomolgus macaques against active tuberculosis and reactivation of latent mycobacterium tuberculosis infection. J Clin Invest. 2012b;122(1):303–14.
181. Pai M, Behr MA, Dowdy D, et al. Tuberculosis. Nat Rev Dis Primers. 2016;2:16076.
182. Sutherland I. The ten-year incidence of clinical tuberculosis following "conversion" in 2550 individuals aged 14–19 years. The Hague: TSRU Progress Report; 1968.
183. Ferebee SH, Mount FW. Tuberculosis morbidity in a controlled trial of the prophylactic use of isoniazid among household contacts. Am Rev Respir Dis. 1962;85:490–510.
184. Vynnycky E, Fine PE. The natural history of tuberculosis: the implications of age-dependent risks of disease and the role of reinfection. Epidemiol Infect. 1997;119:183–201.
185. Reichler MR, Khan A, Sterling TR, et al. Tuberculosis epidemiologic studies consortium task order 2 team. Risk and timing of tuberculosis among close contacts of persons with infectious tuberculosis. J Infect Dis. 2018;218:1000–8.
186. Vega V, Rodriquez S, der Stuyft V, et al. Recurrent TB: a systematic review and meta-analysis of the incidence rates and the proportions of relapses and reinfections. Thorax. 2021;76(5):494–502.
187. Qiu B, Wu Z, Tao B, et al. Risk factors for types of recurrent tuberculosis (reactivation versus reinfection): a global systematic review and meta-analysis. Int J Infect Dis. 2022;116:14–20.
188. Cox H, Kebede Y, Allamuratova S, et al. Tuberculosis recurrence and mortality after successful treatment: impact of drug resistance. PLoS Med. 2006;3(10):e384.
189. Mase SR, Chorda T. Treatment of drug-resistant tuberculosis. Clin Chest Med. 2019;40(4):775–95.

190. Pollard AJ, Bijker EM. A guide to vaccinology: from basic principles to new developments. Nat Rev Immunol. 2021;21:83–100.
191. Lai R, Ogunsole AF, Rakib T, Behar SM. Key advances in vaccine development for tuberculosis—success and challenges. NPJ Vaccines. 2023;8:158.
192. Jenner E. An inquiry into the cause and effects of the variolae vaccinae: a disease discovered in some of the western counties of England, particularly Gloucestershire, and known by the name of the cow pox. Springfield [MA]; 1802.
193. Netea MG, Quintin J, van der Meer JWM. Trained immunity: a memory for innate host defense. Cell Host Microbe. 2011;9:355–61.
194. Kleinnijenhuis J, Quintin J, Preijers F, et al. Bacille Calmette-Guérin induces NOD2-dependent nonspecific protection form reinfection via epigenetic reprogramming of monocytes. PNAS. 2012;109(43):17537–42.
195. Arbues A, Aguilo JI, Gonzalo-Asensio J, et al. Construction, characterization and preclinical evaluation of MTBVAC, the first live-attenuated M. Tuberculosis-based vaccine to enter clinical trials. Vaccine. 2013;31:4867–73.
196. Martin C, Williams A, Hernandez-Pando R, et al. The live *Mycobacterium tuberculosis* phoP mutant strain is more attenuated than BCG and confers protective immunity against tuberculosis in mice and Guinea pigs. Vaccine. 2006;24:3408–19.
197. Aguilar D, Infante E, Martin C, et al. Immunological responses and protective immunity against tuberculosis conferred by vaccination of Balb/C mice with the attenuated *Mycobacterium tuberculosis* (phoP) SO2 strain. Clin Exp Immunol. 2007;147:330–8.
198. Cardona PJ, Asensio JG, Arbues A, et al. Extended safety studies of the attenuated live tuberculosis vaccine SO2 based on phoP mutant. Vaccine. 2009;27:2499–505.
199. Verreck FA, Vervenne RA, Kondova KW, et al. MVA.85A boosting of BCG and an attenuated, phoP deficient *M. Tuberculosis* vaccine both show protective efficacy against tuberculosis in rhesus macaques. PLoS One. 2009;4(4):e5264.
200. Lahey T, Laddy D, Hill K, et al. Immunogenicity and protective efficacy of the DAR-901 booster Vaccine in a murine model of tuberculosis. PLoS One. 2016;11(12):e0168521.
201. Munseri P, Said J, Amour M, et al. DAR-901 vaccine for the prevention of infection with *Mycobacterium tuberculosis* among BCG-immunized adolescents in Tanzania: a randomized controlled, double-blind phase 2b trial. Vaccine. 2020;38(46):7239–45.
202. Vilaplana C, Gil O, Caceres N, et al. Prophylactic effect of a therapeutic vaccine against TB based on fragments of *Mycobacterium tuberculosis*. PLoS One. 2011;6:e20404.
203. Bourinbaiar AS, Batbold U, Efremenko Y, et al. Phase III, placebo-controlled, randomized, double-blind trial of tableted, therapeutic TB vaccine (V7) containing heat-killed *M. vaccae* administered daily for one month. J Clin Tuberc Other Mycobact Dis. 2019;18:100141.
204. Cole ST, Brosch R, Parkill J, et al. Deciphering the biology of *Mycobacterium tuberculosis* from the complete genome sequence. Nature. 1998b;393:537–44.
205. Aagaard C, Hoang TT, Izzo A, et al. Protection and polyfunctional T cells induced by Ag85B-TB10.4/IC31 against *Mycobacterium tuberculosis* is highly dependent on the antigen dose. PLoS One. 2009;4(6):e5930–0.
206. Aichinger MC, Ginzler M, Weghuber J, et al. Adjuvating the adjuvant: facilitated delivery of an immunomodulatory oligonucleotide to TLR9 by a cationic antimicrobial peptide in dendritic cells. Vaccine. 2011;29:426–36.
207. Elvang T, Christensen JP, Billeskov R, et al. CD4 and CD8 T cell responses to the *M. Tuberculosis* Ag85B-TB10.4 promoted by adjuvanted subunit, adenovector or heterologous prime boost vaccination. PLoS One. 2009;4(4):e5139–9.
208. Billeskov R, Elvang TT, Andersen PL, Dietrich J. The HyVac4 subunit vaccine efficiently boosts BCG-primed anti-mycobacterial protective immunity. PLoS One. 2012;7(6):e39909–9.
209. Van Maele L, Fourgeron D, Cayet D, et al. Toll-like receptor 4 signaling in hematopoietic-lineage cells contributes to the enhanced activity of the human vaccine adjuvant AS01. Eur J Immunol. 2019;49(12):2134–45.
210. Brandt L, Skeiky YA, Alderson MR, et al. The protective effect of the Mycobacterium bovis BCG vaccine is increased by coadministration with the *Mycobacterium tuberculosis*

72-kilodalton fusion polyprotein Mtb72F in *M. Tuberculosis*-infected Guinea pigs. Infect Immun. 2004;72:6622–32.
211. Tsenova L, Harbacheuski R, Moreira AL, et al. Evaluation of the Mtb72F polyprotein vaccine in a rabbit model of tuberculous meningitis. Infect Immun. 2006;74:2392–401.
212. Irwin SM, Izzo AA, Dow SW, et al. Tracking antigen-specific CD8 T lymphocytes in the lungs of mice vaccinated with the Mtb72F polyprotein. Infect Immun. 2005;73:5809–16.
213. Tait DR, Hatherill M, Van Der Meeren O, et al. Final analysis of a trial of M72/AS01$_E$ Vaccine to prevent tuberculosis. NEJM. 2019;381:2429–39.
214. Aagaard C, Hoang T, Dietrich J, et al. A multistage tuberculosis vaccine that confers efficient protection before and after exposure. Nat Med. 2011;17(2):189–94.
215. Bertholet S, Ireton GC, Kahn M, et al. Identification of human T cell antigens for the development of vaccines against *Mycobacterium tuberculosis*. J Immunol. 2008;181:7948–57.
216. Coler RN, Bertholet S, Moutaftsi M, et al. Development and characterization of synthetic glucopyranosyl lipid adjuvant system as a vaccine adjuvant. PLoS One. 2011;6:e16333.
217. Jenum S, Tonby K, Rueegg CS, et al. A phase I/II randomized trial of H56:IC31 vaccination and adjunctive cyclooxygenase-2- inhibitor treatment in tuberculosis patients. Nat Comms. 2021;12:6774.
218. Sagawa ZK, Goman C, Frevol A, et al. Safety and immunogenicity of a thermostable ID93 + GLA-SE tuberculosis vaccine candidate in healthy adults. Nat Comms. 2023;14:1138.
219. Behzad H, Huckriede ALW, Haynes L, et al. GLA-SE, a synthetic toll-like receptor 4 agonist, enhances T-cell responses to influenza vaccine in older adults. J Infect Dis. 2012;205(3):466–73.
220. Smaill F, Jeyanathan M, Smieja M, et al. A human type 5 adenovirus–based tuberculosis vaccine induces robust T cell responses in humans despite preexisting anti-adenovirus immunity. Sci Transl Med 2013;5(205):205ra134.
221. Churchyard GJ, Snowden MA, Hokey D, et al. The safety and immunogenicity of an adenovirus type 35-vectored TB vaccine in HIV-infected, BCG-vaccinated adults with $CD4^+$ T cell counts >350 cells/mm^3. Vaccine. 2015;33(15):1890–6.
222. McShane H, Athanm AA, Sander CR, et al. Recombinant modified vaccinia virus Ankara expressing antigen 85A boosts BCG-primed and naturally acquired antimycobacterial immunity in humans. Nat Med. 2004;10(11):1240–4.
223. Tameris MD, Hatherill M, Landry BS, et al. Safety and efficacy of MVA85A, a new tuberculosis vaccine, in infants previously vaccinated with BCG: a randomised, placebo-controlled phase 2b trial. Lancet. 2013;381(9871):1021–8.
224. Hansen SG, Zak DE, Xu G, et al. Prevention of tuberculosis in rhesus macaques by a cytomegalovirus-based vaccine. Nat Med. 2018;24(2):130–43.
225. Zeng J, Jaijyan DK, Yang S, et al. Exploring the potential of cytomegalovirus-based vectors: a review. Viruses. 2023;15(10):2043.
226. Jeyanathan M, Thanthrige-Don N, Afkhami S, et al. Novel chimpanzee adenovirus-vectored respiratory mucosal tuberculosis vaccine: overcoming local anti-human adenovirus immunity for potent TB protection. Mucosal Immunol. 2015;8:1373–87.
227. Afkhami S, Lai R, D'Agostino MR, et al. Single-dose mucosal immunotherapy with chimpanzee adenovirus-based vaccine accelerates tuberculosis disease control and limits its rebound after antibiotic cessation. J Infect Dis. 2019;220:1355–66.
228. Afkhami S, D'Agostino MR, Vaseghi-Shanjani M, et al. Intranasal multivalent adenoviral-vectored vaccine protects against replicating and dormant M.tb in conventional and humanized mice. NPJ Vaccines. 2023;8:25.
229. Stylianou E, Griffiths KL, Poyntz HC, et al. Improvement of BCG protective efficacy with a novel chimpanzee adenovirus and a modified vaccinia Ankara virus both expressing Ag85A. Vaccine. 2015;33:6800–8.
230. Verbeke R, Lentacker I, De Smedt SC, Dewitte H. Three decades of messenger RNA vaccine development. Nano Today. 2019;28:100766.
231. Chaudhary N, Weissman D, Whitehead KN. mRNA vaccines for infectious diseases: principles, delivery, and clinical translation. Nat Rev Drug Discov. 2021;20:817–38.

232. Larsen SE, Erasmus JH, Reese AV, et al. An RNA-based vaccine platform for use against *Mycobacterium tuberculosis*. Vaccine. 2023;11(1):130.
233. Mendoza RU, Dayrit MM, Alfonso CR, Ong MMA. Public trust and the COVID-19 vaccine campaign: lessons from The Philippines as it emerges from the Dengvaxia controversy. Int J Health Plann Manag. 2021;36(6):2048–55.
234. WHO Fact Sheet. Tuberculosis. November 7th, 2023. https://www.who.int/news-room/fact-sheets/detail/tuberculosis#:~:text=TB%20and%20HIV&text=Without%20proper%20treatment%2C%2060%25%20of,died%20of%20HIV%2Dassociated%20TB. Accessed on 21 Feb 2024.
235. Li J, Zhao A, Tang J, et al. Tuberculosis vaccine development: from classic to clinical candidates. European J of Clin Micro and Inf Dis. 2020;39:1405–25.
236. WHO. Safety of BCG vaccination in immunocompromised individuals. January 29th, 2010. https://www.who.int/groups/global-advisory-committee-on-vaccine-safety/topics/bcg-vaccines#:~:text=Use%20of%20BCG%20vaccine%20in%20HIV%2Dinfected%20infants&text=Thus%2C%20BCG%20may%20therefore%20provide,to%20be%20infected%20with%20HIV. Accessed on 21 Feb 2024.
237. Shimizu H, Thorley B, Paladin FJ, et al. Circulation of type 1 vaccine-derived poliovirus in The Philippines in 2001. J Virol. 2004;78(24):13512–21.
238. Ford CB, Lin PL, Chase MR, et al. Use of whole genome sequencing to estimate the mutation rate of Mycobacterium tuberculosis during latent infection. Nat Genet. 2010;43(5):482–8.
239. Walker KB, Brennan MJ, Ho MM, et al. The second Geneva consensus: recommendations for novel live TB vaccines. Vaccine. 2010;28(11):2259–70.
240. TB Vaccine Development Pathway. Preclinical Safety. 2019. https://www.tbvacpathway.org/functions/preclinical-safety. Accessed on 21 Feb 2024.
241. CDC. Historical Vaccine Safety Concerns. 2020. https://www.cdc.gov/vaccinesafety/concerns/concerns-history.html. Accessed 21 Feb 2024.
242. Carapetis J. The cutter incident: how America's first polio vaccine led to the growing vaccine crisis. BMJ. 2006;332(7543):733.
243. Fox GJ, Orlova M, Schurr E. Tuberculosis in newborns: the lessons of the "Lübeck disaster" (1929–1933). PLoS Pathog. 2016;12(1):e1005271.
244. WHO. Annex 1—WHO guidelines on non-clinical evaluation of vaccines. WHO Technical Report Series, No. 927. 2005;
245. Gagneux X, Small PM. Global phylogeography of Mycobacterium tuberculosis and implications for tuberculosis product development. Lancet Infect Dis. 2007;7:328–37.
246. Cooper AM, Dalton DK, Stewart TA, et al. Disseminated tuberculosis in IFN-γ gene-disrupted mice. JEM. 1993;178:2243.
247. Flynn JL, Chan J, Triebold KJ, et al. An essential role of Interferon-γ in resistance to *Mycobacterium tuberculosis* infection. J Exp Med. 1993;178:2249.
248. Lindestam Arlehamn CS, Lewinsohn D, Sette A, Lewinsohn D. Antigens for CD4 and CD8 T cells in tuberculosis. Cold Spring Harb Perspect Med. 2014b;4(7):a018465.
249. Nagai S, Wiker HG, Harboe M, Kinomoto M. Isolation and partial characterization of major protein antigens in the culture fluid of *Mycobacterium tuberculosis*. Infect Immun. 1991;59:372–82.
250. Boesen H, Jensen B, Wilcke T, Andersen P. Human T-cell responses to secreted antigen fractions of *Mycobacterium tuberculosis*. Infect Immun. 1995;63:1491–7.
251. Covert BA, Spencer JS, Orme IM, Belisle JT. The application of proteomics in defining the T cell antigens of *Mycobacterium tuberculosis*. Proteomics. 2001;1:574–86.
252. Andersen P, Doherty TM. TB subunit vaccines—putting the pieces together. Microbes Infect. 2005;7:911–21.
253. Hubbard RD, Flory CM, Collins FM. Immunization of mice with mycobacterial culture filtrate proteins. Clin Exp Immunol. 1992;87:94–8.
254. Pal PG, Horwitz MA. Immunization with extracellular proteins of *Mycobacterium tuberculosis* induces cell-mediated immune responses and substantial protective immunity in a Guinea pig model of pulmonary tuberculosis. Infect Immun. 1992;60:4781–92.

255. Andersen P. The T cell response to secreted antigens of *Mycobacterium tuberculosis*. Immunobiology. 1994;191:537–47.
256. Blythe M, Zhang Q, Vaughan K, et al. An analysis of the epitope knowledge related to mycobacteria. Immunome Res. 2007;3:10.
257. Axelsson-Robertson R, Magalhaes I, Parida SK, et al. The immunological footprint of *Mycobacterium tuberculosis* T-cell epitope recognition. J Infect Dis. 2012;205:S301–15.
258. Schnappinger D, Ehrt S, Voskuil MI, et al. Transcriptional adaptation of *Mycobacterium tuberculosis* within macrophages: insights into the phagosomal environment. J Exp Med. 2003;198:693–704.
259. Wilkinson RJ, Wilkinson KA, De Smet KAL, et al. Human T- and B-cell reactivity to the 16 kDa α-crystallin protein of *Mycobacterium tuberculosis*. Scand J Immunol. 1998;48:403–9.
260. Leyten EMS, Lin MY, Franken KLMC, et al. Human T-cell responses to 25 novel antigens encoded by genes of the dormancy regulon of *Mycobacterium tuberculosis*. Microbes Infect. 2006;8:2052–60.
261. Zu Bentrup KH, Russell DG. Mycobacterial persistence: adaptation to a changing environment. Trends Microbiol. 2001;9:597–605.
262. Yuan Y, Crane DD, Barry CE. Stationary phase-associated protein expression in *Mycobacterium tuberculosis*: function of the mycobacterial α-crystallin homolog. J Bacteriol. 1996;178:4484–92.
263. Florczyk MA, McCue LA, Stack RF, et al. Identification and characterization of mycobacterial proteins differentially expressed understanding and shaking culture conditions, including Rv2623 from a novel class of putative ATP-binding proteins. Infect Immun. 2001;69:5777–85.
264. Monahan IM, Betts J, Banerjee DK, Butcher PD. Differential expression of mycobacterial proteins following phagocytosis by macrophages. Microbiology. 2001;147:459–71.
265. Lewinsohn DA, Swarbrick GM, Park B, et al. Comprehensive definition of human immunodominant CD8 antigens in tuberculosis. NPJ Vaccines. 2019;2(8):1–11.
266. Rogerson BJ, Jung YJ, LaCourse R, et al. Expression levels of Mycobacterium tuberculosis antigen-encoding genes versus production levels of antigen-specific T cells during stationary level lung infection in mice. Immunology. 2006;118:195–201.
267. Baena A, Porcelli SA. Evasion and subversion of antigen presentation by Mycobacterium tuberculosis. Tissue Antigens. 2009;74:189–204.
268. Cole ST, Brosch R, Parkhill J, et al. Deciphering the biology of *Mycobacterium tuberculosis* from the complete genome sequence. Nature. 1998c;396(190):537–44.
269. Lindestam Arlehamn CS, Gerasimova A, Mele F, et al. Memory T cells in latent *Mycobacterium tuberculosis* infection are directed against three antigenic Islands and largely contained in a $CXCR3^{+}CCR6^{+}$ Th1 subset. PLoS Pathog. 2013;9(1):e1003130.
270. Lindestam Arlehamn CS, McKinney DM, Carpenter C, et al. A quantitative analysis of complexity of human pathogen-specific CD4 T cell responses in healthy M. tuberculosis infected South Africans. PLoS Pathog. 2016;12(7):e1005760.
271. Scriba TJ, Carpenter C, Pro SC, et al. Differential recognition of Mycobacterium tuberculosis-specific epitopes as a function of tuberculosis disease history. Am J Respir Crit Care Med. 2017b;196(6):772–81.
272. Ogongo P, Tezera LB, Ardain A, et al. Tissue-resident-like CD4+ T cells secreting IL-17 control Mycobacterium tuberculosis in the human lung. J Clin Invest. 2021;131(10):e142014.
273. Nathan A, Beynor JI, Baglaenko Y, et al. Multimodally profiling memory T cells from a tuberculosis cohort identifies cell state associations with demographics, environment and disease. Nat Immunol. 2021;22(6):781–93.
274. Riou C, Du Bruyn E, Ruzive S, et al. Disease extent and anti-tubercular treatment response correlates with Mycobacterium tuberculosis-specific CD4 T-cell phenotype regardless of HIV-1 status. Clin Transl Immunology. 2020;9(9):e1176.
275. Chen CY, Huang D, Wang RC, et al. A critical role for CD8 T cells in a nonhuman primate model of tuberculosis. PLoS Pathog. 2009;5:e1000392.

276. Flynn JL, Goldstein MM, Triebold KJ, et al. Major histocompatibility complex class I-restricted T cells are required for resistance to Mycobacterium tuberculosis infection. PNAS. 1992;89:12013–7.
277. Woodworth JS, Wu Y, Behar SM. Mycobacterium tuberculosis-specific $CD8^+$ T cells require perforin to kill target cells and provide protection in vivo. J Immunol. 2008;181:8595–603.
278. Winchell CG, Nyquist SK, Chao MC, et al. $CD8^+$ lymphocytes are critical for early control of tuberculosis in macaques. JEM. 2023;220(12):e20230707.
279. Lewinsohn DA, Winata E, Swarbrick GM, et al. Immunodominant tuberculosis CD8 antigens preferentially restricted by HLA-B. PLoS Pathog. 2007;3(9):e127.
280. Yang JD, Mott D, Sutiwisesak R, et al. Mycobacterium tuberculosis-specific CD4+ and CD8+ T cells differ in their capacity to recognize infected macrophages. PLoS Pathog. 2018;14:e1007060.
281. Leddy OK, White FM, Bryson BD. Leveraging immunopeptidomics to study and combat infectious disease. mSystems. 2021;6(4):e00310–21.
282. Leddy OK, White FM, Bryson BD. Immunopeptidomics reveals determinants of *Mycobacterium tuberculosis* antigen presentation on MHC class I. elife. 2023;12:e84070.
283. Bettencourt P, Muller J, Nicastri A, et al. Identification of antigens presented by MHC for vaccines against tuberculosis. Npj Vaccines. 2020;5(2)
284. Ivanyi J. Function and potentials of *M. tuberculosis* epitopes. Front Immunol. 2014;5:107.
285. Rahlwes KC, Dias BRS, Campos PC, et al. Pathogenicity and virulence of Mycobacterium tuberculosis. Virulence. 2023;14(1):2150449.
286. Musvosvi M, Huang H, Wang C, et al. T cell receptor repertoires associated with control and disease progression following *Mycobacterium tuberculosis* infection. Nat Med. 2023;29:258–69.
287. Huang H, Wang C, Rubelt F, et al. Analyzing the *Mycobacterium tuberculosis* immune response by T-cell receptor clustering with GLIPH2 and genome-wide antigen screening. Nat Biotechnol. 2020;38:1194–202.
288. Russell WMS, Burch RL. The principles of humane experimental technique. London, United Kingdom: Methuen; 1959.
289. Gong W, Liang Y, Wu X. Animal models of tuberculosis vaccine research: an important component in the fight against tuberculosis. Biomed Res Int. 2020;2020:4263079.
290. Pena JC, Ho WZ. Monkey models of tuberculosis: lessons learned. Infect Immun. 2015;83(3):852–62.
291. Singh P, Kolloli A, Subbian S. Animal models of tuberculosis. In: Venketaraman V, editor. Understanding the host immune response against Mycobacterium tuberculosis infection. Springer, Cham; 2018. p. 67–97.
292. Lin PL, Rodgers M, Smith L, et al. Quantitative comparison of active and latent tuberculosis in the cynomolgus macaque model. Infect Immun. 2009;77:4631–42.
293. Langermans JA, Andersen P, van Soolingen D, et al. Divergent effect of bacillus Calmette–Guérin (BCG) vaccination on *Mycobacterium tuberculosis* infection in highly related macaque species: Implications for primate models in tuberculosis vaccine research. PNAS 2001;98(20):11497–11502.
294. Darrah PA, Zeppa JJ, Wang C, et al. Airway T cells are a correlate of i.v. Bacille Calmette-Guerin-mediated protection against tuberculosis in rhesus macaques. Cell Host and Microbe. 2023;31(6):962–77.
295. Dijkman K, Sombroek CC, Vervenne RAW, et al. Prevention of tuberculosis infection and disease by local BCG in repeatedly exposed rhesus macaques. Nat Med. 2019;25(2):255–62.
296. Sharpe S, White A, Sarfas C, et al. Alternative BCG delivery strategies improve protection against mycobacterium tuberculosis in non-human primates: protection associated with mycobacterial antigen-specific CD4 effector memory T-cell populations. Tuberculosis (Edinb). 2016b;101:174–90.
297. Verreck FAW, Tchilian EZ, Vervenne RAW, et al. Variable BCG efficacy in rhesus populations: pulmonary BCG provides protection where standard intra-dermal vaccination fails. Tuberculosis (Edinb). 2017b;104:46–57.

298. Liu YE, Darrah PA, Zeppa JJ, et al. Blood transcriptional correlates of BCG-induced protection against tuberculosis in rhesus macaques. Cell Reports Medicine. 2023;4:101096.
299. Larson EC, Ellis-Connell AL, Rodgers MA, et al. Intravenous Bacille Calmette–Guérin vaccination protects simian immunodeficiency virus-infected macaques from tuberculosis. Nat Microbiol 2023;8:2080–2092.
300. Guirado E, Gil O, Cáceres N, et al. Induction of a specific strong polyantigenic cellular immune response after short-term chemotherapy controls bacillary reactivation in murine and Guinea pig experimental models of tuberculosis. Clin Vaccine Immunol. 2008;15:1229–37.
301. Cardona PJ. RUTI: a new chance to shorten the treatment of latent tuberculosis infection. Tuberculosis (Edinb). 2006;86:273–89.
302. Kupz A, Zedler U, Stäber M, Kaufmann S. A mouse model of latent tuberculosis infection to study intervention strategies to prevent reactivation. PLoS One. 2016;11(7):e0158849.
303. Nemeth J, Olson GS, Rothchild AC, et al. Contained *mycobacterium tuberculosis* infection induces concomitant and heterologous protection. PLoS Pathog. 2020;16(7):e1008655.
304. TBVI. TB Vaccine Development Pathway: Stage Gate Criteria for TB Vaccine Development. Accessed on 22 May 2024. https://www.tbvi.eu/wp-content/uploads/2021/06/Stage-Gating-Criteria-Tables-2021.pdf
305. Bill and Melinda Gates Medical Research Institute. Bill & Melinda Gates Medical Research Institute Initiates Phase 3 Clinical Trial of Tuberculosis Vaccine Candidate. Accessed on 15 May 2024. https://www.gatesmri.org/mri-initiates-phase-3-clinical-trial-tuberculosis-vaccine-candidate/
306. Wellcome Trust. The world's first tuberculosis vaccine in 100 years could be in sight. Accessed 15 May 2024. https://wellcome.org/news/worlds-first-tuberculosis-vaccine-100-years-could-be-sight
307. Ji Z, Jian M, Chen T, et al. Immunogenicity and safety of the M72/$AS01_E$ candidate vaccine against tuberculosis: a meta-analysis. Front Immunol. 2019;10:2089.
308. Plotkin SA, Gilbert PB. Nomenclature for immune correlates of protection after vaccination. Clin Infect Dis. 2012;54(11):1615–7.

Part IV

Vaccines Against Tuberculosis in Clinical Trials

Novel Prophylactic TB Vaccines in Clinical Trials

9

Willem A. Hanekom

9.1 Target Populations

The aim of vaccination against TB is control of the epidemic. Mathematical modelling suggests that this control would not be possible without a vaccine that is effective in preventing clinical TB in adolescents and adults [17]. This is because diseased people from these populations spread the pathogen. The Preferred Product Characteristics (PPC) for Novel TB Vaccines from the World Health Organization (WHO) aims for a vaccine with at least 50% efficacy in preventing clinical TB in adolescents and adults [39].

In many geographic settings, HIV infection is a major driver of the TB epidemic [40]. It is therefore important that any novel vaccination strategy targeting adults and adolescents would also accommodate this population, in terms of safety and efficacy.

The WHO PPC also lists ideal characteristics of an infant or childhood vaccine; however, targeting these populations would not nearly be as impactful as vaccinating adolescents and adults [23]. This is because children manifest paucibacillary disease and do not spread the pathogen. The only available current TB vaccine, *Bacillus Calmette-Guerin* (BCG), is ~60% effective in preventing clinical pulmonary TB in the young and ~80% protective against severe forms of clinical TB in this age group [33]. It would be challenging for any novel vaccine to demonstrate superior protection.

This chapter will focus on vaccine candidates that aim to prevent clinical TB in adolescents and adults.

W. A. Hanekom (✉)
Africa Health Research Institute, KwaZulu-Natal, South Africa
e-mail: willem.hanekom@ahri.org

P. J. G. Bettencourt (ed.), *Tuberculosis Vaccines*,
https://doi.org/10.1007/978-3-031-94540-3_9

9.2 Approaches to Clinical Testing of Novel Vaccines

A novel TB vaccine could potentially intervene at various infection or disease stages following exposure to Mtb. First, a vaccine could prevent Mtb infection. Interpretation of trial results with this outcome may be challenging, as the interferon-gamma release assay (IGRA) used as endpoint may revert from positive to negative over time, although in a minority of individuals [4]. Furthermore, it is impossible to know whether prevention of Mtb infection might have occurred only in the 90% of infected persons who would never progresses to clinical TB. Therefore, follow-up studies with clinical TB endpoints are needed to validate potential epidemic impact of a prevention of Mtb infection signal.

The most appropriate and preferred vaccination approach is prevention of clinical TB, usually pulmonary disease. In efficacy trials, it is important to use microbiological confirmation with sputum culture and/or a nuclear amplification test such as GeneXpert to detect Mtb as the endpoint; at least two positive tests are most reliable.

Efficacy trials should ideally focus on populations at large, for translation to ultimate application of the vaccine on a population basis. These studies require large sample sizes, as the incidence of TB is relatively low, even in the highest prevalence settings. Until validated immune correlates of vaccination-induced protection become available [37], these large-scale trials are the only option for efficacy assessment.

On a population basis, a practical sample size for efficacy testing is often possible when IGRA positive individuals only are enrolled, as the risk of developing clinical TB is up to 8 times higher than in IGRA negative persons [29]. Regardless, it is unlikely that regulators would accept evaluation in this population only for registration of a product: safety and immunogenicity data would be required from IGRA negative persons and in those living with HIV (PLWH).

Attempts at accelerating efficacy testing may target subpopulations with a higher incidence of clinical TB than in the general population. One such approach involves prevention of recurrent clinical TB, which occurs in ~4% of people from high prevalence areas after clinical and microbiological cure of TB, within 2 years [45]. Recurrent TB may reflect relapse of disease caused by the same strain that caused the original disease or may be due to reinfection with a new Mtb strain. The potential challenge of this approach, where trials involve vaccination after completion of TB therapy, is that some TB patients may have undefined compromise that places them at risk for recurrent disease. This means that a vaccine candidate that does not show efficacy in this setting may conceivably work in the population at large. Similarly, in settings where the force of infection is higher than in the general population, such as in household contacts of persons with clinical TB, in healthcare workers or in persons deprived of liberty, lack of efficacy in a clinical trial may not necessarily translate to the general population, where the force of infection is lower. A negative result among enrichment approaches—such as those mentioned above—should not preclude testing in the general population.

Globally, ~50% of all TB disease may be asymptomatic [15, 60]. The TB research community is currently learning much about this disease state, which may progress to symptomatic disease or which may self-cure. In the future, it is likely that this endpoint will be incorporated in efficacy trials, with the caveat that an individual vaccine may show differential protective capacity against asymptomatic and symptomatic disease.

A vaccine may also have an indication of improving outcome of clinical TB or long-term outcome after TB has been cured. These would fall within a broad category of host-directed therapy to complement antimicrobials and is beyond the scope of this chapter.

9.3 Overview of the Novel TB Vaccine Clinical Pipeline

The 2025 pipeline of novel TB vaccine currently in clinical development is shown in Table 9.1. The pipeline contains subunit vaccines (adjuvanted protein vaccines), whole cell vaccines, viral-vectored vaccines, and mRNA vaccines (discussed in detail below).

The TB vaccine clinical pipeline is limited when compared with that for other vaccines that target global emergencies, e.g., Covid-19. This reflects limited global investment in TB vaccine discovery and development [54]. Furthermore, classical clinical pipelines of novel products contain an abundance of early phase candidates, compared with later phase candidates—this is appropriate as some products are expected to fail. For TB vaccines, the relative lack of early phase candidates is concerning.

Table 9.1 The current pipeline of novel TB vaccines in clinical trials

Phase 1	Phase 2A	Phase 2B	Phase 3
BNT164a1 and BNT164b1	AEC/BC02	DAR-901	BCG as travel vaccine
TB/FLU-05E	ChAdOx1.85A + MVA85A	RUTI	GamTBvac
H107e/CAF10b	ID93/GLA-SE (QTP101)		Immuvac (MIP)
			VPM1002
			M72/AS01$_{E\text{-}4}$
			MTBVAC

Modified from the Stop TB Partnership Vaccine Group on New TB Vaccines, https://newtbvaccines.org/tb-vaccine-pipeline/clinical-phase/. Orange: Whole cell vaccines. Green: Subunit (protein/adjuvant) vaccines. Blue: Viral vectored vaccines. Grey: mRNA vaccines. Please refer to the narrative for detail about the individual vaccines

The pipeline currently has a lead candidate, the subunit vaccine M72/AS01$_{E-4}$, and a fast-following lead candidate, the whole mycobacterial vaccine MTBVAC (both discussed in detail below). Unfortunately, some candidates in the pipeline are not in active trials currently or do not have clinical data to support testing in later phases.

A common feature of many subunit and viral-vectored vaccines is that they contain so-called immunodominant Mtb antigens. Most of these antigens were identified by screening T cell responses in peripheral blood from people infected with Mtb, without clinical disease. A potential challenge of this approach is that these antigens showed the least variation when multiple global strains of the pathogen were sequenced; other Mtb antigen groups show greater variation [9]. This lack of variation following host immune pressure may suggest that the immune response to these antigens may even pose a relative advantage for the pathogen.

Some "next-generation" vaccines have emerged and are based on advances in understanding protective immunity against the pathogen, including antigen-specific responses that may be important: the subunit vaccines H107e/CAF10b and ID93/GLA-SE and the mRNA vaccines BNT164a1 and BNT164b1 are prototypes of these vaccines (discussed in detail below).

9.4 Novel Subunit TB Vaccines

These vaccines classically contain one or a few protein antigens of Mtb, plus an adjuvant that directs the immune response in a desired direction. As the immune correlates of vaccination-induced protection against TB are not known, most vaccines target a T cell response that is generally thought to be critical for protection: so-called Th1 CD4 cells [3, 48]. In some cases, Th17 cells and CD8 T cells are also targeted.

9.4.1 M72/AS01$_{E-4}$

This candidate was initially developed by GSK and contains a recombinant fusion protein of 2 Mtb antigens, MTB32A and MTB39A. These immunodominant antigens were identified through screening T cell recognition in people with Mtb infection. The non-synthetic adjuvant AS01$_{E-4}$ contains monophosphoryl lipid A (MPL), a toll-like receptor (TLR) 4 agonist, as well as QS-21, a saponin obtained from the soap bark tree, formulated within a cholesterol-containing liposome. There is extensive clinical experience with AS01, which is also a component of the shingles vaccine Shingrix, and of the RTS,S malaria vaccine Mosquirix.

Following extensive preclinical testing, early clinical trials showed an acceptable safety, tolerability, and immunogenicity profile [11, 20, 24, 26, 41]. The only potential concern was large skin reactions at the injection site which occurred in some patients with current or prior clinical TB, who were vaccinated after the intensive treatment phase in a phase 2 trial [16].

The ability of the vaccine to prevent clinical pulmonary TB was evaluated in a phase 2b trial of 3575 young IGRA positive South African adults, who received two doses of the vaccine or placebo [62]. The vaccine showed an efficacy (VE) of 49.7% (95% confidence interval, CI, 2.1–74.2%). This is the first novel TB vaccine that has met efficacy criteria against clinical TB proposed in the WHO PPC. Importantly, a sensitivity analysis was done for this trial, involving stricter— probably more appropriate—endpoint definitions of clinical pulmonary TB: two positive Mtb cultures and/or GeneXperts [56]. The sensitivity analysis resulted in a VE of 68% (95% CI, 25.1–86.3%). This lower limit of the 95% CI is generally thought to be sufficient for licensing of a product; however, an application for licensing was not possible as manufacturing of the product was not ready, and the vaccine had not been tested adequately in IGRA negative persons and in PLWH.

M72/AS01$_{E-4}$ is now being evaluated in a phase 3 trial (NCT06062238, clinicaltrials.gov), with the Gates Medical Research Institute (Gates MRI) as the new license holder and sponsor. Efficacy is being evaluated in 18,000 IGRA positive persons from multiple African and South-East Asian countries. A total of 110 persons with pulmonary clinical TB, diagnosed with two positive sputum tests (see above), is required for the trial to end—likely to be in 2028. Two additional cohorts of 1000 people each, IGRA negative and PLWH, respectively, are being enrolled to evaluate safety and immunogenicity.

9.4.2 GamTBvac

GamTBvac is a vaccine being developed by Gamaleya Research Institute of Epidemiology and Microbiology (Russia) and the Russian Ministry of Health. The candidate contains the immunodominant antigens Ag85A and ESAT6-CFP10, immobilized on dextran, using a dextran-binding domain. The adjuvant consists of this dextran core and cytosine-phosphate-guanine (CPG) oligodeoxynucleotides, which are TLR9 agonists.

The candidate was designed to be used as a booster vaccine after BCG. Acceptable safety, tolerability, and immunogenicity were reported from early clinical trials [61, 64]. Although phase 2b testing has not been reported, GamTBvac is now in a double-blind, placebo-controlled phase 3 trial of ~7000 adults aged 18–40 years in Russia (NCT04975737).

9.4.3 ID-93/GLA-SE (QTP101)

ID93 was initially developed by the Access to Advanced Health Institute (AAHI, USA). The candidate was later acquired by Quratis (South Korea), which renamed it QTP101. A fusion protein contains antigens associated with Mtb virulence, Rv3619, Rv3620, and Rv2608, and an antigen associated with Mtb infection without clinical TB, Rv1813. The adjuvant, GLA-SE, is a squalene emulsion containing the synthetic TLR4 agonist glucopyranosyl lipid A.

ID93/GLA-SE has shown promise in preclinical models and has to date been tested in IGRA negative persons in early phase studies, with acceptable safety, tolerability, and immunogenicity [8, 12, 42, 44]. An ongoing phase 1 trial is testing QTP101 among older adults in South Korea (NCT01927159), while planning for phase 2b testing in South-East Asia is currently underway.

The vaccine is also being evaluated as adjunctive therapy to antimicrobials for clinical TB (NCT06205589).

9.4.4 AEC/BC02

This candidate was developed by Anhui Zifei Longcom Biologic Pharmacy Co, Ltd. (China). The immunodominant Mtb proteins Ag85B, ESAT6 and CFP10 are included—the latter two proteins are fused. The BC02 adjuvant contains BCG-derived unmethylated cytosine-phosphate-guanine (CpG) motifs—TLR9 adjuvants—and aluminum hydroxide—an adjuvant used in many childhood vaccines.

The vaccine is administered in a freeze-dried form and is currently in phase 2a testing in adults, including the elderly (NCT05284812).

9.4.5 H107e/CAF10b

This vaccine was developed by Statens Serum Institute (SSI, Denmark), which has also brought multiple other TB vaccine candidates to clinical testing. The candidate H56/IC31 was most notable among the latter, containing 3 immunodominant proteins, Ag85B, ESAT6, and Rv2660c, together with an adjuvant IC31, which incorporates an 11-mer antibacterial peptide (KLK(5)KLK) and the synthetic oligodeoxynucleotide ODN1a—a TLR9 adjuvant. After showing acceptable tolerability, safety, and immunogenicity in early phase trials [6, 28, 53, 55], the candidate was tested in a prevention of TB recurrence trial at multiple sites in South Africa (NCT03512249). Two doses of the vaccine or placebo was administered after clinical and microbiological cure of clinical TB. No efficacy in preventing recurrent clinical TB was shown during 12 months of follow-up: VE of minus73.8%, 95% CI minus246.9 to 9.8 [18]. Because Mtb isolates from the original episode of clinical TB and from the newly occurring disease were available, relapse and reinfection could be differentiated. There was no VE for reinfection but a suggestion that the vaccine may have increased risk of relapse (3% relapse rate in the vaccine arm and 1.5% in the placebo arm). This candidate is not being developed further.

H107e/CAF10b is a "next-generation" vaccine with a fusion protein that contains multiple Mtb-specific antigens, i.e., antigens not in or not secreted by BCG. These include key components of the ESX-1 secretion system of Mtb, such as multiple copies of ESAT6, and EspI, espA, espC, and PPE68. The other proteins are major secretory proteins of Mtb, i.e., MPT64, MPT70, and MPT83. CAF10b is a potent Th1/Th17 inducing adjuvant and consists of dimethyldioctadecylammonium bromide (DDA), monomycoloyl glycerol (MMG) and CPG, allowing immune activation through the innate receptors MINCLE and TLR9. The vaccine is designed to be used concurrently with BCG, proposing that BCG would have "co-adjuvanting" effect, as has been demonstrated in the mouse, when BCG has been used concurrently with H107e [69]. This co-administration has resulted in protection against pathogen challenge that has been of the best demonstrated to date in the murine model [13].

H107e/CAF10b is currently being evaluated in a first-in-humans clinical trial in South Africa (NCT06050356).

9.5 Novel Whole Bacterial Vaccines

Whole bacterial vaccines have the advantage that many of the 4000 putative proteins of Mtb would be presented to the host following vaccination, averting the need for choosing specific antigens for inclusion in other vaccine platforms. Live attenuated *M. bovis* BCG is the prototype of whole cell vaccines and contains many proteins that is shared with Mtb. Novel whole cell vaccine approaches have involved modification of live BCG, use of other non-tuberculous mycobacteria, some of which have been inactivated, attenuating a virulent Mtb strain and fragmenting whole mycobacteria. Many whole mycobacterial candidates are being developed as potential replacements for BCG in infants as well as for prophylaxis in adolescents and adults.

Novel live bacterial vaccine approaches may pose challenges. First, >100 years of experience with BCG vaccination has shown that vaccine effectiveness is relatively poor in the face of pre-existing mycobacterial immunity, particularly when induced by Mtb infection [30]. Second, as for BCG, the candidates may not be safe in persons with immune compromise due to uncontrolled HIV infection [19]. Third, the vaccines are often administered intradermally, while inadvertent subcutaneous injections may be associated with cold abscesses; intradermal administration is relatively difficult on a population basis outside the newborn period.

9.5.1 MTBVAC

MTBVAC is one of the most promising vaccines currently in late phase clinical testing. The candidate has been developed by Institute Pasteur (France), the University of Zaragosa (Spain), Biofabri (Spain) and IAVI (USA) and is derived from a virulent human clinical isolate of Mtb [32]. Deletion of two genes, phoP and fadD26, has rendered the bacterium as a virulent as BCG. The resulting live attenuated vaccine is void of many virulence-associated cell wall lipids, like phthiocerol dimycocerosates (PDIMs), and is proposed to enhance innate immune responses and improve antigen recognition in vivo.

MTBVAC is administered intradermally as a single dose and has been tested extensively in early phase trials of infants and adults [2, 51, 57, 58]. Tolerability and safety have been acceptable. Immunogenicity has been shown both in mycobacteria-naïve hosts and in persons previously infected with Mtb, whose pre-existing T cell immunity was boosted. In infants, safety has been similar to BCG, while immunogenicity has been superior to BCG.

The vaccine is now being tested in a phase 2b trial of 4300 IGRA positive adolescents and adults in Africa, who will receive one dose of MTBVAC or placebo intradermally (NCT06272812). The endpoint is pulmonary TB diagnosed with 2 sputum tests positive for Mtb. The phase 2b approach has applied lessons from the M72 phase 2b experience, resulting in sample size considerations that may even allow registration if the vaccine is shown to be effective. The phase 2b trial will also collect sputum samples at three times points from all participants, to be evaluated for presence of Mtb after completion of the trial—an assessment of effect on asymptomatic TB. Parallel safety and immunogenicity testing is being completed in IGRA negative adults and PLWH in separate phase 2a trials [47]. A phase 3 trial for prevention of clinical TB in adults is planned for India [47].

MTBVAC is also in a phase 3 trial in infants, aiming to show protection against clinical TB that is superior to BCG (NCT04975178).

MTBVAC still expresses the RD1 region of Mtb, although ESAT6 is not actively secreted. This may result in conversion of ESAT6-containing IGRA tests, including the commonly used Quantiferon Gold In-Tube test [57]. On a population basis, this could pose challenges for diagnosing TB in persons who have received the vaccine.

9.5.2 VPM1002

This candidate has been developed by Max Planck Institute and VPM (Germany), Serum Institute India and the Indian Council of Medical Research (ICMR). The vaccine is a recombinant BCG with a deleted urease C gene, allowing acidification of the intracellular vacuole containing the vaccine, and insertion of the listeriolysin gene from *Listeria monocytogenes* [38]. Listeriolysin punches pores in the vacuolar membrane, allowing antigens to escape and be processed by intracytosolic machinery. The proposed end-result is enhanced immune activation, antigen cross-presentation, and induction of apoptosis and autophagy [7].

VPM1002 is administered intradermally. The candidate has shown tolerability, safety, and immunogenicity patterns that are similar to MTBVAC in infants and in older ages [10, 27].

VPM1002 has been evaluated in two efficacy trials. A prevention of recurrence trial involved 2000 adults in India, who received either VPM1002 or placebo intradermally 2–4 weeks after successful completion of treatment of the initial TB disease (NCT03152903). Follow-up to identify microbiologically confirmed TB disease continued for 12 months. The vaccine had acceptable tolerability and safety, but did not show efficacy: VE was 25.4%, 95% CI of −36.7 to 59.4 [7]. Efficacy was also not shown in any pre-determined secondary outcomes.

The second efficacy trial involved up to 13,000 Indian household contacts of persons with TB disease, who were randomized to receive two doses of either VPM1002, Immuvac (see below) or placebo one month apart. The participants were followed for 36 months to identify TB disease. Results have not been communicated at the time of completion of this chapter.

VPM1002 is also being evaluated in a multi-country "phase 3" trial of prevention of infection in infants, measured by IGRA (NCT04351685). (Phase 3 would be an unusual term for a trial without endpoints that are acceptable to regulators.)

9.5.3 Immuvac

This vaccine has been developed by Cadila (India) and ICMR and contains heat-inactivated *M. indicus pranii* (MIP), a non-tuberculous mycobacterium. After limited early trials, the vaccine has been tested in the phase 3 trial of household contacts of TB disease described above; results are awaited.

The proposed immunomodulatory properties of the candidate is also been exploited in testing as an adjunctive therapy to antimicrobials for clinical TB.

9.5.4 BCG as a Travel Vaccine

A large "phase 3" trial, termed "TIPI", sponsored by the Henry M. Jackson Foundation for the Advancement of Medicine (US) is evaluating efficacy of BCG vaccination in prevention of Mtb infection among BCG-naive travelers to TB-endemic countries (NCT04461379). BCG Tokyo 172, not licensed in the United States, is used for this study which aims to inform public health intervention. (BCG vaccination at birth is not routine in the United States.)

BCG revaccination following routine newborn administration has been evaluated in many clinical trials and epidemiological settings [25]. Overall, minimal or no effect in prevention of Mtb infection or clinical TB has been shown. The most recent reports of such use are from trials of BCG revaccination of Brazil and in South Africa, where no difference in initial and sustained IGRA conversion, respectively, was shown between those who received BCG or placebo [14, 46].

9.5.5 RUTI

This candidate has been developed by Archivel Farma, S.L. (Spain) and is composed of detoxified, nanofragments of the Mtb cell wall, suspended in a liposome. Mtb was grown under stress conditions to generate the vaccine, which contains many antigens of the pathogen.

The vaccine is presented as a dry powder for reconstitution and is administered subcutaneously in a single dose. Acceptable safety and immunogenicity in both PLWH and HIV-negative persons have been demonstrated [36].

The vaccine is currently not being tested for prophylactic indications, but as therapy adjunctive to antimicrobials to improve outcome of disease intervention, regardless of drug susceptibility of the clinical Mtb strain (NCT001136161).

9.5.6 DAR-901

This vaccine has been in the pipeline for a long period, having been developed by Dartmouth's Geisel School of Medicine in collaboration with St Louis University. The DAR-901 vaccine is inactivated *M. obuense*, a non-tuberculous mycobacterium. It was manufactured from the master cell bank of SRL-172, the original vaccine.

The ability of SRL-172 to prevent disseminated TB was tested in phase 3 trial in Tanzanian PLWH with a CD4 T cell count >200/uL [65]. Not all participants were on anti-retroviral therapy. The vaccine or placebo was administered at five time points over a year, and participants followed for up to 5 years. No efficacy was shown against the primary endpoint; however, modest protection against microbiologically confirmed clinical TB was shown: VE 49%, 95% CI, 4 to 61%.

DAR-901 has been tested in a prevention of infection trial, also in Tanzania, involving three vaccine doses. Although the vaccine was safe and immunogenic, the sample size was not adequate for a reliable conclusion of the vaccine effect [35].

The vaccine is not currently in trials.

9.5.7 Vaccae

Although this TB vaccine is not currently in clinical trials, it is worth a mention as results from a phase 3 trial have been reported, although only in a table of a manuscript that focuses on modeling of the vaccine's potential use [31]. The vaccine consists of heat-inactivated *M. vaccae*, a non-tuberculous mycobacterium, and was developed by Anhui Zhifei Longcom Co., Ltd. (China). The phase 3 trial involved 10,000 participants in the age of 15–65 years, who had a tuberculin skin test of ≥15 mm at baseline and who received six doses of the vaccine, 2 weeks apart. After 2 years of follow-up, vaccine efficacy of 54.7% (95% CI, 29.8 to 70.8%) was shown for prevention of microbiologically confirmed TB disease. As for the SLR-172 approach mentioned above, this regimen is generally regarded as unimplementable.

9.6 Novel Viral-Vectored Vaccines

These vaccines exploit the immune stimulatory properties of viruses to induce immunity to specific mycobacterial antigens that are incorporated. The virus is classically engineered to be less virulent than the wild type.

Some of the viral-vectored vaccines are being tested for mucosal use, either by nasal spray or by delivery to the lung through an inhaler device. Mucosal administration may result in an immune response that may differ from parenterally administered vaccines: the developers propose that the mucosal responses would be more appropriate for control of TB [52].

As in any development pipeline, some candidates are expected to fail, as did a replication-deficient adenovirus 35-vectored candidate, AERAS-402, which contained Ag85A, Ag85B, and TB10.4. Although acceptable safety and tolerability was shown in clinical studies, induced immunity was relatively poor in both adults and infants [1, 21].

9.6.1 ChAdOx1.85A and MVA85A

The ChAdOx1.85A and MVA85A vaccine combination regimen is under development by the University of Oxford. Two different viral vectors deliver an immunodominant antigen of Mtb, Ag85A.

The first vector is a chimpanzee adenovirus (ChAdOx1), engineered to be replication deficient. The second vector, a modified vaccinia Ankara virus (MVA) virus, is also replication-deficient and has been used in many commercially available vaccines candidates; the vector, in the smallpox/Mpox vaccine, for example, has a good safety profile and is able to induce strong immune responses [34].

MVA85A as a stand-alone vaccine was one of the earliest novel vaccines developed in the modern era. The vaccine was ultimately tested in a phase 3 trial as a boost to routine newborn BCG vaccination: no additional protection against TB disease was shown [59].

Safety and immunogenicity have been shown in a phase 1 trial where both ChAdOx1.85A and MVA85A were given intramuscularly [68]. Consecutive administration of the two vaccines resulted in a significant boost of the Ag85A-specific T cell response. Intramuscular delivery of the vaccines has also been shown to be safe and immunogenic in a phase 2a trial in Uganda [66]. Additionally, aerosol ChAdOx1.85A was shown to be safe and immunogenic in a phase 1 trail [5].

The developers regard these studies as proof-of-concept and are planning to develop constructs with more antigen inserts for further testing.

9.6.2 TB/FLU-05E

The TB/FLU-05E vaccine is under development by Smorodintsev Research Institute of Influenza (Russia). The recombinant attenuated influenza vector Flu/THSP includes a truncated NS1 protein, NS1(1–124), with the Mtb proteins TB10.4—an immunodominant protein—and HspX, also known as alpha-crystallin, a protein preferentially expressed during Mtb infection in the absence of disease—incorporated in the NS1 open reading frame.

The vaccine is formulated as a liquid nasal spray. After promising findings in preclinical models [49, 50, 63], the vaccine is presumed to be in phase 1 testing, although a "completed" prevention of infection study in 18–50-year olds is listed on clinicaltrials.gov (NCT05945498).

9.7 Novel Nucleic Acid Vaccines

A major advantage of DNA and RNA vaccines over other platforms is ease and rapidity of manufacturing.

mRNA vaccines have found fame during the COVID-19 period, where utility was demonstrated unequivocally. It should be recognized that this success was based on an antibody response, rather than T cell response, generally thought to be important for protection against TB. Furthermore, a relative drawback may be the relatively short duration of protection following mRNA vaccination, although improving longevity of the host response is a focus of intense research interest [43]. The vaccines contain the message for select host proteins; however, the backbone, usually a lipid nanoparticle, is the critical determinant of the character of the induced immune response [22, 67].

9.7.1 BNT164a1 and BNT164b1

These two mRNA vaccines are being developed by BioNTech (Germany). The candidates may be regarded as next-generation novel TB vaccines, given careful selection of the antigens, based on emerging knowledge (as for H107e/CAF10b, for example). Eight antigens are included as four different fusion proteins: antigens associated with Mtb infection without disease ("dormancy"), i.e., VapB47 and Hsp1, those associated with Mtb "resuscitation" from dormancy, i.e., RfpA and RfpD, and more immunodominant antigens often associated with clinical TB, i.e., ESAT6, Ag85B, HBHA, Mtb32A, and Mtb39A. The latter two antigens are also in M72/AS01$_{E-4}$.

The lipid nanoparticle (LNP) carriers differ between the two vaccines: BNT164b1 contains the same nucleoside modification as in the Biontech/Pfizer COVID-19 vaccine—uridine is replaced with 1-methylpseudouridine, proposed to result in reduced innate cell activation and enhanced stability and translation. BNT164a1 contains unmodified uridine, commonly used in BioNTech's oncology platforms, and proposed to have a greater innate and T cell immune response.

Multiple dose levels of the vaccine, given intramuscularly in multiple doses, are currently being evaluated in phase 1 trials in Germany and South Africa (NCT05537038 and NCT05547464).

9.8 Conclusions

The TB vaccine field is hampered by poor funding, incomplete knowledge of protective immunity against TB, suboptimal animal models and a lack of vaccination-induced immune correlates of protection against clinical TB. Regardless, populating the novel TB vaccine pipeline with new candidates is urgent. Vaccine design should be guided by advances in understanding protective immunity against TB and by better understanding of Mtb antigens. These novel candidates could be contingency products for current vaccines that may fail clinical testing or could potentially induce better protection than current vaccines.

M72/AS01$_{E\text{-}4}$ is currently the most promising candidate in clinical testing, having demonstrated 50% protection against clinical TB in an early efficacy trial. If this ultimately translates to 50% effectiveness in a real-world setting, and if successful global roll-out be achieved, the effect on the TB pandemic will be dramatic.

References

1. Abel B, Tameris M, Mansoor N, Gelderbloem S, Hughes J, Abrahams D, Makhethe L, Erasmus M, Kock MD, Van Der Merwe L, Hawkridge A, Veldsman A, Hatherill M, Schirru G, Pau MG, Hendriks J, Weverling GJ, Goudsmit J, Sizemore D, Mcclain JB, Goetz M, Gearhart J, Mahomed H, Hussey GD, Sadoff JC, Hanekom WA. The novel tuberculosis vaccine, AERAS-402, induces robust and polyfunctional CD4+ and CD8+ T cells in adults. Am J Respir Crit Care Med. 2010;181:1407–17.
2. Aguilo N, Uranga S, Marinova D, Monzon M, Badiola J, Martin C. MTBVAC vaccine is safe, immunogenic and confers protective efficacy against mycobacterium tuberculosis in newborn mice. Tuberculosis (Edinb). 2016;96:71–4.
3. Andersen P, Scriba TJ. Moving tuberculosis vaccines from theory to practice. Nat Rev Immunol. 2019;19:550–62.
4. Andrews JR, Hatherill M, Mahomed H, Hanekom WA, Campo M, Hawn TR, Wood R, Scriba TJ. The dynamics of Quantiferon-TB gold in-tube conversion and reversion in a cohort of South African adolescents. Am J Respir Crit Care Med. 2015;191:584–91.
5. Audran R, Karoui O, Donnet L, Soumas V, Fares F, Lovis A, Noirez L, Cavassini M, Fayet-Mello A, Sattti I, Mcshane H, Spertini F. Randomised, double-blind, controlled phase 1 trial of the candidate tuberculosis vaccine ChAdOx1-85A delivered by aerosol versus intramuscular route. J Infect. 2024;89:106205.
6. Bekker LG, Dintwe O, Fiore-Gartland A, Middelkoop K, Hutter J, Williams A, Randhawa AK, Ruhwald M, Kromann I, Andersen PL, Diazgranados CA, Rutkowski KT, Tait D, Miner MD, Andersen-Nissen E, De Rosa SC, Seaton KE, Tomaras GD, Mcelrath MJ, Ginsberg A, Kublin JG, Team HAAP. A phase 1b randomized study of the safety and immunological responses to vaccination with H4:IC31, H56:IC31, and BCG revaccination in Mycobacterium tuberculosis-uninfected adolescents in Cape Town. South Africa EclinicalMedicine. 2020;21:100313.
7. Bruckner SKD. Updates on the VPM1002 clinical trial. TBVI symposium. 2025 Les Diablerets, Switzerland; 2025.
8. Choi YH, Kang YA, Park KJ, Choi JC, Cho KG, Ko DY, Ahn JH, Lee B, Ahn E, Woo YJ, Jung K, Kim NY, Reese VA, Larsen SE, Baldwin SL, Reed SG, Coler RN, Lee H, Cho SN. Safety and immunogenicity of the ID93 + GLA-SE tuberculosis vaccine in BCG-vaccinated healthy adults: A randomized, double-blind, placebo-controlled phase 2 trial. Infect Dis Ther. 2023;12:1605–24.
9. Coscolla M, Copin R, Sutherland J, Gehre F, De Jong B, Owolabi O, Mbayo G, Giardina F, Ernst JD, Gagneux S. M. Tuberculosis T cell epitope analysis reveals paucity of antigenic variation and identifies rare variable TB antigens. Cell Host Microbe. 2015;18:538–48.
10. Cotton MF, Madhi SA, Luabeya AK, Tameris M, Hesseling AC, Shenje J, Schoeman E, Hatherill M, Desai S, Kapse D, Bruckner S, Koen A, Jose L, Moultrie A, Bhikha S, Walzl G, Gutschmidt A, Kotze LA, Allies DL, Loxton AG, Shaligram U, Abraham M, Johnstone H, Grode L, Kaufmann SHE, Kulkarni PS. Safety and immunogenicity of VPM1002 versus BCG in south African newborn babies: a randomised, phase 2 non-inferiority double-blind controlled trial. Lancet Infect Dis. 2022;22:1472–83.

11. Day CL, Tameris M, Mansoor N, Van Rooyen M, De Kock M, Geldenhuys H, Erasmus M, Makhethe L, Hughes EJ, Gelderbloem S, Bollaerts A, Bourguignon P, Cohen J, Demoitie MA, Mettens P, Moris P, Sadoff JC, Hawkridge A, Hussey GD, Mahomed H, Ofori-Anyinam O, Hanekom WA. Induction and regulation of T-cell immunity by the novel tuberculosis vaccine M72/AS01 in South African adults. Am J Respir Crit Care Med. 2013;188:492–502.
12. Day TA, Penn-Nicholson A, Luabeya AKK, Fiore-Gartland A, Du Plessis N, Loxton AG, Vergara J, Rolf TA, Reid TD, Toefy A, Shenje J, Geldenhuys H, Tameris M, Mabwe S, Bilek N, Bekker LG, Diacon A, Walzl G, Ashman J, Frevol A, Sagawa ZK, Lindestam Arlehamn C, Sette A, Reed SG, Coler RN, Scriba TJ, Hatherill M, Team T-S. Safety and immunogenicity of the adjunct therapeutic vaccine ID93 + GLA-SE in adults who have completed treatment for tuberculosis: a randomised, double-blind, placebo-controlled, phase 2a trial. Lancet Respir Med. 2021;9:373–86.
13. Dijkman K, Lindenstrom T, Rosenkrands I, Soe R, Woodworth JS, Lindestam Arlehamn CS, Mortensen R. A protective, single-visit TB vaccination regimen by co-administration of a subunit vaccine with BCG. NPJ Vaccines. 2023;8:66.
14. Dos Santos PCP, Messina NL, De Oliveira RD, Da Silva PV, Puga MAM, Dalcolmo M, Dos Santos G, De Lacerda MVG, Jardim BA, De Almeida EVFF, Curtis N, Andrews JR, Croda J. Effect of BCG vaccination against mycobacterium tuberculosis infection in adult Brazilian health-care workers: a nested clinical trial. Lancet Infect Dis. 2024;24:594–601.
15. Frascella B, Richards AS, Sossen B, Emery JC, Odone A, Law I, Onozaki I, Esmail H, Houben R. Subclinical tuberculosis disease-A review and analysis of prevalence surveys to inform definitions, burden, associations, and screening methodology. Clin Infect Dis. 2021;73:e830–41.
16. Gillard P, Yang PC, Danilovits M, Su WJ, Cheng SL, Pehme L, Bollaerts A, Jongert E, Moris P, Ofori-Anyinam O, Demoitie MA, Castro M. Safety and immunogenicity of the M72/AS01E candidate tuberculosis vaccine in adults with tuberculosis: A phase II randomised study. Tuberculosis (Edinb). 2016;100:118–27.
17. Harris RC, Sumner T, Knight GM, Zhang H, White RG. Potential impact of tuberculosis vaccines in China, South Africa, and India. Sci Transl Med. 2020;12
18. Hatherill M. 2025. Personal communication.
19. Hesseling A, Johnson L, Jaspan H, Cotton M, Whitelaw A, Schaaf H, Fine P, Eley B, Marais B, Nuttall J. Disseminated bacille Calmette-Guerin disease in HIV-infected South African infants. Bull World Health Organ. 2009;87:505–11.
20. Idoko OT, Owolabi OA, Owiafe PK, Moris P, Odutola A, Bollaerts A, Ogundare E, Jongert E, Demoitie MA, Ofori-Anyinam O, Ota MO. Safety and immunogenicity of the M72/AS01 candidate tuberculosis vaccine when given as a booster to BCG in Gambian infants: an open-label randomized controlled trial. Tuberculosis (Edinb). 2014;94:564–78.
21. Kagina BM, Tameris MD, Geldenhuys H, Hatherill M, Abel B, Hussey GD, Scriba TJ, Mahomed H, Sadoff JC, Hanekom WA. The novel tuberculosis vaccine, AERAS-402, is safe in healthy infants previously vaccinated with BCG, and induces dose-dependent CD4 and CD8T cell responses. Vaccine. 2014;32:5908–17.
22. Kim EH, Teerdhala SV, Padilla MS, Joseph RA, Li JJ, Haley RM, Mitchell MJ. Lipid nanoparticle-mediated RNA delivery for immune cell modulation. Eur J Immunol. 2024;54:e2451008.
23. Knight GM, Griffiths UK, Sumner T, Laurence YV, Gheorghe A, Vassall A, Glaziou P, White RG. Impact and cost-effectiveness of new tuberculosis vaccines in low- and middle-income countries. Proc Natl Acad Sci USA. 2014;111:15520–5.
24. Kumarasamy N, Poongulali S, Bollaerts A, Moris P, Beulah FE, Ayuk LN, Demoitie MA, Jongert E, Ofori-Anyinam O. A randomized, controlled safety, and immunogenicity trial of the M72/AS01 candidate tuberculosis vaccine in HIV-positive Indian adults. Medicine (Baltimore). 2016;95:e2459.
25. Lawrence A. Bacillus Calmette-Guerin (BCG) revaccination and protection against tuberculosis: a systematic review. Cureus. 2024;16:e56643.
26. Leroux-Roels I, Forgus S, De Boever F, Clement F, Demoitie MA, Mettens P, Moris P, Ledent E, Leroux-Roels G, Ofori-Anyinam O, Group M S. Improved CD4(+) T cell responses to

mycobacterium tuberculosis in PPD-negative adults by M72/AS01 as compared to the M72/AS02 and Mtb72F/AS02 tuberculosis candidate vaccine formulations: a randomized trial. Vaccine. 2013;31:2196–206.
27. Loxton AG, Knaul JK, Grode L, Gutschmidt A, Meller C, Eisele B, Johnstone H, Van Der Spuy G, Maertzdorf J, Kaufmann SHE, Hesseling AC, Walzl G, Cotton MF. Safety and immunogenicity of the recombinant Mycobacterium bovis BCG vaccine VPM1002 in HIV-unexposed newborn infants in South Africa. Clin vaccine Immunol. 2017;24
28. Luabeya AK, Kagina BM, Tameris MD, Geldenhuys H, Hoff ST, Shi Z, Kromann I, Hatherill M, Mahomed H, Hanekom WA, Andersen P, Scriba TJ, Group HTS, Schoeman E, Krohn C, Day CL, Africa H, Makhethe L, Smit E, Brown Y, Suliman S, Hughes EJ, Bang P, Snowden MA, Mcclain B, Hussey GD. First-in-human trial of the post-exposure tuberculosis vaccine H56:Ic31 in mycobacterium tuberculosis infected and non-infected healthy adults. Vaccine. 2015;33:4130–40.
29. Mahomed H, Machingaidze S, Hanekom WA, Hatherill M, Verver S. Reply: risk of tuberculosis among QuantiFERON converters and nonconverters. Am J Respir Crit Care Med. 2013;187:1140–1.
30. Mangtani P, Abubakar I, Ariti C, Beynon R, Pimpin L, Fine PE, Rodrigues LC, Smith PG, Lipman M, Whiting PF, Sterne JA. Protection by BCG vaccine against tuberculosis: a systematic review of randomized controlled trials. Clin Infect Dis. 2014;58:470–80.
31. Mao JJ, Zang X, Yue WL, Zhai PY, Zhang Q, Li CH, Zhuang X, Liu M, Qin G. Population-level health and economic impacts of introducing Vaccae vaccination in China: a modelling study. BMJ Glob Health. 2023;8
32. Martin C, Marinova D, Aguilo N, Gonzalo-Asensio J. MTBVAC, a live TB vaccine poised to initiate efficacy trials 100 years after BCG. Vaccine. 2021;39:7277–85.
33. Martinez L, Cords O, Liu Q, Acuna-Villaorduna C, Bonnet M, Fox GJ, Carvalho ACC, Chan PC, Croda J, Hill PC, Lopez-Varela E, Donkor S, Fielding K, Graham SM, Espinal MA, Kampmann B, Reingold A, Huerga H, Villalba JA, Grandjean L, Sotgiu G, Egere U, Singh S, Zhu L, Lienhardt C, Denholm JT, Seddon JA, Whalen CC, Garcia-Basteiro AL, Triasih R, Chen C, Singh J, Huang LM, Sharma S, Hannoun D, Del Corral H, Mandalakas AM, Malone LL, Ling DL, Kritski A, Stein CM, Vashishtha R, Boulahbal F, Fang CT, Boom WH, Netto EM, Lemos AC, Hesseling AC, Kay A, Jones-Lopez EC, Horsburgh CR, Lange C, Andrews JR. Infant BCG vaccination and risk of pulmonary and extrapulmonary tuberculosis throughout the life course: a systematic review and individual participant data meta-analysis. Lancet Glob Health. 2022;10:e1307–16.
34. Matusali G, Cimini E, Mazzotta V, Colavita F, Maggi F, Antinori A. Mpox immune response elicited by MVA-BN vaccine over 12 months of follow-up. J Infect. 2024;89:106309.
35. Munseri P, Said J, Amour M, Magohe A, Matee M, Rees CA, Mackenzie T, Tvaroha S, Bailey-Kellogg C, Maro I, Wieland-Alter W, Adams LV, Horsburgh CR, Nakamura K, Arbeit RD, Pallangyo K, Von Reyn CF. DAR-901 vaccine for the prevention of infection with mycobacterium tuberculosis among BCG-immunized adolescents in Tanzania: A randomized controlled, double-blind phase 2b trial. Vaccine. 2020;38:7239–45.
36. Nell AS, D'lom E, Bouic P, Sabate M, Bosser R, Picas J, Amat M, Churchyard G, Cardona PJ. Safety, tolerability, and immunogenicity of the novel antituberculous vaccine RUTI: randomized, placebo-controlled phase II clinical trial in patients with latent tuberculosis infection. PloS One. 2014;9:e89612.
37. Nemes E, Fiore-Gartland A, Boggiano C, Coccia M, D'souza P, Gilbert P, Ginsberg A, Hyrien O, Laddy D, Makar K, Mcelrath MJ, Ramachandra L, Schmidt AC, Shororbani S, Sunshine J, Tomaras G, Yu WH, Scriba TJ, Frahm N, Bcg Correlates Pis Study Team, M. C. P. S. T. The quest for vaccine-induced immune correlates of protection against tuberculosis. Vaccine Insights. 2022;1:165–81.
38. Nieuwenhuizen NE, Kulkarni PS, Shaligram U, Cotton MF, Rentsch CA, Eisele B, Grode L, Kaufmann SHE. The recombinant Bacille Calmette-Guerin vaccine VPM1002: ready for clinical efficacy testing. Front Immunol. 2017;8:1147.

39. World Health Organization, 2018. WHO preferred product characteristics for new tuberculosis vaccines.
40. World Health Organization, 2024. Global Tuberculosis Report.
41. Penn-Nicholson A, Geldenhuys H, Burny W, Van Der Most R, Day CL, Jongert E, Moris P, Hatherill M, Ofori-Anyinam O, Hanekom W, Vaccine Study T, Bollaerts A, Demoitie MA, Kany Luabeya AK, De Ruymaeker E, Tameris M, Lapierre D, Scriba TJ. Safety and immunogenicity of candidate vaccine M72/AS01E in adolescents in a TB endemic setting. Vaccine. 2015;33:4025–34.
42. Penn-Nicholson A, Tameris M, Smit E, Day TA, Musvosvi M, Jayashankar L, Vergara J, Mabwe S, Bilek N, Geldenhuys H, Luabeya AK, Ellis R, Ginsberg AM, Hanekom WA, Reed SG, Coler RN, Scriba TJ, Hatherill M, Team T-S. Safety and immunogenicity of the novel tuberculosis vaccine ID93 + GLA-SE in BCG-vaccinated healthy adults in South Africa: a randomised, double-blind, placebo-controlled phase 1 trial. Lancet Respir Med. 2018;6:287–98.
43. Rodriguez Velasquez S, Biru LE, Hakiza SM, Al-Gobari M, Triulzi I, Dalal J, Varela CBG, Botero Mesa S, Keiser O. Long-term levels of protection of different types of immunity against the omicron variant: a rapid literature review. Swiss Med Wkly. 2024;154:3732.
44. Sagawa ZK, Goman C, Frevol A, Blazevic A, Tennant J, Fisher B, Day T, Jackson S, Lemiale F, Toussaint L, Kalisz I, Jiang J, Ondrejcek L, Mohamath R, Vergara J, Lew A, Beckmann AM, Casper C, Hoft DF, Fox CB. Safety and immunogenicity of a thermostable ID93 + GLA-SE tuberculosis vaccine candidate in healthy adults. Nat Commun. 2023;14:1138.
45. Sauer SM, Mitnick CD, Khan U, Hewison C, Bastard M, Holtzman D, Law S, Khan M, Padayachee S, Ahmed S, Isani AK, Krisnanda A, Vilbrun SC, Bektasov S, Kumsa A, Docteur W, Tintaya K, Mcnicol M, Atshemyan H, Voynilo T, Thwe TT, Seung K, Rich M, Huerga H, Khan P, Franke M. Estimating post-treatment recurrence after multidrug-resistant tuberculosis treatment among patients with and without human immunodeficiency virus: the impact of assumptions about death and missing follow-up. Clin Infect Dis. 2024;78:164–71.
46. Schmidt A. BCG revaccination: lessons learned and implications for the field. Seventh global forum on TB vaccines. Brazil: Rio de Janeiro; 2024.
47. Schrager L 2025. Personal communication.
48. Scriba TJ, Netea MG, Ginsberg AM. Key recent advances in TB vaccine development and understanding of protective immune responses against mycobacterium tuberculosis. Semin Immunol. 2020;50:101431.
49. Sergeeva M, Romanovskaya-Romanko E, Zabolotnyh N, Pulkina A, Vasilyev K, Shurigina AP, Buzitskaya J, Zabrodskaya Y, Fadeev A, Vasin A, Vinogradova TI, Stukova MA. Mucosal influenza vector vaccine carrying TB10.4 and HspX antigens provides protection against mycobacterium tuberculosis in mice and Guinea pigs. Vaccines (Basel). 2021;9
50. Shurygina AP, Zabolotnykh N, Vinogradova T, Khairullin B, Kassenov M, Nurpeisova A, Sarsenbayeva G, Sansyzbay A, Vasilyev K, Buzitskaya J, Egorov A, Stukova M. Preclinical evaluation of TB/FLU-04L-an intranasal influenza vector-based boost vaccine against tuberculosis. Int J Mol Sci. 2023;24
51. Spertini F, Audran R, Chakour R, Karoui O, Steiner-Monard V, Thierry AC, Mayor CE, Rettby N, Jaton K, Vallotton L, Lazor-Blanchet C, Doce J, Puentes E, Marinova D, Aguilo N, Martin C. Safety of human immunisation with a live-attenuated mycobacterium tuberculosis vaccine: a randomised, double-blind, controlled phase I trial. Lancet Respir Med. 2015;3:953–62.
52. Stewart EL, Counoupas C, Quan DH, Wang T, Petrovsky N, Britton WJ, Triccas JA. Lung IL-17A-producing CD4(+) T cells correlate with protection after intrapulmonary vaccination with differentially Adjuvanted tuberculosis vaccines. Vaccines (Basel). 2024;12
53. Suliman S, Luabeya AKK, Geldenhuys H, Tameris M, Hoff ST, Shi Z, Tait D, Kromann I, Ruhwald M, Rutkowski KT, Shepherd B, Hokey D, Ginsberg AM, Hanekom WA, Andersen P, Scriba TJ, Hatherill M, Group HT. Dose optimization of H56:IC31 vaccine for tuberculosis-endemic populations. A double-blind, placebo-controlled, dose-selection trial. Am J Respir Crit Care Med. 2019;199:220–31.
54. Treatment Action Group 2024. Tuberculosis research funding trends 2005–2023.

55. Tait D, Diacon A, Borges AH, Van Brakel E, Hokey D, Rutkowski KT, Hunt DJ, Russell M, Andersen PL, Kromann I, Ruhwald M, Churchyard G, Dawson R. Safety and immunogenicity of the H56:IC31 tuberculosis vaccine candidate in adults successfully treated for drug-susceptible pulmonary tuberculosis: a phase 1 randomized trial. J Infect Dis. 2024;230:1262–70.
56. Tait DR, Hatherill M, Van Der Meeren O, Ginsberg AM, Van Brakel E, Salaun B, Scriba TJ, Akite EJ, Ayles HM, Bollaerts A, Demoitie MA, Diacon A, Evans TG, Gillard P, Hellstrom E, Innes JC, Lempicki M, Malahleha M, Martinson N, Mesia Vela D, Muyoyeta M, Nduba V, Pascal TG, Tameris M, Thienemann F, Wilkinson RJ, Roman F. Final analysis of a trial of M72/AS01(E) vaccine to prevent tuberculosis. N Engl J Med. 2019;381:2429–39.
57. Tameris M, Mearns H, Penn-Nicholson A, Gregg Y, Bilek N, Mabwe S, Geldenhuys H, Shenje J, Luabeya AKK, Murillo I, Doce J, Aguilo N, Marinova D, Puentes E, Rodriguez E, Gonzalo-Asensio J, Fritzell B, Thole J, Martin C, Scriba TJ, Hatherill M, Team MCT. Live-attenuated mycobacterium tuberculosis vaccine MTBVAC versus BCG in adults and neonates: a randomised controlled, double-blind dose-escalation trial. Lancet Respir Med. 2019;7:757–70.
58. Tameris MBS, Rozot V, Imbratta C, Musvosvi M, Murillo Jelsbak I, Geldenhuys H, Shenje J, Luabeya A, Mendelsohn S, Tredoux N, Fisher M, Bilek N, Asma T, Mabwe S, Doce J, Aguilo N, Marinova D, Puentes E, Martin C, Mukherjee R, Scriba T, Hatherill M. Safety, reactogenicity and immunogenicity of MTBVAC in newborns in a TB endemic area: a phase 2a randomized, double-blind, dose-defining trial. BMJ Glob Health. 2023;8
59. Tameris MD, Hatherill M, Landry BS, Scriba TJ, Snowden MA, Lockhart S, Shea JE, Mcclain JB, Hussey GD, Hanekom WA, Mahomed H, Mcshane H. Safety and efficacy of MVA85A, a new tuberculosis vaccine, in infants previously vaccinated with BCG: a randomised, placebo-controlled phase 2b trial. Lancet. 2013;381:1021–8.
60. Teo AKJ, Maclean EL, Fox GJ. Subclinical tuberculosis: a meta-analysis of prevalence and scoping review of definitions, prevalence and clinical characteristics. Eur Respir Rev. 2024;33:230208.
61. Tkachuk AP, Bykonia EN, Popova LI, Kleymenov DA, Semashko MA, Chulanov VP, Fitilev SB, Maksimov SL, Smolyarchuk EA, Manuylov VA, Vasina DV, Gushchin VA, Gintsburg AL. Safety and immunogenicity of the GamTBvac, the recombinant subunit tuberculosis vaccine candidate: A phase II, multi-center, double-blind, randomized. Placebo-Controlled Study. Vaccines (Basel). 2020;8:8.
62. Van Der Meeren O, Hatherill M, Nduba V, Wilkinson RJ, Muyoyeta M, Van Brakel E, Ayles HM, Henostroza G, Thienemann F, Scriba TJ, Diacon A, Blatner GL, Demoitie MA, Tameris M, Malahleha M, Innes JC, Hellstrom E, Martinson N, Singh T, Akite EJ, Khatoon Azam A, Bollaerts A, Ginsberg AM, Evans TG, Gillard P, Tait DR. Phase 2b controlled trial of M72/AS01(E) vaccine to prevent tuberculosis. N Engl J Med. 2018;379:1621–34.
63. Vasilyev K, Shurygina AP, Zabolotnykh N, Sergeeva M, Romanovskaya-Romanko E, Pulkina A, Buzitskaya J, Dogonadze MZ, Vinogradova TI, Stukova MA. Enhancement of the local CD8(+) T-cellular immune response to mycobacterium tuberculosis in BCG-primed mice after intranasal Administration of Influenza Vector Vaccine Carrying TB10.4 and HspX antigens. Vaccines (Basel). 2021;9
64. Vasina DV, Kleymenov DA, Manuylov VA, Mazunina EP, Koptev EY, Tukhovskaya EA, Murashev AN, Gintsburg AL, Gushchin VA, Tkachuk AP. First-in-human trials of GamTBvac, a recombinant subunit tuberculosis vaccine candidate: safety and immunogenicity assessment. Vaccines (Basel). 2019;7
65. Von Reyn CF, Mtei L, Arbeit RD, Waddell R, Cole B, Mackenzie T, Matee M, Bakari M, Tvaroha S, Adams LV, Horsburgh CR, Pallangyo K, Dardar Study G. Prevention of tuberculosis in Bacille Calmette-Guerin-primed, HIV-infected adults boosted with an inactivated whole-cell mycobacterial vaccine. AIDS. 2010;24:675–85.
66. Wajja A, Nassanga B, Natukunda A, Serubanja J, Tumusiime J, Akurut H, Oduru G, Nassuuna J, Kabagenyi J, Morrison H, Scott H, Doherty RP, Marshall JL, Puig IC, Cose S, Kaleebu P, Webb EL, Satti I, Mcshane H, Elliott AM, Team TBS. Safety and immunogenicity of ChAdOx1 85A prime followed by MVA85A boost compared with BCG revaccination among

Ugandan adolescents who received BCG at birth: a randomised, open-label trial. Lancet Infect Dis. 2024;24:285–96.

67. Wang J, Ding Y, Chong K, Cui M, Cao Z, Tang C, Tian Z, Hu Y, Zhao Y, Jiang S. Recent advances in lipid nanoparticles and their safety concerns for mRNA delivery. Vaccines (Basel). 2024;12
68. Wilkie M, Satti I, Minhinnick A, Riste M, Lopez Ramon R, Sheehan S, Manjaly Thomas Z-R, Wright D, Stockdale L, Hamidi A, O'shea MK, Dwivedi K, Behrens HM, Davenne T, Morton J, Vermaak S, Lawrie A, Moss P, Mcshane H. A phase I trial evaluating the safety and immunogenicity of a candidate tuberculosis vaccination regimen, ChAdOx1 85A prime—MVA85A boost in healthy UK adults. Vaccine. 2020;38:779–89.
69. Woodworth JS, Clemmensen HS, Battey H, Dijkman K, Lindenstrom T, Laureano RS, Taplitz R, Morgan J, Aagaard C, Rosenkrands I, Lindestam Arlehamn CS, Andersen P, Mortensen R. A Mycobacterium tuberculosis-specific subunit vaccine that provides synergistic immunity upon co-administration with Bacillus Calmette-Guerin. Nat Commun. 2021;12:6658.

Live-Attenuated Vaccines in Clinical Trials

10

Carlos Martin, Nacho Aguilo, and Jesus Gonzalo-Asensio

Historically, live-attenuated vaccines have played a significant role in immunizing against infectious diseases. The currently successful vaccines have mainly been developed for pathogens that have a stable antigen repertoire and can be controlled by an antibody response [1]. However, in the case of tuberculosis (TB), the mechanisms behind its pathogenicity are not completely understood, and protection against the disease relies primarily on T-cell-mediated rather than antibody-based immunity. The lack of correlation of protection for the study of the efficacy of new vaccine candidates against TB makes it necessary to carry out long and expensive Phase 3 efficacy trials in countries where the disease is endemic [2–4]. As Professor Douglas Young stated "we need new TB vaccines that provide protection against TB, in order to understand the immunology of the disease, and at the same time, we need to know the immunology of TB to develop these new vaccines." In this context, live-attenuated vaccines, containing a greater number of antigens compared to other immunization strategies, endorsed with the cumulative experience of BCG could play a crucial role in tackling TB [2, 5].

C. Martin (✉)
Departamento de Microbiología, Pediatría, Radiología y Salud Pública, Facultad de Medicina, Universidad de Zaragoza, Zaragoza, Spain

CIBERES Enfermedades Respiratorias, Instituto de Salud Carlos III, Madrid, Spain

Servicio de Microbiología, Hospital Universitario Miguel Servet, ISS Aragón, Zaragoza, Spain
e-mail: carlos@unizar.es

N. Aguilo · J. Gonzalo-Asensio
Departamento de Microbiología, Pediatría, Radiología y Salud Pública, Facultad de Medicina, Universidad de Zaragoza, Zaragoza, Spain

CIBERES Enfermedades Respiratorias, Instituto de Salud Carlos III, Madrid, Spain
e-mail: naguilo@unizar.es; jagonzal@unizar.es

P. J. G. Bettencourt (ed.), *Tuberculosis Vaccines*,
https://doi.org/10.1007/978-3-031-94540-3_10

10.1 First Vaccine and Universal Vaccination

The first major scientific breakthrough in vaccines occurred in 1796 when the English doctor Edward Jenner utilized a virus called cowpox, which causes disease in cows, to protect against smallpox, a virus that caused disease in humans. Jenner's revolutionary idea involved inoculating individuals with an infectious virus from animals. The animal version of the virus caused a milder form of the human disease in vaccinated individuals, while providing protection against the severe disease. To eradicate smallpox, it was imperative as universal distribution of the vaccine. In 1803, few years later after Jenner's discovery, the "Royal Philanthropic Vaccine Expedition" embarked from the port of La Coruña in Spain, under the promotion of King Charles IV of Spain. Its purpose was to introduce and distribute the vaccine in America and Asia, where the disease was causing significant mortality [6]. This expedition marked the first global humanitarian mission in history, estimated to have vaccinated over half a million people in the sixteenth century [6]. Jenner wrote, "I cannot imagine that the annals of history will provide a nobler and broader example of philanthropy than this vaccine expedition" [6]. The World Health Organization (WHO) officially declared smallpox eradicated in 1980. Today, smallpox remains the only infectious disease eradicated globally, thanks to the protection conferred by live vaccines and universal vaccination [7].

10.2 The Live-Attenuated Vaccines from Jenner to Pasteur

If we consider Jenner as the inventor of the first vaccine, it was the French biochemist Louis Pasteur who gave the term "vaccine" as a tribute to Jenner and the bovine origin of the first vaccine (from the Latin *vacca*). Pasteur's work on vaccines began nearly 100 years after Jenner's experiments, focusing on attenuation of pathogens for use as vaccines [8].

Initially, Pasteur's research was centered around infectious bacterial diseases affecting animals. He started with *Pasteurella multocida*, the causative agent of fowl cholera, and *Bacillus anthracis*, which is transmitted by spores and causes anthrax in livestock. By using an old culture of the bacteria that had lost its virulence, Pasteur managed to protect chickens from avian cholera and livestock from anthrax. When inoculated with the virulent pathogen, the vaccinated animals survived while the unvaccinated ones died. Pasteur called "attenuation" to the phenomenon which results in the eventual loss of virulence of pathogens, a term that is still used today to refer to vaccines that employ a live-attenuated variant of the pathogen [7, 9].

Next, Pasteur's work focused on the search of vaccines for diseases that affected humans. Pasteur empirically attenuated the rabies virus, a viral zoonosis disease causing rabies in humans due to dog bites that transmits this virus. His rabies vaccine saved the lives of dozens of people, primarily children, and the success of these vaccines led to the establishment of the first Pasteur Institute in 1888 and elevated Pasteur to the status of a national hero [7].

10.3 BCG: The First Vaccine Against TB and Only Authorized TB Vaccine in Use

The last years of the nineteenth century was an interesting time for medical progress. Pasteur had successfully developed a series of attenuated vaccines, and in 1882, the German doctor Robert Koch identified *Mycobacterium tuberculosis* as the causative agent of TB. In this context, at the Pasteur Institute in Lille in 1900, the French doctor Albert Calmette and veterinarian Camille Guérin began a close collaboration with the aim of finding a vaccine against TB. Combining the approaches of Jenner and Pasteur, their initial efforts involved cultivating a virulent strain of *Mycobacterium bovis*, the cause TB in cattle, and weakening its virulence in the laboratory. In the early twentieth century, bovine TB represented a major cause of disease and death in children due to the intake of milk from infected cattle. After 230 subculture passages and 13 years later, *M. bovis*, did not cause disease in various animals, including guinea pigs, monkeys, calves, and horses. This attenuated *M. bovis* strain was named Bacille Calmette-Guérin (BCG) [10, 11].

Genetic sequencing studies has shown that the major cause of attenuation of BCG is due to a loss in the genome region called "region of difference" 1 (RD1) [12]. This region contains among other the gene that codes for ESAT-6 protein, which only when secreted is considered one of the major virulence factors of the *M. tuberculosis* complex. The RD1 deletion contains two other secreted proteins: CFP-10 and PPE68. These three proteins are potent, and highly immunogenic, antigens that are conserved in the strains of the *M. tuberculosis* complex. Accordingly, loss of ESAT-6, CFP-10, and PPE68 in BCG could be a potential cause for the poor protection conferred by BCG against TB [13, 14].

In 1921, a baby, whose mother had died of TB shortly after birth, was the first human to be vaccinated with BCG orally. In the following 6 years, more than 50,000 babies were vaccinated, demonstrating that the live-attenuated BCG vaccine was safe. A significant decrease (more than ten-fold) in mortality of "BCG unvaccinated" (25%) compared to "BCG vaccinated" (less than 2%) was also observed, suggesting a nonspecific effect of BCG that could protect against other infectious diseases [11].

In the late 1920s, the BCG vaccine strain was widely distributed worldwide. The laboratories responsible for maintaining the vaccine conducted successive passages in culture media. These passages were responsible for the emergence of different BCG substrains, which were designated by either laboratory names (such as BCG Pasteur) or geographical names (like BCG Russia, Danish, and Japan). In recent years, comparative studies have been conducted on these BCG substrains, revealing differences in genetic content, morphology, and cell-mediated immune response. These findings align with the WHO's recommendation to preserve lyophilized BCG for vaccine production [11, 15, 16].

Today, 100 years later, BCG is the most widely administered vaccine in the world and is part of the WHO's list of essential medicines [17, 18]. However, its acceptance and recommendation are heterogeneous across countries, with less use in the industrialized world. The main reasons for these differences include lower risk of TB transmission and access to essential healthcare services and treatments, which decrease the chance to develop TB. Undoubtedly, the controversy surrounding the effectiveness of BCG also contributes to its exclusion from the vaccination schedule in countries where TB is not endemic. The BCG vaccine has been shown to be useful against disseminated TB and tuberculous meningitis in childhood, while relatively ineffective against the most common form of the disease in adults, pulmonary TB, which is otherwise responsible for disease transmission [19]. Published studies and different meta-analyses indicate highly variable protection against pulmonary TB, with 80% effectiveness in Native American and British children, and very little protection in studies from Chennai, India, and different studies have suggested that BCG efficacy might vary according to latitude or non-tuberculous mycobacteria exposure [20]. Recent systematic review studies showed that BCG vaccination at birth is effective at preventing TB in young children but is ineffective in adolescents and adults due to an immune waning effect. Immune protection therefore needs to be boosted in older populations [21].

On the other hand, it is also very important to highlight that BCG confers non-specific indirect beneficial effects, through generalized stimulation of the immune system, which may protect against other pathogens. The non-specific effects of BCG and other live-attenuated vaccines were described by Peter Aabey and, currently, this mechanism of action is being studied in-depth by Mihai Netea's team as we will describe later [22]. In a related context, since the 1960s, BCG has demonstrated its value as an immunomodulator, specifically in the chemotherapy of bladder cancer [23].

10.4 TB Vaccine Candidates in Clinical Trials

Among the different TB vaccine candidates in clinical trials, there is a great diversity of platforms and new technologies as diverse as for other infectious diseases. The TB vaccine pipeline include: subunit vaccines (either based on mRNA, viral vectored, or adjuvanted); and whole cell vaccines (either inactivated or live attenuated) [24, 25]. The subunit candidates contain a limited number of antigens and differ in the antigens used for immunization. Subunits candidates are based on major TB antigens such as those belonging to the Ag85 complex, or highly immunogenic antigens as ESAT-6 or CFP-10 missing in BCG, among others. Viral vectors deliver the coding gene(s) for the desired antigen(s). Adjuvanted subunit candidates use new formulations of adjuvants mixed with selected antigenic proteins. The subunit candidate $M72S01_E$ showed efficacy signals in Phase2b clinical trials in participants vaccinated with BCG at birth and previously infected with *M. tuberculosis,* and recently entered in Phase 3 efficacy studies in 2024 [26, 27].

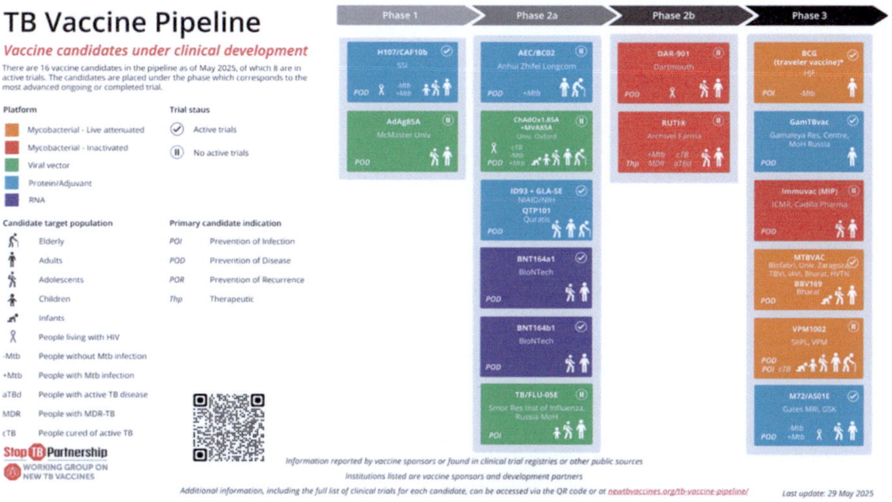

Fig. 10.1 TB vaccine candidates in clinical trials. (Modified from updated the Stop TB Partnership, working Group on New TB vaccines https://newtbvaccines.org/tb-vaccine-pipeline, updated March 2024. The different vaccine platforms and the antigens which they contain are included. Antigens used in formulation are not publicly known)

For an update on the different TB vaccine candidates in clinical trials, the Stop TB Partnership, working Group on New TB vaccines, and the Pipeline Report 2023 Tuberculosis Vaccine from Treatment Action Group, describe the clinical studies carried out and those that are underway (Fig. 10.1) [28, 29].

10.5 Attenuated TB Vaccines in Clinical Trials

In 2015, there were 13 TB vaccine clinical trials undergoing, and six were in Phase 1. In 2024, there are 17 TB vaccine clinical trials for the evaluation of different vaccine platforms [30]. Of the 6 TB vaccine candidates today in Phase 3 efficacy studies, 3 of the vaccine candidates are based on live-attenuated vaccines. One is based on revaccination with BCG, another on a recombinant BCG (VPM1002), and the third on attenuated *M. tuberculosis* (MTBVAC) (Fig. 10.2) [25, 31].

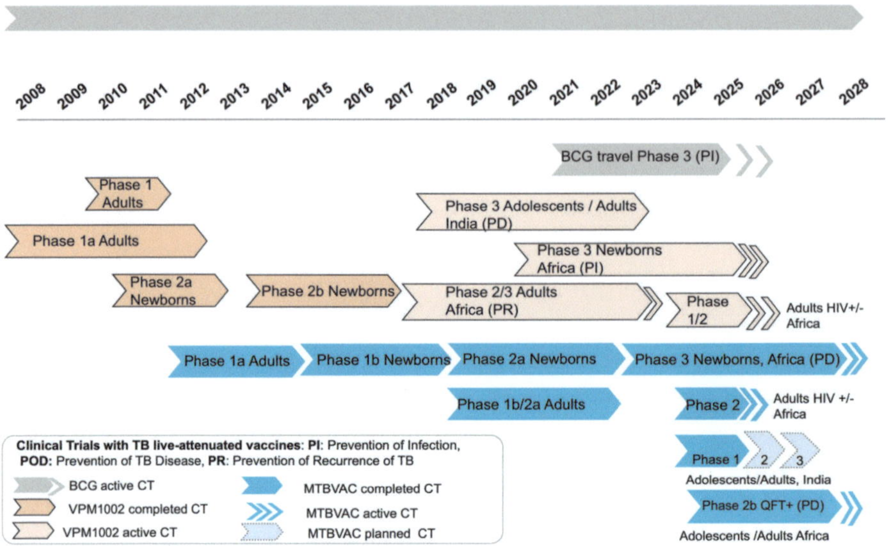

Fig. 10.2 Attenuated TB vaccines in clinical trials. Time line of the clinical trials of the three attenuated vaccine candidates in Phase 3. Revaccination with BCG in grey, the recombinant BCG, VPM1002, in salmon and the attenuated *M. tuberculosis,* MTBVAC, in blue. *PO* prevention of Disease, *PI* Prevention of Infection, *PR* Prevention of TB recurrence

10.6 Attenuated Vaccine *Mycobacterium bovis* BCG

Evidence to date suggests that revaccination with BCG carries minimal risk. A systematic review of the safety of BCG revaccination provided evidence for a small increase in the rate of mild local and systemic reactions, and no serious adverse events were reported in immunocompetent individuals [32]. The effect of BCG revaccination on the incidence of TB has been extensively studied in different trials in school-aged children in Brazil. Revaccination given to children aged 7–14 years in this setting does not provide substantial additional protection [33]. A systematic study of the protection conferred by BCG showed that in the absence of prior *M. tuberculosis* infection or prior sensitization with environmental mycobacteria, it is associated with increased efficacy of BCG against pulmonary TB and possibly against miliary and meningeal TB [20]. The greatest variation in BCG efficacy was seen when the vaccine was administered at school age but not when BCG was administered at birth [34, 35]. Today, even if revaccination with BCG is not systematically recommended due to a lack of proven efficacy of repeated doses for protection against TB, there is a growing interest in the use of revaccination with BCG. This is motivated by results in healthy adolescents which suggest prevention of *M. tuberculosis* infection, or sustained infection, measured as positivity of interferon (IFN)-γ release using QuantiFERON®-TB Gold Test [36, 37]. Although recent studies in Brazil have shown disappointing results, finding no protective effect of revaccination with BCG and placebo against initial or sustained conversion to QFT Plus; Conversion was observed in 34 (3.4%) of 996 participants in the BCG group and 32 (3.2%) of 989 in the placebo group [38, 39].

10.7 BCG in Active Clinical Trials

Phase 2b BCG Revaccination (BCG ReVax). Sponsored by the Bill & Melinda Gates Medical Research Institute, a Phase2b BCG revaccination trial (NCT04152161/ Gates MRI-TBV01-201) is conducted targeting adolescents and children. The trial compares AJVaccines' BCG (substrain Danish 1331) with saline placebo for the prevention of sustained Interferon Gamma Release Assays (IGRA) conversion in 1.936 South African healthy adolescents (Prevention of Infection: PI). This trial studies the repurposing of the existing BCG vaccine conducted to inform policy. No label change or new indication is intended [28]. Results published in New England in 2025 [40] conclude that BCG revaccination in QFT-test negative, HIV-negative adolescents did not provide protection from sustained M. tuberculosis infection.

- *Phase 3 BCG (Travel vaccine) to prevent TB infection (TIPI).* A Phase 3 trial (NCT04453293) is active recruiting with the primary indication: prevention of *M. tuberculosis* infection, or sustained infection (PI), in adults not previously infected with *M. tuberculosis*, healthy adult travelers, 18–65 years of age, exposed to persons with TB in high burden countries. Sponsored by the Henry M. Jackson Foundation for the Advancement of Military Medicine, the trial studies whether a single dose of pre-travel vaccination with BCG can lessen TB infection by producing an immune response when given to adults traveling to countries with a high burden of TB. BCG Japan (substrain Tokyo 172) is compared with a placebo. BCG Japan (Tokyo 172) is used globally, but is not approved for use in the United States, therefore, it is considered experimental. 2000 eligible volunteers will be enrolled. The goals of this study are both public health and scientific. The public health goal of this study is to offer possible protection against TB to U.S. workers traveling abroad to work in countries with a high burden of TB, where there is a risk for multidrug resistant/extensively drug-resistant TB exposure and where effective TB infection control interventions are infrequently fully implemented. A long-term scientific goal is to test the hypothesis that BCG vaccination prevents primary TB infection as measured by IGRA conversion at return from travel visit, as well as sustained conversion at approximately 4–6 months post-return from travel. Rates of IGRA conversion in BCG-vaccinated recipients as compared to placebo recipients will be evaluated. Additionally, this study will collect information regarding exposure to an infection with TB, assessing risk factors for TB infection during the participant's travel. The purpose of this study is not seeking licensure based on this trial [28].

10.8 VPM1002 Recombinant BCG

VPM1002 is a live, genetically modified BCG (recombinant BCG; rBCG) designed to provide better safety and efficacy and to induce a broader immune response against mycobacterial antigens than the original BCG. VPM1001 is based in the inactivation of the urease C gene (*ureC*) being replaced by the gene encoding listeriolysin O (*hly*), a membrane-perforating protein from *Listeria monocytogenes*. The rationale for its design at the Max Planck Institute of Infection Biology in Germany is based on improvement of the optimal pH for Hly activity by construction of a Δ*ureC hly* + rBCG strain that lacks UreC activity [41]. T cells produced abundant type 1 cytokines after restimulation, resulting in ten-fold reduced bacterial burden 90 days after infection. VPM1002 vaccination induces type 17 cytokine response with recruitment of antigen-specific T lymphocytes to the lung upon *M. tuberculosis* infection of rBCG-vaccinated mice and induces apoptosis [42, 43].

10.9 VPM1002 in Clinical Trials

VPM1002 is today in active Phase 3 clinical trials that are sponsored by the Serum Institute of India Private Limited with the development partner(s) Vakzine Projekt Management GmbH. The primary Indication of the trial is prevention of *M. tuberculosis* infection or sustained infection, including other indications as prevention of TB disease (PD) and prevention of TB recurrence (PR). The target populations are adolescents, adults, children, elderly, infants, and people cured of active TB [28].

10.10 VPM1002 Active Clinical Trials

There are three Clinical Trials in Phase 3, and one in Phase 1/2

- *Multicenter Phase 3 to study prevention of TB disease (PD) in adolescents and adults*, sponsored by the Indian Council of Medical Research and registered in India as CTRI/2019/01/017026. This trial evaluates the efficacy, safety, and immunogenicity of VPM1002 and Immuvac MIP (*Mycobacterium indicus pranii* inactivated) [37] vs. placebo in preventing TB disease (pulmonary or extrapulmonary) among 12,721 household contacts (≥six years old, HIV negative) of people with pulmonary TB in India. The study started in 2018 and the primary completion in 2022 [28].
- *Multicenter Phase 3 to study prevention of M. tuberculosis infection (PI), or sustained infection in infants*, sponsored by the Serum Institute of India Pvt. Ltd. and registered in Clinical trials.gov as NCT04351685 PriME. The trial evaluates the efficacy, safety, and immunogenicity of VPM1002 (vs. BCG) in preventing TB infection among 6940 newborns 0–14 days old (HIV-exposed/HIV-negative eligible) in Gabon, Kenya, South Africa, Tanzania, and Uganda. The study started in 2020 and completion is estimated in 2026.
- *Multicenter Phase 2/3 to study prevention of TB recurrence in adults cured of active TB*. This trial is sponsored by the Serum Institute of India Pvt. Ltd. and registered in Clinical trials.gov as NCT03152903. It aims at evaluating efficacy, safety, and immunogenicity of VPM1002 (vs. placebo) in preventing TB disease recurrence (PR) (pulmonary or extrapulmonary) in 2000 HIV-negative adults

ages 18–65 years successfully treated for pulmonary TB in India and Bangladesh. The study started in 2017 and primary completion is estimated in 2024.

- *Phase 1/2 safety/immunogenicity HIV study of VPM1002 and BCG revaccination* (vs. placebo) in 480 HIV-positive and HIV-negative preadolescents of ages 8–14, with and without TB, infection in South Africa. The trial is registered as NCT05539989; IMPAACT 2035/HVTN 604). Trial start is planned for 2024 and study completion is estimated in 2026.

10.11 VPM1002 Completed Clinical Trials

Phase 1 Safety in adults in Germany. Sponsored by Vakzine Projekt Managment GmbH. The trial was registered in Clinical trials.gov as NCT00749034. It consisted of a dose-escalation study about safety and immunogenicity of VPM1002 in comparison with BCG in healthy male volunteers. The study started in 2008 and was completed in 2012, enrolling 80 persons. VPM1002 was safe and immunogenic for B-cell and T-cell responses, and hence brought VPM1002 forward through the clinical trial pipeline [44].

Phase 1 Safety in adults in South Africa. Sponsored by Vakzine Projekt Management GmbH. Trial was registered in Clinical trials.gov as NCT01113281. A dose-escalation study on safety and immunogenicity of VPM1002 compared to BCG was performed in healthy volunteers in South Africa. The study started in 2010 and was completed in 2011. 24 healthy male and female adults, with prior exposure to BCG, received a single vaccination with VPM1002, to demonstrate that the rBCG candidate was safe, well tolerated, and immunogenic [45, 46].

Phase 2a Safety in Infants in South Africa. Sponsored by Vakzine Projekt Management GmbH. Trial was registered in Clinical trials.gov as NCT01479972. This study evaluated safety and immunogenicity of VPM1002 in comparison with BCG in newborn infants in South Africa. Study started in 2011 study and was completed in 2012, enrolling 48 infants. VPM1002 was shown to be safe, well-tolerated, and immunogenic in newborn infants, confirming results from previous trials in adults [45].

Phase 2b in Infants in South Africa. Sponsored by the Serum Institute of India Pvt. Ltd. Trial was registered in Clinical trials.gov as NCT02391415 to evaluate the safety and immunogenicity of VPM1002 in comparison with BCG in HIV-exposed/-unexposed newborn infants in South Africa. Study started in 2015 and was completed in 2017, enrolling 416 infants. VPM1002 was less reactogenic than BCG and was not associated with any serious safety concern. A non-inferiority, double-blind, controlled trial to study safety and immunogenicity of VPM1002 versus BCG in South African newborn babies showed that both vaccines were immunogenic, although responses were higher with the BCG vaccine [47].

10.12 MTBVAC TB Vaccine Candidate Attenuated *M. tuberculosis*

The MTBVAC TB vaccine candidate is based on a rationally attenuated *M. tuberculosis* strain constructed by genetic engineering. Attenuation is achieved by two stable deletions in the *phoP* and *fadD26* genes, conferring PhoPR and PDIM negative phenotypes, while maintaining the rest of the antigens present in the tubercle bacillus, including those absent in the current BCG vaccine due to the loss of the RD1, and other RD regions, responsible for its attenuation.

A quarter of the world's population is estimated to have been in contact with *M. tuberculosis* based on positive tuberculin skin test (TST) or IGRA measured by QuantiFERON®-TB Gold Test (QFT) or enzyme-linked immunosorbent spot (ELISpot) [31]. On average, 5–10% of those who are infected will develop active TB disease over their lifetime. Multiple longitudinal epidemiological studies, however, show that the majority of TB disease manifests soon after infection, with disease rarely occurring more than 2 years after the initial infection [48]. The vast burden of global TB is, therefore, from recently transmitted infection [49]. This is why it is very important to study the host-pathogen immune dynamics of *M. tuberculosis*, as 90% of those infected with TB do not develop TB disease and Individuals with latent TB had a 79% lower risk of progressive TB after reinfection than uninfected individuals [50]. In other words, the initial *M. tuberculosis* infection might confer protection, a hypothesis that fuels the design of live-attenuated vaccines based on *M. tuberculosis*.

MTBVAC was constructed at the University of Zaragoza in collaboration with the Institut Pasteur of Paris, and the Spanish company Biofabri is the sponsor responsible for industrial and clinical development of MTBVAC. Biofabri has partnered with the Indian manufacturer Bharat Biotech. Thus, development partners of MTBVAC are Bharat Biotech, University of Zaragoza, International AIDS Vaccine Initiative (IAVI), Tuberculosis Vaccine Initiative (TBVI), and the HIV Vaccine Trials Network. The primary indication of this vaccine is prevention of TB disease, and the target populations are adolescents, adults, and infants.

10.13 MTBVAC Active Clinical Trials

- *Multicenter Phase 3 to study prevention of TB disease in infants,* sponsored by Biofabri and registered in Clinical trials.gov as NCT04975178. The efficacy, safety, and immunogenicity of MTBVAC compared to BCG will be evaluated in newborns in Sub-Saharan Africa. The final aim is evaluating the efficacy of MTBVAC in preventing TB disease among 7120 newborns (0–7 days old, HIV-exposed/HIV-negative eligible) in South Africa, Senegal, and Madagascar. Study started in 2022 and completion is estimated in 2029.
- *Phase 2 Evaluating the Safety and Immunogenicity of MTBVAC in Adolescents and Adults Living With and Without HIV in South Africa compared to BCG* sponsored by the HIV Vaccine Trials Network. MTBVAC will be tested in 276 HIV-positive and HIV-negative preadolescents aged 8–14 with and without TB

infection in South Africa (NCT05947890). The aim is evaluating the safety and immunogenicity of MTBVAC in adolescents and adults living with and without HIV in South Africa (HVTN605A5421). The study started in 2024 study, and completion is estimated to be 2025.

- *Phase 1 in adolescent adults in India.* Sponsored by Bharat Biotech International Limited in collaboration with Biofabri, this trail aims to evaluate the safety and immunogenicity of MTBVAC (vs. placebo) in adolescents and adults in India. The Phase 1 trial to evaluate the safety and immunogenicity of MTBVAC.

10.14 MTBVAC Clinical Trials in Preparation

- *Phase 2b Study to Evaluate the Efficacy, Safety, and Immunogenicity of MTBVAC in IGRA-Positive Adolescents and Adults Living in a TB Endemic Region* (NCT06272812). Sponsored by the International AIDS Vaccine Initiative (IAVI) in collaboration with Biofabri, this study of MTBVAC will enroll approximately 4300 TB-infected (QFT+), HIV-negative adults and adolescents in Africa previously vaccinated with BCG. Participants will be between 14 and 45 years, living in Sub-Saharan African countries in areas with high TB burden. Participants at 15–20 trial sites will receive a single dose of MTBVAC or placebo. Participants will be followed for 2–3 years to study prevention of TB disease. Study start is planned for 2024, and study completion is estimated to be 2028.
- *Phase 2 and Phase 3 in adolescent adults in India.* Sponsored by Bharat Biotech International Limited in collaboration with Biofabri, this trail aims to evaluate the safety and immunogenicity of MTBVAC (vs. placebo) in adolescents and adults in India and a pivotal safety, immunogenicity, and efficacy trial planned to start in 2025.

10.15 MTBVAC Completed Clinical Trials

Phase 1 Safety in Adults in Lausanne, Switzerland. Sponsored by Biofabri, this trial is registered in Clinical trials.gov as NCT02013245. It consisted of a phase I, double blind, randomized, controlled, dose-escalation study to evaluate the safety and immunogenicity of MTBVAC in comparison with BCG in 36 Elispot TB (ESAT-6, CFP10, PPD)-negative, and HIV- negative adult volunteers. Ages eligible for study inclusion were 18–45 years. MTBVAC showed similar safety to BCG. MTBVAC seemed to be at least as immunogenic as BCG, but the study was not powered to investigate this outcome. Further plans to use more immunogenicity endpoints in a larger number of volunteers (adults and adolescents) were planned, with the aim to thoroughly characterize and potentially distinguish immunogenicity between MTBVAC and BCG in TB-endemic countries. Combined with a safety profile, these data supported advanced clinical development in high-burden TB endemic countries. The study started in 2013 and enrollment was completed in 2014 [51].

Phase 1b Safety in Infants in South Africa. Sponsored by. Biofabri S L, this trial was registered in Clinical trials.gov as NCT02729571. The trial consisted of a randomized, double-blind, dose-escalation clinical trial of the safety, reactogenicity, and immunogenicity of MTBVAC compared to BCG Vaccine SSI, in newborns living in a TB endemic region with a safety arm in adults. MTBVAC had acceptable reactogenicity and induced a durable CD4+ T cell response in infants. The evidence of immunogenicity supported progression of MTBVAC into larger safety and efficacy trials, but also confounded interpretation of tests for *M. tuberculosis* infection, highlighting the need for stringent endpoint definition. The study started in 2015 and was completed in 2018 [52].

Phase 1b/2a Safety and Immunogenicity in Adults in South Africa. Sponsored by the International AIDS Vaccine Initiative (IAVI), this trial is registered in Clinical trials.gov as NCT02933281. This phase 1b/2a randomized, double-blind, active-controlled trial studied the safety, immunogenicity, and dose-escalation in adults with and without latent TB infection in South Africa. Reactogenicity and immunogenicity of MTBVAC was compared to BCG vaccine Japan (Tokyo 172) in 144 enrolled participants. The study started in 2018 and was completed in 2021 [53].

Phase 2a Safety, Immunogenicity, and dose definition of MTBVAC in infants. Sponsored by Biofabri, this trial is registered in Clinical trials.gov as NCT03536117. The aim was to dose-define safety and immunogenicity of MTBVAC in South African neonates living in a high-burden TB-endemic region. Reactogenicity and Immunogenicity of MTBVAC compared to BCG Danish was measured in 99 enrolled participants. The study started in 2019 and was completed in 2022 [54].

10.16 Advantages and Disadvantages of Live-Attenuated TB Vaccines

The development of a new effective vaccine against TB requires innovation in scientific research, exhaustive preclinical studies, and subsequent demonstration of the vaccine's safety, its immunogenicity and finally its effectiveness against the respiratory forms of the disease in different clinical trial [55]. Once a vaccine candidate's safety and efficacy have been demonstrated, subsequent implementation and universal distribution should be part of an integrated approach to disease control [55].

One of the greatest advantages that live-attenuated vaccines against TB present over subunit candidates is the enormous experience acquired in the use, distribution, and administration of BCG. Since BCG was first administered on July 18, 1921, billions of doses have been administered, and today it is estimated that 200 million doses are still administered annually. Its vaccination coverage is close to 90% [21, 31]. BCG is considered a very reactogenic vaccine, producing a scar at the site of inoculation in most cases, but it is safe in immunocompetent people and is administered in the first days after birth. Another great advantage of attenuated vaccines, apart from the experience in use and distribution, is that, unlike subunit vaccines, a single dose is often sufficient.

Numerous epidemiological studies showed a decrease in mortality in babies vaccinated with BCG compared to unvaccinated ones. The initial studies by Calmette and Guérin from 1921 to 1926, vaccinating approximately 50,000 children from tuberculous families with BCG, observed that while mortality in unvaccinated children was approximately 25%, in those vaccinated with BCG mortality decreased to less than 2% [11]. Recent studies in Africa showed similar results, especially in low-weight babies [56]. A seminal study published in 2012 by the laboratory of Mihai Netea, described the Non-Specific Effect (NSE) conferred by BCG, due to an epigenetic modification of genes involved in cellular immunity and metabolic changes, which conferred an immune response to other unrelated pathogens such as bacteria (*Staphylococcus*) or fungi (*Candida albicans*) [57]. Since then, numerous studies have been carried out, and today BCG is the paradigm of NSE conferred by live-attenuated vaccines [22].

The effect of BCG vaccination on conversion of the TST has been widely reported [58]. The IGRA test by QFT or ELISpot, which is based on the stimulation of proteins encoded in the RD1 region that are absent in BCG, such as ESAT-6 and CFP-10, allow the differentiation of BCG vaccinated from previous exposure to *M. tuberculosis*. Live-attenuated vaccines expressing the antigens CFP-10 and ESAT-6, as is the case for some attenuated *M. tuberculosis* and rBCG vaccines, are expected to interfere with IGRA testing, resulting in vaccine-induced IGRA conversion. This phenomenon is analogous to the effect of BCG vaccination on TST conversion, also known as PPD conversion. The TST serves as a marker for cell-mediated immune responses to mycobacteria but is no longer considered as a useful clinical indicator of the effectiveness of vaccination for TB or protective immunity [59, 60]. Clearly, if a live-attenuated vaccine that includes either CFP-10 or ESAT-6 antigens (as several other new TB vaccine candidates do), proves to be effective, the development of an IGRA, or other diagnostic platform, based on alternative antigens would be beneficial for diagnosis of post-vaccination TB exposure [61, 62].

Another potential disadvantage is the use of live-attenuated vaccines in immunocompromised individuals. In a South African multicenter surveillance study, the pooled incidence for disseminated BCG disease in vaccinated children living with HIV was about 900 per 100,000 [63]. Early antiretroviral treatment reduces risk of BCG immune reconstitution adenitis [64]. After a decade of debate regarding the risk-to-benefit ratio of BCG in people living with HIV, the WHO guidelines recommend that adults, children, and neonates living with HIV should receive BCG vaccination if they are stable on antiretroviral therapy. Therefore, it is necessary to carry out safety studies of attenuated vaccines candidates to evaluate the safety and immunogenicity in populations living with HIV [62].

A new vaccine targeting TB in adolescents and adults, rather than in any other age group, is expected to have the most immediate impact on disease transmission and TB control. However, studying the immunogenicity and efficacy of a new TB vaccine candidate in this population, particularly in individuals previously vaccinated with BCG, is highly complex. Factors such as prior BCG vaccination, exposure to environmental mycobacteria, or previous *M. tuberculosis* infections present significant challenges in evaluating the effectiveness of new TB vaccines, as they may obscure or diminish the vaccine's effects.

The most reliable method to determine whether a new TB vaccine outperforms BCG is to conduct efficacy trials in a population without prior exposure, such as newborns, and compare prevention of disease relative to BCG, as a proof of concept. This approach would pave the way for subsequent testing in adolescents and adults, given that widespread implementation in these age groups holds the greatest potential for global TB control.

Potential Conflict of Interest Carlos Martín, Juan Ignacio (Nacho) Aguilo, and Jesús Gonzalo are co-inventors on a patent on Tuberculosis Vaccine held by the University of Zaragoza and Biofabri. Biofabri is an industrial partner of the University of Zaragoza and exclusive licensee and industrial and clinical developer of MTBVAC. The authors declare that they have no other known competing financial interests or personal relationships that could have appeared to influence the work reported here.

References

1. Rappuoli R, Aderem A. A 2020 vision for vaccines against HIV, tuberculosis and malaria. Nature. 2011;473:463–9.
2. Young D, Dye C. The development and impact of tuberculosis vaccines. Cell. 2006;124:683–7.
3. Kamath AT, Fruth U, Brennan MJ, et al. New live mycobacterial vaccines: the Geneva consensus on essential steps towards clinical development. Vaccine. 2005;23:3753–61.
4. Cooper AM. Cell-mediated immune responses in tuberculosis. Annu Rev Immunol. 2009;27:393–422.
5. Martín C, Marinova D, Aguiló N, Gonzalo-Asensio J. MTBVAC, a live TB vaccine poised to initiate efficacy trials 100 years after BCG. Vaccine. 2021;39:7277. https://doi.org/10.1016/j.vaccine.2021.06.049.
6. Franco-Paredes C, Lammoglia L, Santos-Preciado JI. The Spanish royal philanthropic expedition to bring smallpox vaccination to the New World and Asia in the 19th century. Clin Infect Dis. 2005;41:1285–9.
7. Plotkin SA, Plotkin SL. The development of vaccines: how the past led to the future. Nat Rev Microbiol. 2011;9:889–93.
8. Desmond A, Offit PA. On the shoulders of giants—from Jenner's Cowpox to mRNA Covid vaccines. N Engl J Med. 2021;1–3
9. Nature Milestones in Vaccines (2020). https://www.nature.com/collections/hcajdiajij. Accessed 14 Dec 2023.
10. Lange C, Aaby P, Behr MA, Donald PR, Kaufmann SHE, Netea MG, Mandalakas AM. 100 years of Mycobacterium bovis bacille Calmette-Guérin. Lancet Infect Dis. 2021;22:e2–e12.
11. Gheorghiu M, Lagranderie M, Balazuc A-M. Vaccines: a biography. 2009; https://doi.org/10.1007/978-1-4419-1108-7_8.
12. Brosch R, Gordon SV, Garnier T, et al. Genome plasticity of BCG and impact on vaccine efficacy. Proc Natl Acad Sci USA. 2007;104:5596–601.
13. Martín C, Marinova D, Aguiló N, Gonzalo-Asensio J. MTBVAC, a live TB vaccine poised to initiate efficacy trials 100 years after BCG. Vaccine. 2021;39:7277–85.
14. Aguilo N, Gonzalo-Asensio J, Alvarez-Arguedas S, et al. Reactogenicity to major tuberculosis antigens absent in BCG is linked to improved protection against Mycobacterium tuberculosis. Nat Commun. 2017;8:16085.
15. Behr MA (2002) BCG--different strains, different vaccines? Lancet Infect Dis 2:86–92.
16. Keyser A, Troudt JM, Taylor JL, Izzo AA. BCG sub-strains induce variable protection against virulent pulmonary Mycobacterium tuberculosis infection, with the capacity to drive Th2 immunity. Vaccine. 2011;29:9308–15.

17. WHO. WHO BCG Vaccine. https://www.who.int/teams/health-product-and-policy-standards/standards-and-specifications/vaccines-quality/bcg. Accessed 14 Dec 2023.
18. WHO Essential Medicines (2023). https://www.who.int/publications/i/item/WHO-MHP-HPS-EML-2023.03. Accessed 18 Dec 2023.
19. Dockrell HM, Butkeviciute E. Can what have we learnt about BCG vaccination in the last 20 years help us to design a better tuberculosis vaccine? Vaccine. 2021;58:470.
20. Mangtani P, Abubakar I, Ariti C, et al. Protection by BCG vaccine against tuberculosis: a systematic review of randomized controlled trials. Clin Infect Dis. 2014;58:470–80.
21. Martinez L, Cords O, Liu Q, et al. Infant BCG vaccination and risk of pulmonary and extrapulmonary tuberculosis throughout the life course: a systematic review and individual participant data meta-analysis. Lancet Glob Heal. 2022;10:e1307–16.
22. Ziogas A, Bruno M, van der Meel R, Mulder WJM, Netea MG. Trained immunity: target for prophylaxis and therapy. Cell Host Microbe. 2023;31:1776–91.
23. Redelman-Sidi G, Glickman MS, Bochner BH. The mechanism of action of BCG therapy for bladder cancer—a current perspective, vol. 11. Nature Publishing Group; 2014. p. 1–10.
24. Martin C, Aguilo N, Marinova D, Gonzalo-Asensio J. Update on TB vaccine pipeline. Applied Sciences (Switzerland). 2020;10 https://doi.org/10.3390/app10072632.
25. Looney MM, Hatherill M, Musvosvi M, et al. Conference report: WHO meeting report on mRNA-based tuberculosis vaccine development. Vaccine. 2023;41:7060. https://doi.org/10.1016/j.vaccine.2023.10.026.
26. Tait DR, Hatherill M, Meeren OVD, et al. Final analysis of a trial of M72/AS01E vaccine to prevent tuberculosis. N Engl J Med. 2019;381:2429. https://doi.org/10.1056/nejmoa1909953.
27. Meeren OVD, Hatherill M, Nduba V, et al. Phase 2b controlled trial of M72/AS01E vaccine to prevent tuberculosis. N Engl J Med. 2018;379:1621–34.
28. Stop TB Partnership. Working Group on New TB Vaccines (2023). https://newtbvaccines.org/tb-vaccine-pipeline/. Accessed 14 Dec 2023.
29. Frick M (2023) Pipeline Report 2023 Tuberculosis Vaccine.
30. Partnership ST (2023) TB Vaccine Clinical Pipeline 2023. https://newtbvaccines.org/tb-vaccine-pipeline/. Accessed 19 Dec 2023.
31. Innovation 6. TB research and WHO Global Tuberculosis Report 2023. https://www.who.int/teams/global-tuberculosis-programme/tb-reports/global-tuberculosis-report-2023/tb-research-and-innovation. Accessed 14 Dec 2023.
32. Bannister S, Sudbury E, Villanueva P, Perrett K, Curtis N. The safety of BCG revaccination: a systematic review. Vaccine. 2021;39:2736–45.
33. Rodrigues LC, Pereira SM, Cunha SS, et al. Effect of BCG revaccination on incidence of tuberculosis in school-aged children in Brazil: the BCG-REVAC cluster-randomised trial. Lancet. 2005;366:1290–5.
34. Barreto ML, Pilger D, Pereira SM, Genser B, Cruz AA, Cunha SS, Sant'Anna C, Hijjar MA, Ichihara MY, Rodrigues LC (2014) Causes of variation in BCG vaccine efficacy: examining evidence from the BCG REVAC cluster randomized trial to explore the masking and the blocking hypotheses. 1–6.
35. Pereira SM, Barreto ML, Pilger D, Cruz AA, Sant'Anna C, Hijjar MA, Ichihara MY, Santos AC, Genser B, Rodrigues LC. Effectiveness and cost-effectiveness of first BCG vaccination against tuberculosis in school-age children without previous tuberculin test (BCG-REVAC trial): a cluster-randomised trial. Lancet Infect Dis. 2012;12:300–6.
36. Nemes E, Geldenhuys H, Rozot V, et al. Prevention of M. Tuberculosis infection with H4:IC31 vaccine or BCG revaccination. N Engl J Med. 2018;379:138–49.
37. Sable SB, Posey JE, Scriba TJ. Tuberculosis vaccine development: Progress in clinical evaluation. Clin Microbiol Rev. 2019;33:16076.
38. McShane H. Revaccination with BCG: does it work? Lancet Infect Dis. 2024;24:559. https://doi.org/10.1016/s1473-3099(24)00006-9.
39. dos Santos PCP, Messina NL, de Oliveira RD, et al. Effect of BCG vaccination against Mycobacterium tuberculosis infection in adult Brazilian health-care workers: a nested clinical trial. Lancet Infect Dis. 2024;24:594. https://doi.org/10.1016/s1473-3099(23)00818-6.

40. Schmidt AC, Fairlie L, Hellström E, Luabeya Kany Kany A, Middelkoop K, Naidoo K, Nair G, Gela A, Nemes E, Scriba TJ, Cinar A, Frahm N, Mogg R, Kaufman D, Dunne MW, Hatherill M, BCG REVAX Study Team. BCG Revaccination for the prevention of Mycobacterium tuberculosis infection. N Engl J Med. 2025;392:1789–800.
41. Grode L. Increased vaccine efficacy against tuberculosis of recombinant Mycobacterium bovis bacille Calmette-Guerin mutants that secrete listeriolysin. J Clin Invest. 2005;115:2472–9.
42. Desel C, Dorhoi A, Bandermann S, Grode L, Eisele B, Kaufmann SHE. Recombinant BCG ureC hly+ induces superior protection over parental BCG by stimulating a balanced combination of type 1 and type 17 cytokine responses. J Infect Dis. 2011;204:1573–84.
43. Farinacci M, Weber S, Kaufmann SHE. The recombinant tuberculosis vaccine rBCG ΔureC::hly+ induces apoptotic vesicles for improved priming of CD4+ and CD8+ T cells. Vaccine. 2012;30:7608–14.
44. Grode L, Ganoza CA, Brohm C, Weiner J, Eisele B, Kaufmann SHE. Safety and immunogenicity of the recombinant BCG vaccine VPM1002 in a phase 1 open-label randomized clinical trial. Vaccine. 2013;31:1340–8.
45. Loxton AG, Knaul JK, Grode L, et al. Safety and immunogenicity of the recombinant Mycobacterium bovis BCG vaccine VPM1002 in HIV-unexposed newborn infants in South Africa. Clinical and vaccine immunology: CVI; 2017. https://doi.org/10.1128/cvi.00439-16.
46. Kaufmann SH, Cotton MF, Eisele B, Gengenbacher M, Grode L, Hesseling AC, Walzl G. The BCG replacement vaccine VPM1002: from drawing board to clinical trial. Expert Rev Vaccines. 2014;13:619–30.
47. Cotton MF, Madhi SA, Luabeya AK, et al. Safety and immunogenicity of VPM1002 versus BCG in South African newborn babies: a randomised, phase 2 non-inferiority double-blind controlled trial. Lancet Infect Dis. 2022;22:1472. https://doi.org/10.1016/s1473-3099(22)00222-5.
48. Behr MA, Edelstein PH, Ramakrishnan L. Revisiting the timetable of tuberculosis. BMJ (Clinical research ed). 2018;362:k2738.
49. Behr MA, Kaufmann E, Duffin J, Edelstein PH, Ramakrishnan L. Latent tuberculosis: two centuries of confusion. Am J Resp Crit Care. 2021;204:142–8.
50. Andrews JR, Noubary F, Walensky RP, Cerda R, Losina E, Horsburgh CR. Risk of progression to active tuberculosis following reinfection with Mycobacterium tuberculosis. Clin Infect Dis. 2012;54:784–91.
51. Spertini F, Audran R, Chakour R, et al. Safety of human immunisation with a live-attenuated Mycobacterium tuberculosis vaccine: a randomised, double-blind, controlled phase I trial. Lancet Respir Med. 2015;3:953–62.
52. Tameris M, Mearns H, Penn-Nicholson A, et al. Live-attenuated Mycobacterium tuberculosis vaccine MTBVAC versus BCG in adults and neonates: a randomised controlled, double-blind dose-escalation trial. Lancet Respir Med. 2019;7:1–14.
53. Luabella et al. Live-attenuated Mycobacterium tuberculosis vaccine, MTBVAC, in adults with or without M tuberculosis sensitisation: a single-centre, phase 1b-2a, double-blind, dose-escalation, randomised controlled trial. Lancet Glob Health. 2025 Jun;13(6):e1030–e1042.
54. Tameris et al. Safety, reactogenicity, and immunogenicity of MTBVAC in infants: a phase 2a randomised, double-blind, dose-defining trial in a TB endemic setting. EBioMedicine. 2025 Apr;114:105628.
55. Cobelens F, Suri RK, Helinski M, Makanga M, Weinberg AL, Schaffmeister B, Deege F, Hatherill M, Group TVRS. Accelerating research and development of new vaccines against tuberculosis: a global roadmap. Lancet Infect Dis. 2022;22:e108. https://doi.org/10.1016/s1473-3099(21)00810-0.
56. Webb EL, Elliott AM, Arts RJW, et al. BCG-induced non-specific effects on heterologous infectious disease in Ugandan neonates: an investigator-blind randomised controlled trial. Lancet Infect Dis. 2021;388:3027.
57. Kleinnijenhuis JJ, Quintin JJ, Preijers FF, et al. Bacille Calmette-Guerin induces NOD2-dependent nonspecific protection from reinfection via epigenetic reprogramming of monocytes. Proc Natl Acad Sci USA. 2012;109:17537–42.

58. Seddon JA, Paton J, Nademi Z, et al. The impact of BCG vaccination on tuberculin skin test responses in children is age dependent: evidence to be considered when screening children for tuberculosis infection. Thorax. 2016;71:932–9.
59. Ho MM, Southern J, Kang H-N, Knezevic I. WHO Informal Consultation on standardization and evaluation of BCG vaccines Geneva, Switzerland 22–23 September 2009. Vaccine. 2010;28:6945–50.
60. Pittet LF, Fritschi N, Tebruegge M, et al. Bacillus Calmette-Guérin skin reaction predicts enhanced mycobacteria-specific T-cell responses in infants: a post hoc analysis of a randomized controlled trial. Am J Resp Crit Care. 2022;205:830–41.
61. Lange C, Aaby P, Behr MA, Donald PR, Kaufmann SHE, Netea MG, Mandalakas AM. 100 years of Mycobacterium bovis bacille Calmette-Guérin. Lancet Infect Dis. 2022;22:e2–e12.
62. Organization WH. BCG vaccine: WHO position paper, February 2018—recommendations. Vaccine. 2018;36:3408–10.
63. Hesseling A. Disseminated bacille Calmette-Guerin disease in HIV-infected South African infants. Bull World Health Organ. 2009;87:505–11.
64. Rabie H, Violari A, Duong T, et al. Early antiretroviral treatment reduces risk of bacille Calmette-Guérin immune reconstitution adenitis. Int J Tuberc Lung Dis. 2011;15:1194–200.

New Vaccine Strategies Based on Viral Vectors and mRNA

11

Laura Matarazzo and Paulo J. G. Bettencourt

11.1 Introduction

The bacteria *Mycobacterium tuberculosis* (*Mtb*), the causative agent of Tuberculosis (TB), is estimated to have infected 25% of the population worldwide, with 10.8 million new infections and 1.25 million deaths attributed to TB diseases in 2023 [1]. The live attenuated *M. bovis* strain Bacillus Calmette Guerin (BCG) developed in the 1920s, despite its incomplete and variable efficacy, remains the only licensed TB vaccine, as no vaccine candidate have surpassed BCG efficacy in clinical settings to date [2]. Consequently, TB remains the first cause of death by an infectious disease worldwide despite high-coverage of neonatal BCG vaccination programmes in TB-endemic areas. The World Health Organisation alerted on the urge of the situation and the critical role of effective vaccination strategies to achieve rapid reduction in TB incidence and mortality in near future [1].

Viral vector vaccines are based on viruses modified to be avirulent and express genetic sequences encoding for the antigen(s) of interest. mRNA vaccines consist of an RNA fragment encoding the antigen(s) of interest and additional sequences necessary for their translation into the antigenic peptide/protein by the cellular machinery. mRNA vaccines are synthetized in vitro in cell-free processes and usually administered with lipid-based nanocarriers as a delivery system. Those technologies have recently gained significant interest since the COVID-19 pandemics, as both these platforms were used to develop safe, efficient vaccines in a record of time,

L. Matarazzo · P. J. G. Bettencourt (✉)
Universidade Católica Portuguesa, Center for Interdisciplinary Research in Health, Lisbon, Portugal

Universidade Católica Portuguesa, Faculty of Medicine, Lisbon, Portugal
e-mail: pbettencourt@ucp.pt

P. J. G. Bettencourt (ed.), *Tuberculosis Vaccines*,
https://doi.org/10.1007/978-3-031-94540-3_11

initiating a new era in vaccine development, and represent a new hope for diseases for which conventional vaccine technologies failed to provide sufficient protection.

Rather than replacing BCG, one of the most popular strategies currently investigated is to include newly developed TB vaccines in heterologous prime-boost regimens, to boost BCG primary vaccination. Indeed, BCG is very effective to prevent severe forms and reduce mortality in children [3], but induce poor protection against transmission and pulmonary disease in adolescents and adults, with important geographic disparities [4]. Furthermore, BCG-induced protection declines with time and adolescents and adults vaccinated at birth may not be protected anymore [5]. Thus, these groups are a target of choice for boosting vaccination, either by BCG revaccination or heterologous boost with a different vaccine type [6]. In line with these observations, TB viral vector and mRNA vaccines in development are essentially designed to boost pre-existing immunity induced by BCG vaccination, sometimes in heterologous booster vaccination regimens associating different viral vector vaccines encoding the same(s) antigen(s). In this chapter, we present an exhaustive historical review of clinical trials assessing safety, immunogenicity and efficacy of viral vector and mRNA candidate vaccines for prevention of *Mtb* infection and TB disease. Finally, we discuss the successes and failures of these studies, the current challenges, and implications for future TB vaccine development.

11.2 Viral Vector Vaccines

11.2.1 MVA85A

The first viral vector vaccine candidate against TB to reach clinical trials, developed by Helen McShane at the University of Oxford, is a modified vaccinia Ankara (MVA) virus expressing the immunodominant mycobacterial antigen 85A (MVA85A), [7]. The MVA virus belongs to the poxviruses family and was developed as a smallpox vaccine by attenuation of the conventional vaccinia virus by serial passages on avian cells, rendering it unable to replicate in mammalian cells and avirulent in animal models and human [8]. MVA was used as a third-generation smallpox vaccine during the last stage of the smallpox eradication campaign, demonstrating excellent tolerance and immunogenicity. In following years, modifications of MVA viruses by genetic engineering demonstrated that it can efficiently express heterologous genes in mammalian cells and induce a protective immunity associated with high serum antibody levels and strong CD4+ and CD8+ T cell responses against various infectious diseases in animal models, making it a promising tool for vaccine development [9–15].

Intradermal vaccination with MVA85A of healthy volunteers from endemic areas, previously vaccinated with BCG or BCG-naïve, was safe and well tolerated in all age groups [7, 16–19]. A study in healthy UK adults previously vaccinated with BCG demonstrated a dose-dependent effect of MVA85A, with the highest dose of 10^8 PFU inducing higher antigen-specific T cell response and a broader range of Ag85A epitopes detected by IFN-γ ELISPOT compared to the lowest doses (10^7

and 5×10^7) [20]. A higher frequency of reported systemic adverse events was observed in patients receiving the highest vaccine dose, even though this dose was still considered well-tolerated.

MVA85A boost in BCG-vaccinated healthy adults results in higher antigen-specific T cell responses compared to BCG alone [7, 17]. The cell-mediated response to MVA85A boost was analysed by IFN-γ ELISPOT on whole blood samples, showing robust and durable Ag85A-specific T-cell responses in adults [17], adolescents, children [18] and infants [19, 21, 22] from TB endemic areas, with a peak response at Day 7 post-vaccination. Complementary analysis by Intracellular cytokine straining demonstrated that systemic antigen-specific response was predominated by CD4+ T cells expressing IFN-γ and polyfunctional CD4+ T cells co-expressing the Th1 cytokines IFN-γ, TNF-α and IL-2, with a peak at Day 28 [17–19]. Furthermore, those cells mostly display an effector memory phenotype ($CD45RA^-CCR7^-$) [18]. On the other hand, antigen-specific CD8+ T cells producing IFN-γ were inconsistently detected following MVA85A boost [17–19]. The Th17 response was also investigated, revealing a delayed peak of antigen-specific IL-17-producing CD4+ T cells, and CD4+ T cells co-expressing IL-17 and Th1 cytokines were also detected in response to MVA85A vaccination [17–19, 23, 24].

Importantly, age-related differences were observed in the immune response to vaccination. While adults and adolescents had higher pre-existing antigen-specific T cell responses than children and higher T cell response at Day 7 post-vaccination with MVA85A, it is in children and infants that the greatest responsiveness was observed when comparing pre-vaccination and post-vaccination T cell response by IFN-γ ELISPOT assay [19]. In addition, IL-17 producing cells were mostly distinct in children, but in adults they were found on cells co-expressing Th1/Th17 cytokines. Finally, CD8+ T cells producing IFN-γ were detected at low frequency in infants and adults, but not in children and adolescents, and no significant increase of those cells was observed upon MVA85A boost in adults [17–19]. Adjuvating MVA85A with the carrier protein IMX313 was well tolerated but did not significantly improve the immunogenicity of MVA85A vaccine [25].

Of note, the vaccine was also safe and immunogenic in healthy HIV-infected, *Mtb*-infected and *Mtb*/HIV co-infected adults, with a comparable vaccine-induced polyfunctional CD4+ T cell profile, although the response was of lesser magnitude and less durable in HIV-infected group [24, 26–29]. MVA85A prime vaccination was also safe and induced an early modest antigen-specific immune response in HIV-exposed new-borns, which did not enhance or interfere with immunogenicity induced by subsequent BCG vaccination [30].

Follow-up studies evaluated Ag85A-specific T cell response in adults, adolescents, children or infants who received MVA85A vaccine during above-mentioned clinical trials up to 6 years before [24, 31]. These studies showed that polyfunctional, effector memory CD4+ T cells were still detected in most HIV-negative healthy subjects, as well as in HIV-infected individuals under successful antiretroviral therapy, showing the remarkable persistence of the response. However, in untreated HIV-infected individuals, Antigen-specific T cell responses were mostly undetectable 3 to 5 years post-vaccination [31].

In Gambian infants vaccinated with BCG at birth and with MVA85A at 4 months old, significantly higher Ag85A-specific response was observed up to 14 months post-vaccination compared to BCG alone [21]. However, concomitant vaccination with Expanded Program on Immunization (EPI) vaccines and MVA85A in those infants was associated with a significant decrease in MVA85A cellular immune response (humoral responses to the EPI vaccines were not affected) [22]. The presence of alum in EPI vaccines, an adjuvant that mainly induces a Th2 type response, was proposed as the cause of this reduced immunogenicity, which suggest that childhood vaccination schedules may need to be adapted to integrate a T-cell targeting TB vaccine in the vaccination programs [22].

While intradermal (ID) vaccination route was chosen in most clinical trials with MVA85A, alternative routes of administration may present several advantages. A phase I randomized study compared the safety and immunogenicity of 1×10^8 pfu of MVA85A administered by intramuscular (IM) and ID routes in 24 healthy UK adults previously vaccinated with BCG [32]. The Antigen-specific T cells responses and Th1 cytokines expression, as well as serum total IgG level were not significantly different between the two routes in this study, despite a trend for higher immunogenicity with ID route [32]. The incidence of reported systemic adverse events was not significantly different between the two routes. However, IM route induced lower rate of local adverse events such as erythema and swelling at the injection site but higher injection-associated pain [32]. In other studies, aerosol vaccination with MVA85A was assessed for safety and immunogenicity in phase I clinical trials in 12 healthy UK adults [33], and in two UK adults with LTBI [34]. The vaccine was well tolerated in both studies, with no serious vaccine-related adverse events reported [33, 34]. Respiratory adverse events were rare and mild, and systemic adverse events were comparable to those induced by intradermal vaccination [33]. Aerosol vaccination induced comparable systemic antigen-specific T cell responses and higher mucosal (bronchoalveolar lavage) responses than ID vaccination [33]. Another study evaluated the interest of heterologous routes of administration (ID and aerosol) for MVA85A prime-boost protocols in healthy UK adults previously BCG-vaccinated [35]. While aerosol prime—ID boost and ID prime—ID boost regimens were well tolerated, aerosol boost of ID prime vaccination regimen induced more frequent and severe respiratory and systemic adverse events and was thus discontinued. Consistent with previous studies, aerosol MVA85A increased mucosal Ag85A T-cell response and induced comparable systemic cellular response; however, there was no significant difference in the immune response between the group that received the aerosol prime followed by an ID boost, and the group that received both the prime and boost via the intradermal route. Additionally, serum IgG antibodies were only produced in response to the ID vaccination [33–35]. These studies suggest that the aerosol route could be advantageous in TB vaccination strategies, as the boost in mucosal response may prevent more efficiently respiratory infection and transmission of *Mtb* than systemic route of vaccination. Furthermore, the levels of anti-vector antibodies were lower with aerosol vaccination compared to intradermal vaccination, which is interesting for vaccination strategies with repeated administrations, as anti-vector antibodies may decrease vaccine efficacy and tolerance.

Driven by encouraging safety and immunogenicity results from phase I/IIa clinical studies, MVA85A efficacy was assessed in a double-blinded, randomized, placebo-controlled phase IIb clinical trial in healthy infants (aged 2–6 month) from endemic area previously vaccinated with BCG [36]. However, despite modest induction of Ag85A-specific polyfunctional CD4+ T-cell responses, no significant reduction in the incidence rate of TB, *Mtb* infection and QuantiFERON test (QFT) conversion was observed with MVA85A boost compared to placebo [37, 36]. An extended follow-up study of subjects from this trial confirmed the absence of long-term protective efficacy of MVA85A vaccination in infants [38]. Consistently, no significant efficacy was observed in HIV-1 infected adults, as assessed by the incidence of TB diagnostic (defined as culture or GeneXpert *MTB*/RIF positivity, clinical endpoint and/or commencement of antiretroviral therapy) and QFT conversion [28]. Finally, a meta-analysis compiling data from 6 clinical studies based on vaccine efficacy or immunogenicity trials that include measures of clinical efficacy, implicating more than 3800 participants in total, concluded that BCG + MVA85A boost probably has little to no effect on the risk of developing active TB, on the need to start TB treatment and on the risk of developing latent TB compared to BCG alone [39].

11.2.2 AERAS-402

AERAS-402 is another viral vector vaccine developed as a boost for BCG prime vaccination. It is a replication-deficient adenovirus serotype 35 (Ad35) viral vector encoding a fusion protein of the secreted immunodominant *Mtb* antigens Ag85A, Ag85B, and TB10.4. Unlike other adenoviruses such as Ad5, the presence of pre-existing neutralizing antibodies against Ad35, which could impact on vaccine efficacy, is low; in a phase I clinical trial in sub-Saharan Africa, only 5% of participants presented significant levels of anti-Ad35 neutralizing antibodies prior to vaccination [40].

Intramuscular administration of one or two doses of AERAS-402 demonstrated an acceptable safety profile and good immunogenicity in healthy, *Mtb*-uninfected adults previously vaccinated with BCG [40], and in BCG-vaccinated Kenyan adults with positive or negative QuantiFERON test, without evidence of pulmonary TB [41]. AERAS-402 was also safe and immunogenic in healthy infants from endemic region, with dose-dependent T cell responses and local and systemic adverse events (pain, tenderness and erythema at injection site, and mild to moderate systemic adverse events dominated by headache, fever, malaise or myalgia) [42, 43]. A possible association with rhinitis and upper respiratory tract infections was also reported [40, 42]. Of note, the vaccine did not induce severe pulmonary or systemic adverse events (immunogenic post-vaccination Koch-like reaction) when administered to people with prior or active pulmonary TB [44].

AERAS-402 boost induced robust and durable antigen-specific CD4+ and CD8+ T cells responses [40, 42, 43]. CD4+ T cell response was dominated by polyfunctional cells co-expressing IL-2, IFN-γ and TNF-α, but the vaccine did not significantly increase IL-17 expression, unlike BCG and MVA85A [40, 42]. Interestingly, upon single administration of low doses, the response was dominated by monofunctional IFN-γ-expressing CD4+ T cells, while with higher doses and repeated administrations polyfunctional CD4+ T cells (co-expressing IL-2, IFN-γ and TNF-α) were dominant [42]. Furthermore, while MVA85A vaccination resulted in low or undetectable CD8+ T cell response, AERAS-402 induced significant increase of CD8+ T cells expressing IFN-γ and IFN-γ/TNF-α, as well as polyfunctional CD8+ T cells [40, 45, 46]. Of note, no significant boost of T cell responses was observed in patients receiving two high doses of the vaccine compared to a single dose. However, patients who received two high doses were more prone to the development of neutralizing antibodies against Ad35 (83% versus 22% in patients receiving a single dose) [40].

In BCG-vaccinated, HIV-infected South African adults with baseline CD4 counts >350 cells/ml, two-doses vaccination with AERAS-402 was safe and immunogenic, inducing strong Ag85A/B-specific T cell responses dominated by polyfunctional CD4+ T cells and bifunctional (IFN-γ, TNF-α) CD8+ T cells, as well as antibody responses [47]. However, T cell responses were less durable in HIV-infected compared to HIV-uninfected individuals, and the CD8+ T cell response, which is thought to be important for protective immunity against TB, was lower [40, 47, 48]. The vaccine had no impact on CD4+ T cells count nor viral loads, and the safety profile was similar to that of HIV-uninfected adults [40, 47, 48].

Pre-existing anti-mycobacteria immunity may also influence the response to AERAS-402, as a positive correlation was observed between the frequency of pre-existing mycobacteria-specific T cells and the frequency of vaccine-induced T cells [42]. Importantly, a lower response rate and magnitude of CD4+ and CD8+ T cell responses was observed in infants compared to adults [40, 43]. This suggest that different vaccination strategies may be appropriate depending on the target population.

11.2.3 Vaccination Strategies Combining MVA85A with Other Viral Vectors

11.2.3.1 AERAS-402 + MVA85A

In a phase I opened-labelled trial, 40 healthy BCG-vaccinated adults were vaccinated with boost regimens consisting of one or two-doses of AERAS-402 administered intramuscularly followed with one dose of MVA85A administered intradermally, or a third dose of AERAS-402 [45]. Antigen-specific T-cell responses, assessed by IFN-γ ELISPOT between D0 and D203, showed that one or two doses of AERAS-402 followed by one dose of MVA85A, induced stronger and more durable antigen-specific T cell response than three doses of AERAS-402. The one or two-doses AERAS-402 + MVA85A also induced significantly higher frequency of antigen-specific CD4+ and CD8+ T cells expressing intracellular cytokines IL-2, TNF-α and IFN-γ compared to three-doses AERAS-402, and higher magnitude and more durable anti-Ag85A and Ag85B IgG responses in serum. Both vaccine candidates induced mild to moderate adverse events, mostly local (pain, tenderness, erythema), although systemic adverse events were also frequent, such as headache, fever, malaise and myalgia, in a dose-dependent manner, and predominantly related to AERAS-402 [45].

11.2.3.2 ChAdOx1 85A + MVA85A

ChAdOx1 85A (Chimpanzee Adenovirus-vectored Oxford 1) is a replication-deficient simian adenoviral vector expressing Ag85A, which previously demonstrated efficacy in BCG—ChAdOx1 85A—MVA85A regimens in mice [49]. Furthermore, ChAdOx1 vector expressing influenza antigens NP and M1 was safe and immunogenic in clinical settings [50].

In a phase I study in BCG-vaccinated healthy UK adults, ChAdOx1 85A was found to be safe and immunogenic [51]. A single ChAdOx1 85A intramuscular administration induced significant increase of Ag85A-specific T cell response (IFN-γ ELISPOT) at Day 14 and persisted up to Day 168. A second dose at Day 28 did not improve this response, while ChAdOx1 85A prime followed with MVA85A boost administered intramuscularly (at Day 56 after a single ChAdOx1 85A dose or at Day 119 after two ChAdOx1 85A doses), increased the magnitude of these responses compared to ChAdOx1 85A alone [51]. Consistently, intracellular cytokine staining showed that MVA85A boost enhanced the Ag85A-specific polyfunctional CD4+ and CD8+ T cells responses, and antigen-specific IgG response was also detected. Significant increase of ChAdOx1-specific and MVA-specific IgG responses were detected, with higher magnitude of ChAdOx1-specific response after the second dose, and remained significantly elevated up to Day 140 for ChAdOx1 and Day 287 for MVA. The vaccines mostly induce mild or moderate local and systemic adverse events [51].

In a randomized open-label phase IIa trial on healthy Ugandan adolescents aged 12–17 years vaccinated with BCG at birth, the ChAdOx1 85A + MVA85A regimen was compared to BCG revaccination for safety and immunogenicity [52]. In the initial dose-escalation and age de-escalation study with one dose of ChAdOx1 85A, BCG-vaccinated adults and adolescents received a single dose of 5×10^9 or 2.5×10^{10} viral particles intramuscularly, local and systemic reported adverse events were mostly mild to moderate [52]. Severe AEs (one case of myalgia and one case of severe feverishness, headache and malaise) were reported, but resolved by the next visit. Significant increase of Ag85A-specific T-cell response was observed at Day 14 in all groups by IFN-γ ELISPOT and were higher in adolescents than in adults.

Following this first phase, in the randomized trial in adolescents, the peak of INF-γ ELISPOT response was observed at Day 63 post-MVA85A in the ChAdOx1 85A + MVA85A group and Day 14 post-vaccination in the BCG revaccination group [52]. The magnitude of response at the peak was significantly higher in the ChAdOx1 85A–MVA85A group compared to BCG revaccination regarding

Ag85A- and PPD-specific responses, and the AUC was significantly higher in the ChAdOx1 85A–MVA85A group only for Ag85A-specific response. The heterologous boost regimen also induced significantly higher levels of anti-Ag85A-specific (but not anti-PPD) IgG responses in serum at Day 63 and up to Day 224. Higher PPD-specific IgG responses were seen on Day 224 in the BCG revaccination group but not on Day 63, and the AUCs were not significantly different between the two groups. BCG-specific IgG responses were also higher in BCG revaccination group throughout follow-up [52].

Even though this study was not powered to compare protective efficacy between groups against acquisition of latent *Mtb* infection, serologic conversion, assessed by *M. tuberculosis*-specific antigens ESAT-6/CFP-10 ELISpot, was observed in 47% of participants (14/30) in ChAdOx1 85A–MVA85A group and 38% (11/30) in BCG revaccination group. All reverted by the next visit except one participant in ChAdOx1 85A–MVA85A group and three participants in BCG revaccination group, which remain IGRA-positive throughout the duration of the follow-up, with no symptoms or signs of active tuberculosis [52].

This study demonstrated that this ChAdOx1 85A–MVA85A boosting regimen is safe and immunogenic in adolescents from endemic TB area and induce higher Ag85A specific cellular and humoral responses compared to BCG revaccination strategy, supporting further development of heterologous viral-vector BCG-boosting strategy in this target population.

Of note, the potential of ChAdOx1 85A administered by respiratory mucosal route was investigated in a small single-centre, randomized, double-blind and controlled phase I study [53]. The safety and immunogenicity of a single administration of the vaccine by inhaled or intramuscular routes were compared in BCG-vaccinated and BCG-naïve adults with dose-escalation. Both routes of administration were well tolerated, with no serious adverse events reported. Aerosol route induced robust Ag85A-specific humoral and systemic T-cell responses. The systemic T-cell response was stronger upon intramuscular administration; however, inhaled vaccination induced significantly higher mucosal T-cell responses which were dominated by CD4+ T cell co-expressing IFN-γ and IL-17 [53].

11.2.3.3 MVA85A + FP85A

The viral vector candidate vaccine FP85A, consisting of FP9 vector expressing Ag85A, was evaluated in a safety and immunogenicity phase I clinical trial, alone, or in a heterologous prime-boost regimen with MVA85A [54]. FP85A did not induce significant Ag85A-specific T-cell response, and when given prior to MVA85A vaccination, induced a lower immunogenicity compared to MVA85A followed by FP85A. It has been hypothesized by the authors that cross-reactivity of FP9 Antigens was responsible for the decrease of immunogenicity of subsequent MVA85A administration [54].

11.2.4 AdHu5Ag85A

AdHu5Ag85A is a viral vector vaccine based on a recombinant, replication-deficient human type 5 adenovirus expressing Ag85A, developed at McMaster University. AdHu5 vector has been shown as safe and immunogenic in previous clinical trials of HIV and malaria vaccines [55, 56]. However, unlike simian adenoviruses, the high prevalence of pre-existing neutralizing antibodies against human adenoviruses may limit their clinical applications.

In BCG-naïve and BGC-vaccinated healthy adults in Canada, single intramuscular administration was safe and well tolerated and induced strong antigen-specific T-cell responses [57]. Significant increase of Th1 cytokine production, as assessed by IFN-γ, TNF-α and IL-2 ELISA on whole-blood samples and IFN-γ ELISPOT on PBMC, was observed upon stimulation with recombinant Ag85A protein, 6 Ag85A peptide pools or *Mtb* culture filtrate proteins [57, 58]. Of note, high responders were found mostly among previously BCG-vaccinated subjects. Consistently, intracellular cytokine staining flow cytometry showed higher magnitude of antigen-specific polyfunctional CD8+ and CD4+ T-cell in BCG-vaccinated volunteers, while it essentially engages a CD4+ T-cell response in BCG-naïve subjects. Pre-existing anti-AdHu5 antibodies had limited impact on the immunogenicity of the vaccine [57].

Mucosal and systemic vaccination routes were compared in a phase I clinical study evaluating the safety and immunogenicity of single intramuscular or aerosol administration by nebulization at two different doses in healthy adults [59]. Intramuscular and low-dose aerosol administrations induced similar systemic Ag85A-specific polyfunctional T-cell responses, although those cells shrank at 16 weeks in aerosol vaccination group while they remain high upon intramuscular vaccination [59]. In contrast, only aerosol vaccination at both high and low dose induced significant increase of Ag85A-specific polyfunctional CD4+ and CD8+ T-cell in the airways at 2 weeks post-vaccination, with no sign of significant mucosal inflammation, and remain elevated up to 8 weeks post-vaccination. Furthermore, 20% of Ag85A-specific CD4+ and 54% of CD8+ T cells in the airways at 8 weeks were resident memory T-cells, which are critical for mucosal protective immunity [60]. Of note, the low-dose aerosol vaccination was superior to the high-dose in inducing systemic and mucosal T-cell responses, which may be due to immune overactivation of the mucosa with the highest dose. Additionally, RNA-seq analysis revealed that aerosol vaccination induced lasting transcriptional changes in airway macrophages indicative of trained innate immunity. Both routes of administration were safe and well tolerated, with no significant difference on reported respiratory adverse events, and no vaccine-related serious adverse events [59]. Although no significant impact of pre-existing systemic or mucosal anti-AdHu5 neutralizing antibodies on vaccines immunogenicity was found in this study, previous studies with larger sample size identified a negative correlation between anti-AdHu5 antibody levels and vaccine immunogenicity [61, 62].

11.2.5 Influenza A Viral Vector

TB/FLU candidate vaccines are based on an attenuated replication-deficient influenza virus expressing the mycobacterial antigens ESAT-6 (TB/FLU-01 L), a combination of ESAT-6 and Ag85A (TB/FLU-04 L) or a combination of TB10.4 and HspX (TB/FLU-05E). These vaccines were developed for respiratory administration, as a boost to BCG prime vaccination. Safety, immunogenicity, as well as protection against *Mtb* challenge were demonstrated in animal models with TB/FLU-01 L [63, 64], TB/FLU-04 L [65–67] and TB/FLU-05E [68, 69]. A phase I open, randomized and clinical trial evaluated the safety and immunogenicity of TB/FLU-01 L administered by intranasal or sublingual route in healthy BCG-vaccinated adults, intended for immunotherapy of pulmonary tuberculosis (NCT03017378). The safety and immunogenicity of TB/FLU-04 L (NCT02501421) and TB/Flu-05E (NCT05945498) tuberculosis vaccines administered by intranasal route were explored in phase I, double-blind, randomized, placebo-controlled trials in BCG-vaccinated healthy adult. These studies, completed between 2015 and 2023, have no publicly available results.

11.3 mRNA Vaccine Candidates for TB

The high versatility of mRNA platform, allowing for easy design and in vitro synthesis of mRNA from a plasmid template encoding the antigen(s) of interest, supports the fast development and preclinical screening of vaccine candidates [70]. Furthermore, the successful development of the mRNA-based COVID-19 vaccines strongly established the feasibility, as well as the safety and immunogenicity of this technology, leading to the huge pipeline of mRNA vaccines that recently entered phase I/II clinical trials since 2021 (https://clinicaltrials.gov). Two candidate mRNA vaccines against TB, developed by BioNTech (BNT164a1 and BNT164b1), are currently tested in randomized, placebo-controlled, double-blind, dose-escalating phase I/IIa safety/immunogenicity clinical trials in healthy BCG-naïve adults in Germany (NCT05537038) and healthy BCG-vaccinated adults in South Africa (NCT05547464). The antigenic composition of those vaccine candidates has not been publicly disclosed, to this date.

MRNA vaccines against other important pathogens have been developed and are currently being evaluated in clinical trials. For a complete list of clinical trials evaluating mRNA vaccines against infectious diseases, please see the review [71].

11.4 Discussion

Efficient vaccination, conferring protection against pulmonary TB disease in all age groups is essential in the fight against Tuberculosis, as highlighted in the last WHO report [1]. Besides BCG revaccination, two live attenuated (MTBVAC, VPM1002 VPM1002), one inactivated Mycobacteria (Immuvac - MIP), two subunit - protein in adjuvant (M72/AS01E, GamTBvac) have reached phase III of clinical trials [1]

(Table 11.1). As per viral vector vaccines, while the first clinical trial with MVA85A dates from 2002 [7], more than 20 years later and despite encouraging safety and immunogenicity clinical data, only one phase IIb efficacy trial has been conducted, but the candidate vaccine MVA85A did not demonstrate sufficient protective efficacy against pulmonary TB disease [36]. On the other hand, the success story of mRNA vaccines against COVID-19 created a major craze around this novel technology, initiating a new era in the vaccine development field, leading to more than 20 ongoing clinical trials for mRNA vaccines against a wide range of infectious diseases, including Influenza, HIV, Zika, CMV, chikungunya and Malaria [71]. Among them, only two clinical trials evaluating TB candidate vaccines (BNT164a1 and BNT164b1, developed by BioNTech) are being conducted (NCT05537038, NCT05547464), compared to 13 clinical trials for Influenza mRNA vaccines (https://clinicaltrials.gov). The slow pace of TB vaccine development is largely due to the unique specificities of *Mtb* infection and TB disease development, the scarcity of new antigens to be included in vaccine candidates, as well as the absence of well-defined correlates of protection.

The complex biology of *Mtb* and the physiopathology of infection and disease development are inherent challenges to vaccine development [72]. Estimating the transmission rate of *Mtb* and prevalence of latent TB infection is particularly tough, due to the slow growth of *Mtb* in culture, its containment in lung granulomas in a dormant state, associated to poor access to diagnostic in LMIC countries with high TB-burden. This prevalence is estimated to be close to a quarter of the global population, among which 80% are in South-East Asia, Western-Pacific and Africa regions [73]. An estimated 5–10% of infected individuals will progress to active TB disease, in a time frame ranging from a few months to decades. These specificities obviously impact the efficacy assessment of TB vaccine candidates and may as well discourage investments, as, unlike rapidly progressing diseases such as COVID-19 or Influenza, investigators must follow the volunteers for several years. Moreover, suboptimal treatment of TB disease due to poor access to healthcare in LMICs, as well as the lack of observance to long and costly antibiotic treatments with important side effects, favour transmission and emergence of antibiotic-resistant strains. Thus, vaccination remains the most powerful tool in the fight against TB to control transmission and disease.

In high-burden regions, TB pulmonary disease peaks in adolescents and young adults, coinciding with the decline of BCG protection induced by neonatal vaccination, and represent the major cause of transmission. It has been estimated that an adolescent/adult vaccine with 50% efficacy would prevent 76 million TB cases and 8.5 million deaths by 2050, and would have a greater and more immediate impact than an infant vaccine with 80% efficacy [70, 74, 1]. Therefore, administration of boost vaccines in adolescents and young adults appears as a relevant strategy to efficiently control TB disease and transmission [5, 52].

Of note, viral vector vaccines against TB were safe and immunogenic in HIV infected in clinical trials [24, 27, 28, 47]. This is of great importance, as HIV-infected individuals are particularly susceptible to TB disease, which was responsible of an estimated 167,000 deaths among people with HIV in 2022 [1]. However, live attenuated vaccines cannot be used safely in those patients due to risk of

Table 11.1 Ongoing clinical trials evaluating preventive TB vaccine candidates (August 2024)

Vaccine candidate (sponsor)	Type of vaccine	Study design	Study start	Development phase	Status	NCT number
BCG (Bill & Melinda Gates Medical Research Institute)	Live attenuated	Efficacy of BCG revaccination for prevention of *Mtb* sustained infection in healthy adolescents	2019	Phase II	Active, not recruiting	NCT04152161
BCG (Henry M. Jackson Foundation for the Advancement of Military Medicine)	Live attenuated	Pre-travel vaccination of adults traveling to countries with a high TB-burden to Prevent TB infection	2021	Phase III	Recruiting	NCT04453293
BCG (University of Oxford)	Live attenuated	Safety and Immunogenicity of Intradermal vs. aerosol BCG in non-type 2 diabetics	2023	Not applicable	Recruiting	NCT06246851
BCG (University of Oxford)	Live attenuated	Immune Responses to Aerosol BCG Challenge in Healthy UK Adults	2019	Phase I	Active, not recruiting	NCT03912207
MTBVAC (Biofabri, S.L)	Live attenuated	Efficacy, safety and immunogenicity in newborn in Sub-Saharan Africa for prevention against TB disease	2022	Phase III	Recruiting	NCT04975178
MTBVAC (Bharat Biotech International Limited)	Live attenuated (*Mtb*)	Safety, Reactogenicity, Tolerability, and Immunogenicity of *MTB*VAC in healthy Indian adult volunteers	2024	Phase I	Active, not recruiting	NCT06438978

MTBVAC (International AIDS vaccine initiative)	Live attenuated (*Mtb*)	Efficacy, safety and immunogenicity against TB disease in IGRA-positive adolescents and adults in TB endemic region	2024	Phase IIb	Not yet recruiting	NCT06272812
MTBVAC (HIV Vaccine Trials Network)	Live attenuated (*Mtb*)	Safety and immunogenicity of *MTB*VAC in adolescents and adults living with and without HIV in South Africa	2024	Phase II	Recruiting	NCT05947890
VPM1002 (Serum Institute of India Pvt. Ltd.)	Live attenuated (modified BCG)	Efficacy, safety and immunogenicity in healthy newborn, prevention of *Mtb* infection and TB disease	2020	Phase III	Active, not recruiting	NCT04351685
M72/AS01E-4 (Bill and Melinda Gates Research Institute)	Live attenuated (*Mtb*)	Efficacy, safety and immunogenicity in IGRA-positive, IGRA-negative and HIV-positive adolescent and adults for prevention of pulmonary TB disease	2024	Phase III	Recruiting	NCT06062238

(continued)

Table 11.1 (continued)

Vaccine candidate (sponsor)	Type of vaccine	Study design	Study start	Development phase	Status	NCT number
BNT164a1 & BNT164b1 (BioNTech SE)	mRNA	Safety, immunogenicity, dose-finding in healthy BCG-naïve adults for prevention of TB disease	2023	Phase Ia	Active, not recruiting	NCT05537038
BNT164a1 & BNT164b1 (BioNTech SE)	mRNA	Safety, immunogenicity, dose-finding in healthy BCG-vaccinated adults for prevention of TB disease	2023	Phase Ib/IIa	Active, not recruiting	NCT05547464
GamTBvac (Gamaleya Research Institute of Epidemiology and Microbiology, Health Ministry of the Russian Federation)	Subunit recombinant protein	Safety and efficacy for prevention of pulmonary TB disease in healthy BCG-vaccinated adults	2022	Phase III	Recruiting	NCT04975737
H107e/CAF®10b (Statens Serum Institute)	Subunit recombinant protein	Safety, Reactogenicity, and Immunogenicity in healthy adults	2024	Phase Ia	Recruiting	NCT06050356

reactivation. Vaccines conveying efficient protection against TB disease while being safe in HIV patients are thus urgently needed.

The absence of clear correlates of protection is another major limitation in TB vaccine development [75]. Preclinical data in mice and non-human primates provide evidence that increased levels of antigen-specific Th1/Th17 responses in the lung and systemic compartments are associated with protection against *Mtb* infection and/or pulmonary disease [76–78]. In human, high *Mtb* loads in the lungs of TB patients (smear-positive TB) correlates with T cells dysfunction characterized by a decreased frequency of *Mtb*-specific polyfunctional CD4+ T cells compared with patients with latent TB infection and smear-negative TB, and a decrease of the proliferative capacity of both CD4+ and CD8+ T cells [79]. Moreover, an increase of the frequency of polyfunctional T cells was observed following successful anti-TB treatment of patients with smear-positive TB, suggesting that polyfunctional T cells are also essential for the protection against TB in human [79]. However, other studies temper this hypothesis, such as the clinical study showing that the Th1/Th17 cytokine expression profile of CD4+, CD8+ and γδT cells in whole blood samples is not significantly different between BCG-vaccinated infants separated in two groups—protected and not protected [80]. Analysis of lung granuloma formation and bacterial control upon *Mtb* infection in non-human primate models, which is closed to that observed in humans, may help in the identification of factors correlated to efficient bacterial control [81]. In this study, the authors observed that early, high-bacterial burden granulomas promote a type 2 wound healing-like response, whereas late, low-burden granulomas rely on a cytotoxic cellular dominant response, which support the hypothesis that the ability to induce strong CD4+/CD8+ Th1 responses in the lung may be a major factor of vaccine efficacy [81].

Thus, T-cell responses, and particularly polyfunctional Th1 cells co-expressing IFN-γ, TNF-α and IL-2, are chosen as the main parameters to assess the immunogenicity of TB candidate vaccines in most clinical trials [75]. However, although less investigated, the role of B-cells and antibodies should not be neglected [82]. For instance, in macaques, high levels of lung and plasma IgM were strongly correlated to protection against *Mtb* infection after intravenous BCG vaccination [83]. In mouse model, B cells were shown to significantly contribute, along with T cell responses, to protect against *Mtb* infection and control bacterial dissemination upon vaccination with an arabinomanan-Ag85b protein conjugate vaccine [84]. Consistently, serum transfer from LTBI patients or *Mtb*-exposed healthcare workers, but not from patients with active TB, protected mice against *Mtb* challenge [85]. In addition, a clinical study showed that B cells present impaired proliferation, immunoglobulin- and cytokine production in patients with active TB disease or recent *Mtb* infection, which resolved after successful treatment [86]. These studies suggest infection/disease-state differences in the role of B-cells and antibodies. Preclinical and clinical data further suggest that impaired B cell functions during TB disease may impact T-cell responses [87]. This reinforces the evidence that an effective TB vaccine should target both humoral and cellular immune responses.

With the objective of helping the identification of correlates of protection and improving efficacy assessment of vaccine candidates in clinical settings, a human

BCG challenge study was conducted, where BCG-naïve or previously BCG-vaccinated adults were vaccinated intradermally with MVA85A then challenged with intradermal BCG [88]. Bacterial loads in skin biopsies from injection site 2 weeks post-challenge revealed that, also previously BCG-vaccinated patients had lower bacterial loads than BCG-naive, MVA85A vaccination had no added effect on bacterial load reduction [88]. Nonetheless, this study is the first to present a human challenge model able to detect differences in antimycobacterial immunity induced by vaccination, which, in the absence of established correlates of protection, could provide a useful methodology to assess the efficacy of new vaccines and the immune profile of vaccinated subjects.

Overall, identification of clear, validated corelates of protection would greatly accelerate TB vaccine development. The TB Immune Correlates Program, initiated in 2018, provides the strategy and governance structure to enable discovery of correlates of protection from established *Mtb* infection (defined as sustained IGRA conversion) or TB disease through a highly collaborative approach [75].

The rational selection of vaccine antigens is a crucial factor in enhancing the immunogenicity and protective efficacy of TB vaccines. Unlike live attenuated vaccines which contain a wide antigenic repertoire, viral vectors, mRNA, as well as subunit vaccines, encode for a limited number of antigens. Furthermore, *Mtb* is a relatively complex microorganism encoding around 4000 proteins [89]. The major immunodominant secreted *Mtb* antigens Ag85A, Ag85B, ESAT-6, CFP-10 and TB10.4, are over-represented in candidate vaccines, and were sometimes identified decades ago and chosen based on their capacity to induce strong Th1-type responses in ex vivo cell restimulation assays, and protection in animal models [90]. However, more recent data suggest that antigens highly expressed at early stages of infection may lead to T cell exhaustion and dysfunction [91], and that high CD4+ T cell response is not always correlated to protection [92]. New approaches are thus needed to identify relevant target antigens. Targeting antigens from different states of *Mtb* may be a valuable strategy to improve protection. For instance, latency antigens, such as Rv1733c and HspX, present in patients with latent TB infection, but not in patients with TB disease, demonstrated protective efficacy in animal models [93, 94]. Furthermore, BCG vaccination does not induce immune response to those latency antigens [95, 96], which make them interesting candidates for booster vaccines, particularly to improve protection against TB disease development in latently infected patients [90]. Some studies suggest that targeting surface adhesion antigens such as heparin-binding hemagglutinin A (which is also a latency antigen) may prevent bacterial dissemination following intranasal infection [97–100]. Multistage vaccines combining early secretory proteins (such as Ag85A/B, ESAT-6, Hsp65), latency antigens and rfp antigens (which promote the transition from a dormant to an active replicating state of *Mtb*) demonstrated protection in mouse and non-human primate models against infection and pulmonary disease [101–104]. Recently, immunopeptidomics was used to identify BCG and *Mtb* peptides bound to MHC, in infected macrophages very successfully. New antigens were identified and evaluated as pre-clinical vaccine candidates with encouraging results [105, 106]. This is described in greater detail in chapter 6.

Thus, the choice of target antigens is a tough task but essential for achieving optimal protective immune responses. Antigen and epitope screening based on genome-wide strategies are crucial for the identification of novel target antigens for future vaccine development [90].

Comparative clinical studies highlighted that administration of viral vector vaccines by mucosal route induces antigen-specific cellular responses in both the systemic and pulmonary sites, while systemic vaccination induces mostly systemic responses [33–35, 53, 59, 61]. The mucosal route is particularly interesting for respiratory pathogens like *Mtb*, as activation of mucosal immunity may improve protection against infection and transmission of the pathogen. This hypothesis is supported by preclinical studies showing that intranasal administration of viral vector vaccines to BCG-primed or Ag85A DNA-prime animals, induces antigen-specific T cell responses in the lungs and confer superior protection against *Mtb* challenge compared to systemic route [107–109]. Interestingly, anti-vector immunity was lower upon aerosol vaccination compared to the intradermal route in clinical trials [35, 59]. As to mRNA vaccines, intranasal administration was safe and induced protection against SARS-CoV2 or *M. avium* in animal models [110, 111]. Collectively, these data support further development of aerosol vaccines for tuberculosis.

The influence of pre-existing anti-vector immunity—whether arising from natural viral infections or prior vaccinations—on subsequent viral vector vaccine performance remains incompletely understood [112]. While several studies indicate that anti-vector responses, particularly neutralizing antibodies, may diminish the immunogenicity and efficacy of subsequent vaccine administrations [54, 61, 62, 113], others suggest their impact is limited [114, 115]. Strategies to mitigate this risk include selecting vectors with low pre-existing immunity in human populations (e.g., simian rather than human adenoviruses), employing heterologous boosting regimens that combine different viral vectors, or exploring alternative administration routes, such as the respiratory route, which are associated with a reduced development of anti-vector immunity [35, 59, 112].

11.5 Conclusion

Although less clinically advanced than live attenuated and subunit vaccines, viral vector and mRNA vaccines are promising technologies in terms of safety, immunogenicity and cost-effectiveness. Thus, investment in their development should be encouraged to enrich the arsenal against TB and maximize the chances of achieving the objectives of 80% reduction in TB incidence and 90% reduction in TB-associated deaths by 2030 targeted by the End TB Strategy programme [116]. Promoting political and economic commitment towards TB vaccine research, with a particular focus on identification of relevant antigens and establishment of validated correlates of protection for clinical efficacy assessment are key factors to this success.

Competing Interests The author(s) has no competing interests to declare that are relevant to the content of this manuscript.

Ethics Approval The author(s) declares that this manuscript does not include primary research with human participants.

References

1. World Health Organization. Global tuberculosis report 2024. 2024.
2. Bettencourt PJG, Joosten SA, Lindestam Arlehamn CS, Behr MA, Locht C, Neyrolles O. 100 years of the Bacillus Calmette-Guérin vaccine. Vaccine. 2021;39(50):7221–2. https://doi.org/10.1016/j.vaccine.2021.11.038.
3. Schaltz-Buchholzer F, Roth A, de Bree LCJ, Biering-Sørensen S, Timmermann CAG, Monteiro I, Aaby P, Benn CS. Neonatal Bacille Calmette-Guérin vaccination and tuberculin skin test reactions at 2- and 6-months: effects on mortality up to 1 year of age. Vaccine. 2021;39(50):7286–94. https://doi.org/10.1016/j.vaccine.2021.06.077.
4. Wilson ME, Fineberg HV, Colditz GA. Geographic latitude and the efficacy of Bacillus Calmette-Guerin vaccine. Clin Infect Dis. 1995;20(4):982–91. https://doi.org/10.1093/clinids/20.4.982.
5. Abubakar I, Pimpin L, Ariti C, Beynon R, Mangtani P, Sterne J, Fine P, Smith P, Lipman M, Elliman D, Watson J, Drumright L, Whiting P, Vynnycky E, Rodrigues L. Systematic review and meta-analysis of the current evidence on the duration of protection by bacillus Calmette–Guérin vaccination against tuberculosis. Health Technol Assess. 2013;17(37) https://doi.org/10.3310/hta17370.
6. Dalmia N, Ramsay AJ. Prime–boost approaches to tuberculosis vaccine development. Expert Rev Vaccines. 2012;11(10):1221–33. https://doi.org/10.1586/erv.12.94.
7. McShane H, Pathan AA, Sander CR, Keating SM, Gilbert SC, Huygen K, Fletcher HA, Hill AVS. Recombinant modified vaccinia virus Ankara expressing antigen 85A boosts BCG-primed and naturally acquired antimycobacterial immunity in humans. Nat Med. 2004;10(11):1240–4. https://doi.org/10.1038/nm1128.
8. Volz A, Sutter G. Modified vaccinia Virus Ankara. Adv Virus Res. 97:187–243. https://doi.org/10.1016/bs.aivir.2016.07.001.
9. Goonetilleke NP, McShane H, Hannan CM, Anderson RJ, Brookes RH, Hill AVS. Enhanced immunogenicity and protective efficacy against *Mycobacterium tuberculosis* of Bacille Calmette-Guérin vaccine using mucosal administration and boosting with a recombinant modified vaccinia virus Ankara. J Immunol. 2003;171(3):1602–9. https://doi.org/10.4049/jimmunol.171.3.1602.
10. Hirsch VM, Fuerst TR, Sutter G, Carroll MW, Yang LC, Goldstein S, Piatak M, Elkins WR, Alvord WG, Montefiori DC, Moss B, Lifson JD. Patterns of viral replication correlate with outcome in simian immunodeficiency virus (SIV)-infected macaques: effect of prior immunization with a trivalent SIV vaccine in modified vaccinia virus Ankara. J Virol. 1996;70(6):3741–52. https://doi.org/10.1128/jvi.70.6.3741-3752.1996.
11. McShane H, Brookes R, Gilbert SC, Hill AVS. Enhanced immunogenicity of CD4 $^{+}$ T-cell responses and protective efficacy of a DNA-modified vaccinia virus Ankara prime-boost vaccination regimen for murine tuberculosis. Infect Immun. 2001;69(2):681–6. https://doi.org/10.1128/IAI.69.2.681-686.2001.
12. Schneider J, Gilbert SC, Blanchard TJ, Hanke T, Robson KJ, Hannan CM, Becker M, Sinden R, Smith GL, Hill AVS. Enhanced immunogenicity for CD8+ T cell induction and complete

protective efficacy of malaria DNA vaccination by boosting with modified vaccinia virus Ankara. Nat Med. 1998;4(4):397–402. https://doi.org/10.1038/nm0498-397.

13. Sutter G, Wyatt LS, Foley PL, Bennink JR, Moss B. A recombinant vector derived from the host range-restricted and highly attenuated MVA strain of vaccinia virus stimulates protective immunity in mice to influenza virus. Vaccine. 1994;12(11):1032–40. https://doi.org/10.1016/0264-410X(94)90341-7.
14. Williams A, Goonetilleke NP, McShane H, Clark SO, Hatch G, Gilbert SC, Hill AVS. Boosting with poxviruses enhances *Mycobacterium bovis* BCG efficacy against tuberculosis in Guinea pigs. Infect Immun. 2005;73(6):3814–6. https://doi.org/10.1128/IAI.73.6.3814-3816.2005.
15. Wyatt L. Development of a replication-deficient recombinant vaccinia virus vaccine effective against parainfluenza virus 3 infection in an animal model. Vaccine. 1996;14(15):1451–8. https://doi.org/10.1016/S0264-410X(96)00072-2.
16. Brookes RH, Hill PC, Owiafe PK, Ibanga HB, Jeffries DJ, Donkor SA, Fletcher HA, Hammond AS, Lienhardt C, Adegbola RA, McShane H, Hill AVS. Safety and immunogenicity of the candidate tuberculosis vaccine MVA85A in West Africa. PLoS One. 2008;3(8):e2921. https://doi.org/10.1371/journal.pone.0002921.
17. Hawkridge T, Scriba TJ, Gelderbloem S, Smit E, Tameris M, Moyo S, Lang T, Veldsman A, Hatherill M, van der Merwe L, Fletcher HA, Mahomed H, Hill AVS, Hanekom WA, Hussey GD, McShane H. Safety and immunogenicity of a new tuberculosis vaccine, MVA85A, in healthy adults in South Africa. J Infect Dis. 2008;198(4):544–52. https://doi.org/10.1086/590185.
18. Scriba TJ, Tameris M, Mansoor N, Smit E, van der Merwe L, Isaacs F, Keyser A, Moyo S, Brittain N, Lawrie A, Gelderbloem S, Veldsman A, Hatherill M, Hawkridge A, Hill AVS, Hussey GD, Mahomed H, McShane H, Hanekom WA. Modified vaccinia Ankara-expressing Ag85A, a novel tuberculosis vaccine, is safe in adolescents and children, and induces polyfunctional CD4 $^{+}$ T cells. Eur J Immunol. 2010;40(1):279–90. https://doi.org/10.1002/eji.200939754.
19. Scriba TJ, Tameris M, Mansoor N, Smit E, van der Merwe L, Mauff K, Hughes EJ, Moyo S, Brittain N, Lawrie A, Mulenga H, de Kock M, Gelderbloem S, Veldsman A, Hatherill M, Geldenhuys H, Hill AVS, Hussey GD, Mahomed H, et al. Dose-finding study of the novel tuberculosis vaccine, MVA85A, in healthy BCG-vaccinated infants. J Infect Dis. 2011;203(12):1832–43. https://doi.org/10.1093/infdis/jir195.
20. Pathan AA, Minassian AM, Sander CR, Rowland R, Porter DW, Poulton ID, Hill AVS, Fletcher HA, McShane H. Effect of vaccine dose on the safety and immunogenicity of a candidate TB vaccine, MVA85A, in BCG vaccinated UK adults. Vaccine. 2012;30(38):5616–24. https://doi.org/10.1016/j.vaccine.2012.06.084.
21. Odutola AA, Owolabi OA, Owiafe PK, McShane H, Ota MOC. A new TB vaccine, MVA85A, induces durable antigen-specific responses 14 months after vaccination in African infants. Vaccine. 2012;30(38):5591–4. https://doi.org/10.1016/j.vaccine.2012.06.054.
22. Ota MOC, Odutola AA, Owiafe PK, Donkor S, Owolabi OA, Brittain NJ, Williams N, Rowland-Jones S, Hill AVS, Adegbola RA, McShane H. Immunogenicity of the tuberculosis vaccine MVA85A is reduced by coadministration with EPI vaccines in a randomized controlled trial in Gambian infants. Sci Transl Med. 2011;3(88):88ra56. https://doi.org/10.1126/scitranslmed.3002461.
23. de Cassan SC, Pathan AA, Sander CR, Minassian A, Rowland R, Hill AVS, McShane H, Fletcher HA. Investigating the induction of vaccine-induced Th17 and regulatory T cells in healthy, *Mycobacterium bovis* BCG-immunized adults vaccinated with a new tuberculosis vaccine, MVA85A. Clin Vaccine Immunol. 2010;17(7):1066–73. https://doi.org/10.1128/CVI.00047-10.
24. Scriba TJ, Tameris M, Smit E, van der Merwe L, Hughes EJ, Kadira B, Mauff K, Moyo S, Brittain N, Lawrie A, Mulenga H, de Kock M, Makhethe L, Janse van Rensburg E, Gelderbloem S, Veldsman A, Hatherill M, Geldenhuys H, Hill AVS, et al. A phase IIa trial of the new tuberculosis vaccine, MVA85A, in HIV- and/or *Mycobacterium tuberculosis* –

infected adults. Am J Respir Crit Care Med. 2012;185(7):769–78. https://doi.org/10.1164/rccm.201108-1548OC.

25. Minhinnick A, Satti I, Harris S, Wilkie M, Sheehan S, Stockdale L, Thomas Z-RM, Lopez-Ramon R, Poulton I, Lawrie A, Vermaak S, Le Vert A, Del Campo J, Hill F, Moss P, McShane H. A first-in-human phase 1 trial to evaluate the safety and immunogenicity of the candidate tuberculosis vaccine MVA85A-IMX313, administered to BCG-vaccinated adults. Vaccine. 2016;34(11):1412–21. https://doi.org/10.1016/j.vaccine.2016.01.062.
26. Dieye TN, NDiaye BP, Dieng AB, Fall M, Britain N, Vermaak S, Camara M, Diop-Ndiaye H, Ngom-Gueye NF, Diaw PA, Toure-Kane C, Sow PS, Mboup S, McShane H. Two doses of candidate TB vaccine MVA85A in antiretroviral therapy (ART) naïve subjects gives comparable immunogenicity to one dose in ART+ subjects. PLoS One. 2013;8(6):e67177. https://doi.org/10.1371/journal.pone.0067177.
27. Minassian AM, Rowland R, Beveridge NER, Poulton ID, Satti I, Harris S, Poyntz H, Hamill M, Griffiths K, Sander CR, Ambrozak DR, Price DA, Hill BJ, Casazza JP, Douek DC, Koup RA, Roederer M, Winston A, Ross J, et al. A phase I study evaluating the safety and immunogenicity of MVA85A, a candidate TB vaccine, in HIV-infected adults. BMJ Open. 2011;1(2):e000223. https://doi.org/10.1136/bmjopen-2011-000223.
28. Ndiaye BP, Thienemann F, Ota M, Landry BS, Camara M, Dièye S, Dieye TN, Esmail H, Goliath R, Huygen K, January V, Ndiaye I, Oni T, Raine M, Romano M, Satti I, Sutton S, Thiam A, Wilkinson KA, et al. Safety, immunogenicity, and efficacy of the candidate tuberculosis vaccine MVA85A in healthy adults infected with HIV-1: a randomised, placebo-controlled, phase 2 trial. Lancet Respir Med. 2015;3(3):190–200. https://doi.org/10.1016/S2213-2600(15)00037-5.
29. Sander CR, Pathan AA, Beveridge NER, Poulton I, Minassian A, Alder N, Van Wijgerden J, Hill AVS, Gleeson FV, Davies RJO, Pasvol G, McShane H. Safety and immunogenicity of a new tuberculosis vaccine, MVA85A, in *Mycobacterium tuberculosis* –infected individuals. Am J Respir Crit Care Med. 2009;179(8):724–33. https://doi.org/10.1164/rccm.200809-1486OC.
30. Nemes E, Hesseling AC, Tameris M, Mauff K, Downing K, Mulenga H, Rose P, van der Zalm M, Mbaba S, Van As D, Hanekom WA, Walzl G, Scriba TJ, McShane H, Hatherill M, Abrahams C, Abrahams D, Africa H, Baartman V, et al. Safety and immunogenicity of newborn MVA85A vaccination and selective, delayed Bacille Calmette-Guerin for infants of human immunodeficiency virus-infected mothers: a phase 2 randomized, controlled trial. Clin Infect Dis. 2018;66(4):554–63. https://doi.org/10.1093/cid/cix834.
31. Tameris M, Geldenhuys H, Luabeya AK, Smit E, Hughes JE, Vermaak S, Hanekom WA, Hatherill M, Mahomed H, McShane H, Scriba TJ. The candidate TB vaccine, MVA85A, induces highly durable Th1 responses. PLoS One. 2014;9(2):e87340. https://doi.org/10.1371/journal.pone.0087340.
32. Meyer J, Harris SA, Satti I, Poulton ID, Poyntz HC, Tanner R, Rowland R, Griffiths KL, Fletcher HA, McShane H. Comparing the safety and immunogenicity of a candidate TB vaccine MVA85A administered by intramuscular and intradermal delivery. Vaccine. 2013;31(7):1026–33. https://doi.org/10.1016/j.vaccine.2012.12.042.
33. Satti I, Meyer J, Harris SA, Thomas Z-RM, Griffiths K, Antrobus RD, Rowland R, Ramon RL, Smith M, Sheehan S, Bettinson H, McShane H. Safety and immunogenicity of a candidate tuberculosis vaccine MVA85A delivered by aerosol in BCG-vaccinated healthy adults: a phase 1, double-blind, randomised controlled trial. Lancet Infect Dis. 2014;14(10):939–46. https://doi.org/10.1016/S1473-3099(14)70845-X.
34. Riste M, Marshall J, Satti I, Harris S, Wilkie M, Lopez Ramon R, Wright D, Wittenberg R, Vermaak S, Powell Doherty R, Lawrie A, Conlon C, Cosgrove C, Gleeson F, Lipman M, Moss P, Perrin F, Dedicoat M, Bettinson H, McShane H. Phase I trial evaluating the safety and immunogenicity of candidate TB vaccine MVA85A, delivered by aerosol to healthy M.tb-infected adults. Vaccine. 2021;9(4):396. https://doi.org/10.3390/vaccines9040396.
35. Manjaly Thomas Z-R, Satti I, Marshall JL, Harris SA, Lopez Ramon R, Hamidi A, Minhinnick A, Riste M, Stockdale L, Lawrie AM, Vermaak S, Wilkie M, Bettinson H, McShane

H. Alternate aerosol and systemic immunisation with a recombinant viral vector for tuberculosis, MVA85A: a phase I randomised controlled trial. PLoS Med. 2019;16(4):e1002790. https://doi.org/10.1371/journal.pmed.1002790.

36. Tameris MD, Hatherill M, Landry BS, Scriba TJ, Snowden MA, Lockhart S, Shea JE, McClain JB, Hussey GD, Hanekom WA, Mahomed H, McShane H. Safety and efficacy of MVA85A, a new tuberculosis vaccine, in infants previously vaccinated with BCG: a randomised, placebo-controlled phase 2b trial. Lancet. 2013;381(9871):1021–8. https://doi.org/10.1016/S0140-6736(13)60177-4.
37. Andrews JR, Nemes E, Tameris M, Landry BS, Mahomed H, McClain JB, Fletcher HA, Hanekom WA, Wood R, McShane H, Scriba TJ, Hatherill M. Serial QuantiFERON testing and tuberculosis disease risk among young children: an observational cohort study. Lancet Respir Med. 2017;5(4):282–90. https://doi.org/10.1016/S2213-2600(17)30060-7.
38. Bunyasi EW, Luabeya AKK, Tameris M, Geldenhuys H, Mulenga H, Landry BS, Scriba TJ, Schmidt B-M, Hanekom WA, Mahomed H, McShane H, Hatherill M. Impact of isoniazid preventive therapy on the evaluation of long-term effectiveness of infant MVA85A vaccination. Int J Tuberc Lung Dis. 2017;21(7):778–83. https://doi.org/10.5588/ijtld.16.0709.
39. Kashangura R, Jullien S, Garner P, Johnson S. MVA85A vaccine to enhance BCG for preventing tuberculosis. Cochrane Database Syst Rev. 2019;2019(4):CD012915. https://doi.org/10.1002/14651858.CD012915.pub2.
40. Abel B, Tameris M, Mansoor N, Gelderbloem S, Hughes J, Abrahams D, Makhethe L, Erasmus M, de Kock M, van der Merwe L, Hawkridge A, Veldsman A, Hatherill M, Schirru G, Pau MG, Hendriks J, Weverling GJ, Goudsmit J, Sizemore D, et al. The novel tuberculosis vaccine, AERAS-402, induces robust and polyfunctional CD4 $^{+}$ and CD8 $^{+}$ T cells in adults. Am J Respir Crit Care Med. 2010;181(12):1407–17. https://doi.org/10.1164/rccm.200910-1484OC.
41. Walsh DS, Owira V, Polhemus M, Otieno L, Andagalu B, Ogutu B, Waitumbi J, Hawkridge A, Shepherd B, Pau MG, Sadoff J, Douoguih M, McClain JB. Adenovirus type 35-vectored tuberculosis vaccine has an acceptable safety and tolerability profile in healthy, BCG-vaccinated, QuantiFERON®-TB Gold (+) Kenyan adults without evidence of tuberculosis. Vaccine. 2016;34(21):2430–6. https://doi.org/10.1016/j.vaccine.2016.03.069.
42. Kagina BMN, Tameris MD, Geldenhuys H, Hatherill M, Abel B, Hussey GD, Scriba TJ, Mahomed H, Sadoff JC, Hanekom WA, Mansoor N, Hughes J, de Kock M, Whatney W, Africa H, Krohn C, Veldsman A, Kany ALK, Douoguih M, et al. The novel tuberculosis vaccine, AERAS-402, is safe in healthy infants previously vaccinated with BCG, and induces dose-dependent CD4 and CD8T cell responses. Vaccine. 2014;32(45):5908–17. https://doi.org/10.1016/j.vaccine.2014.09.001.
43. Tameris M, Hokey DA, Nduba V, Sacarlal J, Laher F, Kiringa G, Gondo K, Lazarus EM, Gray GE, Nachman S, Mahomed H, Downing K, Abel B, Scriba TJ, McClain JB, Pau MG, Hendriks J, Dheenadhayalan V, Ishmukhamedov S, et al. A double-blind, randomised, placebo-controlled, dose-finding trial of the novel tuberculosis vaccine AERAS-402, an adenovirus-vectored fusion protein, in healthy, BCG-vaccinated infants. Vaccine. 2015;33(25):2944–54. https://doi.org/10.1016/j.vaccine.2015.03.070.
44. van Zyl-Smit RN, Esmail A, Bateman ME, Dawson R, Goldin J, van Rikxoort E, Douoguih M, Pau MG, Sadoff JC, McClain JB, Snowden MA, Benko J, Hokey DA, Rutkowski KT, Graves A, Shepherd B, Ishmukhamedov S, Kagina BMN, Abel B, et al. Safety and immunogenicity of adenovirus 35 tuberculosis vaccine candidate in adults with active or previous tuberculosis. A randomized trial. Am J Respir Crit Care Med. 2017;195(9):1171–80. https://doi.org/10.1164/rccm.201603-0654OC.
45. Sheehan S, Harris SA, Satti I, Hokey DA, Dheenadhayalan V, Stockdale L, Manjaly Thomas Z-R, Minhinnick A, Wilkie M, Vermaak S, Meyer J, O'Shea MK, Pau MG, Versteege I, Douoguih M, Hendriks J, Sadoff J, Landry B, Moss P, McShane H. A phase I, open-label trial, evaluating the safety and immunogenicity of candidate tuberculosis vaccines AERAS-402 and MVA85A, administered by prime-boost regime in BCG-vaccinated healthy adults. PLoS One. 2015;10(11):e0141687. https://doi.org/10.1371/journal.pone.0141687.

46. Sivakumaran D, Blatner G, Bakken R, Hokey D, Ritz C, Jenum S, Grewal HMS. A 2-dose AERAS-402 regimen boosts CD8+ polyfunctionality in HIV-negative, BCG-vaccinated recipients. Front Immunol. 2021;12:673532. https://doi.org/10.3389/fimmu.2021.673532.
47. Churchyard GJ, Snowden MA, Hokey D, Dheenadhayalan V, McClain JB, Douoguih M, Pau MG, Sadoff J, Landry B. The safety and immunogenicity of an adenovirus type 35-vectored TB vaccine in HIV-infected, BCG-vaccinated adults with CD4+ T cell counts ˃350 cells/mm3. Vaccine. 2015;33(15):1890–6. https://doi.org/10.1016/j.vaccine.2015.02.004.
48. Hoft DF, Blazevic A, Stanley J, Landry B, Sizemore D, Kpamegan E, Gearhart J, Scott A, Kik S, Pau MG, Goudsmit J, McClain JB, Sadoff J. A recombinant adenovirus expressing immunodominant TB antigens can significantly enhance BCG-induced human immunity. Vaccine. 2012;30(12):2098–108. https://doi.org/10.1016/j.vaccine.2012.01.048.
49. Stylianou E, Griffiths KL, Poyntz HC, Harrington-Kandt R, Dicks MD, Stockdale L, Betts G, McShane H. Improvement of BCG protective efficacy with a novel chimpanzee adenovirus and a modified vaccinia Ankara virus both expressing Ag85A. Vaccine. 2015;33(48):6800–8. https://doi.org/10.1016/j.vaccine.2015.10.017.
50. Antrobus RD, Coughlan L, Berthoud TK, Dicks MD, Hill AVS, Lambe T, Gilbert SC. Clinical assessment of a novel recombinant simian adenovirus ChAdOx1 as a vectored vaccine expressing conserved Influenza A antigens. Mol Ther. 2014;22(3):668–74. https://doi.org/10.1038/MT.2013.284.
51. Wilkie M, Satti I, Minhinnick A, Harris S, Riste M, Ramon RL, Sheehan S, Thomas Z-RM, Wright D, Stockdale L, Hamidi A, O'Shea MK, Dwivedi K, Behrens HM, Davenne T, Morton J, Vermaak S, Lawrie A, Moss P, McShane H. A phase I trial evaluating the safety and immunogenicity of a candidate tuberculosis vaccination regimen, ChAdOx1 85A prime—MVA85A boost in healthy UK adults. Vaccine. 2020;38(4):779–89. https://doi.org/10.1016/j.vaccine.2019.10.102.
52. Wajja A, Nassanga B, Natukunda A, Serubanja J, Tumusiime J, Akurut H, Oduru G, Nassuuna J, Kabagenyi J, Morrison H, Scott H, Doherty RP, Marshall JL, Puig IC, Cose S, Kaleebu P, Webb EL, Satti I, McShane H, et al. Safety and immunogenicity of ChAdOx1 85A prime followed by MVA85A boost compared with BCG revaccination among Ugandan adolescents who received BCG at birth: a randomised, open-label trial. Lancet Infect Dis. 2023;24:285. https://doi.org/10.1016/S1473-3099(23)00501-7.
53. Audran R, Karoui O, Donnet L, Soumas V, Fares F, Lovis A, Noirez L, Cavassini M, Fayet-Mello A, Satti I, McShane H, Spertini F. Randomised, double-blind, controlled phase 1 trial of the candidate tuberculosis vaccine ChAdOx1-85A delivered by aerosol versus intramuscular route. J Infect. 2024;89(2):106205. https://doi.org/10.1016/j.jinf.2024.106205.
54. Rowland R, Pathan AA, Satti I, Poulton ID, Matsumiya MML, Whittaker M, Minassian AM, O'Hara GA, Hamill M, Scott JT, Harris SA, Poyntz HC, Bateman C, Meyer J, Williams N, Gilbert SC, Lawrie AM, Hill AVS, McShane H. Safety and immunogenicity of an FP9-vectored candidate tuberculosis vaccine (FP85A), alone and with candidate vaccine MVA85A in BCG-vaccinated healthy adults. Hum Vaccin Immunother. 2013;9(1):50–62. https://doi.org/10.4161/hv.22464.
55. Priddy FH, Brown D, Kublin J, Monahan K, Wright DP, Lalezari J, Santiago S, Marmor M, Lally M, Novak RM, Brown SJ, Kulkarni P, Dubey SA, Kierstead LS, Casimiro DR, Mogg R, DiNubile MJ, Shiver JW, Leavitt RY, et al. Safety and immunogenicity of a replication-incompetent adenovirus type 5 HIV-1 Clade B *gag/pol/nef* vaccine in healthy adults. Clin Infect Dis. 2008;46(11):1769–81. https://doi.org/10.1086/587993.
56. Tamminga C, Sedegah M, Regis D, Chuang I, Epstein JE, Spring M, Mendoza-Silveiras J, McGrath S, Maiolatesi S, Reyes S, Steinbeiss V, Fedders C, Smith K, House B, Ganeshan H, Lejano J, Abot E, Banania GJ, Sayo R, et al. Adenovirus-5-vectored P. falciparum vaccine expressing CSP and AMA1. Part B: safety, immunogenicity and protective efficacy of the CSP component. PLoS One. 2011;6(10):e25868. https://doi.org/10.1371/journal.pone.0025868.
57. Smaill F, Jeyanathan M, Smieja M, Medina MF, Thanthrige-Don N, Zganiacz A, Yin C, Heriazon A, Damjanovic D, Puri L, Hamid J, Xie F, Foley R, Bramson J, Gauldie J, Xing Z. A human type 5 adenovirus–based tuberculosis vaccine induces robust T cell responses in

humans despite preexisting anti-adenovirus immunity. Sci Transl Med. 2013;5(205):205ra134. https://doi.org/10.1126/scitranslmed.3006843.

58. Jeyanathan M, Damjanovic D, Yao Y, Bramson J, Smaill F, Xing Z. Induction of an immune-protective T-cell repertoire with diverse genetic coverage by a novel viral-vectored tuberculosis vaccine in humans. J Infect Dis. 2016;214(12):1996–2005. https://doi.org/10.1093/infdis/jiw467.
59. Jeyanathan M, Fritz DK, Afkhami S, Aguirre E, Howie KJ, Zganiacz A, Dvorkin-Gheva A, Thompson MR, Silver RF, Cusack RP, Lichty BD, O'Byrne PM, Kolb M, Medina MFC, Dolovich MB, Satia I, Gauvreau GM, Xing Z, Smaill F. Aerosol delivery, but not intramuscular injection, of adenovirus-vectored tuberculosis vaccine induces respiratory-mucosal immunity in humans. JCI Insight. 2022;7(3):e155655. https://doi.org/10.1172/jci.insight.155655.
60. Szabo PA, Miron M, Farber DL. Location, location, location: tissue resident memory T cells in mice and humans. Science Immunol. 2019;4(34):eaas9673. https://doi.org/10.1126/sciimmunol.aas9673.
61. Wu S, Huang J, Zhang Z, Wu J, Zhang J, Hu H, Zhu T, Zhang J, Luo L, Fan P, Wang B, Chen C, Chen Y, Song X, Wang Y, Si W, Sun T, Wang X, Hou L, Chen W. Safety, tolerability, and immunogenicity of an aerosolised adenovirus type-5 vector-based COVID-19 vaccine (Ad5-nCoV) in adults: preliminary report of an open-label and randomised phase 1 clinical trial. Lancet Infect Dis. 2021;21(12):1654–64. https://doi.org/10.1016/S1473-3099(21)00396-0.
62. Zhu F-C, Guan X-H, Li Y-H, Huang J-Y, Jiang T, Hou L-H, Li J-X, Yang B-F, Wang L, Wang W-J, Wu S-P, Wang Z, Wu X-H, Xu J-J, Zhang Z, Jia S-Y, Wang B-S, Hu Y, Liu J-J, et al. Immunogenicity and safety of a recombinant adenovirus type-5-vectored COVID-19 vaccine in healthy adults aged 18 years or older: a randomised, double-blind, placebo-controlled, phase 2 trial. Lancet. 2020;396(10249):479–88. https://doi.org/10.1016/S0140-6736(20)31605-6.
63. Sereinig S, Stukova M, Zabolotnyh N, Ferko B, Kittel C, Romanova J, Vinogradova T, Katinger H, Kiselev O, Egorov A. Influenza virus NS vectors expressing the *Mycobacterium tuberculosis* ESAT-6 protein induce $CD4^+$ Th1 immune response and protect animals against tuberculosis challenge. Clin Vaccine Immunol. 2006;13(8):898–904. https://doi.org/10.1128/CVI.00056-06.
64. Stukova MA, Sereinig S, Zabolotnyh NV, Ferko B, Kittel C, Romanova J, Vinogradova TI, Katinger H, Kiselev OI, Egorov A. Vaccine potential of influenza vectors expressing Mycobacterium tuberculosis ESAT-6 protein. Tuberculosis. 2006;86(3–4):236–46. https://doi.org/10.1016/j.tube.2006.01.010.
65. Buzitskaya Z, Stosman K, Khairullin B, Kassenov M, Nurpeisova A, Abylai Sansyzbay A, Shurygina A-P, Aleksandrov A, Sivak K, Stukova M. A new intranasal influenza vector-based vaccine TB/FLU-04L against tuberculosis: preclinical safety studies. Drug Research. 2022;72(05):255–8. https://doi.org/10.1055/a-1785-3936.
66. Shurygina A-P, Zabolotnykh N, Vinogradova T, Khairullin B, Kassenov M, Nurpeisova A, Sarsenbayeva G, Sansyzbay A, Vasilyev K, Buzitskaya J, Egorov A, Stukova M. Preclinical evaluation of TB/FLU-04L—an intranasal influenza vector-based boost vaccine against tuberculosis. Int J Mol Sci. 2023;24(8):7439. https://doi.org/10.3390/ijms24087439.
67. Stosman K, Sivak K, Aleksandrov A, Buzitskaya Z, Rassokha T, Stukova M. Preclinical safety evaluation: acute and repeated-dose toxicity of a new intranasal recombinant vector vaccine TB/FLU-04L against tuberculosis. Drug Res. 2022;72(04):215–9. https://doi.org/10.1055/a-1771-5985.
68. Sergeeva M, Romanovskaya-Romanko E, Zabolotnyh N, Pulkina A, Vasilyev K, Shurigina AP, Buzitskaya J, Zabrodskaya Y, Fadeev A, Vasin A, Vinogradova TI, Stukova MA. Mucosal influenza vector vaccine carrying TB10.4 and HspX antigens provides protection against Mycobacterium tuberculosis in mice and Guinea pigs. Vaccine. 2021;9(4):394. https://doi.org/10.3390/vaccines9040394.
69. Vasilyev K, Shurygina A-P, Zabolotnykh N, Sergeeva M, Romanovskaya-Romanko E, Pulkina A, Buzitskaya J, Dogonadze MZ, Vinogradova TI, Stukova MA. Enhancement of the local CD8+ T-cellular immune response to Mycobacterium tuberculosis in BCG-primed

mice after intranasal administration of influenza vector vaccine carrying TB10.4 and HspX antigens. Vaccine. 2021;9(11):1273. https://doi.org/10.3390/vaccines9111273.
70. Looney MM, Hatherill M, Musvosvi M, Flynn J, Kagina BM, Frick M, Kafuko Z, Schmidt A, Southern J, Wilder-Smith A, Tippoo P, Paradkar V, Popadić D, Scriba TJ, Hanekom W, Giersing B. Conference report: WHO meeting summary on mRNA-based tuberculosis vaccine development. Vaccine. 2023;41(48):7060–6. https://doi.org/10.1016/j.vaccine.2023.10.026.
71. Matarazzo L, Bettencourt PJG. mRNA vaccines: a new opportunity for malaria, tuberculosis and HIV. Front Immunol. 2023;14:1172691. https://doi.org/10.3389/fimmu.2023.1172691.
72. Yang H, Lei X, Chai S, Su G, Du L. From pathogenesis to antigens: the key to shaping the future of TB vaccines. Front Immunol. 2024;15:1440935. https://doi.org/10.3389/fimmu.2024.1440935.
73. Houben RMGJ, Dodd PJ. The global burden of latent tuberculosis infection: a re-estimation using mathematical modelling. PLoS Med. 2016;13(10):e1002152. https://doi.org/10.1371/journal.pmed.1002152.
74. Portnoy A, Clark RA, Quaife M, Weerasuriya CK, Mukandavire C, Bakker R, Deol AK, Malhotra S, Gebreselassie N, Zignol M, Sim SY, Hutubessy RCW, Baena IG, Nishikiori N, Jit M, White RG, Menzies NA. The cost and cost-effectiveness of novel tuberculosis vaccines in low- and middle-income countries: A modeling study. PLoS Med. 2023;20(1):e1004155. https://doi.org/10.1371/journal.pmed.1004155.
75. Nemes E, Fiore-Gartland A, Boggiano C, Coccia M, D'Souza P, Gilbert P, Ginsberg A, Hyrien O, Laddy D, Makar K, McElrath MJ, Ramachandra L, Schmidt C, Shotorbani S, Sunshine J, Tomaras G, Yu W-H, Scriba TJ, Frahm N. The quest for vaccine-induced immune correlates of protection against tuberculosis. Vaccine Insights. 2022;1(3):165–81. https://doi.org/10.18609/vac/2022.027.
76. Darrah PA, Zeppa JJ, Maiello P, Hackney JA, Wadsworth MH, Hughes TK, Pokkali S, Swanson PA, Grant NL, Rodgers MA, Kamath M, Causgrove CM, Laddy DJ, Bonavia A, Casimiro D, Lin PL, Klein E, White AG, Scanga CA, et al. Prevention of tuberculosis in macaques after intravenous BCG immunization. Nature. 2020;577(7788):95–102. https://doi.org/10.1038/s41586-019-1817-8.
77. Derrick SC, Yabe IM, Yang A, Morris SL. Vaccine-induced anti-tuberculosis protective immunity in mice correlates with the magnitude and quality of multifunctional CD4 T cells. Vaccine. 2011;29(16):2902–9. https://doi.org/10.1016/j.vaccine.2011.02.010.
78. Dijkman K, Sombroek CC, Vervenne RAW, Hofman SO, Boot C, Remarque EJ, Kocken CHM, Ottenhoff THM, Kondova I, Khayum MA, Haanstra KG, Vierboom MPM, Verreck FAW. Prevention of tuberculosis infection and disease by local BCG in repeatedly exposed rhesus macaques. Nat Med. 2019;25(2):255–62. https://doi.org/10.1038/s41591-018-0319-9.
79. Day CL, Abrahams DA, Lerumo L, Janse van Rensburg E, Stone L, O'rie T, Pienaar B, de Kock M, Kaplan G, Mahomed H, Dheda K, Hanekom WA. Functional capacity of *Mycobacterium tuberculosis* -specific T cell responses in humans is associated with mycobacterial load. J Immunol. 2011;187(5):2222–32. https://doi.org/10.4049/jimmunol.1101122.
80. Kagina BMN, Abel B, Scriba TJ, Hughes EJ, Keyser A, Soares A, Gamieldien H, Sidibana M, Hatherill M, Gelderbloem S, Mahomed H, Hawkridge A, Hussey G, Kaplan G, Hanekom WA. Specific T cell frequency and cytokine expression profile do not correlate with protection against tuberculosis after Bacillus Calmette-Guérin vaccination of newborns. Am J Respir Crit Care Med. 2010;182(8):1073–9. https://doi.org/10.1164/rccm.201003-0334OC.
81. Gideon HP, Hughes TK, Tzouanas CN, Wadsworth MH, Tu AA, Gierahn TM, Peters JM, Hopkins FF, Wei J-R, Kummerlowe C, Grant NL, Nargan K, Phuah JY, Borish HJ, Maiello P, White AG, Winchell CG, Nyquist SK, Ganchua SKC, et al. Multimodal profiling of lung granulomas in macaques reveals cellular correlates of tuberculosis control. Immunity. 2022;55(5):827–846.e10. https://doi.org/10.1016/j.immuni.2022.04.004.
82. Achkar JM, Prados-Rosales R. Updates on antibody functions in Mycobacterium tuberculosis infection and their relevance for developing a vaccine against tuberculosis. Curr Opin Immunol. 2018;53:30–7. https://doi.org/10.1016/j.coi.2018.04.004.

83. Irvine EB, O'Neil A, Darrah PA, Shin S, Choudhary A, Li W, Honnen W, Mehra S, Kaushal D, Gideon HP, Flynn JL, Roederer M, Seder RA, Pinter A, Fortune S, Alter G. Robust IgM responses following intravenous vaccination with Bacille Calmette–Guérin associate with prevention of Mycobacterium tuberculosis infection in macaques. Nat Immunol. 2021;22(12):1515–23. https://doi.org/10.1038/s41590-021-01066-1.
84. Prados-Rosales R, Carreño L, Cheng T, Blanc C, Weinrick B, Malek A, Lowary TL, Baena A, Joe M, Bai Y, Kalscheuer R, Batista-Gonzalez A, Saavedra NA, Sampedro L, Tomás J, Anguita J, Hung S-C, Tripathi A, Xu J, et al. Enhanced control of Mycobacterium tuberculosis extrapulmonary dissemination in mice by an arabinomannan-protein conjugate vaccine. PLoS Pathog. 2017;13(3):e1006250. https://doi.org/10.1371/journal.ppat.1006250.
85. Li H, Wang X, Wang B, Fu L, Liu G, Lu Y, Cao M, Huang H, Javid B. Latently and uninfected healthcare workers exposed to TB make protective antibodies against *Mycobacterium tuberculosis*. Proc Natl Acad Sci. 2017;114(19):5023–8. https://doi.org/10.1073/pnas.1611776114.
86. Joosten SA, van Meijgaarden KE, del Nonno F, Baiocchini A, Petrone L, Vanini V, Smits HH, Palmieri F, Goletti D, Ottenhoff THM. Patients with tuberculosis have a dysfunctional circulating B-cell compartment, which normalizes following successful treatment. PLoS Pathog. 2016;12(6):e1005687. https://doi.org/10.1371/journal.ppat.1005687.
87. Tsai C-Y, Oo M, Peh JH, Yeo BCM, Aptekmann A, Lee B, Liu JJJ, Tsao W-S, Dick T, Fink K, Gengenbacher M. Splenic marginal zone B cells restrict Mycobacterium tuberculosis infection by shaping the cytokine pattern and cell-mediated immunity. Cell Rep. 2024;43(7):114426. https://doi.org/10.1016/j.celrep.2024.114426.
88. Harris SA, Meyer J, Satti I, Marsay L, Poulton ID, Tanner R, Minassian AM, Fletcher HA, McShane H. Evaluation of a human BCG challenge model to assess antimycobacterial immunity induced by BCG and a candidate tuberculosis vaccine, MVA85A, alone and in combination. J Infect Dis. 2014;209(8):1259–68. https://doi.org/10.1093/infdis/jit647.
89. Cole ST, Brosch R, Parkhill J, Garnier T, Churcher C, Harris D, Gordon SV, Eiglmeier K, Gas S, Barry CE, Tekaia F, Badcock K, Basham D, Brown D, Chillingworth T, Connor R, Davies R, Devlin K, Feltwell T, et al. Deciphering the biology of Mycobacterium tuberculosis from the complete genome sequence. Nature. 1998;393(6685):537–44. https://doi.org/10.1038/31159.
90. Coppola M, Ottenhoff TH. Genome wide approaches discover novel Mycobacterium tuberculosis antigens as correlates of infection, disease, immunity and targets for vaccination. Semin Immunol. 2018;39:88–101. https://doi.org/10.1016/j.smim.2018.07.001.
91. Moguche AO, Musvosvi M, Penn-Nicholson A, Plumlee CR, Mearns H, Geldenhuys H, Smit E, Abrahams D, Rozot V, Dintwe O, Hoff ST, Kromann I, Ruhwald M, Bang P, Larson RP, Shafiani S, Ma S, Sherman DR, Sette A, et al. Antigen availability shapes T cell differentiation and function during tuberculosis. Cell Host Microbe. 2017;21(6):695–706.e5. https://doi.org/10.1016/j.chom.2017.05.012.
92. Ernst JD, Cornelius A, Desvignes L, Tavs J, Norris BA. Limited antimycobacterial efficacy of epitope peptide administration despite enhanced antigen-specific CD4 T-cell activation. J Infect Dis. 2018;218(10):1653–62. https://doi.org/10.1093/infdis/jiy142.
93. Coppola M, van den Eeden SJF, Wilson L, Franken KLMC, Ottenhoff THM, Geluk A. Synthetic long peptide derived from Mycobacterium tuberculosis latency antigen Rv1733c protects against tuberculosis. Clin Vaccine Immunol. 2015;22(9):1060–9. https://doi.org/10.1128/CVI.00271-15.
94. Shi C, Chen L, Chen Z, Zhang Y, Zhou Z, Lu J, Fu R, Wang C, Fang Z, Fan X. Enhanced protection against tuberculosis by vaccination with recombinant BCG over-expressing HspX protein. Vaccine. 2010;28(32):5237–44. https://doi.org/10.1016/j.vaccine.2010.05.063.
95. Geluk A, Lin MY, van Meijgaarden KE, Leyten EMS, Franken KLMC, Ottenhoff THM, Klein MR. T-cell recognition of the HspX protein of *Mycobacterium tuberculosis* correlates with latent *M. tuberculosis* infection but not with *M. bovis* BCG vaccination. Infect Immun. 2007;75(6):2914–21. https://doi.org/10.1128/IAI.01990-06.
96. Lin MY, Geluk A, Smith SG, Stewart AL, Friggen AH, Franken KLMC, Verduyn MJC, van Meijgaarden KE, Voskuil MI, Dockrell HM, Huygen K, Ottenhoff THM, Klein MR. Lack

of immune responses to *Mycobacterium tuberculosis* DosR regulon proteins following *Mycobacterium bovis* BCG vaccination. Infect Immun. 2007;75(7):3523–30. https://doi.org/10.1128/IAI.01999-06.

97. Fukui M, Shinjo K, Umemura M, Shigeno S, Harakuni T, Arakawa T, Matsuzaki G. Enhanced effect of BCG vaccine against pulmonary *Mycobacterium tuberculosis* infection in mice with lung Th17 response to mycobacterial heparin-binding hemagglutinin adhesin antigen. Microbiol Immunol. 2015;59(12):735–43. https://doi.org/10.1111/1348-0421.12340.
98. Guerrero GG, Debrie A-S, Locht C. Boosting with mycobacterial heparin-binding haemagglutinin enhances protection of Mycobacterium bovis BCG-vaccinated newborn mice against M. tuberculosis. Vaccine. 2010;28(27):4340–7. https://doi.org/10.1016/j.vaccine.2010.04.062.
99. Kohama H, Umemura M, Okamoto Y, Yahagi A, Goga H, Harakuni T, Matsuzaki G, Arakawa T. Mucosal immunization with recombinant heparin-binding haemagglutinin adhesin suppresses extrapulmonary dissemination of Mycobacterium bovis bacillus Calmette-Guérin (BCG) in infected mice. Vaccine. 2008;26(7):924–32. https://doi.org/10.1016/j.vaccine.2007.12.005.
100. Rouanet C, Debrie A-S, Lecher S, Locht C. Subcutaneous boosting with heparin binding haemagglutinin increases BCG-induced protection against tuberculosis. Microbes Infect. 2009;11(13):995–1001. https://doi.org/10.1016/j.micinf.2009.07.005.
101. Aagaard C, Hoang T, Dietrich J, Cardona P-J, Izzo A, Dolganov G, Schoolnik GK, Cassidy JP, Billeskov R, Andersen P. A multistage tuberculosis vaccine that confers efficient protection before and after exposure. Nat Med. 2011;17(2):189–94. https://doi.org/10.1038/nm.2285.
102. Geluk A, van den Eeden SJF, van Meijgaarden KE, Dijkman K, Franken KLMC, Ottenhoff THM. A multistage-polyepitope vaccine protects against Mycobacterium tuberculosis infection in HLA-DR3 transgenic mice. Vaccine. 2012;30(52):7513–21. https://doi.org/10.1016/j.vaccine.2012.10.045.
103. Hansen SG, Zak DE, Xu G, Ford JC, Marshall EE, Malouli D, Gilbride RM, Hughes CM, Ventura AB, Ainslie E, Randall KT, Selseth AN, Rundstrom P, Herlache L, Lewis MS, Park H, Planer SL, Turner JM, Fischer M, et al. Prevention of tuberculosis in rhesus macaques by a cytomegalovirus-based vaccine. Nat Med. 2018;24(2):130–43. https://doi.org/10.1038/nm.4473.
104. Hu Z, Xia J, Wu J, Zhao H, Ji P, Gu L, Gu W, Chen Z, Xu J, Huang X, Ma J, Chen A, Li J, Shu T, Fan X-Y. A multistage Sendai virus vaccine incorporating latency-associated antigens induces protection against acute and latent tuberculosis. Emerg Microbes Infect. 2024;13(1):2300463. https://doi.org/10.1080/22221751.2023.2300463.
105. Bettencourt P, Müller J, Nicastri A, Cantillon D, Madhavan M, Charles PD, Fotso CB, Wittenberg R, Bull N, Pinpathomrat N, Waddell SJ, Stylianou E, Hill AVS, Ternette N, McShane H. Identification of antigens presented by MHC for vaccines against tuberculosis. NPJ Vaccines. 2020;5(1):2. https://doi.org/10.1038/s41541-019-0148-y.
106. Almujri SS, Stylianou E, Nicastri A, Satti I, Korompis M, Li S, et al. MetE: a promising protective antigen for tuberculosis vaccine development. Front Immunol. 2025;16:1593263. https://doi.org/10.3389/fimmu.2025.1593263.
107. Forbes EK, Sander C, Ronan EO, McShane H, Hill AVS, Beverley PCL, Tchilian EZ. Multifunctional, high-level cytokine-producing Th1 cells in the lung, but not spleen, correlate with protection against *Mycobacterium tuberculosis* aerosol challenge in mice. J Immunol. 2008;181(7):4955–64. https://doi.org/10.4049/jimmunol.181.7.4955.
108. Wang J, Thorson L, Stokes RW, Santosuosso M, Huygen K, Zganiacz A, Hitt M, Xing Z. Single mucosal, but not parenteral, immunization with recombinant adenoviral-based vaccine provides potent protection from pulmonary tuberculosis. J Immunol. 2004;173(10):6357–65. https://doi.org/10.4049/jimmunol.173.10.6357.
109. Xing Z, McFarland CT, Sallenave J-M, Izzo A, Wang J, McMurray DN. Intranasal mucosal boosting with an adenovirus-vectored vaccine markedly enhances the protection of BCG-

primed Guinea pigs against pulmonary tuberculosis. PLoS One. 2009;4(6):e5856. https://doi.org/10.1371/journal.pone.0005856.
110. Baldeon Vaca G, Meyer M, Cadete A, Hsiao CJ, Golding A, Jeon A, Jacquinet E, Azcue E, Guan CM, Sanchez-Felix X, Pietzsch CA, Mire CE, Hyde MA, Comeaux ME, Williams JM, Sung JC, Carfi A, Edwards DK, Bukreyev A, Bahl K. Intranasal mRNA-LNP vaccination protects hamsters from SARS-CoV-2 infection. Sci Adv. 2023;9(38) https://doi.org/10.1126/sciadv.adh1655.
111. Touray BJB, Hanafy M, Phanse Y, Hildebrand R, Talaat AM. Protective RNA nanovaccines against Mycobacterium avium subspecies hominissuis. Front Immunol. 2023;14:1188754. https://doi.org/10.3389/fimmu.2023.1188754.
112. Wallace R, Bliss CM, Parker AL. The immune system—A double-edged sword for adenovirus-based therapies. Viruses. 2024;16(6):973. https://doi.org/10.3390/v16060973.
113. Kim J, Kim C, Lee JA, Lee SJ, Lee KH, Kim JH, Ahn JY, Jeong SJ, Ku NS, Yeom J-S, Song YG, Choi JY. Immunogenicity differences of the ChAdOx1 nCoV-19 vaccine according to pre-existing adenovirus immunity. Vaccine. 2023;11(4):784. https://doi.org/10.3390/vaccines11040784.
114. Byazrova MG, Astakhova EA, Minnegalieva AR, Sukhova MM, Mikhailov AA, Prilipov AG, Gorchakov AA, Filatov AV. Anti-Ad26 humoral immunity does not compromise SARS-COV-2 neutralizing antibody responses following Gam-COVID-Vac booster vaccination. Npj Vaccines. 2022;7(1):145. https://doi.org/10.1038/s41541-022-00566-x.
115. Smaill F, Xing Z. Human type 5 adenovirus-based tuberculosis vaccine: is the respiratory route of delivery the future? Expert Rev Vaccines. 2014;13(8):927–30. https://doi.org/10.1586/14760584.2014.929947.
116. World Health Organization. The end TB strategy. 2015.

Systems Immunology and *Omics* Data from Developing Countries Are Needed to Inform Vaccine Development

12

Tufária Mussá

12.1 Diversity of the Human Immune System

Genetic diversity has significantly influenced the evolution of the human immune system [1, 2]. Alleles that are predominantly deleterious due to loss of function are often associated with increased risk for infectious and non-infectious diseases [2]. In this context, genetic variants enriched with population-specific signals of natural selection, particularly among Europeans with Neandertal ancestry, play a role in the variability of transcriptional responses to inflammatory and infectious challenges [1].

Research by Bellamy et al. (1998) demonstrated that West Africans who were heterozygous for two natural resistance-associated macrophage protein 1 (NRAMP1) polymorphisms, one in intron 4 and another in the 3′ untranslated region, were notably overrepresented among tuberculosis patients compared to those with the more common NRAMP1 genotype [3]. In the context of Alzheimer's disease, the process of β-amyloid metabolism, primarily influenced by Apoliprotein E (APOE) variants, has been identified as a significant factor contributing to the disease's overall modulation [4]. Additionally, Belloy et al. (2019) revealed that APOE4 represents a strong risk factor for Alzheimer's disease in Japanese populations, a moderate risk in Caucasians, a low risk for African Americans, and little to no risk for Hispanic populations [5].

From these examples, it can be argued that the occurrence, frequency, and distribution of specific alleles within the population are shaped by purifying selection, genetic drift, and migration [2, 6, 7]. One advantage of certain genetic variants is their ability

T. Mussá (✉)
Department of Microbiology, Faculty of Medicine of Eduardo Mondlane University, Maputo, Mozambique

P. J. G. Bettencourt (ed.), *Tuberculosis Vaccines*,
https://doi.org/10.1007/978-3-031-94540-3_12

to confer protection and resilience [4], leading to positive selection,[1] which results in the emergence of new organisms or genetic characteristics, as observed in *E. coli* [9] and Severe Acute Respiratory Syndrome Coronavirus 2 (SARS-CoV-2) [10].

In their investigation of positive selection signals related to coronary artery disease (CAD) across global populations, Byars et al. (2017) utilized novel methods to quantify the relationships between polygenic selection signals and genetic risk for CAD. They identified new candidate adaptive *loci* consistently associated with male and female reproductive traits, suggesting that selection may have targeted these traits due to their direct effects on fitness [11]. Moreover, genetic variants have been shown to impact human immunity and host defence, influenced by selection pressures from microbes, age, and inter-individual characteristics [2, 6, 7, 12]. Genetic pressures often lead to the accumulation of variants in innate immune genes, resulting in high allele frequencies through regulated processes that require distinguishing changing amino acid sequences [6, 13].

In a study examining subjects with active tuberculosis (TB) and their contacts from high-income and low-income countries, the protein signature of active TB patients was characterized by an accumulation of proteins related to complement activation, inflammation, and immune response modulation. Notably, there was also a decrease in a small subset of proteins, including apolipoprotein A and serotransferrin, indicating the significance of lipid transport and iron assimilation in disease progression [14]. Additionally, differences in genetic adaptation are expected, as multiple pathways can lead to resistance against infectious pathogens in populations with specific comorbidities [15]. Environmental and non-environmental factors, including time between sampling, age, sex, circadian cycle, genetics, microbiota, bacterial dysbiosis, and viral infections, can influence genetic profiles and immune system responses [16–18]. These responses generally relate to changes in immune system components due to perturbations from these factors, which may provide insights into individual and inter-individual sensitivities, including predictions of responsiveness or non-responsiveness to vaccines [10, 18–20].

On the other hand, infectious diseases exert selective pressure on human populations. Individuals with genetic variations that confer resistance to specific pathogens tend to have a survival advantage, leading to an increased prevalence of these traits. Examples include the sickle cell trait, which provides resistance to malaria, and certain HLA alleles that enhance immune responses to viral infections [2, 21]. As pathogens adapt to survive against host immune defenses and antibiotic treatments, they undergo genetic changes that can increase their virulence or alter transmission dynamics. For example, *Mycobacterium tuberculosis* (Mtb) has developed various mutations that allow it to evade the immune response or persist in host tissues, impacting public health [22].

Environmental factors such as nutrition, sanitation, pollution, and climate significantly impact immune system function and gene expression. Poor environmental

[1] Positive selection occurs when specific alleles provide a survival or reproductive advantage to individuals (with favorable traits that enhance their fitness) in a given environment. As a result, these advantageous alleles become more common in the population over generations due to the differential reproductive success of organisms that carry them [8].

conditions can exacerbate susceptibility to infections and influence genetic adaptations. For example, malnutrition can weaken immune responses, making populations more vulnerable to infectious diseases and potentially shaping genetic diversity related to immune function [23]. Additionally, environmental changes like urbanization and land use can alter the dynamics of infectious diseases, creating new exposures for populations [24]. This, in turn, drives natural selection and genetic changes in both hosts and pathogens. The presence of zoonotic reservoirs and vectors in specific environments leads to unique pathogen-host interactions, further affecting the genetic landscape of the population [25].

12.2 System Biology and TB Vaccine

Despite being largely curable, TB remains a significant global cause of morbidity and mortality. Control of TB infection relies heavily on $CD4^+$ T cells and cytokines such as IL-12, IFN-γ, and TNF [26]. However, the host and pathogen factors determining susceptibility to TB remain poorly understood. Systems biology offers a powerful approach to understanding the complex interplay between host and pathogen, informing the development of improved vaccines, treatments, and diagnostic tools. Specifically in TB vaccine development, systems biology integrates high-throughput *omics* technologies with computational modeling to provide a comprehensive understanding of the immune response [27]. Integrating data from various *omics* platforms clarifies how pathogen virulence factors interact with host immune mechanisms, which is crucial for identifying vaccine targets and biomarkers of susceptibility and vaccine response [28, 29]. For example, transcriptomics reveals gene expression changes in immune cells, proteomics identifies involved proteins, and metabolomics highlights metabolic shifts during infection and vaccination [30–33].

Integrating diverse data types allows researchers to develop computational models that predict population-specific responses to TB vaccines, considering genetic and environmental factors [30, 34, 35]. These models can simulate various vaccination scenarios, guiding the design of targeted clinical trials, and tailoring vaccines to diverse genetic backgrounds improving the likelihood of successful trials [36, 37]. Analyzing immune profiling data across populations and correlating it with clinical outcomes identifies biomarkers predictive of protective immunity. These biomarkers can be used for patient stratification in clinical trials or to predict vaccine efficacy in real-world settings [38–41].

Tuberculosis vaccination elicits an immune response characterized by T cell activation and differentiation [42]. The use of systems biology approaches offers valuable insights into this response, revealing details of T cell repertoire diversity, clonal expansion, and the cytokine environment, and single-cell technologies further dissect the heterogeneity of T cell responses and their correlation with vaccine efficacy[43, 44]. This understanding can inform the development of improved TB vaccines, particularly combination strategies. Additionally, by modeling the synergistic effects of different vaccine components, including antigens and adjuvants, researchers can design more effective formulations [45, 46]. These systems biology approaches hold significant promise for advancing TB prevention strategies, including the development of multi-valent vaccines targeting diverse aspects of the immune response.

Employing systems biology in TB vaccine research enhances the inclusion of diverse populations in studies. It also allows analyzing of genetic variability across different ethnic groups, and researchers can develop vaccines that take genomic differences into account, thereby improving efficacy for various demographics. Initiatives focused on generating more robust datasets from underrepresented populations can further refine vaccine design, ultimately leading to better health outcomes worldwide [47].

12.2.1 System Biology and Targets for TB Vaccine

High-throughput sequencing of the Mtb genome through Whole Genome Sequencing (WGS) and Next-Generation Sequencing (NGS) has significantly advanced the identification of novel antigenic targets. By analyzing a variety of Mtb strains that may differ geographically, researchers can investigate virulence factors, surface proteins, and immunogenic epitopes. For instance, genome studies have identified several protective antigens, such as Ag85A, Ag85B, and ESAT-6, which are crucial for eliciting strong immune responses [48, 49]. Additionally, WGS enables the detection of genetic variations and mutations in Mtb that could influence host immune responses, facilitating the search for effective vaccine candidates. NGS technologies also provide high-throughput analysis of T cell receptor (TCR) repertoires and immunoglobulin genes, allowing for a comprehensive study of immune responses in vaccinated and infected individuals. By comparing genomic data from diverse Mtb strains, researchers can identify conserved and unique genetic elements that may serve as potential vaccine targets [50–52].

Proteomics has played a crucial role in identifying specific Mtb proteins recognized by the host immune system. This can be achieved through two main approaches: Mass Spectrometry, which analyses the Mtb proteome to identify proteins that elicit immune responses during infection and in specific host environments, and serological proteomics, which examines serum samples from TB patients and vaccinated individuals to detect antibody responses against Mtb proteins. Such studies facilitate the discovery of biomarkers associated with protective immunity, aiding in the evaluation of vaccine efficacy and the stratification of individuals based on their predicted immune responses [53]. By assessing immune responses to these proteins in infected individuals, researchers can determine which antigens are most likely to induce protective immunity. Identification of immunodominant antigens through proteomic technologies also supports the selection of candidates for subunit vaccines. Notably, antigens such as Ag85A and Early Secreted Antigen 6 kDa (ESAT-6) have been recognized for their potential in vaccine formulations [48, 50, 54].

12.2.2 System Biology and Vaccine-Induced Immunity

Genomics allows the profiling of immune cell gene expression before and after vaccination. This analysis helps identify specific gene expression signatures associated with robust immune responses, enhancing our understanding of what constitutes protective immunity. Studying the transcriptomes of vaccinated individuals reveals key immune pathways activated in response to TB vaccination, thereby facilitating the identification of biomarkers that predict vaccine efficacy [55–57]. Additionally, genomic studies investigating genetic diversity within populations identify variations in immune response-related genes, such as HLA alleles. Understanding these variations enables the tailoring of vaccine strategies to improve efficacy across different demographic groups. Research indicates that individuals from diverse genetic backgrounds exhibit varying immune responses to TB vaccines, underscoring the importance of comprehending how genetic and environmental factors interact to shape immunity [58–62].

Other approaches, such as RNA sequencing, are employed to profile gene expression in immune cells from individuals who have received TB vaccines. This technique elucidates the molecular pathways activated upon vaccination. Understanding transcriptional signatures associated with protective immunity can lead to the identification of biomarkers predicting vaccination outcomes. The most advanced technique, Single-Cell RNA Sequencing, allows for examination of gene expression at the single-cell level within immune populations, providing detailed insights into heterogeneous responses. By uncovering distinct immune cell subsets responding to vaccination, researchers can identify pathways crucial for developing effective immunity [63, 64].

In vitro immunological assays, including enzyme-linked immunosorbent assays (ELISAs), flow cytometry, and other techniques, measure cytokine production, Tcell activation, and antibody responses to TB antigens. These assays generate essential data on the immunogenicity of vaccine candidates and their mechanisms of action [65–67].

Animal models, such as mice, guinea pigs, and non-human primates, are employed to evaluate the efficacy and safety of vaccine candidates before human trials. These animal studies are crucial for understanding the pre-clinical immune response and the overall effectiveness of vaccine formulations [68].

Phase I/II clinical trials assess the safety and immunogenicity of human vaccine candidates. The genomic and proteomic data collected during these trials refine our understanding of immune responses. Biomarkers identified through these trials can stratify populations and customize vaccination strategies based on individual susceptibility and immune characteristics. Longitudinal studies are also conducted to track immune responses over time in vaccinated individuals, examining changes in gene expression [69–72].

12.2.3 System Biology for Novel TB Vaccine Strategies

When integrating genomic and proteomic data with systems biology, researchers can model the immune response and predict outcomes based on individual genetic profiles. This method enhances the design of vaccines that are more likely to be effective across diverse populations. Omics technologies contribute to the development of combination vaccines that target multiple immune pathways simultaneously, thus providing broader protection against tuberculosis [28, 36, 38, 50, 53]. To achieve this, bioinformatics tools analyze various *omics* data (genomic, proteomic, and transcriptomic) to identify patterns in immune responses and correlate them with vaccine outcomes [31, 32, 73]. With multi-*omics* data, researchers can more accurately predict vaccine efficacy and tailor candidate selection to optimize immune responses. Furthermore, vaccine design platforms, which include computational modeling and simulations, are used to predict how different antigens will interact with the immune system. This approach aids in the rational design of new vaccines by identifying optimal combinations of antigens and adjuvants to enhance the immune response against TB [28, 30, 35, 41, 58].

The lack of comprehensive data from developing countries significantly affects TB vaccine research and the subsequent efficacy of vaccines in these regions [30, 34, 35, 61, 74].

Historically, many vaccine trials have occurred primarily in high-income countries, leading to a limited understanding of how vaccines perform in the diverse genetic backgrounds and environmental conditions of developing countries [75, 76]. Consequently, vaccine effectiveness and safety may vary significantly between populations due to genetic, immunological, and environmental differences. In these areas, omics technologies are often underutilized due to technological and financial barriers, restricting the exploration of genetic factors influencing vaccine responses. Without comprehensive *omics* data, researchers struggle to understand variations in immune responses or efficacy in specific populations, leading to knowledge gaps that hinder effective vaccine design [42, 58]. Diverse immune responses to TB vaccines, influenced by genetic and environmental factors, must be thoroughly studied to ensure research findings are applicable globally [12, 37, 61, 76–78].

Though recent TB vaccine trials have sought to include more diverse populations, data gaps persist in developing countries. *Omics* technologies have provided valuable insights, but these studies often focus on cohorts from high-income regions. For instance, the recent M72/AS01E vaccine trial, which included populations from South Africa and Kenya, provided crucial insights into immune responses within African cohorts [79, 80].

To rectify these disparities, research initiatives must emphasize collaboration and capacity-building in developing countries, including training local researchers in *omics* technologies, and integrating local populations into vaccine research. Adopting a more inclusive model of vaccine research will facilitate the development of vaccines that are safe and effective across various demographic groups [81, 82].

Systems biology offers a comprehensive framework for TB vaccine research by integrating diverse data types and computational methods. This interdisciplinary approach enhances the understanding of host-pathogen interactions, predicts immune responses, identifies biomarkers, and informs the creation of effective vaccines tailored to diverse populations. As research advances, systems biology will be pivotal in developing innovative strategies to combat TB, aiming for improved vaccination outcomes worldwide.

12.2.4 System Immunology and TB Vaccine Development

System immunology, genetic diversity, and *omics* technologies are essential for understanding disease susceptibility and vaccine responsiveness, particularly regarding complex diseases such as TB. System immunology focuses on a holistic analysis of immune responses, enabling the identification of biomarkers for susceptibility and vaccine responsiveness, rather than examining isolated components [27, 56].

Genetic diversity within populations reveals significant genetic differences that can inform tailored vaccine strategies, improving efficacy and minimizing adverse effects [60, 83]. For instance, polymorphisms in genes associated with the immune system, such as those related to cytokines or antigen presentation, can greatly influence individual responses to infections and vaccines [84]. Variations in immune-related genes, particularly those encoding major histocompatibility complex (MHC) proteins, cytokines, and receptors, can notably affect how individuals respond to Mtb. These genetic variations can lead to differences in antigen presentation, cytokine production, and overall immune efficacy, all critical for a robust TB vaccine response [58, 60, 76, 84]. Certain MHC class II alleles are associated with better control of TB infection, enhancing the presentation of TB antigens to T cells. Understanding which alleles confer resistance can guide vaccine development, allowing the inclusion of specific antigens that are most effectively presented by prevalent MHC variants across different populations [85–87]. Furthermore, polymorphisms in cytokine genes have been linked to varied immune responses in TB variants. Those variants that boost pro-inflammatory responses may offer better protection, while anti-inflammatory variants may increase susceptibility [88, 89].

Omics technologies also play a crucial role in identifying key molecules involved in disease susceptibility and adverse vaccine responses. Genomic studies of Mtb can reveal virulence factors and immunogenic proteins vital for mounting an effective immune response. This information aids in the selection of antigens for vaccines that are likely to elicit strong and long-lasting responses [38, 60, 90, 91].

Proteomic analyses further enhance our understanding by identifying specific proteins recognized by the host immune system in TB. Discovering biomarkers of vaccine efficacy can lead to improved predictions of suboptimal responses to vaccination, which can inform necessary modifications to vaccine formulations [14, 53, 92].

Additionally, metabolomic studies provide insights into metabolic changes in host cells during TB infection and after vaccination. Understanding these metabolic pathways can guide the design of adjuvants that enhance vaccine efficacy by optimizing immune metabolism [93–95]. Identification of these molecules and biomarkers can be instrumental in predicting vaccine responsiveness, ultimately enabling more effective and targeted vaccine strategies [16, 96, 97].

Integration of systems immunology, genetic analysis, and *omics* data enables researchers to model the immune landscape and enhance the vaccine development process, considering variability in genetic backgrounds and immune responses [20, 35, 98]. By leveraging these approaches, researchers can gain deeper insights into the factors contributing to disease susceptibility and variations in vaccine responses.

This comprehensive strategy not only enhances vaccine effectiveness across diverse populations but also supports the development of personalized immunization strategies that address intrinsic genetic differences. Aligning vaccine strategies with the genetic landscape and immune response profiles of different populations can lead to improved vaccination outcomes and ultimately help control the spread of TB.

12.3 *Omics* and Current TB Vaccines

The TB vaccines, such as Bacillus Calmette- Guérin (BCG), H4:IC31, and M72/AS01E, highlight the potential of *omics* technologies to enhance our understanding of vaccine efficacy and identify biomarkers for susceptibility.

Bacillus Calmette-Guérin has been the only widely used vaccine for TB for nearly a century, demonstrating varying degrees of efficacy in preventing TB across different populations and geographic locations. Research has revealed that distinct gene expression profiles following BCG vaccination correlate with protective immune responses. Transcriptomic analyses have identified specific pathways and genes linked to robust immunity. Furthermore, omics approaches have highlighted potential biomarkers that could predict vaccine responses, aiding in the development of tailored booster strategies or additional vaccines to enhance BCG effectiveness [37, 41].

The H4:IC31 vaccine, a fusion protein comprising two TB antigens (Ag85B and TB10.4) combined with the IC31 adjuvant, aims to improve immune responses beyond BCG. It has shown promise in clinical trials by preventing infections, similar to the effects of BCG revaccination [99, 100]. For instance, a phase 2a trial of the candidate vaccine H4:IC31 compared to BCG revaccination involved 990 adolescents aged 12–17 years in a high-transmission setting in South Africa, all of whom had previously received neonatal BCG vaccination. The results indicated that BCG revaccination prevented sustained Mtb infection, with an efficacy of 45.5% (95% CI 6.4–68.1) [70, 100]. Studies employing proteomic analyses have evaluated the immune responses elicited by the H4:IC31 vaccine, identifying specific proteins associated with vaccine-induced immunity and revealing how responses differ among individuals with varying genetic backgrounds [37, 101, 102]. Genetic analyses within clinical trial populations can identify polymorphisms that may influence vaccine efficacy, informing the design of follow-up studies and aiding in selection based on genetic susceptibility.

The M72/AS01E is a novel vaccine candidate targeting specific TB antigens. In a phase 3 trial of the M72/AS01E candidate vaccine versus placebo included 3575 adults aged 18–50 with confirmed Mtb infection but without disease. The vaccine appeared to protect against progression to pulmonary tuberculosis disease for at least 36 months, showing an efficacy of 49.7% (90% CI 12.1–71.2) [70, 79, 103]. Additionally, data from the M72 vaccine trials revealed immunological signatures that predict vaccine efficacy [104, 105]. By integrating transcriptomic profiles with clinical outcomes, researchers identified immune response correlates that distinguish individuals who respond favorably to the vaccine. Additionally, omics approaches have identified potential biomarkers to stratify trial participants based on their likelihood of developing TB, enabling targeted vaccine strategies [79].

The emergence of new pathogens and the exponential increase in strain-specific genome sequencing data have prompted a growing search for answers to understand host-pathogen interactions [31, 63, 106].

In recent years, many candidates for TB vaccines have been evaluated in clinical trials, but it appears that progress is still slow. However, the expectation of utilization of *omics* data, at population and cellular levels, will provide invaluable insights for the stratification of individuals with similar syndromes but different underlying conditions. This approach will enhance disease diagnosis and expedite the development of new vaccines, drugs, and therapeutics, ultimately leading to optimal strategies for intervention delivery.

12.4 *Omics* Data from Developing Countries

Developing countries in sub-Saharan Africa, South America, and East Asia are widely recognized as hotspots for emerging and re-emerging infectious diseases [107]. These regions contribute significantly to global statistics for TB, Human Immunodeficiency Virus (HIV), malaria, and other diseases [108], which threatens the achievement of the Sustainable Development Goals (SDGs), particularly SDG 3 [109]. The interplay of infectious diseases, environmental factors, and the rise of antimicrobial resistance has influenced genetic dynamics and driven the adaptation of hosts, vectors, and pathogens [107, 110]. This scenario was notably highlighted by the emergence of the SARS-CoV-2 virus [10], underscoring a global need for information sharing to accelerate research and development of tools, therapies, surveillance, and monitoring platforms. Additionally, there is an urgent requirement to thoroughly understand the host immune system and pathogen biology to effectively counter future threats.

Despite these challenges, endemic infections and non-infectious diseases continue to prevail, while numerous clinical, epidemiological, and implementation science studies are underway in developing countries. Unfortunately, neglected tropical and infectious diseases often receive inadequate attention in these research efforts [110, 111].

As well as population genetic diversity affecting immune response differences, potentially leading to pathogen variability [10, 15, 112], generation of *omics* data from developing countries is increasingly recognized as crucial for advancing vaccine development, particularly for diseases like TB. However, the absence of this data presents significant challenges that can hinder the creation of effective and context-specific vaccines. Limited region-specific *omics* data obstructs understanding of how TB manifests in diverse populations, complicating targeted vaccine development. Often, developing countries harbor different strains of Mtb that may respond variably to vaccines. Without adequate data, these strain differences may remain uncharacterized, resulting in less effective vaccine formulations [60, 84, 113, 114].

Populations in developing countries often display extensive genetic diversity, which can significantly influence immune responses to TB and vaccination. Gaining insights into this genetic diversity through *omics* data can reveal crucial biomarkers and genetic predispositions vital for tailored vaccines [3, 76, 84, 115]. Furthermore, environmental conditions such as nutrition, co-infections, and pollutants, commonly found in developing countries can considerably impact immune responses. *Omics* data can help clarify how these factors interact with genetic predispositions to affect vaccine efficacy [3, 76, 84, 115].

The practical challenges of generating omics data in certain countries are linked to three main factors. First, there is limited access to high-throughput technologies, inadequate funding, and a lack of infrastructure for complex data analysis. Second, there is a shortage of trained personnel capable of conducting omics studies or analyzing and interpreting complex data, which leads to reliance on external collaborations that can be logistically complicated. Third, ensuring ethical standards in research involving human subjects complicates the collection of samples and data, especially in resource-limited settings. Despite these challenges, successful initiatives, such as multicenter collaborations and investments in local research facilities, have emerged to bolster capacity. For instance, programs focused on integrating *omics* by providing training and resources are beginning to take shape [74, 82, 116].

Examining the impact of environmental and genetic differences on vaccine responses is essential to consider various factors. Exposure to other pathogens, nutritional status, and socioeconomic conditions can significantly alter the effectiveness of TB vaccines. The diversity of microbiota across different regions may influence immune system training, which affects vaccination responses. Continuous exposure to non-tuberculous mycobacteria or other infections can also modulate the immune landscapes of populations, further impacting vaccine efficacy [117, 118].

In developing countries, genetic variability among populations plays a critical role in immune responses. For instance, specific alleles in genes related to immune function, such as HLA genes, may alter the recognition of vaccine antigens. Variations in immune-related genes can lead to differences in the magnitude and quality of Tcell and antibody responses [119]. Consequently, individuals from certain genetic backgrounds may either benefit from a vaccine or experience heightened adverse effects [15, 85, 120].

Other factors to consider in developing countries are co-infections (e.g., with HIV or malaria), nutritional status, and urban versus rural living conditions greatly impact immune system function. For instance, malnutrition can impair immune response effectiveness, thereby reducing the efficacy of TB vaccines in vulnerable populations [121]. Additionally, cultural practices and health-seeking behaviors can influence vaccine immunogenicity. Variations in healthcare utilization may affect the timing and dosage of vaccinations, complicating further outcomes [121–123]. Therefore, without context-specific *omics* data from diverse populations, vaccine candidates may fail to elicit adequate immune responses. This could lead to vaccines performing well in clinical trials conducted in developed countries but proving ineffective in endemic regions [124]. Furthermore, the absence of localized *omics* data means that biomarkers linked to susceptibility and vaccine responsiveness may remain unidentified. The knowledge gap restricts the ability to tailor vaccines to specific populations, potentially leading to higher rates of TB infection and morbidity.

Overall, the lack of omics data from developing countries represents a significant barrier to effective TB vaccine development. This limitation hampers the understanding of local genetic diversity and environmental influences on immune responses. To optimize vaccine efficacy and customize strategies for diverse populations, there is an urgent need to build infrastructure, foster collaboration, and invest in training on *omics* technologies in these regions. Addressing these challenges will enhance global TB control efforts and lead to more effective vaccines that meet local needs. Additionally, omics data from clinical studies conducted in developing countries should be analyzed with consideration for the epidemiology, nutrition, specific comorbidities, and genetic backgrounds of the participant populations to inform research and development effectively.

12.5 The Impact of NCD on TB Vaccine Development

Non-communicable Diseases (NCDs) pose emerging challenges to health systems in sub-Saharan Africa, which have traditionally focused on managing infectious diseases, as well as maternal, neonatal, and child mortality. To address the health transition needs in these countries, detailed epidemiological and omics data on infectious diseases and NCDs is needed. NCDs, which include cardiovascular diseases, diabetes, cancer, and chronic respiratory diseases, result from complex interactions among predisposing, environmental, and genetic factors [125, 126]. In addition, the prevalence of NCDs is increasing in developing countries, driven by factors such as urbanization, lifestyle changes, and a rise in risk factors like smoking and obesity. The coexistence of TB and NCDs complicates disease management, as individuals with NCDs may be more susceptible to TB infection, and those with TB may be at higher risk for developing NCDs. This interplay underscores the necessity for integrated *omics* approaches that account for variations in metabolic, genomic, and immune responses among individuals with both conditions.

Omics technologies can deepen our understanding of how these diseases interact at the molecular level. By identifying shared biomarkers that indicate susceptibility to either NCDs or TB, researchers can gain insights into the pathophysiological mechanisms involved. For instance, chronic inflammation associated with NCDs may affect the immune response during TB infection [127, 128]. Identifying such biomarkers could inform preventive measures and treatment strategies.

The dual burden of NCDs and TB places significant strain on healthcare resources and funding, potentially shifting focus away from TB vaccine development. As countries prioritize NCD management due to their rising prevalence and economic impact, investments in TB vaccination programs may be delayed. Moreover, individuals with NCDs often exhibit altered immune responses, which can compromise vaccine efficacy. Therefore, understanding how pre-existing conditions affect immune responses to TB vaccines is vital and *omics* research can shed light on how NCDs may modulate vaccine-induced immunity. For this achievement a strategic solution might involve developing combinatorial vaccines that address TB and NCDs. Research into how the metabolic pathways affected by NCDs intersect with TB pathology could uncover innovative vaccine targets [124, 129].

To effectively tackle the dual burden, integrated healthcare approaches are necessary, incorporating considerations for both NCDs and TB within public health initiatives. This could include screening for TB among individuals with NCDs and vice versa, thereby enabling more comprehensive care strategies. Supporting interdisciplinary research that brings together specialists in infectious and chronic diseases can promote a better understanding of how to optimize vaccine strategies for populations affected by both health burdens.

Ultimately, addressing the dual burden of NCDs and TB requires an integrated approach that leverages *omics* technologies. These tools can provide essential insights for vaccine development tailored to the unique immunological and metabolic profiles of affected populations. A holistic response is crucial for improving health outcomes, advancing vaccine strategies, and reducing the incidence and impact of both TB and NCDs.

12.6 *Omics* and TB Resistance

Infectious diseases, particularly TB, along with environmental factors and the rise of antimicrobial resistance (AMR), significantly influence genetic changes in pathogens. This dynamic interaction shapes the genomic landscapes of both pathogens and their hosts, presenting challenges for treatment and prevention strategies. Infectious diseases create selective pressures that affect both pathogens and humans, prompting pathogens to evolve rapidly in response to immune defenses and treatment regimens. These evolutionary changes can lead to genetic adaptations that enhance virulence, infectivity, or resistance [130, 131].

Mycobacterium tuberculosis, for example, displays significant genetic variability, which has resulted in the emergence of drug-resistant strains. Genetic mutations in the bacterial genome, driven by antibiotic exposure, increase the organism's survival in hostile environments, contributing to the evolution of multi-drug resistant (MDR) strains [132]. In regions with a high burden of TB and challenging socioeconomic conditions, Mtb can evolve quickly in response to environmental stresses such as malnutrition, overcrowding, and co-infections with HIV. These environmental adaptations may involve metabolic changes that enable survival in diverse host nutrient environments [130, 131].

The widespread use and misuse of antibiotics have resulted in the emergence of AMR in various pathogens, including Mtb. Resistance develops through genetic mutations, horizontal gene transfer, and the selective pressure imposed by antibiotic treatments [130]. In the case of tuberculosis, several specific genetic changes have been documented. For instance, (1) the *rpo*B gene that encodes the β-subunit of RNA polymerase, and mutations such as S450L can confer resistance to rifampicin, a key drug used to treat TB [131, 133]; (2) the katG gene that encodes the catalase-peroxidase enzyme, and the S315T mutation in *kat*G are associated with high-level resistance to isoniazid, rendering many standard treatment regimens ineffective [134]; and (3) mutations in the *em*bB gene, responsible for the synthesis of mycolic acids in the bacterial cell wall, can confer resistance to ethambutol [135].

Moreover, the misuse and overuse of antibiotics have resulted in the selection of resistant strains of bacteria. Genetic variations enabling antibiotic resistance, often through plasmids or chromosomal mutations, can spread widely within bacterial populations. Major pathogens such as *Escherichia coli* and *Streptococcus pneumoniae* have developed resistance through mechanisms like beta-lactamase production and modifications of target sites [136].

The emergence of AMR also compels human populations to adapt, potentially influencing genetics linked to immune function and overall health. Individuals with specific genetic backgrounds may exhibit varying responses to infections caused by resistant strains, impacting public health outcomes. The increased incidence of infections with resistant strains necessitates changes in treatment protocols, which may lead to shifts in population genetics over time [137].

Overall, infectious diseases, environmental factors, and the rise of antimicrobial resistance collectively shape the genetics of human populations and pathogens. This dynamic interaction underscores the importance of understanding genetic variations in relation to disease susceptibility, host-pathogen interactions, and the ongoing challenges posed by AMR.

12.7 The Need of *Omics* Data to Inform Vaccine Development

Vaccines represent one of the most effective medical technologies, offering hope for reducing the burden or even eradicating certain infectious diseases. However, current vaccines are only available for approximately one-tenth of infectious pathogens affecting humans, and effective vaccines are still lacking for two of the world's top three infectious diseases: TB and HIV.

Traditional vaccine design approaches, such as using live or killed microorganisms, are often unfeasible due to safety, efficacy, and scalability concerns. As a result, research is increasingly focusing on subunit and genetic vaccines. A primary challenge in producing these vaccines lies in selecting appropriate antigens, which has prompted the need for genome-specific models to identify epitope-containing regions of pathogens [98, 138–140]. Technological advances have greatly enhanced our understanding of this complexity. In this context, *omics* technologies provide a high-throughput and cost-effective means to measure immune response signatures [18].

Various *omics* platforms have been employed in systems vaccinology [97], including genomics, transcriptomics, proteomics, metabolomics, epigenomics, and microbiomics, as well as single-cell level analyses [18, 27, 141]. Continuous improvements in these platforms enable scientists to utilize more robust bioinformatics tools for developing novel diagnostics and personalized therapies for diseases and vaccines [98]. For instance, Weiner et al. (2018) designed a model with ten features to predict TB progression, facilitating the determination of whether specific metabolomic signatures are associated with the disease [138]. Integration of *omics* technologies into TB vaccine research has yielded comprehensive insights into biological systems and advanced the field. These technologies aid in identifying novel antigens, understanding immune responses, and optimizing vaccine formulations. For example, whole-genome sequencing of Mtb has uncovered genetic variations linked to virulence and drug resistance, highlighting potential vaccine targets [142]. Analyzing the proteins expressed by Mtb also assists in identifying potential vaccine candidates, while understanding the immune proteome correlates immune responses with protection [143].

Moreover, examining gene expression profiles during infection can reveal host-pathogen interaction dynamics, informing vaccine design aimed at specific immune pathways [144]. Studying metabolites produced during TB infection can suggest biomarkers for disease progression and vaccine efficacy [93, 130, 138]. By integrating data from various *omics* approaches scientists can have a holistic view of TB and the immune response, facilitating rational vaccine development [16, 53, 57]. These examples demonstrate that *omics* technologies hold significant promise for enhancing TB vaccine development and leading to more effective preventive strategies. However, the development of novel adjuvants and delivery systems based on *omics* findings, along with personalized vaccine approaches that identify specific immune correlates of protection, remains crucial in the search for solutions to TB.

12.8 Conclusions and Future Directions

The ongoing challenges posed by TB highlight the need for continuous innovation in vaccine research. Future steps in TB vaccine development should prioritize enhancing both the efficacy and safety of vaccines, with the integration of *omics* technologies playing a crucial role in advancing this field. Completion of ongoing clinical trials, such as those evaluating M72/AS01E or MVA85A, is essential for establishing efficacy across diverse demographics, especially in high-burden regions. Additionally, research efforts must include varied populations, particularly those with comorbidities such as HIV and diabetes [105, 126, 145].

Regarding specific actions, for short- or long-term research innovative vaccine candidates, including live-attenuated and subunit vaccines that target specific antigens, need further investigation. Exploring heterologous prime-boost strategies could enhance immune responses [146]. Identifying specific immune correlates that predict protection against TB will aid development of more effective vaccines, necessitating persistent research to define these correlates through population-based studies [33, 65]. It is also vital to design and test vaccines targeting high-risk populations, including individuals with co-existing conditions such as HIV and diabetes, to ensure broad applicability and effectiveness [124].

Utilizing transcriptomic analyses allows researchers to investigate gene expression levels related to effective immune responses to TB vaccines, aiding the identification of relevant biomarkers for assessing vaccine-induced immunity [147]. This approache can uncover proteins involved in the immune response to TB, leading to the discovery of novel biomarkers for vaccine efficacy and patient prognostics [41, 148].

Investigating metabolic changes in response to TB vaccination through metabolomics can provide valuable insights into the metabolic pathways that prime the immune system, potentially resulting in innovative adjuvants or combination therapies [42, 60, 95, 124]. Combining various *omics* data within a systems biology framework leads to a comprehensive understanding of the immune response to Mbt.

In the context of the epidemiological transition and the re-emergence of infectious pathogens, along with the rising burden of NCDs and antimicrobial resistance, the immune systems of human populations evolve to become more resilient against these threats. Following this line of research, robust platforms must be developed to analyze *omics* data obtained from clinical studies in developing countries. This will play an essential role not only in predicting the effectiveness of vaccines and drugs and informing personalized medicine but also in disease prevention and a better understanding of host-pathogen interactions [13, 73, 97, 139, 149].

Conflict of Interest The author declares that the research was conducted without any commercial or financial relationships that could be construed as a potential conflict of interest.

Competing Interests The author(s) has no competing interests to declare that are relevant to the content of this manuscript.

Ethics Approval The author(s) declares that this manuscript does not include primary research with human participants.

References

1. Quach H, Rotival M, Pothlichet J, et al. Genetic adaptation and neandertal admixture shaped the immune system of human populations. Cell. 2016;167:643–656.e17.
2. Quintana-Murci L. Understanding rare and common diseases in the context of human evolution. Genome Biol. 2016;17:225.
3. Bellamy R, Ruwende C, Corrah T, McAdam KPWJ, Whittle HC, Hill AVS. Variations in the *NRAMP1* gene and susceptibility to tuberculosis in West Africans. N Engl J Med. 1998;338:640–4.
4. Tesi N, van der Lee SJ, Hulsman M, et al. Immune response and endocytosis pathways are associated with the resilience against Alzheimer's disease. Transl Psychiatry. 2020;10:332.

5. Belloy ME, Napolioni V, Greicius MD. A quarter century of APOE and Alzheimer's disease: progress to date and the path forward. Neuron. 2019;101:820–38.
6. Azad AK, Lloyd C, Sadee W, Schlesinger LS. Challenges of immune response diversity in the human population concerning new tuberculosis diagnostics, therapies, and vaccines. Front Cell Infect Microbiol. 2020;10:139.
7. Benton ML, Abraham A, LaBella AL, Abbot P, Rokas A, Capra JA. The influence of evolutionary history on human health and disease. Nat Rev Genet. 2021;22:269–83.
8. Koropoulis A, Alachiotis N, Pavlidis P. Detecting positive selection in populations using genetic data. Methods Mol Biol. 2020;2090:87–123.
9. Pearson ER. Personalized medicine in diabetes: the role of 'omics' and biomarkers. Diabet Med. 2016;33:712–7.
10. Maiti AK. The African-American population with a low allele frequency of SNP rs1990760 (T allele) in IFIH1 predicts less IFN-beta expression and potential vulnerability to COVID-19 infection. Immunogenetics. 2020;72:387–91.
11. Byars SG, Huang QQ, Gray L-A, Bakshi A, Ripatti S, Abraham G, Stearns SC, Inouye M. Genetic loci associated with coronary artery disease harbor evidence of selection and antagonistic pleiotropy. PLoS Genet. 2017;13:e1006328.
12. Klebanov N. Genetic predisposition to infectious disease. Cureus. 2018; https://doi.org/10.7759/cureus.3210.
13. Corona E, Chen R, Sikora M, Morgan AA, Patel CJ, Ramesh A, Bustamante CD, Butte AJ. Analysis of the genetic basis of disease in the context of worldwide human relationships and migration. PLoS Genet. 2013;9:e1003447.
14. Mateos J, Estévez O, González-Fernández Á, et al. Serum proteomics of active tuberculosis patients and contacts reveals unique processes activated during Mycobacterium tuberculosis infection. Sci Rep. 2020;10:3844.
15. Nédélec Y, Sanz J, Baharian G, et al. Genetic ancestry and natural selection drive population differences in immune responses to pathogens. Cell. 2016;167:657–669.e21.
16. Yu J, Peng J, Chi H. Systems immunology: integrating multi-omics data to infer regulatory networks and hidden drivers of immunity. Curr Opin Syst Biol. 2019;15:19–29.
17. Chu X, Zhang B, Koeken VACM, Gupta MK, Li Y. Multi-omics approaches in immunological research. Front Immunol. 2021;12:668045.
18. Unterman A, Sumida TS, Nouri N, et al. Single-cell multi-omics reveals dyssynchrony of the innate and adaptive immune system in progressive COVID-19. Nat Commun. 2022;13:440.
19. Brodin P, Davis MM. Human immune system variation. Nat Rev Immunol. 2017;17:21–9.
20. Zhou W, Sailani MR, Contrepois K, et al. Longitudinal multi-omics of host–microbe dynamics in prediabetes. Nature. 2019;569:663–71.
21. Kerner G, Neehus A-L, Abel L, Casanova J-L, Patin E, Laval G, Quintana-Murci L. Genetic adaptation to pathogens and increased risk of inflammatory disorders in post-Neolithic Europe 2022.07.02.498543. 2022.
22. Sebastian J, Thomas A, Levine C, Shrestha R, Levy S, Safi H, Pentakota SR, Kumar P, Alland D. Origin and dynamics of Mycobacterium tuberculosis subpopulations that predictably generate drug tolerance and resistance. MBio. 2022;13:e0279522.
23. Health NRC (US) C on D and. Genetics and nutrition. Diet and health: implications for reducing chronic disease risk. 1989.
24. Church DL. Major factors affecting the emergence and re-emergence of infectious diseases. Clin Lab Med. 2004;24:559–86.
25. Richard L, Aenishaenslin C, Zinszer K. Zoonoses and social determinants of health: a consultation of Canadian experts. One Health. 2020;12:100199.
26. O'Garra A, Redford PS, McNab FW, Bloom CI, Wilkinson RJ, Berry MPR. The immune response in tuberculosis. Annu Rev Immunol. 2013;31:475–527.
27. Dhillon BK, Smith M, Baghela A, Lee AHY, Hancock REW. Systems biology approaches to understanding the human immune system. Front Immunol. 2020;11:1683.
28. Borah K, Xu Y, McFadden J. Dissecting host-pathogen interactions in TB using systems-based omic approaches. Front Immunol. 2021;12:762315.

29. Raman K, Bhat AG, Chandra N. A systems perspective of host-pathogen interactions: predicting disease outcome in tuberculosis. Mol BioSyst. 2010;6:516–30.
30. Duffy FJ, Weiner J, Hansen S, et al. Immunometabolic signatures predict risk of progression to active tuberculosis and disease outcome. Front Immunol. 2019;10:527.
31. Estévez O, Anibarro L, Garet E, et al. An RNA-seq based machine learning approach identifies latent tuberculosis patients with an active tuberculosis profile. Front Immunol. 2020;11:1470.
32. Silver RF, Xia M, Storer CE, et al. Distinct gene expression signatures comparing latent tuberculosis infection with different routes of Bacillus Calmette-Guérin vaccination. Nat Commun. 2023;14:8507.
33. Wang J, Fan X-Y, Hu Z. Immune correlates of protection as a game changer in tuberculosis vaccine development. NPJ Vaccines. 2024;9:1–13.
34. Doherty M, Wallis RS, Zumla A, WHO-Tropical Disease Research/European Commission joint expert consultation group. Biomarkers for tuberculosis disease status and diagnosis. Curr Opin Pulm Med. 2009;15:181–7.
35. Krishnan S, Queiroz ATL, Gupta A, et al. Integrative multi-omics reveals serum markers of tuberculosis in advanced HIV. Front Immunol. 2021;12:676980.
36. Cheng P, Jiang F, Wang G, Wang J, Xue Y, Wang L, Gong W. Bioinformatics analysis and consistency verification of a novel tuberculosis vaccine candidate HP13138PB. Front Immunol. 2023; https://doi.org/10.3389/fimmu.2023.1102578.
37. Moorlag SJCFM, Folkman L, ter Horst R, et al. Multi-omics analysis of innate and adaptive responses to BCG vaccination reveals epigenetic cell states that predict trained immunity. Immunity. 2024;57:171–187.e14.
38. Guha P, Dutta S, Murti K, Charan JK, Pandey K, Ravichandiran V, Dhingra S. The integration of omics: a promising approach to personalized tuberculosis treatment. Med Omics. 2024;12:100033.
39. Kaufmann SHE, Fortune S, Pepponi I, Ruhwald M, Schrager LK, Ottenhoff THM. TB biomarkers, TB correlates and human challenge models: new tools for improving assessment of new TB vaccines. Tuberculosis. 2016;99:S8–S11.
40. Khan N, Das A. Can the personalized medicine approach contribute in controlling tuberculosis in general and India in particular? Precis Clin Med. 2020;3:240–3.
41. Yong YK, Tan HY, Saeidi A, Wong WF, Vignesh R, Velu V, Eri R, Larsson M, Shankar EM. Immune biomarkers for diagnosis and treatment monitoring of tuberculosis: current developments and future prospects. Front Microbiol. 2019; https://doi.org/10.3389/fmicb.2019.02789.
42. Zhuang L, Yang L, Li L, Ye Z, Gong W. Mycobacterium tuberculosis: immune response, biomarkers, and therapeutic intervention. MedComm. 2024;5:e419.
43. Kong L, Moorlag SJCFM, Lefkovith A, et al. Single-cell transcriptomic profiles reveal changes associated with BCG-induced trained immunity and protective effects in circulating monocytes. Cell Rep. 2021;37:110028.
44. Li W, Moorlag SJCFM, Koeken VACM, et al. A single-cell view on host immune transcriptional response to in vivo BCG-induced trained immunity. Cell Rep. 2023;42:112487.
45. Cooper AM, Mayer-Barber KD, Sher A. Role of innate cytokines in mycobacterial infection. Mucosal Immunol. 2011;4:252–60.
46. Morris S, Kelley C, Howard A, Li Z, Collins F. The immunogenicity of single and combination DNA vaccines against tuberculosis. Vaccine. 2000;18:2155–63.
47. Lu G, Shan S, Zainab B, Ayaz Z, He J, Xie Z, Rashid U, Zhang D, Mehmood Abbasi A. Novel vaccine design based on genomics data analysis: a review. Scand J Immunol. 2021;93:e12986.
48. Chugh S, Bahal RK, Dhiman R, Singh R. Antigen identification strategies and preclinical evaluation models for advancing tuberculosis vaccine development. NPJ Vaccines. 2024;9:1–21.
49. Timpson NJ, Greenwood CMT, Soranzo N, Lawson DJ, Richards JB. Genetic architecture: the shape of the genetic contribution to human traits and disease. Nat Rev Genet. 2018;19:110–24.

50. Bibi S, Ullah I, Zhu B, Adnan M, Liaqat R, Kong W-B, Niu S. In silico analysis of epitope-based vaccine candidate against tuberculosis using reverse vaccinology. Sci Rep. 2021;11:1249.
51. Gagneux S, Small PM. Global phylogeography of Mycobacterium tuberculosis and implications for tuberculosis product development. Lancet Infect Dis. 2007;7:328–37.
52. Jia X, Yang L, Dong M, et al. The bioinformatics analysis of comparative genomics of Mycobacterium tuberculosis Complex (MTBC) provides insight into dissimilarities between intraspecific groups differing in host association, virulence, and epitope diversity. Front Cell Infect Microbiol. 2017; https://doi.org/10.3389/fcimb.2017.00088.
53. Hoffmann E, Machelart A, Song O-R, Brodin P. Proteomics of Mycobacterium infection: moving towards a better understanding of pathogen-driven immunomodulation. Front Immunol. 2018; https://doi.org/10.3389/fimmu.2018.00086.
54. Gopinath V, Raghunandanan S, Gomez RL, Jose L, Surendran A, Ramachandran R, Pushparajan AR, Mundayoor S, Jaleel A, Kumar RA. Profiling the proteome of *Mycobacterium tuberculosis* during dormancy and reactivation*. Mol Cell Proteomics. 2015;14:2160–76.
55. Kathirvel M, Mahadevan S. The role of epigenetics in tuberculosis infection. Epigenomics. 2016;8:537–49.
56. Lai R, Ogunsola AF, Rakib T, Behar SM. Key advances in vaccine development for tuberculosis—success and challenges. NPJ Vaccines. 2023;8:1–10.
57. Thomas SS, Abhinand K, Menon AM, Nair BG, Kumar GB, Arun KB, Edison LK, Madhavan A. Epigenetic mechanisms induced by Mycobacterium tuberculosis to promote its survival in the host. Int J Mol Sci. 2024;25:11801.
58. Barreiro LB, Tailleux L, Pai AA, Gicquel B, Marioni JC, Gilad Y. Deciphering the genetic architecture of variation in the immune response to Mycobacterium tuberculosis infection. Proc Natl Acad Sci. 2012;109:1204–9.
59. Hoseinpour R, Hasani A, Baradaran B, et al. Tuberculosis vaccine developments and efficient delivery systems: a comprehensive appraisal. Heliyon. 2024;10:e26193.
60. Kanabalan RD, Lee LJ, Lee TY, Chong PP, Hassan L, Ismail R, Chin VK. Human tuberculosis and *Mycobacterium tuberculosis* complex: a review on genetic diversity, pathogenesis and omics approaches in host biomarkers discovery. Microbiol Res. 2021;246:126674.
61. Kimman TG, Vandebriel RJ, Hoebee B. Genetic variation in the response to vaccination. Community Genet. 2007;10:201–17.
62. Lai R, Gong DN, Williams T, et al. Host genetic background is a barrier to broadly effective vaccine–mediated protection against tuberculosis. J Clin Invest. 2024; https://doi.org/10.1172/JCI167762.
63. Wang L, Ma H, Wen Z, et al. Single-cell RNA-sequencing reveals heterogeneity and intercellular crosstalk in human tuberculosis lung. J Infect. 2023;87:373–84.
64. Wen Z, Wang L, Ma H, et al. Integrated single-cell transcriptome and T cell receptor profiling reveals defects of T cell exhaustion in pulmonary tuberculosis. J Infect. 2024;88:106158.
65. Peralta Alvarez MP, Marshall JL, Tanner R. Correlates of protection from tuberculosis. In: Christodoulides M, editor. Vaccines for neglected pathogens: strategies, achievements and challenges: focus on leprosy, leishmaniasis, melioidosis and tuberculosis. Cham: Springer International Publishing; 2023. p. 99–137.
66. Teixeira HC, Abramo C, Munk ME. Immunological diagnosis of tuberculosis: problems and strategies for success. J Bras Pneumol. 2007;33:323–34.
67. Tuaillon E, Mwyia M, Bollore K, et al. Combination of serological and cytokine release assays for improved diagnosis of childhood tuberculosis in Zambia (PROMISE-TB). Int J Infect Dis. 2024; https://doi.org/10.1016/j.ijid.2024.107248.
68. Li H, Li H. Animal models of tuberculosis. In: Christodoulides M, editor. Vaccines for neglected pathogens: strategies, achievements and challenges: focus on leprosy, leishmaniasis, melioidosis and tuberculosis. Cham: Springer International Publishing; 2023. p. 139–70.
69. Li J, Zhao A, Tang J, Wang G, Shi Y, Zhan L, Qin C. Tuberculosis vaccine development: from classic to clinical candidates. Eur J Clin Microbiol Infect Dis. 2020;39:1405–25.

70. Venkatesan P. Progress in tuberculosis vaccine research. Lancet Microbe. 2021;2:e12.
71. Zhou F, Zhang D. Recent advance in the development of tuberculosis vaccines in clinical trials and virus-like particle-based vaccine candidates. Front Immunol. 2023; https://doi.org/10.3389/fimmu.2023.1238649.
72. Progress in tuberculosis vaccine research – The Lancet Microbe. https://www.thelancet.com/journals/lanmic/article/PIIS2666-5247(20)30228-7/fulltext. Accessed 28 May 2022
73. Chung R-H, Kang C-Y. A multi-omics data simulator for complex disease studies and its application to evaluate multi-omics data analysis methods for disease classification. Gigascience. 2019;8:giz045.
74. Lang TA, White NJ, Hien TT, et al. Clinical research in resource-limited settings: enhancing research capacity and working together to make trials less complicated. PLoS Negl Trop Dis. 2010;4:e619.
75. Tientcheu LD, Koch A, Ndengane M, Andoseh G, Kampmann B, Wilkinson RJ. Immunological consequences of strain variation within the Mycobacterium tuberculosis complex. Eur J Immunol. 2017;47:432–45.
76. van Tong H, Velavan TP, Thye T, Meyer CG. Human genetic factors in tuberculosis: an update. Trop Med Int Health. 2017;22:1063–71.
77. Chowdhury D, Zhou X, Li B, Zhang Y, Cheung WK, Lu A, Zhang L. Editorial: predicting high-risk individuals for common diseases using multi-omics and epidemiological data. Front Genet. 2021;12:737598.
78. Haks MC, Bottazzi B, Cecchinato V, et al. Molecular signatures of immunity and immunogenicity in infection and vaccination. Front Immunol. 2017; https://doi.org/10.3389/fimmu.2017.01563.
79. Tait DR, Hatherill M, Van Der Meeren O, et al. Final analysis of a trial of M72/AS01 $_E$ vaccine to prevent tuberculosis. N Engl J Med. 2019;381:2429–39.
80. Ullah I, Bibi S, Ul Haq I, et al. The systematic review and meta-analysis on the immunogenicity and safety of the tuberculosis subunit vaccines M72/AS01E and MVA85A. Front Immunol. 2020; https://doi.org/10.3389/fimmu.2020.01806.
81. Bowsher G, Papamichail A, El Achi N, Ekzayez A, Roberts B, Sullivan R, Patel P. A narrative review of health research capacity strengthening in low and middle-income countries: lessons for conflict-affected areas. Glob Health. 2019;15:23.
82. Ogundahunsi OAT, Vahedi M, Kamau EM, Aslanyan G, Terry RF, Zicker F, Launois P. Strengthening research capacity—TDR's evolving experience in low- and middle-income countries. PLoS Negl Trop Dis. 2015;9:e3380.
83. Kurtz SL, Baker RE, Boehm FJ, et al. Multiple genetic loci influence vaccine-induced protection against Mycobacterium tuberculosis in genetically diverse mice. PLoS Pathog. 2024;20:e1012069.
84. Wodelo W, Wampande EM, Andama A, Kateete DP, Ssekatawa K. Polymorphisms in immune genes and their association with tuberculosis susceptibility: an analysis of the African population. TACG. 2024;17:33–46.
85. Chihab LY, Kuan R, Phillips EJ, et al. Expression of specific HLA class II alleles is associated with an increased risk for active tuberculosis and a distinct gene expression profile. HLA. 2023;101:124–37.
86. Duarte R, Carvalho C, Pereira C, et al. HLA class II alleles as markers of tuberculosis susceptibility and resistance. Rev Port Pneumol. 2011;17:15–9.
87. Wamala D, Buteme HK, Kirimunda S, Kallenius G, Joloba M. Association between human leukocyte antigen class II and pulmonary tuberculosis due to mycobacterium tuberculosis in Uganda. BMC Infect Dis. 2016;16:23.
88. Meenakshi P, Ramya S, Shruthi T, Lavanya J, Mohammed HH, Mohammed SA, Vijayalakshmi V, Sumanlatha G. Association of -1β +3954 C/T and -10-1082 G/A cytokine gene polymorphisms with susceptibility to tuberculosis. Scand J Immunol. 2013;78:92–7.
89. Selvaraj P, Alagarasu K, Harishankar M, Vidyarani M, Nisha Rajeswari D, Narayanan PR. Cytokine gene polymorphisms and cytokine levels in pulmonary tuberculosis. Cytokine. 2008;43:26–33.

90. Liston A, Humblet-Baron S, Duffy D, Goris A. Human immune diversity: from evolution to modernity. Nat Immunol. 2021;22:1479–89.
91. Moreno-Molina M, Shubladze N, Khurtsilava I, et al. Genomic analyses of Mycobacterium tuberculosis from human lung resections reveal a high frequency of polyclonal infections. Nat Commun. 2021;12:2716.
92. Graw S, Chappell K, Washam CL, Gies A, Bird J, Robeson MS, Byrum SD. Multi-omics data integration considerations and study design for biological systems and disease. Mol Omics. 2021;17:170–85.
93. Chaiyachat P, Kaewseekhao B, Chaiprasert A, Kamolwat P, Nonghanphithak D, Phetcharaburanin J, Sirichoat A, Ong RT-H, Faksri K. Metabolomic analysis of Mycobacterium tuberculosis reveals metabolic profiles for identification of drug-resistant tuberculosis. Sci Rep. 2023;13:8655.
94. Diray-Arce J, Conti MG, Petrova B, Kanarek N, Angelidou A, Levy O. Integrative metabolomics to identify molecular signatures of responses to vaccines and infections. Metabolites. 2020;10:492.
95. Rawat BS, Kumar D, Soni V, Rosenn EH. Therapeutic potentials of immunometabolomic modulations induced by tuberculosis vaccination. Vaccine. 2022;10:2127.
96. Davis MM, Tato CM, Furman D. Systems immunology: just getting started. Nat Immunol. 2017;18:725–32.
97. Pulendran B, Li S, Nakaya HI. Systems vaccinology. Immunity. 2010;33:516–29.
98. Rapin N, Kesmir C, Frankild S, Nielsen M, Lundegaard C, Brunak S, Lund O. Modelling the human immune system by combining bioinformatics and systems biology approaches. J Biol Phys. 2006;32:335–53.
99. Bekker L-G, Garrett N, Goga A, et al. Effectiveness of the Ad26.COV2.S vaccine in healthcare workers in South Africa (the Sisonke study): results from a single-arm, open-label, phase 3B, implementation study. Lancet. 2022;399:1141–53.
100. Nemes E, Geldenhuys H, Rozot V, et al. Prevention of *M. tuberculosis* infection with H4:IC31 vaccine or BCG revaccination. N Engl J Med. 2018;379:138–49.
101. Cho T, Khatchadourian C, Nguyen H, Dara Y, Jung S, Venketaraman V. A review of the BCG vaccine and other approaches toward tuberculosis eradication. Hum Vaccin Immunother. 2021;17:2454–70.
102. Geldenhuys H, Mearns H, Miles DJC, et al. The tuberculosis vaccine H4:IC31 is safe and induces a persistent polyfunctional CD4 T cell response in South African adults: a randomized controlled trial. Vaccine. 2015;33:3592–9.
103. Ji Z, Jian M, Chen T, et al. Immunogenicity and safety of the M72/AS01E candidate vaccine against tuberculosis: a meta-analysis. Front Immunol. 2019;10:2089.
104. Ginsberg AM. Designing tuberculosis vaccine efficacy trials – lessons from recent studies. Expert Rev Vaccines. 2019;18:423–32.
105. Van Der Meeren O, Hatherill M, Nduba V, et al. Phase 2b controlled trial of M72/$AS01_E$ vaccine to prevent tuberculosis. N Engl J Med. 2018;379:1621–34.
106. Norsigian CJ, Fang X, Palsson BO, et al. Pangenome Flux Balance Analysis Toward Panphenomes. 2020 May 1. In: Tettelin H, Medini D, editors. The Pangenome: Diversity, Dynamics and Evolution of Genomes [Internet]. Cham (CH): Springer; 2020. Available from: https://www.ncbi.nlm.nih.gov/books/NBK558827/ https://doi.org/10.1007/978-3-030-38281-0_10.
107. Coker RJ, Hunter BM, Rudge JW, Liverani M, Hanvoravongchai P. Emerging infectious diseases in southeast Asia: regional challenges to control. Lancet. 2011;377:599–609.
108. WHO. State of inequality: HIV, tuberculosis and malaria. 2021. https://www.who.int/publications-detail-redirect/9789240039445. Accessed 21 Mar 2022
109. The Global fund. Fighting pandemics and building a healthier and more equitable world. In: Fighting pandemics and building a healthier and more equitable world. 2022. https://www.theglobalfund.org/en/strategy/. Accessed 21 Mar 2022
110. Cassini A, Colzani E, Pini A, et al. Impact of infectious diseases on population health using incidence-based disability-adjusted life years (DALYs): results from the Burden of

Communicable Diseases in Europe study, European Union and European Economic Area countries, 2009 to 2013. Eurosurveillance. 2018; https://doi.org/10.2807/1560-7917.ES.2018.23.16.17-00454.

111. Furuse Y. Analysis of research intensity on infectious disease by disease burden reveals which infectious diseases are neglected by researchers. Proc Natl Acad Sci USA. 2019;116:478–83.
112. Wang T, Antonacci-Fulton L, Howe K, et al. The Human Pangenome Project: a global resource to map genomic diversity. Nature. 2022;604:437–46.
113. Otchere ID, Aboagye SY, Arthur PK, Asante-Poku A. Viewpoint of multi-omics potential in tuberculosis research: identifying biomarkers for biomanufacturing of efficient control tools. Front Trop Dis. 2024; https://doi.org/10.3389/fitd.2024.1443248.
114. Zhang J, Heng S, Le Moullec S, Refregier G, Gicquel B, Sola C, Guillard B. A first assessment of the genetic diversity of Mycobacterium tuberculosis complex in Cambodia. BMC Infect Dis. 2011;11:42.
115. Bellamy R, Beyers N, McAdam KP, et al. Genetic susceptibility to tuberculosis in Africans: a genome-wide scan. Proc Natl Acad Sci USA. 2000;97:8005–9.
116. Alemayehu C, Mitchell G, Nikles J. Barriers for conducting clinical trials in developing countries- a systematic review. Int J Equity Health. 2018;17:37.
117. Isidori AM, Hasenmajer V, Sciarra F, Venneri MA. Environmental impact on immune system. In: Pivonello R, Diamanti-Kandarakis E, editors. Environmental endocrinology and endocrine disruptors: endocrine and endocrine-targeted actions and related human diseases. Cham: Springer International Publishing; 2020. p. 1–33.
118. MacGillivray DM, Kollmann TR. The role of environmental factors in modulating immune responses in early life. Front Immunol. 2014; https://doi.org/10.3389/fimmu.2014.00434.
119. Li F, Dang W, Du Y, Xu X, He P, Zhou Y, Zhu B. Tuberculosis vaccines and T cell immune memory. Vaccine. 2024;12:483.
120. Zimmermann P, Curtis N. Factors that influence the immune response to vaccination. Clin Microbiol Rev. 2019;32: https://doi.org/10.1128/cmr.00084-18.
121. Ockenga J, Fuhse K, Chatterjee S, Malykh R, Rippin H, Pirlich M, Yedilbayev A, Wickramasinghe K, Barazzoni R. Tuberculosis and malnutrition: the European perspective. Clin Nutr. 2023;42:486–92.
122. Buregyeya E, Kulane A, Colebunders R, Wajja A, Kiguli J, Mayanja H, Musoke P, Pariyo G, Mitchell EMH. Tuberculosis knowledge, attitudes and health-seeking behaviour in rural Uganda. Int J Tuberc Lung Dis. 2011;15:938–42.
123. Ehsanul Huq KATM, Moriyama M, Zaman K, et al. Health seeking behaviour and delayed management of tuberculosis patients in rural Bangladesh. BMC Infect Dis. 2018;18:515.
124. Zhuang L, Ye Z, Li L, Yang L, Gong W. Next-generation TB vaccines: progress, challenges, and prospects. Vaccine. 2023;11:1304.
125. Novelli G, Biancolella M, Latini A, Spallone A, Borgiani P, Papaluca M. Precision medicine in non-communicable diseases. High Throughput. 2020;9:3.
126. Chikowore T, Kamiza AB, Oduaran OH, Machipisa T, Fatumo S. Non-communicable diseases pandemic and precision medicine: is Africa ready? EBioMedicine. 2021;65:103260.
127. Cohen IR, Efroni S. The immune system computes the state of the body: crowd wisdom, machine learning, and immune cell reference repertoires help manage inflammation. Front Immunol. 2019; https://doi.org/10.3389/fimmu.2019.00010.
128. Zumla A, Rao M, Parida SK, Keshavjee S, Cassell G, Wallis R, Axelsson-Robertsson R, Doherty M, Andersson J, Maeurer M. Inflammation and tuberculosis: host-directed therapies. J Intern Med. 2015;277:373–87.
129. Mahjabeen A, Hasan MZ, Rahman MT, Islam MA, Khan RT, Kaiser MS. Genetic insights into the connection between pulmonary TB and non-communicable diseases: an integrated analysis of shared genes and potential treatment targets. PLoS One. 2024;19:e0312072.
130. Wheeler PR, Ratledge C. Metabolism of Mycobacterium tuberculosis. In: Tuberculosis. John Wiley & Sons, Ltd; 1994. p. 353–85.

131. Zhang Y, Yew WW. Mechanisms of drug resistance in Mycobacterium tuberculosis. Int J Tuberc Lung Dis. 2009;13:1320–30.
132. Allué-Guardia A, García JI, Torrelles JB. Evolution of drug-resistant Mycobacterium tuberculosis strains and their adaptation to the human lung environment. Front Microbiol. 2021; https://doi.org/10.3389/fmicb.2021.612675.
133. Yue J, Shi W, Xie J, Li Y, Zeng E, Wang H. Mutations in the rpoB gene of multidrug-resistant Mycobacterium tuberculosis isolates from China. J Clin Microbiol. 2003;41:2209–12.
134. Bollela VR, Namburete EI, Feliciano CS, Macheque D, Harrison LH, Caminero JA. Detection of katG and inhA mutations to guide isoniazid and ethionamide use for drug-resistant tuberculosis. Int J Tuberc Lung Dis. 2016;20:1099–104.
135. Bakuła Z, Napiórkowska A, Bielecki J, Augustynowicz-Kopeć E, Zwolska Z, Jagielski T. Mutations in the embB gene and their association with ethambutol resistance in multidrug-resistant Mycobacterium tuberculosis clinical isolates from Poland. Biomed Res Int. 2013;2013:167954.
136. Murray CJL, Ikuta KS, Sharara F, et al. Global burden of bacterial antimicrobial resistance in 2019: a systematic analysis. Lancet. 2022;399:629–55.
137. Seung KJ, Keshavjee S, Rich ML. Multidrug-resistant tuberculosis and extensively drug-resistant tuberculosis. Cold Spring Harb Perspect Med. 2015;5:a017863.
138. Weiner J, Maertzdorf J, Sutherland JS, et al. Metabolite changes in blood predict the onset of tuberculosis. Nat Commun. 2018;9:5208.
139. Kotliarov Y, Sparks R, Martins AJ, et al. Broad immune activation underlies shared set point signatures for vaccine responsiveness in healthy individuals and disease activity in patients with lupus. Nat Med. 2020;26:618–29.
140. Global coalition to accelerate COVID-19 clinical research in resource-limited settings. Lancet. 2020;395:1322–25
141. Sharp G, Relton C. Epigenetics and noncommunicable diseases. 2017. https://doi.org/10.2217/epi-2017-0045.
142. Meehan CJ, Goig GA, Kohl TA, et al. Whole genome sequencing of Mycobacterium tuberculosis: current standards and open issues. Nat Rev Microbiol. 2019;17:533–45.
143. Liu H, Su L, Zhu T, et al. Comparative analysis on proteomics profiles of intracellular and extracellular M.tb and BCG from infected human macrophages. Front Genet. 2022; https://doi.org/10.3389/fgene.2022.847838.
144. Stanley SA, Cox JS. Host-pathogen interactions during Mycobacterium tuberculosis infections. Curr Top Microbiol Immunol. 2013;374:211–41.
145. Kostova D, Chaloupka FJ, Frieden TR, Henning K, Paul J, Osewe PL, Asma S. Noncommunicable disease risk factors in developing countries: policy perspectives. Prev Med. 2017;105:S1–3.
146. Tameris MD, Hatherill M, Landry BS, et al. Safety and efficacy of MVA85A, a new tuberculosis vaccine, in infants previously vaccinated with BCG: a randomised, placebo-controlled phase 2b trial. Lancet. 2013;381:1021–8.
147. Fletcher HA. Profiling the host immune response to tuberculosis vaccines. Vaccine. 2015;33:5313–5.
148. Goletti D, Petruccioli E, Joosten SA, Ottenhoff THM. Tuberculosis biomarkers: from diagnosis to protection. Infect Dis Rep. 2016;8:6568.
149. Noble AJ, Purcell RV, Adams AT, Lam YK, Ring PM, Anderson JR, Osborne AJ. A final frontier in environment-genome interactions? Integrated, multi-omic approaches to predictions of non-communicable disease risk. Front Genet. 2022;13:831866.

Part V

Public Health and Societal Challenges for the Development of Tuberculosis Vaccines

Public Health Strategies and Prevention of Tuberculosis

13

Frank Cobelens

13.1 Principles and Evolution of Tuberculosis Control

In much of the industrialized world, tuberculosis (TB) mortality had been declining since the second half of the nineteenth century when, in the 1950s, the availability of effective antituberculosis combination treatment boosted public health interventions to control the disease. By the end of the twentieth century, early diagnosis and prompt treatment, often combined with large-scale chest radiology screening programs, had brought down the reported TB incidence by 10–20 fold [1]. But while the industrialized world considered tuberculosis a problem of the past, the disease remained rampant elsewhere. There, treatment was often not available or extremely long and ineffective with low cure rates.

13.1.1 The DOTS Strategy

Modern global TB control started with the DOTS approach that was piloted in the 1970s and 1980s in Tanzania and several other low-income countries under the leadership of Karel Styblo (1921–1998). The DOTS principles were simple and aimed at scalability and affordability in resource-poor settings that had a shortage of health facilities, medical specialists, and microbiology laboratories (Table 13.1). The pilots were hugely effective: TB cure rates increased from around 40% to almost 80% at a cost of US$ 10 per treatment [2]. Based on a cost per disability-adjusted life year (DALY) saved of about $1 to $3, the 1993 World Development

F. Cobelens (✉)
Department of Global Health, Amsterdam University Medical Centres Location University of Amsterdam, Amsterdam, The Netherlands

Amsterdam Institute for Global Health and Development, Amsterdam, The Netherlands
e-mail: f.cobelens@aighd.org; f.g.cobelens@amsterdamumc.nl

P. J. G. Bettencourt (ed.), *Tuberculosis Vaccines*,
https://doi.org/10.1007/978-3-031-94540-3_13

Table 13.1 Principles of global tuberculosis control: The original DOTS Strategy's core components and their rationale

Principle	Key rationale
Treatment with standard drug regimens that include isoniazid and rifampicin	Allowed shortening treatment from 6 to 9 months ("short course") Resulted in quick sputum conversion, abrogating transmission In combination with DOT, prevented development of drug resistance Easy to train, monitor and supply, allowing for non-specialist treatment
Standard monitoring and reporting of treatment outcomes	Allowed quality assurance and early identification of problems (e.g., resistance) Allowed comparisons between health facilities
Case detection by sputum smear microscopy	Does not require extensive lab training or infrastructure Positive sputum smear associated with morbidity and mortality Smear-positive pulmonary TB contributes 50–60% of the cases, but 90–95% of transmission
Continuous supply of quality-assured drugs	Prevents treatment interruptions, treatment failure, and development of drug resistance
Government commitment	Necessary for scale-up and sustained implementation

DOT: treatment directly observed by a health worker during the first 2 months

Report declared "chemotherapy for tuberculosis one of the most cos-effective of all (health) interventions" [3].

In 1994, the World Health Organization adopted the DOTS approach as the basis for its global TB control strategy [4]. Worldwide, countries established or revised national TB control programs (NTPs) to implement the DOTS Strategy. NTPs, generally under the Ministry of Health, were and still are responsible for support to health facilities, public health tasks, and reference laboratory functions. Most NTPs took the classical public health approach of a "vertical" program with their own targets, supply and reporting systems, and in some countries even separate DOTS clinics. Much effort was spent on expanding population coverage of TB services under the new strategy ("DOTS expansion") [4].

13.1.2 Beyond the DOTS Strategy

During the early years of DOTS, several gaps in the strategy became apparent. Awareness grew that public health efforts alone would not be sufficient to diagnose and treat all TB patients, and that other healthcare sectors and professionals needed to be involved. This resulted in a wide range of "public-private mix" pilots and models in which roles and responsibilities for TB control were divided and activities were aligned between the public and the private sector [5]. The HIV epidemic increasingly posed major challenges for TB control which required additions to the standard DOTS approach [6]. Among people living with HIV (PLWH), TB incidence was three to ten times higher than in the HIV negative population, smear-negative pulmonary and extrapulmonary TB were much more common, and mortality was high despite anti-TB treatment [7, 8]. A third problem that increasingly required attention was that of drug resistance, in particular multidrug-resistant TB (MDR-TB, defined as resistance to at least isoniazid and rifampicin) [9]. While DOTS was effective in preventing drug resistance where almost all circulating strains of *M. tuberculosis* were still fully susceptible, it did little to prevent further development and spread of MDR-TB where there were already moderate to high levels of drug resistance, such as in Eastern Europe and Central Asia after the dissolution in the 1990s of the Soviet Union and the accompanying collapse of its public health system [10]. An outbreak in 2006 in South Africa of MDR-TB in which the *M. tuberculosis* strains had additional resistance to fluoroquinolones and aminoglycosides, the most effective second-line drugs (extensively drug resistant TB or XDR-TB), made clear that global TB control could no longer ignore the problem of drug resistance [11].

The WHO's Stop TB Strategy (2006–2015), inspired by the Millennium Development Goals, therefore, emphasized additional interventions to prevent, diagnose, and treat TB-HIV co-infection, diagnose smear-negative pulmonary TB, scale-up drug resistance testing, and provide effective second-line treatment for MDR-TB patients, as well as involvement of all healthcare providers in TB control [12]. It also called for massive investments in research and development.

During this decade, new tools, products, and interventions became available that allowed major improvements in TB control in resource-poor settings. Rapid PCR-based drug resistance testing allowed early identification of MDR-TB, preventing exposure to ineffective drug regimens and continued transmission [13]. Cartridge-based PCR testing of sputum allowed rapid diagnosis without the requirement of sophisticated lab infrastructure [14]. Bedaquiline and delamanid, the first new anti-TB drugs since 40 years, received regulatory approval, allowing shortened, more effective and less toxic treatment of MDR- and XDR-TB [15, 16]. Antiretroviral treatment and isoniazid preventive treatment proved effective in preventing TB among PLWH [17, 18]. Donor funding, among others through the Global Fund to fight AIDS, Tuberculosis, and Malaria, enabled scale-up of these new tools in low-income countries and an expanding reach of TB control [19]. Strengthened surveillance and implementation of national TB prevalence surveys in several countries improved targeting new interventions and provided more robust estimates of the TB burden [20].

13.1.3 End-TB: Focus on Elimination

Despite these improvements, major challenges remained. A continued large gap between the numbers of TB patients diagnosed and notified, and the numbers of new TB disease episodes that occurred according to WHO estimates, showed that much more needed to be done to "find the missing cases" [21]. TB incidence remained very high, and increasingly, studies confirmed that this was strongly related to poverty, poor access to diagnosis and treatment, and other social determinants [22]. TB low-incidence countries were successful in preventing TB by preventive treatment of high-risk groups, but this was hardly implemented in high-incidence countries. The classical public health frame became increasingly questioned, calling for a human rights-based approach in which the patient was no longer a "TB case" but a human being with individual rights, needs, and preferences who should be given a voice.

WHO's End TB Strategy that started in 2015 embraced these needs and developments [23]. Inspired by the Sustainable Development Goals (SDGs), and taking a human rights-based approach, it called for more focus on prevention through TB preventive treatment and vaccination, systematic screening of contacts of TB patients and other high-risk groups, community and civil society engagement, universal health coverage, social protection and poverty alleviation, and a step up in research and innovation. The End TB Strategy implied a paradigm shift in TB control, as it was the first to aim to not just reduce morbidity and mortality, but to eliminate TB as a health problem at global level, for which the WHO as well as the SDGs set ambitious targets (Table 13.2). The End TB Strategy received political support from countries worldwide in two United Nations High-Level Meetings on TB held in 2018 and 2023, affirming its principles and targets, and committing funding for the efforts needed [24].

Thereby global TB control that started as a basic, public health-driven approach to early diagnosis and treatment, over time evolved to become an all-encompassing patient-centered elimination strategy.

Table 13.2 The World Health Organization's End TB Strategy—milestones and targets

	Milestones		Targets	
	2020	2025	2030 (SDG[a])	2035 (End TB)
Reduction in number of TB deaths compared with 2015	35%	75%	90%	95%
Reduction in TB incidence rate compared with 2015	20%	50%	80%	90%
TB-affected families facing catastrophic costs due to TB	0%	0%	0%	0%

Adapted from World Health Organization (2015). The End TB Strategy: Brochure [81]

[a]The United Nations Sustainable Development Goals (SDGs) include ending the TB epidemic by 2030 under Goal 3

13.2 Tuberculosis Prevention

In addition to BCG vaccination, which is described in detail in other chapters, there are currently three prevention strategies for TB: infection control, treatment of pulmonary TB disease, and TB preventive therapy. While complementary, they are very different in scope and level of implementation.

13.2.1 Infection Control

M. tuberculosis is transmitted by aerosols, primarily in closed, ill-ventilated spaces [25], and infectious individuals may have few recognizable symptoms [26]. As a result, most transmission in the community goes unnoticed, and opportunities for prevention of transmission through infection control measures are in practice limited to controlled high-transmission settings such as hospitals. These measures include administrative controls such as triaging and separation of (presumed) infectious individuals, environmental controls, such as face mask wearing for those who are potentially infectious and germicidal ultraviolet radiation, and personal protection measures such as FFP2 masks for directly exposed healthcare workers [27].

13.2.2 Treatment as Prevention

The basis of the sequential global TB control strategies has been early treatment of infectious patients with a drug regimen that makes them non-infectious, with the expectation that this reduces *M. tuberculosis* transmission. Thereby TB control not only aims at reducing TB morbidity and mortality, but also at preventing new infections. Supported by mathematical modeling, WHO's initial DOTS Strategy set targets for national TB programs with regard to case detection (the proportion of new pulmonary TB cases that would be diagnosed and started on treatment) and cure rate (later treatment success rate: the proportion of patients who completed treatment and if tested were sputum smear-negative at the end) that should be met to see the reduction that had been observed in the industrialized world [28]. However, despite decades of early diagnosis and treatment, only limited reductions have been observed at global level, and strong reductions that occurred in some countries were primarily associated with economic growth (e.g., China) or scale-up of antiretroviral treatment (e.g., South Africa) rather than with TB control efforts [29]. This suggests that with current control strategies, too many people with TB disease are diagnosed late or not at all, and/or that socio-economic deprivation is too strong a driver of *M. tuberculosis* transmission, or of progression to TB disease, for its effect to be overcome by early treatment of infectious individuals.

13.2.3 Tuberculosis Preventive Treatment Regimens

For decades, tuberculosis preventive treatment (TPT) has been an important TB control measure in countries with low TB incidence [30]. Trials done in several countries in the 1950s and 1960s had shown that daily monotherapy with isoniazid was effective in preventing TB disease [31, 32]. The duration of preventive treatment in the initial trials was 12 months, showing an overall protective efficacy of around 90% if more than 80% of the doses had been taken [33]. Later, shorter durations of 6–9 months were recommended, although 6 months of isoniazid appeared to be less effective than 12 months and 9 to 10 months appeared to offer the best balance between duration and effectiveness [34].

Isoniazid prophylaxis gradually became part of routine TB control in North America, Europe, and Australia, generally in a targeted approach of testing people with high risk of *M. tuberculosis* infection for latent TB infection (LTBI) and preventive treatment of those tested positive [35]. Testing for LTBI was initially done by tuberculin skin testing (TST), and now commonly by interferon-gamma release assays (IGRA). Short-course options for prophylaxis became available that proved equally effective to 6 months of isoniazid, mainly in trials among PLWH [36]. These include daily rifampicin for 3 months, daily isoniazid-rifampicin for 3 months, and daily rifampicin-pyrazinamide for 3 months, although the latter combination was withdrawn because of reports of severe liver injury [37]. More recently, the inclusion of rifapentin, a long-acting rifamycin, allowed a 3 months course taken weekly or even a 1 month course taken daily, both in combination with high dose isoniazid [38, 39].

13.2.4 Preventive Treatment in Low-Incidence Settings

Targeted TPT, although often with alternative drug regimens, is still the mainstay of TB prevention in most low-incidence countries. Although countries differ in their approach, the most common target populations are close contacts of infectious pulmonary TB patients, healthcare workers, PLWH, people initiating anti-TNF treatment, receiving dialysis, or preparing for organ or hematological transplant, prisoners, immigrants from countries with a high TB burden, homeless people, and people who use drugs [40]. Cost-effectiveness studies of targeted TPT have shown varied results, depending on the target groups studied, the LTBI diagnostic used, and the local TB epidemiology [41]. Even in recently infected individuals, the majority of those with a positive TST or IGRA do not develop TB, resulting in a number needed to treat to prevent a single case of TB disease of 20–50 [42]. In addition, while TPT is generally well tolerated, all combinations carry a risk of hepatoxicity. The benefit of TPT, therefore, needs to be balanced against the individual risk profile [40].

13.2.5 Preventive Treatment in High-Incidence Settings

In high-incidence countries, TPT was for years restricted to PLWH and children up to 5 years old who are close contacts of infectious TB patients, and largely by isoniazid prophylaxis [43]. This restricted indication was based on prioritizing diagnosis and treatment of TB patients, cost-effectiveness, epidemiological considerations about high reinfections rates, feasibility, and concerns about the potential for selection of drug resistant *M. tuberculosis* strains, even though trials had not shown significant increase in isoniazid resistance [44]. For these same reasons, the uptake of TPT was slow, even for PLWH for whom trials had shown it provided additional protection when combined with antiretroviral therapy irrespective of TST or IGRA testing [17, 45], as well as for exposed children for whom it was clearly recommended by the WHO [46]. With the WHO's End-TB's elimination goals and arrival of effective and safe rifapentin-based short-course prophylaxis, many countries are expanding TPT beyond these initial target populations. In addition to these, the 2020 WHO guidelines recommend providing TPT to all household contacts of infectious TB patients regardless of age, selected high-risk contacts of MDR-TB patients and, if the health system can afford it, all other target populations indicated for TPT in low-incidence countries [27].

The level of implementation of these expanded indications for TPT is still highly variable. A major cost-effectiveness concern is the need for LTBI testing. While this is not considered necessary prior to starting TPT in PLWH and child contacts of infectious TB patients, guidelines do recommend LTBI testing for other target groups. IGRA are generally too expensive to use in low-income settings, and TPT is too non-specific. New skin test reagents based on the antigens used in IGRA offer a potential solution [47], although even with these novel skin tests the number needed to treat to prevent a single case of TB disease may remain prohibitively high [48].

13.2.6 Preventive Treatment in TB Vaccine Trials

The need and expanded indications for TPT for populations with high TB incidence, such as PLWH and close contacts of infectious TB patients, poses an ethical obligation to provide TPT to participants in phase 2 or 3 trials of novel TB vaccines and has implications for trial design [49].

13.3 Organization of Tuberculosis Control

Although in most countries the private sector plays an increasingly important role, TB control is generally regarded a government task, executed or at least orchestrated by a national TB program through a number of core responsibilities (Table 13.3). Here we describe the typical organization of TB control in a low- or middle income, TB high-incidence country.

Table 13.3 Core responsibilities of a national tuberculosis control program

Support to clinics
Provide and maintain diagnostic equipment
Provide drugs for treatment
Train staff, regular supervision
Procurement and supply
Public health tasks
Surveillance of TB
Monitoring of treatment and outcomes
Community screening
Preventive treatment
Public campaigns and education
Reference laboratory
Laboratory quality assurance
Drug resistance testing

13.3.1 Diagnosis

Since access to adequate TB diagnosis is essential for successful control, much effort has been put into expanding the number of health facilities capable of diagnosing TB in patients who report with TB-suggestive symptoms such as persistent cough, low-grade fever, and unexplained weight loss. Microbiological confirmation is considered important, for which molecular tests are nowadays the first-line diagnostic. The WHO has endorsed a number of molecular tests that can be used at near point-of-care, such as the GeneXpert MTB/RIF and Ultra systems, the TB-LAMP assay, and the Truenat MTB and MTB and MTB Plus systems [50]. These tests are generally done on sputum for pulmonary TB, and on other body fluids for extrapulmonary TB. Because of their superior sensitivity, microscopic smear examination has been largely abandoned except for treatment monitoring. Mycobacterial culture is hardly used for diagnosing TB, because it is slow (at least 2–3 weeks) and requires specialized laboratory expertise as well as expensive equipment and/or special biosafety measures.

Access to rapid diagnosis close to the patient (e.g., at the community level) increases the numbers of patients diagnosed with TB and of patients initiated on treatment [51]. However, not all clinics have molecular diagnostic systems, therefore, often sputum samples are transported by roving couriers to a lab (e.g., at the district level) where the test can be run. Chest X-rays can aid in the diagnosis, although the availability is different in different health systems. If the molecular test remains negative but the chest X-ray or the patient's history suggests TB, the physician may choose to start treatment regardless. This is generally referred to as "clinical diagnosis" (as opposed to microbiologically confirmed diagnosis).

For patient groups in whom TB is difficult to diagnose because they often don't produce sputum, notably PLWH and children, additional diagnostic options exist. Lateral flow testing for lipoarabinomannan (LAM) in urine has relatively high sensitivity in PLWH with CD4 counts below 100 cells/ml [52]. In young children, gastric aspiration increases the sensitivity. Recently, good experience has been reported with molecular testing on stool [53].

13.3.2 Drug Resistance Testing

Most first-line molecular diagnostic systems test not only for presence of *M. tuberculosis*, but also for mutations in resistance genes, in particular for rifampicin [50]. Because rifampicin is the key drug defining multidrug resistance and response to first-line treatment, this allows immediate triaging of the patient to first-line treatment for susceptible TB, or second-line treatment for rifampicin resistant or MDR-TB. There is generally no resistance screening for other anti-tuberculosis drugs, although in some epidemiological settings additional testing for isoniazid resistance is being introduced because of intermediate-level rifampicin resistance that is not detected by first-line molecular tests [54].

If rifampicin resistance is detected, the patient is referred for diagnostic workup for MDR-TB and second-line treatment. This includes testing for additional first- and second-line drug resistance to determine the treatment regimen, generally at a specialized or reference laboratory. Most additional resistance testing is done by molecular assays that detect specific mutations in resistance genes and produce results within 24–48 hours, although resistance to some drugs, such as bedaquiline, can currently only be detected by phenotypic drug resistance testing. This requires biosafety three level and results may take several weeks. Increasingly, reference laboratories are introducing whole genome sequencing which allows testing for a broad range of resistance-conferring mutations [55].

13.3.3 First-Line Treatment

First-line treatment for rifampicin-susceptible TB is generally through ambulatory care unless the patient is severely ill. It is provided as close as possible to the patient's home, often by a dedicated physician or nurse in a district-level or community-level clinic. Patients are to be counselled prior to treatment initiation about their disease, what they can expect from the treatment in terms of benefit and harm, dosing schedules, adherence, and what to do in case of adverse events. Standard combinations of anti-tuberculosis drugs are used for standard durations [56]. Most used is 2 months of rifampicin (R), isoniazid (H), pyrazinamide (Z), and ethambutol (E) followed by 4 months of R and H (2RHZE/2RH) taken daily. A recent alternative recommended for some cases is a 4-months regimen consisting of 2 months of HZ plus rifapentin (P) and moxifloxacin (M), followed by 2 months of HPM (2HPMZ/2HPM). Different regimens exist for children. First-line TB drugs are in principle taken as fixed-dose combinations in age- and weight-dependent dose bands, which simplifies treatment, reduces the daily number of pills, and allows easy stock-keeping and supply. Monitoring for adverse reactions is generally passive based on signs and symptoms; laboratory monitoring is indicated for patients with specific clinical conditions or risks.

Adherence to treatment is important and can be compromised, in particular, after the first weeks when patients start feeling better. In the early days of the DOTS Strategy, patients needed to take their medication witnessed by a health worker. This directly observed therapy (DOT) approach has been gradually abandoned, because it is considered non-patient-centered and studies have shown limited added benefit with regard to treatment outcomes [57]. Several alternative approaches to enhancing treatment adherence are being used, including treatment support by family members, video-observed treatment, pill boxes that provide signals and/or record pill taking, and mobile phone messaging [58].

Standardized monitoring of treatment outcomes is a core component of global TB control. Clinical progress is measured after 2 months of treatment and toward the end of the scheduled treatment duration, primarily by microscopic sputum smear examination. While this can only be used for patients who were sputum smear positive at the start of treatment, this method is preferred since treatment monitoring with molecular assays will yield many false-positives due to detecting DNA from non-viable bacilli. A positive smear at month two is reason for review of treatment adherence and drug resistance testing. A positive smear at the end of treatment is designated treatment failure and reason for drug resistance testing and referral for first- or second-line retreatment [56].

13.3.4 Second-Line Treatment

Second-line treatment for drug-resistant TB is generally provided by specialized facilities. It may be started in hospital to monitor initial drug tolerance, followed by ambulatory treatment. Initially, second-line treatment regimens were 18–24 months duration with 5–8 drugs including injectables such as kanamycin, amikacin, and capreomycin with high levels of toxicity. The availability of new and repurposed drugs has allowed massive shortening of treatment and all-oral regimens. Currently, first choice is 6 months of bedaquiline, pretomanid, linezolid, and moxifloxacin (BPaLM), with various alternative options in case of drug resistance or contra-indications [59]. Monitoring for adverse reactions is more intensive than for first-line treatment and includes routine laboratory and electrocardiograph monitoring depending on the drug combinations. Adherence is similarly important as for first-line treatment; treatment outcome monitoring is also standardized.

13.3.5 Systematic Screening

Systematic screening (previously called *active case finding*) for pulmonary TB has become increasingly important to complement diagnostic efforts for patients reporting to health facilities with TB-suggestive symptoms (*passive case finding*). Systematic screening is targeted at specific populations where a high prevalence of undiagnosed TB disease can be expected. Depending on the epidemiological setting these may include close contacts of infectious TB patients, in- and outpatients in health facilities, PLWH, prisoners, homeless persons, miners exposed to silica dust, and refugees, but also high-prevalence communities such as in urban slums or settlements for internally displaced persons [60]. The common principle is that a screening step, if positive, is followed by a diagnostic confirmation step. There are several approaches to the screening step. Asking for TB-suggestive symptoms such as persistent cough is simple and inexpensive, and often used in screening of in- or outpatients. The sensitivity is, however, low (many false negatives), as surveys have shown that the majority of undiagnosed TB patients do not have such typical symptoms [26]. The specificity is, however, also low (many false positives), resulting in high costs for the diagnostic confirmation step [60]. Chest X-ray screening has much higher sensitivity and specificity, but for long its feasibility in low- and middle-income settings was limited due to high cost and the need for trained professionals to interpret the images. The increasing availability of low-cost portable digital X-ray systems and developments in artificial intelligence-based detection of TB abnormalities have recently made chest X-ray screening much more feasible and affordable [61, 62], and many NTPs have started scaling-up this approach. Community-wide sputum testing with a rapid molecular assay has a high case detection yield and in addition can reduce TB transmission [63], but is often neither feasible nor affordable. Tongue swabbing for mycobacteria potentially combined with pooled molecular testing may be an alternative approach that potentially allows large-scale screening without need for X-ray [64].

13.3.6 Comorbidities

Several health conditions increase morbidity and mortality due to TB. Those with largest impact on a global scale are HIV, diabetes mellitus, alcohol use disorders, tobacco smoking, and undernutrition. Other comorbidities include chronic respiratory disease, COVID-19, mental and drug use disorders, viral hepatitis, and iatrogenic immune suppression (e.g., renal dialysis, organ transplant, anti-TNF-alpha treatment) [65]. Increasingly TB control seeks to include specific measures targeting these conditions.

Uncontrolled HIV infection is the strongest known risk factor for progression from TB infection to disease [40] and a major cause of mortality among TB patients, off as well as on treatment [66]. Key interventions to address HIV-TB coinfection among PLWH are initiating early antiretroviral therapy, systematic screening and prompt TB treatment, and TB preventive therapy. Among TB patients these are provider-initiated testing for HIV, and effective linkage to antiretroviral therapy and other HIV care among those tested positive [67]. This requires integrated delivery of TB and HIV services: close collaboration between designated TB and HIV focal workers at health facilities, as well as between disease control programs at various levels in the health system (local, regional, national, and global).

Diabetes increases the risk of TB disease two- to threefold and carries an increased risk of mortality during TB treatment and of recurrent TB following treatment completion [68, 69]. Key interventions to address this comorbidity include early diagnosis of TB among people with diabetes, in some settings complemented with systematic TB screening, and detection and management of diabetes, including stringent glycemic control, among TB patients.

Alcohol-use disorders increase the risk of TB disease threefold and affect TB treatment adherence [70, 71]. Key interventions among TB patients with alcohol disorders include regular clinical monitoring, psychological support, and alcohol cessation counselling. Tobacco smoking increases the risk of TB twofold, increasing both the risk of infection and the risk of progression to disease, and is associated with TB treatment failure [72–74]. Key interventions among TB patients are screening for tobacco use and tobacco cessation. Undernutrition measured as low body mass index (BMI) increases the risk of TB disease threefold [75], while TB disease itself may cause wasting leading to low BMI. Given the high prevalence of undernutrition in resource-poor settings it is the most important comorbidity contributing to the TB epidemic, with an estimated one-fifth of global TB incidence attributable to undernutrition. A community-randomized trial of nutritional supplementation showed 39% efficacy in preventing TB disease in an undernourished population [76]. Key interventions include systematic screening for TB in undernourished populations, and nutritional status assessment and nutritional support for TB patients.

13.3.7 Preventive Treatment

See Prevention Strategies.

13.3.8 Surveillance

Since the DOTS Strategy, surveillance has played an important role to plan and target TB control activities, identify populations with high risk of TB or poor TB treatment outcomes, and detect flaws in the control response. TB surveillance in high incidence setting rests on two pillars: routine reporting and surveys.

Routine reporting of TB in most countries is based on mandatory notification to the public health authorities. Case notification is generally done when TB treatment is initiated. The standard case reporting system that has existed since the beginning of the DOTS Strategy is paper-based recording in clinics, with aggregate quarterly reporting to district and national level. Standard reporting data stratification includes disease location (pulmonary/extrapulmonary), new versus previously treated disease, laboratory confirmation, age, and gender. In the past decade, several countries have moved from aggregate paper-based reporting to individual patient electronic reporting, either as a stand-alone digital reporting system or integrated in a national electronic health management information system. The second component is the standard treatment outcome reporting. This was initially also done on a quarterly aggregate basis and is increasingly being integrated into electronic reporting systems. Often separate, the third is the reporting system for patients diagnosed with rifampicin-resistant or MDR-TB. Most rapid molecular diagnostic systems routinely store data for each test run, and this source of information is also increasingly used for surveillance purposes, both of drug-susceptible and of drug-resistant TB.

Surveys (systematic cross-sectional data collections on a representative sample of the target population) often complement routine data and can be implemented for a variety of purposes. Drug resistance surveys, often at national level, were held at 5–10 years intervals in most countries, but have increasingly become obsolete because rapid molecular tests provide direct resistance data for all diagnosed TB patients, and all patients with rifampicin resistance are meant to get routine testing for additional drug resistance.

Several countries have implemented national prevalence surveys to obtain an estimate of the TB burden in the country and collect information on variation by region, age groups, and gender, as well as on health-seeking behavior of those with TB-suggestive symptoms. These surveys are almost exclusively based on population screening for TB-suggestive symptoms combined with chest X-ray screening, and sputum laboratory testing of those screened positive on either. Because of this screening algorithm, national prevalence surveys also allow estimation of the burden of asymptomatic pulmonary TB, that is, without the screening symptom [26, 77]. Examples of other surveys that are done regularly include those to measure catastrophic costs to households due to TB, those to understand community TB knowledge, practice and preferences, and surveys of TB-associated stigma.

Routine reporting data and often also survey data are shared with the WHO on a regular basis and included in global estimations, such as in the annual Global Tuberculosis Report.

13.3.9 Social Protection

TB is strongly associated with poverty. Studies have shown that TB patients and their household members may incur catastrophic costs, defined as costs associated with diagnosis and management exceeding 20% of the annual pre-TB household income [78]. These costs can be directly or indirectly related to diagnosis and treatment, and also include opportunity costs. Although in principle TB diagnostic testing and treatment are offered for free, patients may in practice incur directly related costs, for example, for hospital admission or additional laboratory testing before diagnosis or during treatment [79]. Because in many resource-poor settings health insurance coverage tends to be low, these costs need to be made out-of-pocket [80]. Indirect costs include, for example, costs for transport to the health facility and extra food. Opportunity costs may relate to loss of work and income, not being able provide childcare, and home care needed by family members. The household financial burden tends to be highest for patients with drug resistance or with TB-HIV co-infection [78]. Zero catastrophic cost is among the core targets of the End TB Strategy. TB control efforts are, therefore, increasingly addressing poverty and social protection. These include a variety of measures, such as nutrition support during TB treatment, financial support (e.g., cash transfers) to TB-affected households and expanding universal health coverage including health insurance.

13.3.10 Actors in TB Control

Effective TB control requires engagement and collaborations of various actors in and beyond the health sector. Health facilities, government-owned, or private including faith-based, are the primary providers of TB diagnosis among patients seeking care, and of treatment of TB disease. These services are supported by NTPs, the key public health actors in TB control. In addition to the NTP's core responsibilities (Table 13.3) this can, for example, be a public-private collaboration in which a private health facility provides clinical care to TB patients while the NTP facilitates their treatment adherence, monitors treatment outcomes, screens their household members for TB disease, and provides TB preventive treatment if indicated. Similarly, private health facilities and laboratories may be contracted to do systematic screening for TB disease in designated populations. Communities and civil society organizations are often involved, for example, in identifying people with TB-suggestive symptoms, raising awareness about TB and its treatment, as well as in setting agendas for patient-centered prevention and care. Professional organizations, along with the NTPs, are important for developing clinical guidelines and continuous medical and other health professional education. Additional stakeholders within the health sectors include other disease control programs such as those for HIV/AIDS and alcohol and tobacco control, national immunization programs that are responsible for neonatal BCG vaccination, and national regulatory authorities that are responsible for pharmacovigilance of TB drugs and vaccines. Important stakeholders outside the health sector are the education, social protection, and judicial sectors, as well as ministries of finance responsible for budget allocation.

Competing Interests The author(s) has no competing interests to declare that are relevant to the content of this manuscript.

Ethics Approval The author(s) declares that this manuscript does not include primary research with human participants.

References

1. Styblo K. Overview and epidemiologic assessment of the current global tuberculosis situation with an emphasis on control in developing countries. Rev Infect Dis. 1989;11(Suppl 2):S339–46.
2. Murray CJ, DeJonghe E, Chum HJ, Nyangulu DS, Salomao A, Styblo K. Cost effectiveness of chemotherapy for pulmonary tuberculosis in three sub-Saharan African countries. Lancet. 1991;338:1305–8.

3. World development report 1993: investing in health. In: World Bank. https://documents.worldbank.org/en/publication/documents-reports/documentdetail/468831468340807129/World-development-report-1993-investing-in-health. Accessed 27 Jan 2024.
4. An expanded DOTS framework for effective tuberculosis control. Int J Tuberc Lung Dis. 2002;6:378–88.
5. Uplekar M. Involving private health care providers in delivery of TB care: global strategy. Tuberculosis (Edinb). 2003;83:156–64.
6. Harries AD, Zachariah R, Corbett EL, Lawn SD, Santos-Filho ET, Chimzizi R, Harrington M, Maher D, Williams BG, De Cock KM. The HIV-associated tuberculosis epidemic – when will we act? Lancet. 2010;375:1906–19.
7. Harries AD, Hargreaves NJ, Kemp J, Jindani A, Enarson DA, Maher D, Salaniponi FM. Deaths from tuberculosis in sub-Saharan African countries with a high prevalence of HIV-1. Lancet. 2001;357:1519–23.
8. Frieden TR, Sterling TR, Munsiff SS, Watt CJ, Dye C. Tuberculosis. Lancet. 2003;362:887–99.
9. Pablos-Méndez A, Raviglione MC, Laszlo A, et al. Global surveillance for antituberculosis-drug resistance, 1994-1997. World Health Organization-International Union against Tuberculosis and Lung Disease Working Group on anti-tuberculosis drug resistance surveillance. N Engl J Med. 1998;338:1641–9.
10. Espinal MA, Kim SJ, Suarez PG, Kam KM, Khomenko AG, Migliori GB, Baéz J, Kochi A, Dye C, Raviglione MC. Standard short-course chemotherapy for drug-resistant tuberculosis: treatment outcomes in 6 countries. JAMA. 2000;283:2537–45.
11. Gandhi NR, Moll A, Sturm AW, Pawinski R, Govender T, Lalloo U, Zeller K, Andrews J, Friedland G. Extensively drug-resistant tuberculosis as a cause of death in patients co-infected with tuberculosis and HIV in a rural area of South Africa. Lancet. 2006;368:1575–80.
12. Implementing the WHO stop TB strategy: a handbook for national tuberculosis control programmes. Geneva: World Health Organization; 2008.
13. Morgan M, Kalantri S, Flores L, Pai M. A commercial line probe assay for the rapid detection of rifampicin resistance in Mycobacterium tuberculosis: a systematic review and meta-analysis. BMC Infect Dis. 2005;5:62.
14. Boehme CC, Nicol MP, Nabeta P, et al. Feasibility, diagnostic accuracy, and effectiveness of decentralised use of the Xpert MTB/RIF test for diagnosis of tuberculosis and multidrug resistance: a multicentre implementation study. Lancet. 2011;377:1495–505.
15. Gler MT, Skripconoka V, Sanchez-Garavito E, et al. Delamanid for multidrug-resistant pulmonary tuberculosis. N Engl J Med. 2012;366:2151–60.
16. Diacon AH, Pym A, Grobusch MP, et al. Multidrug-resistant tuberculosis and culture conversion with bedaquiline. N Engl J Med. 2014;371:723–32.
17. A trial of early antiretrovirals and isoniazid preventive therapy in Africa. New England J Med. 2015;373:808–22.
18. Samandari T, Agizew TB, Nyirenda S, et al. 6-month versus 36-month isoniazid preventive treatment for tuberculosis in adults with HIV infection in Botswana: a randomised, double-blind, placebo-controlled trial. Lancet. 2011;377:1588–98.
19. Atun R, Silva S, Knaul FM. Innovative financing instruments for global health 2002-15: a systematic analysis. Lancet Glob Health. 2017;5:e720–6.
20. National tuberculosis prevalence surveys 2007-2016. https://www.who.int/publications-detail-redirect/9789240022430. Accessed 16 Oct 2023.
21. World Health Organization Global tuberculosis control. Geneva: World Health Organization; 2011.
22. Lönnroth K, Castro KG, Chakaya JM, Chauhan LS, Floyd K, Glaziou P, Raviglione MC. Tuberculosis control and elimination 2010-50: cure, care, and social development. Lancet. 2010;375:1814–29.
23. Uplekar M, Weil D, Lonnroth K, et al. WHO's new end TB strategy. Lancet. 2015;385:1799–801.
24. United Nations High-Level Meeting on TB | Stop TB Partnership. https://www.stoptb.org/advocate-to-endtb/united-nations-high-level-meeting-tb. Accessed 28 Jan 2024.

25. Riley RL, Mills CC, Nyka W, Weinstock N, Storey PB, Sultan LU, Riley MC, Wells WF. Aerial dissemination of pulmonary tuberculosis. A two-year study of contagion in a tuberculosis ward. 1959. Am J Epidemiol. 1995;142:3–14.
26. Frascella B, Richards AS, Sossen B, Emery JC, Odone A, Law I, Onozaki I, Esmail H, Houben RMGJ. Subclinical tuberculosis disease – a review and analysis of prevalence surveys to inform definitions, burden, associations and screening methodology. Clin Infect Dis. 2020; https://doi.org/10.1093/cid/ciaa1402.
27. WHO operational handbook on tuberculosis: module 1: prevention: infection prevention and control. https://www.who.int/publications-detail-redirect/9789240078154. Accessed 28 Jan 2024.
28. Dye C, Garnett GP, Sleeman K, Williams BG. Prospects for worldwide tuberculosis control under the WHO DOTS strategy. Directly observed short-course therapy. Lancet. 1998;352:1886–91.
29. Dye C, Lönnroth K, Jaramillo E, Williams BG, Raviglione M. Trends in tuberculosis incidence and their determinants in 134 countries. Bull World Health Organ. 2009;87:683–91.
30. Salazar-Austin N, Dowdy DW, Chaisson RE, Golub JE. Seventy years of tuberculosis prevention: efficacy, effectiveness, toxicity, durability, and duration. Am J Epidemiol. 2019;188:2078–85.
31. Comstock GW, Ferebee SH, Hammes LM. A controlled trial of community-wide isoniazid prophylaxis in Alaska. Am Rev Respir Dis. 1967;95:935–43.
32. Mount FW, Ferebee SH. Preventive effects of isoniazid in the treatment of primary tuberculosis in children. N Engl J Med. 1961;265:713–21.
33. Ferebee SH. Controlled chemoprophylaxis trials in tuberculosis. A general review. Bibl Tuberc. 1970;26:28–106.
34. Comstock GW. How much isoniazid is needed for prevention of tuberculosis among immunocompetent adults? Int J Tuberc Lung Dis. 1999;3:847–50.
35. Targeted tuberculin testing and treatment of latent tuberculosis infection. This official statement of the American Thoracic Society was adopted by the ATS Board of Directors, July 1999. This is a joint statement of the American Thoracic Society (ATS) and the Centers for Disease Control and Prevention (CDC). This statement was endorsed by the Council of the Infectious Diseases Society of America. (IDSA), September 1999, and the sections of this statement. Am J Respir Crit Care Med. 2000;161:S221–47.
36. Akolo C, Adetifa I, Shepperd S, Volmink J. Treatment of latent tuberculosis infection in HIV infected persons. Cochrane Database Syst Rev. 2010;2010:CD000171.
37. Centers for Disease Control and Prevention (CDC), American Thoracic Society. Update: adverse event data and revised American Thoracic Society/CDC recommendations against the use of rifampin and pyrazinamide for treatment of latent tuberculosis infection – United States, 2003. MMWR Morb Mortal Wkly Rep. 2003;52:735–9.
38. Swindells S, Ramchandani R, Gupta A, et al. One month of Rifapentine plus isoniazid to prevent HIV-related tuberculosis. N Engl J Med. 2019;380:1001–11.
39. Sterling TR, Villarino ME, Borisov AS, et al. Three months of rifapentine and isoniazid for latent tuberculosis infection. N Engl J Med. 2011;365:2155–66.
40. Getahun H, Matteelli A, Chaisson RE, Raviglione M. Latent mycobacterium tuberculosis infection. N Engl J Med. 2015;372:2127–35.
41. Diel R, Lampenius N, Nienhaus A. Cost effectiveness of preventive treatment for tuberculosis in special high-risk populations. PharmacoEconomics. 2015;33:783–809.
42. Zhou G, Luo Q, Luo S, et al. Interferon-γ release assays or tuberculin skin test for detection and management of latent tuberculosis infection: a systematic review and meta-analysis. Lancet Infect Dis. 2020;20:1457–69.
43. Getahun H, Matteelli A, Abubakar I, Hauer B, Pontali E, Migliori GB. Advancing global programmatic management of latent tuberculosis infection for at risk populations. Eur Respir J. 2016;47:1327–30.
44. Balcells ME, Thomas SL, Godfrey-Faussett P, Grant AD. Isoniazid preventive therapy and risk for resistant tuberculosis. Emerging Infect Dis. 2006;12:744–51.

45. Rangaka MX, Wilkinson RJ, Boulle A, et al. Isoniazid plus antiretroviral therapy to prevent tuberculosis: a randomised double-blind, placebo-controlled trial. Lancet. 2014;384:682–90.
46. Hamada Y, Sidibe A, Matteelli A, Dadu A, Aziz MA, Del Granado M, Nishikiori N, Floyd K, Getahun H. Policies and practices on the programmatic management of latent tuberculous infection: global survey. Int J Tuberc Lung Dis. 2016;20:1566–71.
47. Hamada Y, Kontsevaya I, Surkova E, et al. A systematic review on the safety of mycobacterium tuberculosis-specific antigen-based skin tests for tuberculosis infection compared with tuberculin skin tests. Open Forum Infect Dis. 2023;10:ofad228.
48. Goscé L, Allel K, Hamada Y, Korobitsyn A, Ismail N, Bashir S, Denkinger CM, Abubakar I, White PJ, Rangaka MX. Economic evaluation of novel Mycobacterium tuberculosis specific antigen-based skin tests for detection of TB infection: a modelling study. PLOS Glob Public Health. 2023;3:e0002573.
49. Rangaka MX, Frick M, Churchyard G, et al. Clinical trials of tuberculosis vaccines in the era of increased access to preventive antibiotic treatment. Lancet Respir Med. 2023;11:380–90.
50. Rapid Communication: molecular assays as initial tests for the diagnosis of tuberculosis and rifampicin resistance. https://www.who.int/publications-detail-redirect/9789240000339. Accessed 28 Jan 2024.
51. Cattamanchi A, Reza TF, Nalugwa T, et al. Multicomponent strategy with decentralized molecular testing for tuberculosis. N Engl J Med. 2021;385:2441–50.
52. Shah M, Ssengooba W, Armstrong D, Nakiyingi L, Holshouser M, Ellner JJ, Joloba M, Manabe YC, Dorman SE. Comparative performance of urinary lipoarabinomannan assays and Xpert MTB/RIF in HIV-infected individuals. AIDS. 2014;28:1307–14.
53. Segala FV, Papagni R, Cotugno S, et al. Stool Xpert MTB/RIF as a possible diagnostic alternative to sputum in Africa: a systematic review and meta-analysis. Front Public Health. 2023;11:1117709.
54. Barilar I, Fernando T, Utpatel C, et al. Emergence of bedaquiline-resistant tuberculosis and of multidrug-resistant and extensively drug-resistant Mycobacterium tuberculosis strains with rpoB Ile491Phe mutation not detected by Xpert MTB/RIF in Mozambique: a retrospective observational study. Lancet Infect Dis. 2023; S1473-3099(23)00498-X.
55. Use of targeted next-generation sequencing to detect drug-resistant tuberculosis. https://www.who.int/publications-detail-redirect/9789240078079. Accessed 28 Jan 2024.
56. WHO consolidated guidelines on tuberculosis: module 4: treatment: drug-susceptible tuberculosis treatment. https://www.who.int/publications-detail-redirect/9789240048126. Accessed 25 Jan 2024.
57. Karumbi J, Garner P. Directly observed therapy for treating tuberculosis. Cochrane Database Syst Rev. 2015;2015:CD003343.
58. Alipanah N, Jarlsberg L, Miller C, Linh NN, Falzon D, Jaramillo E, Nahid P. Adherence interventions and outcomes of tuberculosis treatment: a systematic review and meta-analysis of trials and observational studies. PLoS Med. 2018;15:e1002595.
59. WHO operational handbook on tuberculosis. Module 4: treatment – drug-resistant tuberculosis treatment, 2022 update. https://www.who.int/publications-detail-redirect/9789240065116. Accessed 25 Jan 2024.
60. WHO consolidated guidelines on tuberculosis: module 2: screening: systematic screening for tuberculosis disease. https://www.who.int/publications-detail-redirect/9789240022676. Accessed 7 Dec 2023.
61. Jo Y, Kagujje M, Johnson K, Dowdy D, Hangoma P, Chiliukutu L, Muyoyeta M, Sohn H. Costs and cost-effectiveness of a comprehensive tuberculosis case finding strategy in Zambia. PLoS One. 2021;16:e0256531.
62. Gelaw SM, Kik SV, Ruhwald M, et al. Diagnostic accuracy of three computer-aided detection systems for detecting pulmonary tuberculosis on chest radiography when used for screening: analysis of an international, multicenter migrants screening study. PLOS Glob Public Health. 2023;3:e0000402.
63. Marks GB, Nguyen NV, Nguyen PTB, et al. Community-wide screening for tuberculosis in a high-prevalence setting. N Engl J Med. 2019;381:1347–57.

64. Lima F, Santos AS, Oliveira RD, Silva CCR, Gonçalves CCM, Andrews JR, Croda J. Oral swab testing by Xpert® MTB/RIF ultra for mass tuberculosis screening in prisons. J Clin Tuberc Other Mycobact Dis. 2020;19:100148.
65. Framework for collaborative action on tuberculosis and comorbidities. https://www.who.int/publications-detail-redirect/9789240055056. Accessed 25 Jan 2024.
66. Ford N, Matteelli A, Shubber Z, Hermans S, Meintjes G, Grinsztejn B, Waldrop G, Kranzer K, Doherty M, Getahun H. TB as a cause of hospitalization and in-hospital mortality among people living with HIV worldwide: a systematic review and meta-analysis. J Int AIDS Soc. 2016;19:20714.
67. WHO | WHO policy on collaborative TB/HIV activities: guidelines for national programmes and other stakeholders. In: WHO. http://www.who.int/tb/publications/2012/tb_hiv_policy_9789241503006/en/index.html. Accessed 24 May 2012.
68. Baker MA, Harries AD, Jeon CY, Hart JE, Kapur A, Lönnroth K, Ottmani S-E, Goonesekera SD, Murray MB. The impact of diabetes on tuberculosis treatment outcomes: a systematic review. BMC Med. 2011;9:81.
69. Jeon CY, Murray MB. Diabetes mellitus increases the risk of active tuberculosis: a systematic review of 13 observational studies. PLoS Med. 2008;5:e152.
70. Ragan EJ, Kleinman MB, Sweigart B, Gnatienko N, Parry CD, Horsburgh CR, LaValley MP, Myers B, Jacobson KR. The impact of alcohol use on tuberculosis treatment outcomes: a systematic review and meta-analysis. Int J Tuberc Lung Dis. 2020;24:73–82.
71. Lönnroth K, Williams BG, Stadlin S, Jaramillo E, Dye C. Alcohol use as a risk factor for tuberculosis – a systematic review. BMC Public Health. 2008;8:289.
72. Siddiqi K, Keding A, Marshall A-M, et al. Effect of quitting smoking on health outcomes during treatment for tuberculosis: secondary analysis of the TB & tobacco trial. Thorax. 2022;77:74–8.
73. Lin H-H, Ezzati M, Murray M. Tobacco smoke, indoor air pollution and tuberculosis: a systematic review and meta-analysis. PLoS Med. 2007;4:e20.
74. Nijenbandring de Boer R, de Oliveira e Souza Filho JB, Cobelens F, Ramalho DDP, Campino Miranda PF, de Logo K, Oliveira H, Mesquita E, Oliveira MM, Kritski A. Delayed culture conversion due to cigarette smoking in active pulmonary tuberculosis patients. Tuberculosis (Edinb). 2014;94:87–91.
75. Lönnroth K, Williams BG, Cegielski P, Dye C. A consistent log-linear relationship between tuberculosis incidence and body mass index. Int J Epidemiol. 2010;39:149–55.
76. Bhargava A, Bhargava M, Meher A, et al. Nutritional supplementation to prevent tuberculosis incidence in household contacts of patients with pulmonary tuberculosis in India (RATIONS): a field-based, open-label, cluster-randomised, controlled trial. Lancet. 2023;402:627–40.
77. Stuck L, van Haaster AC, Kapata-Chanda P, Klinkenberg E, Kapata N, Cobelens F. How "subclinical" is subclinical tuberculosis? An analysis of National Prevalence Survey Data from Zambia. Clin Infect Dis. 2022;75:842–8.
78. Ghazy RM, El Saeh HM, Abdulaziz S, Hammouda EA, Elzorkany AM, Khidr H, Zarif N, Elrewany E, Abd ElHafeez S. A systematic review and meta-analysis of the catastrophic costs incurred by tuberculosis patients. Sci Rep. 2022;12:558.
79. van den Hof S, Collins D, Hafidz F, Beyene D, Tursynbayeva A, Tiemersma E. The socioeconomic impact of multidrug resistant tuberculosis on patients: results from Ethiopia, Indonesia and Kazakhstan. BMC Infect Dis. 2016;16:470.
80. Lönnroth K, Glaziou P, Weil D, Floyd K, Uplekar M, Raviglione M. Beyond UHC: monitoring health and social protection coverage in the context of tuberculosis care and prevention. PLoS Med. 2014;11:e1001693.
81. The End TB Strategy: Brochure. https://www.who.int/publications/m/item/the-end-tb-strategy-brochure. Accessed 28 Jan 2024.

14 Technological Advances Applied to TB Vaccine Development: How Can AI Contribute to the Development of New TB Vaccines?

João Santos Pereira and David Pires

14.1 Introduction

Tuberculosis (TB) has followed human beings since the out-of-Africa migration. Its etiological agent is the bacterium *Mycobacterium tuberculosis*, identified by Robert Koch in 1882. Today, it remains one of the deadliest diseases caused by a single infectious agent, having caused 1.3 million deaths in 2022 [1], only surpassed by COVID-19. The BCG vaccine, developed in 1921, is the only vaccine ever licensed for TB and only protects against severe forms of the disease in children, with its efficacy decreasing against pulmonary TB, particularly in adults [2]. Traditional vaccine development is a costly and lengthy process usually following a sequence of steps ranging from pathogen isolation to identification of its antigens, formulation of the vaccine, preclinical tests in animal models, and finally, clinical trials [3, 4].

Several promising vaccine candidates have recently been proposed and are undergoing clinical trials. This increase in available data creates several opportunities for associating the results from preclinical studies with clinical trial outcomes. This increase in available data comes when artificial intelligence and machine learning provide tools for handling and analysing massive datasets and discovering interactions that human eyes and minds would miss. Some of these tools are already

J. S. Pereira (✉)
Universidade Católica Portuguesa, Católica Medical School, Center for Interdisciplinary Research in Health, Rio de Mouro, Portugal
e-mail: jmspereira@ucp.pt

D. Pires
Universidade Católica Portuguesa, Católica Medical School, Center for Interdisciplinary Research in Health, Rio de Mouro, Portugal

Host-Pathogen Interactions Unit, Research Institute for Medicines (iMed.ULisboa), Faculty of Pharmacy, Universidade de Lisboa, Lisbon, Portugal

P. J. G. Bettencourt (ed.), *Tuberculosis Vaccines*,
https://doi.org/10.1007/978-3-031-94540-3_14

being employed in distinct steps of vaccine development, such as antigen selection, epitope prediction, adjuvant identification, and immunogen design [4].

Whether our generation will be the one to close the chapter of human tuberculosis remains to be known. Still, the exponential possibilities that new digital technologies are opening should propel us to start planning the road for future development and implementation of an effective TB vaccine, while also addressing the common challenges faced by introducing a novel vaccine.

14.2 Artificial Intelligence and Machine Learning

Artificial Intelligence (AI) refers to the simulation of human intelligence in machines programmed to think, learn, and problem-solve. AI systems can perform tasks that typically require human intelligence, such as visual perception, speech recognition, decision-making, and language translation. Machine Learning (ML) is a subset of AI that involves training algorithms on large datasets to recognise patterns and make decisions with minimal or no human intervention. ML models may improve over time as they are exposed to more data. Whereas both terms are often used interchangeably, such a distinction is key in highlighting some of the more technical aspects that underlie the algorithms involved.

AI has greatly evolved over the past few years, notably through the increase in computational processing and storage capacity available. Algorithms have also evolved, taking advantage of such capacity by having a greater number of parameters. For instance, Deep Learning is a subset of ML that uses neural networks with multiple layers of "digital neurons" that mimic the processing of the human brain: the addition of layers, which are computationally expensive, allows such programs to model increasingly complex patterns in large datasets. Such deep neural networks are behind one of the most impactful models launched up to the present date: ChatGPT.

The launch of ChatGPT (short for Chat Generative Pre-trained Transformer) in November 2022 was a watershed moment for AI technology and, most importantly, for the public awareness of its potential. It is a type of Large Language Model (LLM) that was specifically designed for generating human-like text based on a given prompt after being trained on vast datasets using large-scale, deep learning techniques. Although the public had already seen the rise of virtual assistants and chatbots—notably Siri (Apple), Cortana (Microsoft), and Alexa (Amazon)—the use cases for these were limited. With ChatGPT, the public was faced with a model that was able to process far more complex inputs, integrating data from its vast training database to generate apparently original and coherent texts. The long-held promise of AI models that could add clear value to their users was finally accomplished.

Of course, many other models, with impressive capabilities and scope of action, were being developed and have been launched in the meantime. The list and specifications of these are beyond the scope of this text. The key aspect is that there was an inflexion point in public perception and general use of AI in later 2022. Although ML algorithms were already present in most systems before this date, even in basic home appliances, AI became ubiquitous, and the acceptance of its use grew significantly with the advent of such advanced AI technologies. This shift was marked by the increasing integration of AI in everyday life, from improved virtual assistants to personalised recommendations on streaming platforms and social media. As AI demonstrated its capability to improve efficiency, enhance user experiences, and solve complex problems, public and industry confidence in its potential solidified, leading to its widespread adoption across various sectors, notably in healthcare.

Alan Turing's famous test was proposed in 1950 to assess if a machine could present an intelligent behaviour indistinguishable from that of a human. No model has passed it yet. Whereas one group of experts says it is only a matter of time until such a "singularity" event occurs, another states that, despite their impressive feats, AI models will never be a match for human general intelligence. One thing is certain though: the potential of these models is still in its infancy.

14.3 What Is the Role of AI in Health?

The role of AI in healthcare has expanded rapidly, transforming how medical professionals diagnose, treat, and manage diseases. AI technologies are being integrated into various aspects of healthcare, from fundamental research to patient management and hospital workflows. The applications are as vast as the broad scope of the field.

The use of ML algorithms in health has a long history. An early example from the 1990s is the development of computer-aided diagnosis (CAD) systems for medical imaging, particularly in mammography for breast cancer detection. These early CAD systems used ML algorithms to analyse digitised mammogram images to detect signs of breast cancer, such as microcalcifications and masses. The algorithms were trained on large datasets of annotated images, learning to identify patterns associated with cancerous tissues. Although rudimentary compared to today's AI technologies, these algorithms represented a significant advancement at the time and paved the way for more sophisticated diagnostic tools. Today, AI algorithms, particularly those based on deep learning, are increasingly used to analyse medical images and identify patterns that may be too subtle for the human eye to detect.

In fact, diagnostics is a natural application of AI in health, as it can be seen as a complex pattern detection problem. Beyond imaging, models have been created to analyse patient data and try to come up with a diagnostic answer. An example of this is IBM's Watson model, which famously won the *Jeopardy!* quiz show in 2011, an important milestone in the evolution of language models. Its speed of response and the ability to understand subtle context cues proved that such programs could read, analyse, and learn from natural language to the extent that human-like decisions were made possible. The model was repurposed and commercially deployed for healthcare applications, notably as a Clinical Decision Support System (CDSS). These systems use patient data to produce advice regarding health care, interacting with clinicians to reach better diagnoses. Although originally idealised as autonomous systems that would make decisions instead of clinicians, they have evolved to become “discussion partners” and not final decision-makers.

Another model that was able to beat humans at a complex game was Google DeepMind’s AlphaGo. After beating a professional *Go* player in 2016, this model—which also uses deep learning methods—was further enhanced and generalised. A version of it called AlphaFold was deployed in 2020 and represented a significant advancement in the problem of protein folding. Improved versions released thereafter have seen a progressive enhancement of performance metrics across various benchmarks. This has been of great importance for simulating new compounds and accelerating the discovery of drug and vaccine candidates.

By analysing vast datasets, AI can, therefore, accelerate drug and vaccine research and development, identifying potential drug candidates more quickly and accurately than conventional methods. ML models can predict how different compounds will interact with biological targets, helping to streamline the drug development process. The advancement of personalised medicine is also facilitated by these algorithms, making it possible to analyse diverse types of data, from genetic information to medical history, in order to tailor therapies to individual patients. As diverse biological compounds and environments can be simulated *in silico*, it is therefore possible to optimise treatment efficacy and minimise side effects while reducing testing time and costs.

Furthermore, AI is also improving patient care and management by monitoring patients in real-time. This can be done by analysing data from wearable devices and electronic health records to provide insights into a patient’s condition, predict potential complications, and recommend timely interventions. This continuous monitoring is the cornerstone of any preventive and predictive healthcare system, tackling risk factors before diseases appear. It is also beneficial for managing chronic diseases and prognostic factors and ensuring early detection of changes in a patient’s condition, which can prevent hospitalisations and improve quality of life.

Healthcare operations are also impacted, notably patient flow and administrative tasks. The use of AI models can reduce costs while increasing the efficiency of the system. For instance, predictive analytics can forecast patient admissions, enabling better resource allocation and minimising waiting times. For public health, AI models are paramount to predict disease outbreaks, track the spread of infections, and develop strategies for managing pandemics, as seen during the COVID-19 crisis.

As AI continues to evolve, its integration into healthcare is expected to deepen. Concerns about ethics and human involvement in any decision process are also increasing, with the European Union presenting the AI Act in 2023, a first regulation on AI. Regardless of the improvement of the models, it is unlikely that AI will replace human decision-making in healthcare any time soon. The question lies in whether humans will be more “in the loop”, with AI models seen as partners in the process, or “on the loop”, with humans acting solely as occasional overseers of autonomous systems. It will depend greatly on the context, of course, with the possibility that humans will be "out of the loop" in some low-risk, low-impact applications. Whatever the scenario, everyone working in healthcare will need to adjust to a new, AI-driven paradigm.

14.4 Current Challenges in Vaccination

Vaccines played a fundamental role in human healthcare during the twentieth century. More recently, the COVID-19 pandemic reminded humanity how this preventive strategy has shaped how we deal with human pathogens. Nevertheless, vaccine research, development, and implementation still face significant challenges, from preclinical research to logistical and socio-political areas. The vastness of unresolved problems may as well represent an unexplored pool of opportunities for new AI models to intervene and help researchers, industrial pipelines, and policymakers.

On the scientific side, vaccine research must deliver robust, ample, and durable immunity against diverse pathogens, each with its complexity. Characterisation of the pathogen leads to the identification of antigens with immunogenic properties. Integrating this with our knowledge of the immune system and antigen presentation allows the selection of the best epitopes. Other immunogenic components might be added during the design process to trigger the desired immune response. These will imitate the invading pathogen while not harming the individual. All these processes occur on a trial-and-error empirical basis and are thus time-consuming.

Translating preclinical data from the bench to clinical trials remains a critical challenge. Many promising vaccine candidates do not resist the trial of the natural infection outside the controlled laboratory environment [5]. This is particularly true for rapidly evolving pathogens such as the Influenza virus and HIV [3, 4] and those with sophisticated evasion mechanisms such as *Mycobacterium tuberculosis* (Mtb) [6]. Pathogen variability and high mutation rates continuously force researchers to develop updated versions and booster shots of current vaccines. Improved strategies for antigen discovery and iterative approaches to vaccine design could help screen for the best candidate epitopes that generate strong immune responses while being less likely to suffer mutations, thus guaranteeing long-term effectiveness and concomitantly predicting safeness [7]. While knowledge of the genome and proteome of the pathogen is paramount to selecting the best candidate antigens, its integration with data from our immune system is necessary to prioritise epitopes according to the desired immune cell response [8]. For the specific case of tuberculosis, antigen variability poses a less significant challenge since Mtb evolution rate is lower than in other pathogens. However, the lack of clear immune correlates of protection makes it difficult to predict whether a vaccine will be effective in humans [8, 9]. The immune response against TB involves several actors of the immune system, including innate cells and T and B cells, and it has been difficult to single out which factors are strongly associated with the control of the infection [10]. Furthermore, the immune factors and responses necessary to prevent infection might differ from the ones needed to control it once established. The selection of the best antigens and epitopes also suffers from the innate biases of the researchers, often opting for well-studied antigens.

This uncertainty at the starting point of vaccine development slows antigen screening. Insights from many decades of administration of the Bacille Calmette-Guérin (BCG) vaccine have also demonstrated how variable a TB vaccine can be in its efficacy, particularly in adults [10–13]. And while live or attenuated vaccines are able to produce a strong immune response by themselves, subunit vaccines have the added necessity of an adjuvant that stimulates immune receptors to boost the response to the vaccine [10]. Several of these adjuvant molecules, based on aluminium salts, proteins, nucleic acids, liposomes or others, are being applied in vaccine clinical trials [14, 15] and the choice for those improving vaccine efficacy would benefit from better data integration and analysis. As for viral vectored vaccines, there is no need for an adjuvant since the vector triggers a strong immune response [16]. The downside is this strong response against the vector might limit their repeated use, and there could be preexisting immunity against it in the population, possibly rendering the vector useless. The stability of the vaccine is also an essential matter of research. Distinct molecules and vector combinations have particular needs for storage and transport conditions, as we learned from COVID-19 mRNA vaccines [17, 18].

Mycobacterium tuberculosis is thought to reside dormant in a large proportion of the human population. Developing a vaccine that prevents reactivation or eliminates latent bacilli is an additional problem. Difficulties in identifying asymptomatic infected individuals confound the ability of vaccine candidates to prevent infection [10].

The consequence of these challenges in TB vaccine research is a costly and lengthy vaccine development process. Translation of vaccine candidates from the lab to clinical trials and eventual commercialisation has a high failure rate [4], with most candidates failing the clinical trials due to a lack of efficacy or safety concerns [19–21]. The complexity of TB vaccine clinical trials is furthered by the lack of clear biomarkers of disease progression that force researchers to wait for actual disease outcomes, leading to long follow-up periods to assess efficacy and safety. Moreover, there is a necessity to conduct the trials in high-burden settings that are often resource-limited and lack training of non-clinical staff on vaccine handling [22]. Significant progress has been made in countries such as Uganda, where several clinical trials have been conducted for diseases such as HIV, Ebola, and COVID-19, thanks to the training of specialised teams [23]. Still, logistical, ethical, and regulatory challenges need to be overcome. The population in these regions often suffers from other comorbidities that constitute confounding factors complicating data interpretation, such as HIV co-infection [22]. Limited funding opportunities exacerbate these challenges, slowing the progression of promising candidates through the pipeline, and investors are discouraged by the high failure rates [4, 21].

As promising candidates appear from the clinical trials pipeline, the challenges for implementing new vaccines continue on the manufacturing, logistical, ethical, and regulatory fronts [24]. Intellectual property issues may affect low-income countries, representing a substantial portion of TB cases. These may lack the resources necessary for vaccine production. Implementing TB vaccination programs in resource-limited settings also faces logistical questions [25] for maintaining adequate cold-chain conditions from storage to distribution [26]. The additional burden from integrating a new vaccine program into existing healthcare systems, including vaccine administration and subsequent surveillance, must also be carefully considered to ensure its complementarity to existing TB control measures without conflicting or draining excessive resources. These logistical difficulties, together with supply chain disruptions caused by natural disasters, geopolitical conflicts, or other pandemics, will affect the equitable distribution of vaccines, especially to remote regions [27]. Safe introduction of these new vaccines, considering the uncertain risk profiles of the recipients and their informed consent, must also be accomplished [28, 29]. Navigating the regulatory landscape and the different standards across countries can potentially delay the rollout of new vaccines [19]. This could be mitigated by regulatory harmonisation and global coordination between governments and other stakeholders [23, 30].

The final recipients of the vaccine pipeline are the patients and the general public. Vaccine acceptance and hesitancy are concepts of the highest importance for the success of a new vaccine program. Public trust can be affected by scepticism towards new vaccines due to cultural beliefs, the spread of misinformation amplified by social media or the activity of anti-vaccine movements, distrust of public officials and historical grievances against healthcare establishments. Tuberculosis is also associated with stigma and discrimination, which might discourage individuals from participating in vaccination programs. Routine vaccination might be preferable to mass vaccination campaigns that draw additional stigma against the patients and suffer from precarious implementation due to limited healthcare resources [31].

New technologies have emerged as a potential solution to some of these challenges. The COVID-19 pandemic has shown how digital health investments can strengthen health systems, but ensuring these technologies are effectively integrated into a broader health system strengthening strategy remains a challenge [32].

Addressing these issues requires a multifaceted approach involving advancements in vaccine design, capacity building in resource-limited settings, community engagement, and integrating advanced technologies. These efforts are essential to overcoming the barriers to successful vaccine research, development, and implementation globally.

14.5 AI in Vaccine Research and Development

Developing new drugs is a lengthy and expensive process. An estimate of the average costs for the development of a drug accepted by the Food and Drug Administration (FDA) stands at $648 million (US dollars), with an average lead time of 7.3 years [33]. Moreover, an important proportion of newly developed drugs fail before reaching the preclinical phase, largely due to intolerable side effects, toxicological issues, or unpredictable drug interactions. Because of these challenges, the pharmaceutical industry tends to focus more on enhancing and producing existing drugs to minimise financial risks. However, there remains a pressing need for new active substances and vaccines. This is where AI models can rebalance the financial return eq.

AI models, such as the previously mentioned AlphaFold, have been used by scientists to discover novel drugs and chart all known proteins [34, 35]. It is a clear example of *in silico* biology, which relies on computational methods to simulate and solve biological problems. The emergence of *in silico* biology dates back to the 1980s, with the first characterisation of biological experiments carried out entirely in a simulated computer environment. As biological problems may be too costly and time-consuming to solve with traditional *in vivo* or *in vitro* methods due to the complex interplay of many variables, this field has greatly benefited from the enhancement of AI models. In particular, *in silico* studies have been performed to assess the safety, efficacy, toxicity effects, and interactions of drugs and vaccines [36, 37].

The use of such digital models is effective in tackling problems that were once thought intractable. For instance, it is now possible to predict how a pathogen might evolve [38, 39], helping researchers develop effective vaccines against future strains or scour vast databases in search of the right compound to research or develop. Antigenic variation models have been applied to predict how virus such as SARS-CoV-2, influenza or HIV evolve in response to our immune system and escape neutralising antibodies [38, 39]. Indeed, identifying targets worth working on has been one of the greatest AI boons for vaccine development, impacting all stages, from identifying antigens and adjuvants to aiding the actual market launch, not forgetting the challenges of clinical trials.

It is worth underlining that, during the COVID-19 pandemic, AI played a central role in accelerating the development of Pfizer-BioNTech and Moderna mRNA-based vaccines. These were developed in record time using AI-driven antigen design and clinical trial optimisation [40, 41]. This marked a key paradigm shift in vaccine development, reducing multiple-year lead times to months or even weeks. In line with this success, the implementation of AI and ML solutions is one of the recommendations of the secretariat of the "100 Days Mission" [42], an initiative to prepare a global response to a future pandemic that produced diagnostics, therapeutics and vaccines in 100 days following detection. Companies and researchers cannot ignore the power of algorithms to analyse large datasets of biological and clinical data and find patterns that point to the highest likelihood of success.

14.5.1 Identification of Antigens

Vaccine development typically starts with the isolation and characterisation of the target pathogen. Antigens must then be identified that both elicit an optimal immune response and avoid causing side effects. Once selected, these immunogens must be stable, safe, and suitable for mass production. Such a process can be resource-intensive and is often done on a trial-and-error basis.

The application of AI in efficiently identifying antigens and subsequent immunogen design is evident. This can be achieved by analysing large genomic, proteomic, and other biological information datasets in a process of virtual screening. This process simulates the interaction of these libraries' candidates with target molecules (e.g. immune system components), making it possible to identify antigens that could elicit an immune response.

AI algorithms have been instrumental in identifying novel antigens using ML algorithms, such as deep learning and random forests, with successful applications, for example, in malaria vaccines [43]. To achieve this, it is fundamental to analyse vast genomic sequences, protein structures, and immune interactions, which is only made possible by utilising advanced computational techniques.

AI models can thus prioritise antigens for experimental validation, reducing the time and cost associated with traditional antigen discovery. Additionally, AI-powered generative models and molecular dynamics simulations have enhanced the design of immunogens, focusing on improving their stability, immunogenicity, and antigenic coverage. This is especially challenging in highly mutable antigens such as the influenza virus. Even in such a scenario, improved antigenicity and cross-reactivity were possible in novel immunogens proposed by generative ML algorithms [44].

Such digital models allow exploring parametric spaces with many different variables. Including information regarding the structural behaviour—both in terms of dynamics and stability—of possible candidates further enhances the ability to accurately predict their suitability. The inclusion of information on molecular dynamics simulations is an important addition, otherwise intractable without recourse to ML. This was also demonstrated in the refinement of the SARS-CoV-2 spike protein for COVID-19 vaccines [45]. These simulations allow for unprecedented detail at the atomic level, permitting the precise design of immunogens that interact more effectively with immune receptors, boosting vaccine efficacy.

14.5.2 Reverse Vaccinology

The pathogen's genome may provide fundamental clues to finding the most adequate immunogens through reverse vaccinology. Digital models have been developed to predict the immunogenic proteome from the structural features, amino acid chemical properties or sequence of each gene/protein. These features include the presence of epitopes exposed on the bacterial surface for host immune recognition, antigenicity, sequence conservation across isolates, expression during infection, and similarity to host proteins [46, 47].

Such features can be extracted and then computationally analysed through a filtering approach using decision trees. Each sequence is passed through a series of filters, which will depend on the measurements made of the protein features or on computationally derived probabilities based, for example, on molecular dynamics. Different trees can be obtained by using different types and numbers of filters. Vaccine candidates sharing a specific feature, or sets thereof, can be obtained by applying cut-off points in these filters.

The aforementioned filtering approach does not require sophisticated, if any, ML models. An alternative approach entails the application of ML classification algorithms trained with known immunogenic and non-immunogenic vaccine candidates. This can be done, for instance, using support vector machines (SVMs), a supervised learning algorithm that classifies inputs based on a previously learnt labelled dataset of cases. These methods are more complex, though they can potentially provide more subtle classifications of candidates while avoiding discarding options altogether, as happens with filtering. Moreover, many more features can be analysed simultaneously, detecting patterns that may be elusive to the human mind. The performance will only be as good as the training data provided, which is a key challenge, especially if only a limited number of candidates with known, robust relevant properties is available.

Typical of ML methods, applications may stack both approaches, with a first step relying on a feature extraction similar to the filtering approach above. The ML algorithm would then work with the output thereof, only using the highlighted characteristics. An example of this is Vaxign2 [48, 49] which combines filtering and machine learning workflows (from Vaxign and Vaxign-ML, respectively). Some of these methods have already been used to identify Mtb antigens or to evaluate the antigenicity of Mtb vaccine candidates [50–53]. A more thorough review of the different reverse vaccinology methods can be found in Dalsass et al. and Kaushik et al. [54, 55].

14.5.3 Identification of Epitopes

The adequate prioritisation of targets for vaccine development is especially important when developing epitope-based vaccines. The *in silico* approach to this requires searching antigen protein databases, analysing interactions, and characterising the epitopes recognised by both T cells and B cells, and analysing antigenicity and homology [56]. The prediction of epitopes is based on sequences and structure and not on pathological mechanisms. Moreover, in vaccine design, one must avoid peptide sequences similar to those of human peptides. For this to be possible, reliable antigenic protein data must be available, such as those provided by the National Center of Biotechnology Information (NCBI), UniProt, or Protein Data Bank (PDB). Again, it is worth mentioning that any AI model is only as good as the data it uses.

After protein data is analysed, further tools can be deployed for 3D protein analysis and modelling using such available programs as MODELLER [57]. This allows for the simulation of protein interactions through protein docking. Molecular docking is also performed, ensuring vaccine candidates can generate stable immune responses. Predictive models can also be used to predict antigenicity based on simple scores, though empirical ML-based assessments will likely become more robust than such rule-based methods.

Whereas 3D models have shown great promise, not all target antigens have known 3D structures. Moreover, determining such structures is a cost-intensive endeavour. This is especially true for B-cell epitopes, often discontinuous and presenting a complex folded structure. In such cases, simpler linear sequence-based prediction models often compare the tendency of amino acids to become epitopes relative to amino acids that form the antigens. ML algorithms are of great importance here in order to distinguish epitope and non-epitope antigenic structures based on structural differences and physicochemical characteristics: the more of these characteristics are assessed, the more accurate the model becomes [56]. Improvements using SVMs have been introduced to improve accuracy. Still, such methods have limited performance as they rely on continuous structures, which are rarer in B-cell epitopes. Algorithms using 3D protein structures are required—and are being developed—to achieve better accuracy and predictive power despite the aforementioned limitations.

T-cell epitope prediction is simpler, as such epitopes' structure is short and linear. Here, motif-based methods can be deployed. At its most basic, these methods require having a library of patterns, each called a motif, against which candidate sequences are compared. These methods can be enhanced by ML algorithms, which not only allow for multiple classifications at the same time, but can also assign different weights to binding and non-binding subsets of peptide sequences. The prediction of T-cell epitopes can also benefit from other classification algorithms, such as SVMs and molecular dynamics methods. The latter rely on the parameters of the structure of the receptor-ligand complex to calculate the free binding energy of the candidate.

It is worth noting that the application of the aforementioned methods is relatively simple, as there is a diverse array of publicly available programs that can be used "off the shelf". For instance, the immune epitope database (IEDB) presents a versatile, user-friendly interface for analysing epitome characteristics and for many different prediction analyses. Another set of tools, NetMHC [58] and NetMHCII [59], are neural networks that predict the binding of peptides to the corresponding MHC class I or II molecules. These were trained on a vast set of peptide sequences and binding affinities to each corresponding MHC molecule. The accuracy of such tools, however, is never perfect, as biological systems are inherently dynamic and unpredictable. Small changes in 3D conformations, sequences, residues, context, and so on, may lead to erroneous conclusions. Methods that combine basic, linear prediction tools with more advanced ML algorithms, while taking advantage of molecular dynamics and 3D structures, are most promising. The computation power required for these is vast, though that is a hurdle that is becoming ever easier to overcome.

14.5.4 Identification of Adjuvants

Adjuvants are fundamental components in vaccine formulation, enhancing the immune response to antigens [4]. Once again, AI models have proven useful to ensure these adjuvants fulfil their role in promoting robust and long-lasting protective immune responses [60].

An adjuvant must present with both optimal safety and efficacy, presenting with low toxicity, high stability, and immunogenicity. Their interplay with the immune system is of particular concern, making them a challenging immunomodulation problem. Researchers are faced with the daunting task of choosing the most adequate compounds from vast libraries of chemical and biological options. AI can step in to predict the immunomodulatory effects of such molecules and compounds based on known features and properties. This can be done through virtual screening, already mentioned above, which can be coupled with docking simulations and structure-based models to elicit more robust formulations.

Whereas virtual screening looks at biological characteristics and binding affinities to scour large datasets and find adequate candidates, docking simulations are key in accounting for immunomodulatory effects. This is done by creating models that predict how potential adjuvants react between themselves as well as with immune receptors. AutoDock [61] and Deepchem [62] are some of the tools used to this effect when combined with ML models.

Structural analyses can then be added to the mix in order to further optimise the design of adjuvant formulations [63]. From these structures, predictive models aim to infer the physical, chemical, biological, and toxic properties of compounds. Quantitative structure-activity relationship (QSAR) modelling is one of the most popular tools used for drug discovery and compound optimisation [64] using statistical and ML techniques to relate the chemical structures of potential adjuvants to their activity. DeepTox [65], on the other hand, is a tool used to predict compound toxicity using deep learning methods. A review of the different models and tools and the respective adjuvants identified using them can be found in Zhang et al. [64].

14.5.5 Clinical Trials

As mentioned before, AI also presents great potential for the improvement of all administrative processes surrounding healthcare. In particular, AI-powered virtual assistants are making regulatory compliance, logistics, and bureaucratic management simpler. This is of particular relevance for clinical trials, where patient recruitment, trial design, monitoring and analysis can all be enhanced by AI models.

For instance, AI can optimise the recruitment process for clinical trials by identifying suitable candidates based on genetic profiles, medical history, and other relevant data. This can lead to improved recruitment efficiency, as well as better sample representativeness and more adequate assignment strategies. AI models can also monitor participants' responses and side effects in real-time, adjusting protocols to improve safety and efficacy. This is especially critical in the postmarketing surveillance stage. Moreover, it can analyse vast amounts of data generated from these trials to identify patterns that traditional analysis methods might miss. Communication with the regulatory bodies and docketing is also highly enhanced. Finally, algorithms can also simulate possible scenarios and predict potential outcomes: the contrast between reality and simulation can provide important coordinates and point to potential future results or avoidable bottlenecks. This is invaluable for identifying optimal end-points.

The Universal Immune System Simulator (UISS) is an example of a computational framework of the immune system that can be used to simulate clinical trials and that has been recently expanded to simulate the immune system of virtual patients in response to tuberculosis, vaccination, and treatment [66]. UISS has been applied to predict the efficacy of vaccine candidates for COVID-19, influenza and tuberculosis [66–69]. All of the above can lead to quicker, successful processes or highlight potential issues early on so that "go/no go" decisions can be made before spending too many resources. Most importantly, scientists and support staff can be released from too much paperwork and focus on the most important elements: the patients and the science. This said, such models are not meant as wholesale substitutes for traditional preclinical and clinical methods. AI complements, enhances, and optimises, thus ensuring full regulatory compliance coupled with the highest safety and transparency standards. Animal and human testing will still be of paramount importance in the foreseeable future (Table 14.1).

Table 14.1 Tools mentioned in this chapter

Tool Name	Function	References
AlphaFold	Protein structure prediction	[34, 35]
EVEscape	Antibody escape predictions	[39]
Vaxign2	Epitope prediction	[48, 49]
MODELLER	Protein structure prediction	[57]
NetMHC	Epitope prediction	[58, 59]
AutoDock	Prediction of drug-receptor binding	[61]
Deepchem	Drug candidate prediction	[62]
DeepTox	Toxicity prediction	[65]
Universal Immune System Simulator	Immune system simulation	[66–69]

14.6 AI in Vaccine Deployment

Once a successful vaccine candidate is identified and duly validated through a clinical trial, its deployment to the public is required. That entails several steps where AI may also be of relevance, especially by using multiple AI algorithms, datasets, and digital strategies in an integrated manner. Such integration, if well achieved, can lead to flexible processes that are fine-tuned to the market's specific requirements.

For instance, AI can optimise vaccine manufacturing processes, ensuring efficiency, consistency, and scalability, all at a lower cost. From automating quality control processes to predicting potential issues before they arise, AI tools are now ubiquitous in production settings, notably when high precision is required. Real-time feedback mechanisms can also be implemented, thus allowing for quick reaction times whenever it is required to adjust dosages, delivery systems, or formulations due to e.g. environmental or regulatory changes.

Supply chain management is also affected, not only to ensure optimal manufacturing capability tailored to public demand, but also downstream, ensuring smooth distribution logistics so that vaccines are delivered efficiently and equitably, even in remote areas. For more sensitive compounds, AI-powered sensors can monitor the conditions (notably temperature and humidity) in which vaccines are stored and transported, ensuring they remain effective until they reach the point of use.

Population dynamics may be challenging to interpret in order to define vaccination strategies and priorities. AI models can analyse demographic data to target vaccine awareness campaigns more effectively to increase vaccination rates in specific populations. These models may also be able to predict where vaccine-preventable diseases might emerge, allowing for proactive efforts to avoid outbreaks. Moreover, within the scope of the postmarketing surveillance mentioned above, AI can continuously monitor the effectiveness of vaccines in real-world conditions, providing insights for necessary updates or booster shots.

Such vaccination strategies no longer need to be "one size fits all", with AI models allowing for some degree of personalisation. At a basic level, this allows researchers to deploy multiple formulations and/or delivery systems, quickly identifying the optimal strategy with real-time feedback. At a more individual level, it is possible to consider designing personalised vaccination strategies based on an individual's genetic makeup, health status, and risk factors. Personalised cancer vaccines targeting tumour neoantigens specific for each patient are already undergoing clinical trials [70–72]. This could lead to more effective vaccination campaigns, especially in populations with varying susceptibility to TB. Although such tailor-made solutions may still take some time to implement, herd immunity can be effectively tackled by adjusting strategies to different locations, socio-economic status, and education levels. This is only made possible by algorithms tuned to a vast array of exposure and demographic variables coupled with the continuous monitoring of the effectiveness of different strategies.

Concerns about ethics can also be allayed using algorithms. For instance, models can be tuned to ensure vaccines are distributed equitably, especially in low- and middle-income countries. Their ability to handle complex data makes them ideal for considering factors like vulnerability and access to healthcare, which may be hard to assess without recourse to ML. Another major concern, seen during the COVID-19 pandemic, is infodemics, where false or misleading information abound, especially in digital environments. AI-driven tools can help identify and counter vaccine misinformation, improving public trust and uptake.

14.7 Limitations in Current AI Technologies

No matter how good the AI model is, its outputs will only be as good as the data used for its training. An issue with generalist AI models available is that this training data is too broad, which may lead to unwarranted conclusions when tasked with specific, expert prompts. Additionally, if one forces a model to extrapolate from its original data parameters, the result will likely be nonsensical or at least mathematically questionable. Creativity, although apparent in some algorithms, still solely pertains to human thought. An option is to train such ML algorithms using very specific datasets, thus limiting such negative outcomes. This was done with IBM's Watson when applied to health applications.

Data is, therefore, a key asset in the AI world. However, datasets are often heterogeneous, fragmented, or even biased. The use of biased data is of special concern, as its inclusion in training ML algorithms will only perpetuate such a bias. Data needs to be humanly monitored to ensure its quality. Moreover, large-scale datasets are less likely to be biased. However, a lack of clear data standards that would harmonise different datasets makes it very hard to achieve proper scale. Science will truly benefit from AI if broad collaborative efforts are achieved, entailing large amounts of data sharing between institutions and ambitious interdisciplinary projects. Vaccine design entails complex and diverse challenges that require such broad horizons and openness.

Another key asset in the AI world is computational power. Access to high-performance computing is fundamental to deploying more complex and accurate models. Such access is often expensive, energy-hungry, and restricted by a limited number of gate-keepers (companies or states that own the computers accessed by Cloud protocols). Once again, collaboration is paramount to overcome such barriers and ensure proper scale.

Such broad-scale efforts must always ensure compliance with data protection regulations (e.g. with the General Data Protection Regulation), as well as with strict ethical guidelines. Informed consent must be obtained where risks and benefits are clearly presented, as well as the intended use of the data. The latter is of particular relevance for research projects, as "recycled data" cannot be used if the original scope changed in the meantime. Data must then be stored, anonymised, and encrypted to ensure digital security. Public acceptance and cooperation during research and development stages critically rely on this.

Regulatory agencies, notably the European Medicines Agency (EMA) and the Food and Drug Administration (FDA) also have strict procedures and processes that must be followed. Whereas the inclusion of AI tools within these guidelines is slowly occurring, advancements in AI-driven technologies will necessarily outpace the speed of regulatory updates, posing both a serious challenge and a compliance risk that must be mitigated through rigor and transparency.

Transparency may be the main challenge at the moment. Most of the more complex AI algorithms, especially within the generative and deep learning fields, present conclusions that may be impossible to explain strictly logically. Why was such a solution favoured over another one? This simple question may not be obvious, leading to serious accountability and auditing concerns. Efforts are underway to include explanation mechanisms in critical AI systems, especially ones that require regulatory oversight. Domain knowledge should also be included in such models to ensure conclusions remain within the realm of biological plausibility. Therefore, transparency, accountability, and reliability are keywords that are unavoidable when working with AI in vaccine development.

It is important to underline that *in silico* testing will not, and cannot, fully replace *in vivo* testing. Regardless of the quality of the AI model, the complexity of a biological system requires any new compound to be tested in real biological conditions. Unexpected side effects, toxicity, or lack of efficacy may be present that were not predicted by the algorithms. As more promising compounds will reach this stage, however, such negative outcomes will likely be reduced, greatly improving the return on investment of pharmaceutical projects while reducing development times.

14.8 Prospects

Despite the recent rise of more generalist and adaptable models, the field of AI in health and science will still rely heavily on expert systems. These simulate the decision-making abilities of a human expert using a set of facts and rules about a specific domain (a knowledge base) coupled with an inference engine to apply that knowledge using logical rules. Such systems typically do not require training, with their rules defined *a piori* by human experts. This limits the range of outputs, avoiding erroneous conclusions while still being able to explore a vast set of possibilities far more efficiently than what is humanly possible. On the other hand, the underlying rules can still be explored and expanded on using ML algorithms, which learn directly from data and detect complex patterns that may prove too elusive for the human mind. The interplay between these two forms of AI—expert systems and ML—will help balance a risk-averse application rationale when deployed for public use, coupled with an exploratory, data-driven perspective when looking out for new findings.

Research and development efforts will doubtlessly rely on AI models, notably ML-based, to explore datasets and parse vast amounts of data to find patterns and novel approaches to known problems. In fact, these models may even help identify hitherto unknown problems, challenging commonly accepted rules and definitions. The speed of scientific discovery will further increase with the shortening of the cycles of generating hypotheses and their testing *in silico*. Scientific dead ends will be reduced in the process, saving resources to test more plausible avenues further.

For vaccine development, as well as for its posterior market deployment, AI will surely be a key asset across all stages. A healthy level of scepticism and prudence is required, though. Data is king when it comes to AI, so data sources must be carefully considered and monitored. Models that use incomplete, biased, or generic data should not be relied upon for serious scientific work. The same goes for algorithmic design: whereas many tools are available, only the ones with peer-reviewed publications detailing their contents, rationale, validation methods and limitations should be considered as relevant. Although more technical, validation methods should also be carefully assessed to identify potential sources of bias or blind spots that the authors may not have acknowledged or even detected.

The offer of AI tools is ever-increasing, encompassing all aspects of both scientific research and development and daily life. From writing a grant or a scientific publication to a virtual research assistant, from models that quickly generate and select novel hypotheses to explore to programs that replicate wet-laboratory conditions *in silico*, scientists must be ready and willing to incorporate new ways of working in order to stay relevant and impactful. A proficient user may not need to know how to code an AI model or be an expert in the intricacies of ML software development. Still, basic training is required to avoid becoming passive users of tools that seem to surpass one's understanding. Any AI model will have specific definitions, parameters, use cases and limitations. None should be used, especially in science, without *at least* some knowledge of these. AI will not replace the human mind anytime soon, provided humanity does not become mindless while using it.

Competing Interests The author(s) has no competing interests to declare that are relevant to the content of this manuscript.

Ethics Approval The author(s) declares that this manuscript does not include primary research with human participants.

References

1. World Health Organization. Global tuberculosis report 2023. Geneva; 2023.
2. Lange C, Aaby P, Behr MA, Donald PR, Kaufmann SHE, Netea MG, Mandalakas AM. 100 years of Mycobacterium bovis bacille Calmette-Guérin. Lancet Infect Dis. 2022;22:e2–e12.
3. Brisse M, Vrba SM, Kirk N, Liang Y, Ly H. Emerging concepts and technologies in vaccine development. Front Immunol. 2020;11:583077.
4. Olawade DB, Teke J, Fapohunda O, Weerasinghe K, Usman SO, Ige AO, Clement David-Olawade A. Leveraging artificial intelligence in vaccine development: a narrative review. J Microbiol Methods. 2024;224:106998.
5. Valkenburg SA, Leung NHL, Bull MB, Yan L, Li APY, Poon LLM, Cowling BJ. The hurdles from bench to bedside in the realization and implementation of a universal influenza vaccine. Front Immunol. 2018;9:390431.
6. Evans TG, Schrager L, Thole J. Status of vaccine research and development of vaccines for tuberculosis. Vaccine. 2016;34:2911–4.
7. Kaufmann SHE, Juliana McElrath M, Lewis DJM, Del Giudice G. Challenges and responses in human vaccine development. Curr Opin Immunol. 2014;28:18–26.

8. Jiang F, Sun T, Cheng P, Wang J, Gong W. A summary on tuberculosis vaccine development—where to go? J Pers Med. 2023;13:408.
9. Checkley AM, McShane H. Tuberculosis vaccines: progress and challenges. Trends Pharmacol Sci. 2011;32:601–6.
10. Lai R, Ogunsola AF, Rakib T, Behar SM. Key advances in vaccine development for tuberculosis-success and challenges. NPJ Vaccines. 2023;8:158.
11. Usman MM, Ismail S, Teoh TC. Vaccine research and development: tuberculosis as a global health threat. Cent Eur J Immunol. 2017;42:196–204.
12. Dockrell HM. Towards new TB vaccines: what are the challenges? Pathog Dis. 2016;74:ftw016.
13. Mangtani P, Abubakar I, Ariti C, et al. Protection by BCG vaccine against tuberculosis: a systematic review of randomized controlled trials. Clin Infect Dis. 2014;58:470–80.
14. Wang H, Wang S, Fang R, Li X, Xing J, Li Z, Song N. Enhancing TB vaccine efficacy: current progress on vaccines, adjuvants and immunization strategies. Vaccines (Basel). 2023; https://doi.org/10.3390/vaccines12010038.
15. Stewart E, Triccas JA, Petrovsky N. Adjuvant strategies for more effective tuberculosis vaccine immunity. Microorganisms. 2019;7:255. https://doi.org/10.3390/microorganisms7080255.
16. Hu Z, Lu SH, Lowrie DB, Fan XY. Research advances for virus-vectored tuberculosis vaccines and latest findings on tuberculosis vaccine development. Front Immunol. 2022;13:895020. https://doi.org/10.3389/FIMMU.2022.895020.
17. Oude Blenke E, Örnskov E, Schöneich C, Nilsson GA, Volkin DB, Mastrobattista E, Almarsson Ö, Crommelin DJA. The storage and in-use stability of mRNA vaccines and therapeutics: not a cold case. J Pharm Sci. 2023;112:386–403.
18. Uddin MN, Roni MA. Challenges of storage and stability of mRNA-based COVID-19 vaccines. Vaccines (Basel). 2021;9:1033. https://doi.org/10.3390/VACCINES9091033.
19. Buckland BC. The process development challenge for a new vaccine. Nat Med. 2005;11(Suppl 1):16–9.
20. Metz B, Van Den Dobbelsteen G, Van Els C, Van Der Gun J, Levels L, Van Der Pol L, Rots N, Kersten G. Quality-control issues and approaches in vaccine development. Expert Rev Vaccines. 2009;8:227–38.
21. Fletcher HA, Voss G, Casimiro D, Neyrolles O, Williams A, Kaufmann SHE, McShane H, Hatherill M. Progress and challenges in TB vaccine development. F1000Res. 2018;7:199. https://doi.org/10.12688/F1000RESEARCH.13588.1.
22. Brennan MJ, Morris SL, Sizemore CF. Tuberculosis vaccine development: research, regulatory and clinical strategies. Expert Opin Biol Ther. 2004;4:1493–504.
23. Naluyima P, Mwesigwa B, Tindikahwa A, Mugamba S, Ssensamba JT, Musingye E, Mirembe G, Kibuuka H, Wabwire-Mangen F. Developing capacity for implementation and evaluation of vaccine trials in Uganda: perspective of the Makerere University Walter Reed Project. Afr Health Sci. 2022;22:34–41.
24. Forman R, Shah S, Jeurissen P, Jit M, Mossialos E. COVID-19 vaccine challenges: what have we learned so far and what remains to be done? Health Policy. 2021;125:553.
25. Arora NK, Lal AA, Hombach JM, Santos JI, Bhutta ZA, Sow SO, Greenwood B. The need for targeted implementation research to improve coverage of basic vaccines and introduction of new vaccines. Vaccine. 2013;31(Suppl 2):B129–36.
26. Belton S, Schultz R, Speare T. Vaccine cold chain in remote environments: culturally appropriate training opportunities, an evaluation. J Pharm Pract Res. 2023;53:147–51.
27. Eckermann S. Globally optimal trial design and risk sharing arrangements are key to avoiding opportunity costs of delay and enabling equitable, feasible and effective global vaccine research and implementation in current or future pandemics. Front Public Health. 2022;10:1085319. https://doi.org/10.3389/FPUBH.2022.1085319/PDF.
28. Boulanger RF, Komparic A, Dawson A, Upshur REG, Silva DS. Developing and implementing new TB technologies: key informants' perspectives on the ethical challenges. J Bioeth Inq. 2020;17:65–73.

29. Deen JL, Clemens JD. Issues in the design and implementation of vaccine trials in less developed countries. Nat Rev Drug Discov. 2006;5:932–40.
30. Chinyenze K, Nduati E, Muturi-Kioi V. Accelerating HIV vaccine development through meaningful engagement of local scientists and communities. Curr Opin HIV AIDS. 2023;18:284–9.
31. Pelzer PT, Seeley J, Sun FY, et al. Potential implementation strategies, acceptability, and feasibility of new and repurposed TB vaccines. PLoS Global Public Health. 2022;2:e0000076.
32. do Nascimento N, Sichel A, Waugaman A, et al. Learning from digital health investments during COVID-19 vaccine program implementation: a research collaboration and theory of change. Oxford Open Digital Health. 2024;2:i7–i15.
33. Prasad V, Mailankody S. Research and development spending to bring a single cancer drug to market and revenues after approval. JAMA Intern Med. 2017;177:1569–75.
34. Jumper J, Evans R, Pritzel A, et al. Highly accurate protein structure prediction with AlphaFold. Nature. 2021;596(7873):583–9.
35. Abramson J, Adler J, Dunger J, et al. Accurate structure prediction of biomolecular interactions with AlphaFold 3. Nature. 2024;630(8016):493–500.
36. Saldanha L, Langel Ü, Vale N. In Silico studies to support vaccine development. Pharmaceutics. 2023;15:654. https://doi.org/10.3390/PHARMACEUTICS15020654.
37. Sarkar B, Ullah MA, Araf Y, Islam NN, Zohora US. Immunoinformatics-guided designing and in silico analysis of epitope-based polyvalent vaccines against multiple strains of human coronavirus (HCoV). Expert Rev Vaccines. 2021;21:1.
38. Han W, Chen N, Xu X, et al. Predicting the antigenic evolution of SARS-COV-2 with deep learning. Nat Commun. 2023;14(1):1–14.
39. Thadani NN, Gurev S, Notin P, Youssef N, Rollins NJ, Ritter D, Sander C, Gal Y, Marks DS. Learning from prepandemic data to forecast viral escape. Nature. 2023;622:818–25.
40. Aileni M, Rohela GK, Jogam P, Soujanya S, Zhang B. Biotechnological perspectives to combat the COVID-19 pandemic: precise diagnostics and inevitable vaccine paradigms. Cells. 2022;11:1182.
41. Saravanan V, Chagaleti BK, Narayanan PL, et al. Discovery and development of COVID-19 vaccine from laboratory to clinic. Chem Biol Drug Des. 2024;103:e14383.
42. International Pandemic Preparedness Secretariat. 100 days mission – implementation report 2023. London; 2024.
43. Wistuba-Hamprecht J, Reuter B, Fendel R, Hoffman SL, Campo JJ, Felgner PL, Kremsner PG, Mordmüller B, Pfeifer N. Machine learning prediction of malaria vaccine efficacy based on antibody profiles. PLoS Comput Biol. 2024;20:e1012131. https://doi.org/10.1371/JOURNAL.PCBI.1012131.
44. Kim DN, McNaughton AD, Kumar N. Leveraging artificial intelligence to expedite antibody design and enhance antibody–antigen interactions. Bioengineering. 2024;11:185.
45. Singh A, Thakur M, Sharma LK, Chandra K. Designing a multi-epitope peptide based vaccine against SARS-CoV-2. Sci Rep. 2020;10(1):1–12.
46. Delany I, Rappuoli R, Seib KL. Vaccines, reverse vaccinology, and bacterial pathogenesis. Cold Spring Harb Perspect Med. 2013;3:a012476. https://doi.org/10.1101/CSHPERSPECT.A012476.
47. Sette A, Rappuoli R. Reverse vaccinology: developing vaccines in the era of genomics. Immunity. 2010;33:530–41.
48. Ong E, Cooke MF, Huffman A, Xiang Z, Wong MU, Wang H, Seetharaman M, Valdez N, He Y. Vaxign2: the second generation of the first web-based vaccine design program using reverse vaccinology and machine learning. Nucleic Acids Res. 2021;49:W671–8.
49. Ong E, Wang H, Wong MU, Seetharaman M, Valdez N, He Y. Vaxign-ML: supervised machine learning reverse vaccinology model for improved prediction of bacterial protective antigens. Bioinformatics. 2020;36:3185–91.

50. Teahan B, Ong E, Yang Z. Identification of mycobacterium tuberculosis antigens with vaccine potential using a machine learning-based reverse vaccinology approach. Vaccines (Basel). 2021;9:1098. https://doi.org/10.3390/VACCINES9101098/S1.
51. Al Tbeishat H. Novel in Silico mRNA vaccine design exploiting proteins of M. tuberculosis that modulates host immune responses by inducing epigenetic modifications. Sci Rep. 2022;12(1):1–19.
52. Arega AM, Dhal AK, Pattanaik KP, Nayak S, Mahapatra RK. An immunoinformatics-based study of Mycobacterium tuberculosis region of difference-2 uncharacterized protein (Rv1987) as a potential subunit vaccine candidate for preliminary ex vivo analysis. Appl Biochem Biotechnol. 2024;196:2367–95.
53. Hossain MS, Azad AK, Chowdhury PA, Wakayama M. Computational identification and characterization of a promiscuous T-cell epitope on the extracellular protein 85B of Mycobacterium spp. for peptide-based subunit vaccine design. Biomed Res Int. 2017;2017:1. https://doi.org/10.1155/2017/4826030.
54. Dalsass M, Brozzi A, Medini D, Rappuoli R. Comparison of open-source reverse vaccinology programs for bacterial vaccine antigen discovery. Front Immunol. 2019;10:113. https://doi.org/10.3389/FIMMU.2019.00113.
55. Kaushik R, Kant R, Christodoulides M. Artificial intelligence in accelerating vaccine development – current and future perspectives. Front Bacteriol. 2023; https://doi.org/10.3389/fbrio.2023.1258159.
56. Yurina V, Adianingsih OR. Predicting epitopes for vaccine development using bioinformatics tools. 2022. https://doi.org/10.1177/25151355221100218.
57. Janson G, Grottesi A, Pietrosanto M, Ausiello G, Guarguaglini G, Paiardini A. Revisiting the "satisfaction of spatial restraints" approach of MODELLER for protein homology modeling. PLoS Comput Biol. 2019;15:e1007219.
58. Andreatta M, Nielsen M. Gapped sequence alignment using artificial neural networks: application to the MHC class I system. Bioinformatics. 2016;32:511–7.
59. Jensen KK, Andreatta M, Marcatili P, Buus S, Greenbaum JA, Yan Z, Sette A, Peters B, Nielsen M. Improved methods for predicting peptide binding affinity to MHC class II molecules. Immunology. 2018;154:394–406.
60. Alawam AS, Alwethaynani MS. Construction of an aerolysin-based multi-epitope vaccine against Aeromonas hydrophila: an in silico machine learning and artificial intelligence-supported approach. Front Immunol. 2024;15:1369890.
61. Morris GM, Ruth H, Lindstrom W, Sanner MF, Belew RK, Goodsell DS, Olson AJ. AutoDock4 and AutoDockTools4: automated docking with selective receptor flexibility. J Comput Chem. 2009;30:2785.
62. Altae-Tran H, Ramsundar B, Pappu AS, Pande V. Low data drug discovery with one-shot learning. ACS Cent Sci. 2017;3:283–93.
63. Goetz M, Thotathil N, Zhao Z, Mitragotri S. Vaccine adjuvants for infectious disease in the clinic. Bioeng Transl Med. 2024;9:e10663.
64. Zhang WY, Zheng XL, Coghi PS, Chen JH, Dong BJ, Fan XX. Revolutionizing adjuvant development: harnessing AI for next-generation cancer vaccines. Front Immunol. 2024;15:1438030.
65. Mayr A, Klambauer G, Unterthiner T, Hochreiter S. DeepTox: toxicity prediction using deep learning. Front Environ Sci. 2016;3:167215.
66. Pennisi M, Russo G, Sgroi G, et al. Predicting the artificial immunity induced by RUTI® vaccine against tuberculosis using universal immune system simulator (UISS). BMC Bioinformatics. 2019;20:504. https://doi.org/10.1186/S12859-019-3045-5.
67. Russo G, Pennisi M, Fichera E, Motta S, Raciti G, Viceconti M, Pappalardo F. In silico trial to test COVID-19 candidate vaccines: a case study with UISS platform. BMC Bioinformatics. 2020;21:527. https://doi.org/10.1186/S12859-020-03872-0.

68. Russo G, Di Salvatore V, Sgroi G, Parasiliti Palumbo GA, Reche PA, Pappalardo F. A multi-step and multi-scale bioinformatic protocol to investigate potential SARS-CoV-2 vaccine targets. Brief Bioinform. 2022;23:1–9.
69. Russo G, Crispino E, Maleki A, Di Salvatore V, Stanco F, Pappalardo F. Beyond the state of the art of reverse vaccinology: predicting vaccine efficacy with the universal immune system simulator for influenza. BMC Bioinformatics. 2023;24:1–22.
70. Dolgin E. Personalized cancer vaccines pass first major clinical test. Nat Rev Drug Discov. 2023;22:607–9.
71. Weber JS, Carlino MS, Khattak A, et al. Individualised neoantigen therapy mRNA-4157 (V940) plus pembrolizumab versus pembrolizumab monotherapy in resected melanoma (KEYNOTE-942): a randomised, phase 2b study. Lancet. 2024;403:632–44.
72. Rojas LA, Sethna Z, Soares KC, et al. Personalized RNA neoantigen vaccines stimulate T cells in pancreatic cancer. Nature. 2023;618(7963):144–50.

15 From Cutting-edge Science to Innovative Finance: The Road to TB Vaccine Implementation

José Manuel Durão Barroso

Hopefully, by this point, readers have a burgeoning sense of the incredible ingenuity and tenacity it has taken for vaccine researchers to get to this stage of TB vaccine development. More than 100 years since Albert Calmette and Jean-Marie Camille Guerin developed the Bacille Calmette–Guerin (BCG) vaccine against tuberculosis (TB), the world now stands on the cusp of having a new vaccine against one of the oldest diseases of humanity.

A pivotal phase 3 clinical trial of the M72/AS01 candidate TB vaccine, funded by Wellcome and the Bill & Melinda Gates Foundation, will test the safety and efficacy of the vaccine in countries with high rates of TB, including Indonesia, Kenya, Malawi, Mozambique, South Africa, Vietnam, and Zambia.[1] Meanwhile, there are at least 15 other candidate TB vaccines under active clinical development.[2]

If proven safe and effective in the phase 3 trial, M72 could become not only the world's first vaccine against TB since the BCG, but crucially it would be the first to protect adolescents and adults, who make up the majority of cases, from pulmonary TB.

The impact could be enormous. TB remains one of the world's biggest infectious killers, and is the 13th most common cause of death overall, rising to the seventh most common cause of death in low-income and middle-income countries.[3] The

[1] https://wellcome.org/news/worlds-first-tuberculosis-vaccine-100-years-could-be-sight

[2] https://www.who.int/publications/i/item/9789240064690

[3] https://www.who.int/news-room/fact-sheets/detail/the-top-10-causes-of-death

J. M. D. Barroso (✉)
Gavi, the Vaccine Alliance, Global Health Campus, Le Grand-Saconnex, Switzerland
e-mail: jmbarroso@gavi.org

P. J. G. Bettencourt (ed.), *Tuberculosis Vaccines*,
https://doi.org/10.1007/978-3-031-94540-3_15

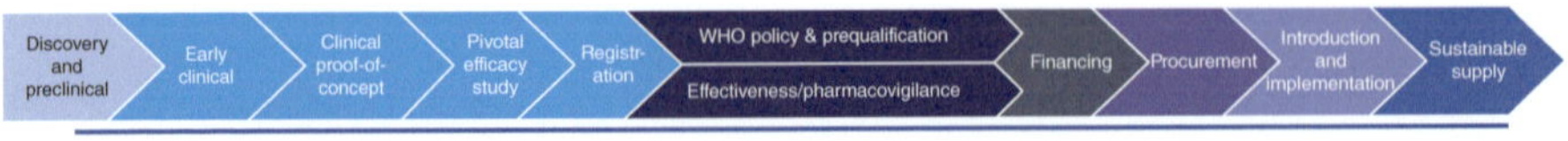

Fig. 15.1 Model vaccine development and implementation pathway

disease claims around 1.5 million lives every year, and often destroys the livelihoods of more than 10 million people who are newly diagnosed with the disease each year.[4] The disease remains the leading killer of people living with HIV, causing one in three deaths.

But as Fig. 15.1 shows, positive phase 3 clinical trial results, whilst certainly momentous, would only get us to the half-way point in the journey of a TB vaccine from concept to implementation.

After the gruelling years of research, development and clinical testing comes a different but no less challenging journey: that of financing, procuring, and implementing a new TB vaccine at the scale required to ensure equitable access and save millions of lives.

In this chapter, I will briefly discuss the status of TB control efforts to date and the growing need for a vaccine; discuss the challenging funding landscape for vaccine research and implementation; and outline potential pathways and challenges to financing and implementing a WHO prequalified TB vaccine.

In so doing I will draw extensively on my experience as Chair of the Board of Gavi, the Vaccine Alliance. In December 2023, the Gavi Board voted to include TB on the Alliance's shortlist for its 2024 Vaccine Investment Strategy, which will eventually determine the new vaccines that the Alliance plans to introduce in Gavi-supported countries.

15.1 Stalling Progress: The Case for a New Safe and Effective TB Vaccine

Research suggests that the bacterial pathogen that causes TB, *Mycobacterium tuberculosis*, has probably plagued humanity for three million years,[5] and the disease has been a subject of scholarly inquiry since antiquity, with the earliest written mentions appearing in India more than 3000 years ago, and China more than 2000 years ago.[6] The ancient Romans knew it as *tabes*, the ancient Greeks as *phthisis*, and it was referred to as *schachepeth* in ancient Hebrew.[7] Indeed, WHO estimates that TB is highly likely to rank as the leading infectious cause of death throughout human history, claiming over a billion lives during the past two centuries.

[4] https://www.who.int/news-room/fact-sheets/detail/tuberculosis

[5] https://www.thelancet.com/journals/laninf/article/PIIS1473-3099(05)70230-9/abstract

[6] https://www.cdc.gov/tb/worldtbday/history.htm

[7] https://www.gavi.org/vaccineswork/5-ancient-diseases-and-what-ancients-said-about-them

The question, then, is why has a scourge of the ancient world persisted into modernity?

Unlike many infectious diseases, TB has commanded high-level political commitment for several decades. And that commitment has brought some notable success.

Set up in 2002, the Global Fund to Fight AIDS, Tuberculosis and Malaria galvanised TB prevention and treatment efforts. The Global Fund provides three-quarters of all international financing for TB control, and has invested US$ 9.2 billion in TB prevention and treatment over the past two decades.[8] In countries where the Global Fund invests, the Fund reports, TB deaths dropped by 16% between 2002 and 2021.

More effective diagnosis and treatment of TB saved an estimated 58 million lives between 2000 and 2018. Indeed, the 2015 Millennium Development Goal (MDG) target to "stop the increase in incidence and halve the mortality of TB between 1990 and 2015" was achieved early.

But although the MDG target was reached when looked at from a global perspective, in the African region and India, which are hardest hit by the disease, TB has proven to be a much tougher nut to crack.

The past decade has been defined by the world's failure, despite best efforts, to get within touching distance of the targets set by the End TB Strategy, which was adopted by WHO Member States in May 2014 as part of the successors to the MDGs, the Sustainable Development Goals (SDGs). The official SDG 3.3 target related to communicable diseases aims to "end the epidemics of AIDS, tuberculosis, malaria and neglected tropical diseases and combat hepatitis, water-borne diseases and other communicable diseases."

The End TB strategy translates the SDG 3.3 target into hard numbers, aiming to reduce TB incidence by 80% and TB deaths by 90% by 2030 compared with 2015. But as WHO's Global Strategy for TB Research and Innovation[9] makes clear, "an enormous gap persists ... between current reality and the SDG vision." Figure 15.2[10] lays bare the size of the challenge.

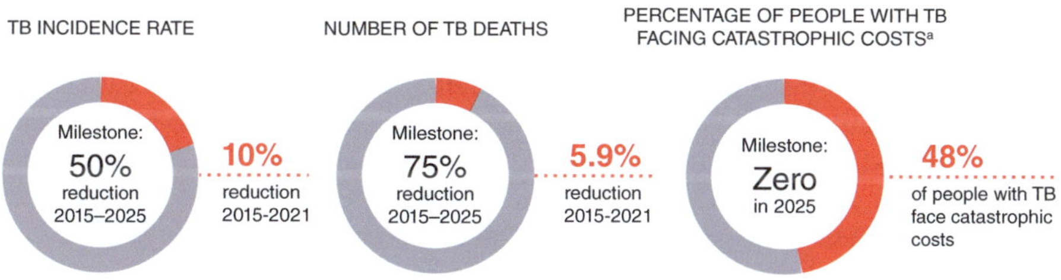

Fig. 15.2 Progress against the End TB 2025 milestones. (Figure adapted from Global Tuberculosis Report 2022)

[8] https://www.theglobalfund.org/en/tuberculosis/

[9] https://www.who.int/teams/global-tuberculosis-programme/research-innovation/development-of-a-global-strategy-for-tb-research-and-innovation

[10] Global Tuberculosis Report 2022

The number of people who died from TB actually increased in 2021 for the second consecutive year, and the number of people falling ill with TB increased to an estimated 10.6 million in 2022.[11]

The causes of this backsliding are complex, with a host of interacting factors including the effects of the COVID-19 pandemic on already fragile health systems. In parallel, the inexorable rise of multi-drug resistant TB—a subset of the broader problem of antimicrobial resistance—has created additional complexity to the successful treatment of the disease. An estimated 490,000 people worldwide developed MDR-TB in 2016 according to WHO,[12] and the problem is increasing.

Such is the urgency of the situation that the annual decline in global tuberculosis incidence will need to accelerate to 17% each year between 2024 and 2030 for the End TB goals to be reached.

At the second ever UN High-Level Meeting on the Fight Against Tuberculosis, held in September 2023, Member States used the meeting's political declaration to voice their concern[13] that "while it has been 30 years since the World Health Organization declared tuberculosis a global emergency, the global tuberculosis epidemic still is a critical challenge in all regions and affects every country of the world and disproportionately affects developing countries."

In the same declaration, the UN's Member States recognised that reaching the 2030 End TB target will require a technological breakthrough by 2025, bringing the need to rapidly prequalify, fund and implement any new safe and effective TB vaccine to the forefront of TB control efforts.

15.2 Renewed Global Coordination Collides with a Challenging Funding Landscape

In light of the centuries-long toll of TB on health and prosperity, and the key role of vaccination in the control of infectious diseases, it may seem strange that research into new methods of TB control have been comparatively underfunded, with vaccine research in particular suffering from chronic under-investment.

The most recent report[14] into TB research funding trends by the Stop TB Partnership found that the US$ 4.7 billion funding for research during 2018–2022 was less than half of the US$ 10 billion pledged by world leaders at the first United Nations High-Level Meeting on TB in 2018. The report's authors concluded that "current R&D funding levels are insufficient to produce and roll out the new tools needed to find, treat, and prevent the 10 million new cases of TB each year."

[11] https://apps.who.int/gb/ebwha/pdf_files/EB154/B154_10-en.pdf

[12] https://www.who.int/news-room/questions-and-answers/item/tuberculosis-multidrug-resistant-tuberculosis-(mdr-tb)

[13] https://www.who.int/activities/preparing-for-the-un-high-level-meeting-on-the-fight-against-tuberculosis%2D%2D2023

[14] https://www.treatmentactiongroup.org/wp-content/uploads/2023/12/tb_research_funding_2023.pdf

The report also found that although spending on research for TB drugs and diagnostics undershot targets set by the partnership's *2018–2022 Global Plan to End TB* by 75% and 35%, respectively, the shortfall was greatest for vaccine research, which was a full 80% short of the target. According to WHO, the average annual investment in TB vaccine research over the past 5 years has been only US$ 115 million, compared with a target of US$ 790 million per year set by the Stop TB Partnership's plan.

TB research has also suffered from a lack of diversity in its funding sources. The generosity of the United States National Institutes of Health and the Bill & Melinda Gates Foundation accounted for over half of TB research funding in 2022.

To put these figures into context, the phase 3 trial of the M72 candidate vaccine alone will cost around US$ 550 million, with Wellcome providing up to US$ 150 million and the Bill & Melinda Gates Foundation funding the remainder of about US$ 400 million.

The slow progress and relative lack of funding for TB vaccine research and implementation prompted WHO's Director General Dr. Tedros Adhanom Ghebreyesus, in January 2023, to propose the establishment of a TB Vaccine Accelerator Council to "create and catalyse high-level alignment between funders, global agencies, governments, and end users on the important challenges in TB vaccine development."

The aim of the Council, which was established in September 2023 with Gavi as a member of the Principal Group, is to apply some of the lessons from the COVID-19 response and inject a sense of urgency and collective purpose into the development and implementation of TB vaccines. As Dr. Tedros noted when the Council was announced, "one of the most important lessons from the response to the COVID-19 pandemic is that innovative health interventions can be delivered fast if they are prioritised politically and financed adequately."

Gavi, the Vaccine Alliance, played a key role as a co-lead of COVAX, the vaccine pillar of the global response to COVID-19. Between its establishment in April 2020 and its sunsetting at the end of 2023, COVAX distributed almost 2 billion doses of COVID-19 vaccines to 146 countries, averting the deaths of an estimated 2.7 million people in lower-income countries.

COVAX was the largest and most complex emergency response in the history of global health, and was the only dependable source of COVID-19 vaccines for hundreds of millions of people around the world. And although the challenges presented by TB and COVID-19 are different, the lessons pf COVAX can provide a useful guide when we think about TB. The urgent, up-front investment, innovative financing, engagement with the private sector, and links with communities that were so vital during the pandemic are just as critical for the success of TB vaccines, and they are concepts that go to the heart of the mission of Gavi, the Vaccine Alliance.

15.3 The Potential Role of Gavi in Assuring Equitable Access to a Future TB Vaccine

15.3.1 A Brief History of Gavi, the Vaccine Alliance

Gavi was established in 2000 in large part to kick-start the stalling progress on global immunisation rates that prevailed throughout the late 1990s. The organisation was founded on the fundamental principle that all lives are equal, and access to life-saving vaccines should never be a function of geographical or economic circumstance.

Since then, Gavi has helped to vaccinate over one billion children with routine vaccines in the world's poorest countries, alongside enabling billions of critical vaccinations during campaigns, emergencies, and pandemics.

In total, Gavi has enabled roughly 6 billion vaccinations around the world, protecting children and adults against 19 infectious diseases and preventing more than 17 million future deaths.[15] Basic immunisation coverage in Gavi-supported countries has increased from 59% to 80% since 2000, and the Alliance is on track to immunise 300 million children between 2021 and 2025, preventing a projected 7–eight million deaths and generating an estimated US$ 80–100 billion in economic benefits.

As an alliance, Gavi brings together four core international partners—the World Health Organization, UNICEF, the World Bank, and the Bill & Melinda Gates Foundation—and many more global, regional, and national public and private organisations and institutes as part of an extended alliance.

In addition to its four core partners, Gavi works with implementing countries, donors including philanthropies and national governments, private sector foundations and corporate partners; non-governmental organisations, advocacy groups, professional and community associations, faith-based organisations and academia; vaccine manufacturers, including those in emerging markets; and research and technical health institutes.

Gavi pools the demand for vaccines from the world's 54 poorest countries[16] (Box 15.1), representing more than half of the world's birth cohort, to achieve economies of scale and send a clear signal to manufacturers that there is a large, predictable, and viable market for the vaccines that Gavi supports.

At the same time, Gavi plans its activities and raises funds in 5-year cycles (known as strategic periods), delivering predictable and long-term support that provides countries with the confidence and security to establish vaccine programmes for the long term, and giving manufacturers the confidence to invest in sustainable production capacity.

---

[15] https://www.gavi.org/sites/default/files/programmes-impact/our-impact/Gavi-Facts-and-figures-October-2023.pdf

[16] https://www.gavi.org/types-support/sustainability/eligibility

All countries pay a share of the cost of their Gavi-supported vaccines. As a country's income grows, its **co-financing** payments gradually increase to cover the full cost of vaccines.

15.3.2 The Vital Role of Health Systems for Immunity, and Vice Versa

Gavi's support for immunisation extends beyond vaccines themselves. The essential public health functions that underpin immunisation—supply chain management and infrastructure, data systems, leadership and coordination, and community engagement—are also the backbone of effective and resilient primary healthcare systems. This means that investments in these essential functions not only have immediate payoffs for immunisation, but also yield crucial benefits in terms of universal health coverage and global health security.

In 2016, Gavi launched a health system and immunisation strengthening framework, and in 2023 updated its policy on the health system and immunisation strengthening[17] to ensure that all of the Alliance's health system strengthening activities are aligned and better able to boost routine immunisation and support new vaccine launches.

Box 15.1: Eligibility for Gavi Support

Gavi supports the world's poorest countries, and, therefore, bases eligibility for Gavi support on national income. In 2023, countries are eligible for Gavi support if their most recent gross national income per capita, according to World Bank data,[18] was less than or equal to US$ 1730. The eligibility threshold is adjusted for inflation on an annual basis.

Governments who receive Gavi support co-finance vaccines by financing a fraction of the needed doses. As national income levels grow, co-financing levels for governments increase, and Gavi's support tapers. A full explanation of the mechanics of co-financing are set out in Gavi's co-financing policy.[19] The policy remains under periodic review, and may be amended in response to changing global and national economic and epidemiological realities.

In 2023, 54 countries were eligible to apply for new vaccine support from Gavi, down from 74 countries when Gavi was first launched in 2000, when the eligibility threshold was set at US$ 1000.

---

[17] https://www.gavi.org/sites/default/files/programmes-impact/Gavi-Health-Systems-and-Immunisation-Strengthening-Policy.pdf

[18] https://www.gavi.org/sites/default/files/document/guidelines/GNI-per-capita.pdf

[19] https://www.gavi.org/programmes-impact/programmatic-policies/co-financing-policy

15.3.3 TB and the Gavi Portfolio: The Vaccine Investment Strategy

At the beginning of 2024, Gavi supported vaccines against 19 infectious diseases (Fig. 15.3); up from four diseases in 2000, with vaccines against malaria the most recent to have been added to Gavi's portfolio.

Gavi's disease prevention focus and vaccine portfolio have evolved over time, moving from vaccines focused on routine infant immunisation to prevent endemic disease to include vaccines that target other age groups, such as HPV, as well as vaccines that support outbreak, epidemic, and pandemic preparedness and response.

So how does Gavi choose which vaccines to support, and how might Gavi assess a potential TB vaccine? The answers lie in Gavi's Vaccine Investment Strategy (VIS) process.

Led by Gavi's Policy team, the VIS process is a full evaluation of the value of vaccines, including their impact on mortality and morbidity, but also their social and economic benefits and other factors.

The VIS is an 18-month process initiated once every 5 years to support the long-term strategic planning of immunisation programmes, and align with Gavi's forthcoming 5-year strategic period.

The process takes place in three stages, the first of which aims to produce a longlist of potential investments drawing on a WHO analysis of the vaccine landscape. For the 2024 VIS, which will support Gavi's sixth 5-year strategic period from January 2026 to the end of 2030, the longlist was compiled based on the following inclusion criteria:

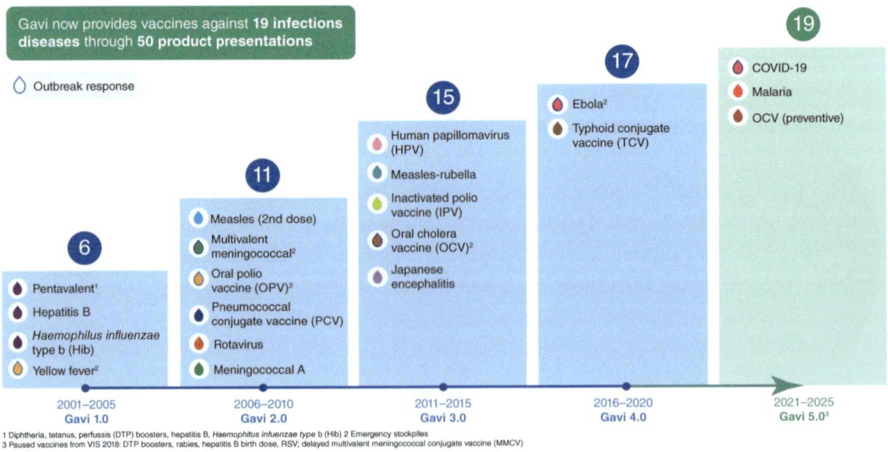

Fig. 15.3 The evolution of Gavi's vaccine portfolio

- Immunisation products of relevance to Gavi-eligible countries with expected licensure by 2030
- Vaccines not currently in Gavi's portfolio but of relevance to Gavi-eligible countries, or incremental investments for Gavi-supported vaccines

A second key output of phase 1 is to develop evaluation frameworks (Fig. 15.4) against which the longlist of products can be analysed during phase 2 of the VIS, during which the longlist is narrowed down through comparisons of candidate vaccines not only with each other, but with vaccines in Gavi's existing portfolio. The results of this narrowing down of candidates to a shortlist, drawing on insights from the VIS Steering Committee and other external consultations, is then put before Gavi's Board for approval.

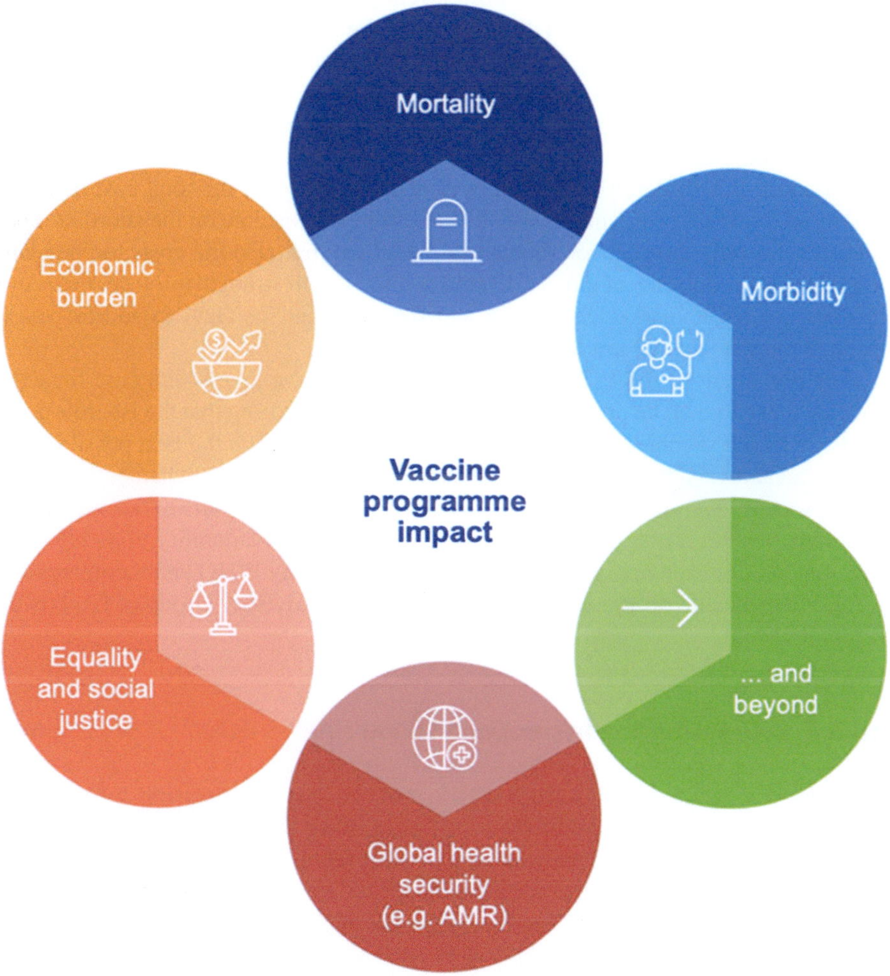

Fig. 15.4 High-level considerations for vaccine impact evaluations

At the meeting of Gavi's Board in December 2023, we considered the results of phase 2 of the VIS 2024 process, and recommended that, amongst others, vaccines against TB be included on the Alliance's shortlist of candidates to progress to phase 3 of the VIS process.

This third and final phase of the VIS process will involve the development of detailed investment cases for VIS shortlist candidates. This includes more detailed modelling of health and economic impacts, in addition to sophisticated demand forecasting. Phase 3 of the process will draw on detailed consultations with a broad range of disease experts, academics, and others to yield the most accurate estimates and projections possible of the potential costs and benefits of investments in each shortlisted candidate.

The feasibility of implementing new vaccination programmes is also considered during phase 3. This includes an assessment of how challenging it would be to reach age or population groups that are not currently part of existing vaccination programmes and services, which will be of particular relevance for a TB vaccine that also targets adolescents and adults. It also takes into consideration the potential need to re-train health workers and ensures the necessary surveillance and diagnostics capacity to understand the evolving burden of the disease and confirm or rule out suspected cases.

Based on this in-depth additional evidence and analysis, the total cost of introducing vaccination programmes is calculated for each vaccine on the shortlist. This includes not only the costs of vaccine procurement, but also the costs to Gavi and implementing countries of any associated health system strengthening needed. And last but not least, market challenges and the potential for Gavi to address these through market shaping are examined.

The end result of the VIS process is a comprehensive investment case for each vaccine that can then be presented to the Gavi Board, ensuring that the Board's decisions on which vaccines to support in the future are based on the best possible evidence and analysis. At this stage any decision by the Board about whether to support a new vaccine is in principle. In practice, whether Gavi supports a vaccine is also contingent on several key external factors, including the availability of an effective vaccine that has been pre-qualified (a type of approval) by WHO and recommended for use in a vaccine programme by WHO's Strategic Advisory Group of Experts on Immunisation.

15.3.4 Estimating the Impact of a TB Vaccine

Although we can't pre-empt Gavi's VIS process, nor any decision by the Gavi Board, we can look at some of the types of existing data that may be taken into consideration during a VIS analysis for TB vaccines.

For example, a recent WHO commissioned study[20] estimates that, over 25 years, a TB vaccine that is 50% effective in preventing disease (50% is usually the

[20] https://www.who.int/publications/i/item/9789240064690

threshold WHO uses to approve or "prequalify" a vaccine—a pre-requisite for Gavi support) among adolescents and adults could "avert up to 76 million new TB cases, 8.5 million deaths, 42 million courses of antibiotic treatment and US$ 6.5 billion in costs faced by TB affected households, especially for the poorest and most vulnerable".

A vaccine that is 75% effective could avert up to 110 million new TB cases and 12.3 million deaths of the same 25-year period. The study further suggests that based on an assumed cost of US$ 5 per dose, every US$ 1 invested in a 50% effective vaccine could generate an economic return of US$ 7 in terms of averted health costs and increased productivity.

So we can see that on the basis of the most recent WHO analysis, TB vaccines for adolescents and adults are expected by to have a marked positive impact on health in countries that are currently supported by Gavi, and are likely to be good value for money in terms of procurement costs.

Thanks to the work of the Global Fund and others, robust data are available on TB burden in most countries. But a full understanding of the overall cost and the potential size of the market for any TB vaccine will also depend on further clarity around the recommended vaccination strategy.

15.4 Implementation Considerations

15.4.1 Lessons from Malaria

Should the Gavi Board recommend that TB be added to Gavi's portfolio for support, there are still several important considerations before new vaccines reach target populations.

Gavi can only fund vaccines that have been recommended for use and prequalified by WHO. And any vaccine introduction programme requires meticulous planning and preparation, including at the community level in countries that wish to introduce the vaccine. Here, the experience of recent malaria vaccine introductions is instructive.

After decades of research, the RTS,S malaria vaccine was rolled out on 22 January 2024, when a child in Cameroon became the first to receive the vaccine in a non-pilot country. Burkina Faso followed suit in February. It was a moment of triumph, but it came on the back of many years of painstaking planning and a huge pilot programme, the Malaria Vaccine Implementation Programme (MVIP). There are many more years of painstaking work ahead to ensure that countries, manufacturers, and health systems are ready to meet the huge demand for the vaccine.

Coordinated by WHO and funded by Gavi, the Global Fund, and Unitaid, the MVP was designed to evaluate the public health use of the RTS,S vaccine in Ghana, Kenya, and Malawi. As the first vaccine of its kind, it was important to ensure that not only could RTS,S be introduced without having a detrimental impact on other immunisation services, but also that it would not have any negative effect on the use of other essential anti-malaria interventions, such as bed nets, insecticide spraying, and seasonal chemoprophylaxis.

Since 2019, nearly two million children at risk of malaria have been reached with the malaria vaccine across the three countries that took part in the MVP. The results were exactly what was hoped for, with malaria vaccine implementation resulting in a substantial fall in severe malaria hospitalisations and a 13% drop in all-cause child mortality.

It is possible that the type of large-scale implementation pilot that was successful for the malaria vaccine would also be recommended for any newly approved TB vaccine. And although a TB vaccine will be a powerful new weapon, like malaria, effective TB prevention and control relies on a multifaceted and multi-disciplinary package of public health measures that includes active case finding, integrated TB and HIV service delivery, increased use rapid diagnostic tests and expanded use of chest radiography, clinical care pathways, community engagement and interventions that lower barriers to access care, and effective supply chain management to ensure uninterrupted supplies of essential diagnostics and therapeutics.

Ensuring that these measures are in place wherever the vaccine is introduced will require careful coordination between national governments, civil society organisations and implementing partners, key funders such as the Global Fund and Gavi, and other Alliance partners.

As the declaration of the 2023 UN high-level meeting made clear, "ending tuberculosis requires accelerating progress towards universal health coverage, particularly through strong and sustainable primary health care, with multisectoral approaches that address tuberculosis determinants, that engages people affected by tuberculosis and civil society, and reaches people with tuberculosis, or at risk of tuberculosis, with equitable and affordable access to high-quality services, close to their everyday environments, enabling them to fully enjoy the benefits of scientific advances, and free of financial hardship."

15.4.2 Supply, Demand, and Co-financing

Co-financing arrangements that outline the costs that any countries participating in TB introductions with Gavi support will be expected to pay, and any additional support available from Gavi and other partners would have to be determined for any new introduction. A key question for Gavi will be country eligibility for Gavi support, given the high burden of disease, and therefore likely very high vaccine demand, in middle-income countries.

15.5 Funding Remains the Key Battle Ground in the Fight Against TB

The political declaration of the UN high-level meeting on TB was at pains to note that overall international funding for TB has stagnated since 2018, and stressed "the importance of adequately replenishing voluntary international financing mechanisms," of which Gavi and the Global Fund are perhaps the most critical for the chances of TB control in the future.

Assuming that one or more of the TB vaccines in the most advanced stages of development are found to be effective, they would most likely be licensed towards the end of Gavi's sixth strategic period in 2030. Most introductions of the TB vaccine would, therefore, be likely to take place during Gavi's seventh strategic period from 2031 onwards, but programme design, in close collaboration with key partners, such as the Global Fund, would need to take place throughout the 2026–2030 time frame.

Competing Interests The author(s) has no competing interests to declare that are relevant to the content of this manuscript.

Ethics Approval The author(s) declares that this manuscript does not include primary research with human participants.